BIOPSYCHOSOCIAL ASSESSMENT IN CLINICAL HEALTH PSYCHOLOGY

Forthcoming

Biofeedback: A Practitioner's Guide, Fourth Edition
Edited by Mark S. Schwartz and Frank Andrasik

Biopsychosocial Assessment in Clinical Health Psychology

edited by

Frank Andrasik
Jeffrey L. Goodie
Alan L. Peterson

THE GUILFORD PRESS
New York   London

© 2015 The Guilford Press
A Division of Guilford Publications, Inc.
72 Spring Street, New York, NY 10012
www.guilford.com

Printed in the United States of America

This book is printed on acid-free paper.

Last digit is print number: 9   8   7   6   5   4   3   2   1

The authors have checked with sources believed to be reliable in their efforts to
provide information that is complete and generally in accord with the standards
of practice that are accepted at the time of publication. However, in view of the
possibility of human error or changes in behavioral, mental health, or medical
sciences, neither the authors, nor the editors and publisher, nor any other party
who has been involved in the preparation or publication of this work warrants
that the information contained herein is in every respect accurate or complete,
and they are not responsible for any errors or omissions or the results obtained
from the use of such information. Readers are encouraged to confirm the
information contained in this book with other sources.

Library of Congress Cataloging-in-Publication Data

Biopsychosocial assessment in clinical health psychology / edited by Frank
Andrasik, Jeffrey L. Goodie, Alan L. Peterson.
    p. ; cm.
   Includes bibliographical references and indexes.
   ISBN 978-1-4625-1773-2 (hardcover : alk. paper)
   I. Andrasik, Frank, 1949– , editor.   II. Goodie, Jeffrey L., editor.
III. Peterson, Alan L., editor.
   [DNLM: 1. Psychology, Clinical—methods.   2. Behavioral Medicine—
methods.   3. Psychology, Medical—methods.   WM 105]
   RC454.4
   616.89—dc23
                                                        2014037257

About the Editors

Frank Andrasik, PhD, is Distinguished Professor and Chair of Psychology at the University of Memphis. He is Editor-in-Chief of *Applied Psychophysiology and Biofeedback*, Associate Editor of *Cephalalgia*, and past Editor-in-Chief of *Behavior Therapy*. Dr. Andrasik's primary areas of research include behavioral medicine, pain (with a particular focus on recurrent headache disorders), stress, and biofeedback and applied psychophysiology. He has published extensively and delivered numerous presentations in the United States and abroad on these topics. Dr. Andrasik is a past president of the Association for Behavioral and Cognitive Therapies (2009–2010) and the Association for Applied Psychophysiology and Biofeedback (1993–1994).

Jeffrey L. Goodie, PhD, ABPP, is Associate Professor in the Department of Family Medicine and the Department of Medical and Clinical Psychology at the Uniformed Services University of the Health Sciences. Dr. Goodie's research, clinical, and teaching interests focus on behavioral health assessments and interventions in primary care settings, disaster behavioral health, and community resilience. He is coauthor of the book *Integrated Behavioral Health in Primary Care: Step-by-Step Guidance for Assessment and Intervention*.

Alan L. Peterson, PhD, ABPP, is Professor and Chief of the Division of Behavioral Medicine in the Department of Psychiatry at the University of Texas Health Science Center at San Antonio. He is Director of the STRONG STAR Consortium and the Consortium to Alleviate PTSD. Dr. Peterson served previously as Chair of the Department of Psychology and Clinical Health Psychology Fellowship Program Director at Wilford Hall Medical Center in San Antonio, Texas. His research and publications focus on posttraumatic stress disorder, tobacco cessation, pain management, weight management, insomnia, temporomandibular disorders, tic disorders, aerophagia, and blepharospasm.

Contributors

Michelle C. Acosta, PhD, is Principal Investigator and Administrative Director of the Center for Technology and Health at the National Development and Research Institutes, Inc. Her research focuses on technology-based adaptations of evidence-based substance abuse interventions that may improve the reach, acceptability, and potency of these treatments in vulnerable populations.

Frank Andrasik, PhD (See "About the Editors").

Thomas M. Atkinson, PhD, is Assistant Attending Behavioral Scientist at Memorial Sloan-Kettering Cancer Center, where he serves as a psychometrician and outcomes researcher with expertise in quantitative and qualitative methodology. His current line of independent research focuses on the exploration of the psychometric properties of existing patient-reported outcome measures for the purposes of evaluating their use for inclusion in clinical trials and regulatory review, as well as methods for assessing the reliability between various reports of adverse events (i.e., clinicians vs. clinicians, clinicians vs. patients).

Jessica Barnack-Tavlaris, PhD, is Assistant Professor in the Department of Psychology at the College of New Jersey. Her current research focuses on reproductive and sexual health promotion and people's awareness and attributions of health disparities.

Melanie K. Bean, PhD, is Assistant Professor of Pediatrics at the Children's Hospital of Richmond (CHoR) at Virginia Commonwealth University and Director of Clinical and Behavioral Services at the Healthy Lifestyles Center, CHoR's comprehensive pediatric obesity treatment and research center. Dr. Bean conducts psychological assessments and interventions with patients with obesity and other endocrine disorders within the Division of Endocrinology and Metabolism. She conducts presurgical assessments and both pre- and postsurgical treatment for adolescents as part of the bariatric surgery program at CHoR. Her research in pediatric obesity has been funded by the American Cancer Society, the American Heart Association, and the National Institutes of Health, among others.

Cynthia D. Belar, PhD, ABPP, is past Executive Director of the Education Directorate of the American Psychological Association (APA). She is also Professor Emerita at the University of Florida Health Sciences Center, where she directed the doctoral program. Former roles have included President, APA Division 38; President, American Board of Health Psychology; Chair, Council of University Directors of Clinical Psychology; and Chair, Association of Psychology Postdoctoral and Internship Centers. She has chaired national conferences on internship training, the scientist-practitioner model, and postdoctoral education and training in professional psychology. Her experience as chief psychologist at the Los Angeles Kaiser Permanente Medical Center in the 1980s led to her commitment to health care reform.

James A. Blumenthal, PhD, ABPP, is J. P. Gibbons Professor of Psychiatry and Behavioral Sciences in the Division of Behavioral Medicine at Duke University Medical Center. Dr. Blumenthal is the recipient of several awards, including an honorary doctorate from Uppsala University, the Michael L. Pollack Established Investigator Award, and Outstanding Contributions to Health Psychology from the American Psychological Association (APA; Division 38). He is former president of the American Psychosomatic Society and Division 38, Health Psychology, of the APA.

Krysten Williams Bold, MS, is a PhD candidate in clinical psychology at Rutgers, The State University of New Jersey. She has interests in addiction research and health psychology, particularly the use of drug self-administration paradigms and intensive longitudinal data to understand the proximal factors that influence momentary decisions to smoke. She is also interested in addiction treatment development and evaluation.

Adam D. Bramoweth, PhD, is a Research Health Science Specialist at the VISN 4 Mental Illness Research, Education, and Clinical Center, VA Pittsburgh Healthcare System, and a Visiting Instructor in Psychiatry at the University of Pittsburgh School of Medicine. Dr. Bramoweth's research is focused on behavioral sleep medicine, the relationship between chronic insomnia and health care utilization, and the implementation and dissemination of behavioral treatments for insomnia.

Antoinette R. Brundige, MA, is licensed as a Psychological Associate through the Texas State Board of Examiners of Psychologists. She works as a Project Coordinator in the Division of Behavioral Medicine, Department of Psychiatry, School of Medicine, the University of Texas Health Science Center at San Antonio. Ms. Brundige has contributed to research projects in areas including weight management, tobacco cessation, Tourette syndrome, and posttraumatic stress disorder in the military population.

Lisa M. Buckloh, PhD, is a Pediatric Psychologist at Nemours Children's Clinic–Jacksonville in the Division of Psychology and Psychiatry and Assistant Professor of Psychology at the Mayo Clinic College of Medicine. She specializes in the assessment and treatment of children with diabetes, disorders of sex development, and elimination disorders. Her research has focused on psychological factors and interventions for youth with types 1 and 2 diabetes mellitus and their families.

Dawn C. Buse, PhD, is Associate Professor in the Department of Neurology at Albert Einstein College of Medicine of Yeshiva University and Assistant Professor in the Clinical Health Psychology Doctoral Program at Ferkauf Graduate School of Psychology of Yeshiva University. She is a licensed clinical psychologist, Director of Behavioral Medicine for the Montefiore Headache Center in New York City, and a Fellow of the American Headache Society. She has authored or coauthored more than 100 publications in scientific journals and books, presented more than 220 scientific abstracts, and coauthored manuscripts that have won the American Headache Society Wolff Award and the Italian Society for the Study of Headaches Enrico Greppi Award. At the Montefiore Headache Center, Dr. Buse provides clinical care to individuals using biobehavioral techniques.

Jan Busschbach, PhD, is Professor of Health Related Quality of Life and Head of the Section of Medical Psychology and Psychotherapy in the Department of Psychiatry at the Erasmus MC in Rotterdam. He is a senior investigator at the Viersprong Institute for Studies on Personality Disorders. His main research interests are health-related quality of life and the cost-effectiveness of psychotherapy, as well as the operationalization of arguments other than cost effectiveness in reimbursement decisions, such as distributional and ethical arguments. He has considerable experience in the validation of quality-of-life instruments. Dr. Busschbach is a member of the Medication Commission of the National Health Care Insurance Board in The Netherlands, which determines reimbursement. He is Chair of the EuroQoL Research Foundation, and he validated the EQ-5D-3L health questionnaire in The Netherlands.

Laura K. Campbell, PhD, is a Behavioral Medicine Psychologist in the Division of Psychiatry at Geisinger Health System. Her research interests broadly include coping with and adaptation to chronic health conditions throughout adolescence and adulthood, and the neurocognitive sequelae of medical illness, with studies published in *Pediatric Diabetes*, the *International Journal of Dia-*

betes Mellitus, *Pediatric Blood and Cancer*, and the *Journal of Pediatric Psychology*.

Dean G. Cruess, PhD, is Professor in the Department of Psychology and the Department of Medicine at the University of Connecticut. He is an Associate Editor of the journal *Biological Psychology*. Dr. Cruess's research interests focus on the effects of mental health within the context of medical illnesses, including HIV/AIDS.

William W. Deardorff, PhD, ABPP, is board certified in clinical health psychology and is a Fellow of the American Psychological Association. Dr. Deardorff is coauthor of 10 books and numerous scientific articles and book chapters in the area of clinical health psychology. He is the founder of *BehavioralHealthCE.com*, a multidisciplinary continuing education website focusing on health care integration.

Patricia M. Dubbert, PhD, is a health psychologist and investigator at the Mental Illness Research, Education, and Clinical Center and the Geriatric Research, Education, and Clinical Center at the Central Arkansas Veterans Healthcare System and at the Department of Psychiatry, University of Arkansas for Medical Sciences, Little Rock, Arkansas. Her research interests include assessment and promotion of physical activity and other healthy lifestyle behaviors for improving physical and mental health in older adults.

Barry A. Edelstein, PhD, is the Eberly Family Distinguished Professor of Clinical Psychology in the Department of Psychology at West Virginia University. His research interests include anxiety and decision making in older adults. His clinical work focuses on the assessment of older adults in long-term care and the development of interventions to manage problem behaviors.

Monica Escamilla, PsyD, is a family psychologist at the Polytrauma Rehabilitation Center at the Audie L. Murphy VA Hospital in San Antonio, Texas. Her interests include training in couple and family therapy, multicultural treatment approaches, and the treatment and assessment of posttraumatic stress disorder.

Amy Fiske, PhD, CBSM, is Associate Professor and Director of Clinical Training in the Department of Psychology at West Virginia University and a Faculty Affiliate of the WVU Injury Control Research Center. She is past president of the Society for Clinical Geropsychology. Her research focuses on depression and suicidal behavior in older adults.

Jeanne Gabriele, PhD, is Evidence-Based Psychotherapy Coordinator at the G. V. (Sonny) Montgomery VA Medical Center in Jackson, Mississippi, and Assistant Professor in the Department of Psychiatry and Human Behavior at the University of Mississippi Medical Center. Dr. Gabriele is a licensed psychologist who provides treatments for individuals with depression, posttraumatic stress disorder, insomnia, chronic pain, and obesity. Her research interests include individual and organizational factors that influence the adoption and implementation of evidence-based practice, social support and health promotion, physical activity and mental health, and weight loss/weight maintenance.

Luz Garcini, MS, is a Ford Fellow and a doctoral student at the San Diego State University–University of California, San Diego, Joint Doctoral Program in Clinical Psychology. Her primary research interests include Latino immigrant health and the development of community-based interventions for health promotion and disease prevention among underserved populations, including undocumented Latino immigrants.

Robert J. Gatchel, PhD, ABPP, is Distinguished Professor and Chairman of the Department of Psychology at the University of Texas at Arlington and an internationally recognized expert on chronic pain management and disability. Dr. Gatchel has authored approximately 300 peer-reviewed papers on pain management and serves on the editorial boards of several academic journals, including *Spine, Journal of Occupational Rehabilitation, Pain Practice, Journal of Applied Biobehavioral Research, Spine Journal,* and *Practical Pain Management.* He has won numerous awards over his career, including the Elizabeth H. Penn Professorship in Clinical Psychology at the University of Texas Southwestern Medical Center at Dallas, the Texas Psychological Association Outstanding Contribution to Science and Lifetime Achievement Awards, the American Psychological Association (APA) Division 38 Outstanding Contributions to Clinical Health Psychology Award, and the APA Award for Distinguished Professional Contributions to Applied Research.

Douglas P. Gibson, PsyD, MPH, is the owner and lead psychologist of MedPsych of Virginia, a neuropsychology and forensic psychology practice in Reston, Virginia. He was Associate Professor of Psychiatry and Surgery at Virginia

Commonwealth University until 2012. Dr. Gibson has published in the areas of neurocognitive functioning and quality of life in medical patients as well as posttraumatic stress disorder in combat soldiers. Additionally, he serves as a Major and Chief Behavioral Science Officer for the Virginia Army National Guard.

Alan G. Glaros, PhD, is Professor in the School of Dentistry at the University of Missouri–Kansas City. Dr. Glaros is past president of the Association for Applied Psychophysiology and Biofeedback (AAPB) and the 2009 recipient of the Distinguished Scientist Award from AAPB. He maintains an active research program in facial pain, particularly temporomandibular disorders, and he has published more than 50 peer-reviewed works in behavioral dentistry.

Amy Goetzinger, PhD, is a clinical psychologist and Assistant Clinical Professor in the Department of Anesthesiology at the University of North Carolina at Chapel Hill. She works with chronic-pain patients, and her research examines the impact of physical trauma and/or injury on psychological adjustment to acute pain and progression to chronic pain. Dr. Goetzinger is a member of the Society of Behavioral Medicine, the American Psychological Association, the Society of Biological Psychiatry, and the International Association for the Study of Pain.

Linda Gonder-Frederick, PhD, is Associate Professor in the Department of Neurobehavioral Sciences and Psychiatry and Clinical Director of the Behavioral Medicine Center at the University of Virginia. She has been involved in diabetes research for more than 25 years, with a focus on the development of behavioral interventions and understanding fear of hypoglycemia in patients and their families. Dr. Gonder-Frederick has published more than 145 articles and book chapters and serves as associate editor, editorial board member, and reviewer for several scientific journals.

Jeffrey L. Goodie, PhD, ABPP (see "About the Editors").

Christine E. Gould, PhD, is a clinical psychologist in the Geriatric Research, Education, and Clinical Center at the VA Palo Alto Health Care System and an Instructor (affiliated) in the Department of Psychiatry and Behavioral Sciences at Stanford University School of Medicine. Her research focuses on late-life anxiety and medical comorbidity.

Mekhala Gunaratne, MA, is a research coordinator in the Psychosocial Medicine Lab in the Department of Psychology at Ryerson University.

Deborah L. Haller, PhD, ABPP, is Professor of Clinical Psychology at the Icahn School of Medicine at Mount Sinai in New York, having previously been Professor of Clinical Psychology (in Psychiatry) at Columbia University College of Physicians and Surgeons and Chair of the Division of Psychiatric Research at St. Luke's–Roosevelt Hospital. As a Fellow of the American Academy of Clinical Health Psychology, her research has focused on medical populations with comorbid addiction and psychiatric problems, including those who are pregnant, have chronic pain, have HIV/AIDS, require organ transplant, or are morbidly obese. Dr. Haller teaches and supervises trainees to deliver evidence-based interventions for substance abuse, both psychological and pharmacological. In 2003, she received the Distinguished Mentor Award from Virginia Commonwealth University.

Abigail Herron, DO, is the Director of Psychiatry at the Institute for Family Health and Assistant Professor of Psychiatry at the Icahn School of Medicine at Mt. Sinai. Until recently, she was the Director of the Fellowship in Addiction Medicine at the Addiction Institute of New York at Mt. Sinai St. Luke's and Roosevelt Hospitals. Her interests include co-occurring addictive and mental health disorder, pharmacological treatment strategies, and medical education.

Susan Himes, PhD, is a clinical research psychologist and Clinical Assistant Professor in the Department of Psychiatry and Human Behavior at Lifespan Physician Group in Providence, Rhode Island, and the Warren Alpert Medical School of Brown University. Her research interests include treatments for binge eating, postbariatric surgery adherence, and mood dysregulation in obesity.

Benson M. Hoffman, PhD, is Assistant Professor in the Department of Psychiatry and Behavioral Sciences at Duke University Medical Center, where he specializes in the assessment and treatment of organ transplant patients and contributes to research on the effects of behavioral interventions for depression, cognition, and health. He is a member of the Society of Behavioral Medicine, the American Psychological Association, and the American Psychosomatic Society.

David Houghton, MS, is a doctoral student in clinical psychology at Texas A&M University. His research interests include cognitive-behavioral and acceptance-based behavioral interventions for anxiety and substance use disorders. His current research also investigates the mediational roles of experiential avoidance and valued living in smoking cessation, with a focus on informing theory-driven treatment applications.

Solam Huey, PhD, is a practicing clinical health psychologist at the James J. Peters VA Medical Center, Bronx, New York, where she is the Health Behavior Coordinator and the Cochair of the Health Promotion and Disease Prevention Program Committee. Dr. Huey is also the Lead Psychologist for the Bariatric Surgery and Smoking and Tobacco Use Cessation Programs, and an active contributing psychologist in the Primary Care–Mental Health Integration and National Weight Management Programs.

Christopher L. Hunter, PhD, ABPP, is the Department of Defense Program Manager for Behavioral Health in Primary Care. He has served as Chair for the Society of Behavioral Medicine's Integrated Primary Care Special Interest Group and has been a Collaborative Family Healthcare Association board member. He also served as a member of the American Psychological Association (APA) President Initiated Inter-Organizational Work Group Initiative on Competencies for Psychological Practice in Primary Care. In 2002 he received the Arthur W. Melton Early Career Achievement Award from APA Division 19, Military Psychology, for his work on integrated behavioral health in primary care service and training. He has published several research articles and book chapters in primary care psychology and is the lead author of the book *Integrated Behavioral Health in Primary Care: Step-by-Step Guidance for Assessment and Intervention.*

Iman Hussain, BS, is a Research Analyst at the Centre for Addiction and Mental Health in Toronto. She investigates Internet-based interventions and community prevention research. She is interested in exploring the biopsychosocial model in treating mental health disorders and addictions in women.

Seth C. Kalichman, PhD, is Professor in the Psychology Department at the University of Connecticut and Director of the Southeast HIV/AIDS Research and Evaluation Project. His research focuses on social and behavioral aspects of AIDS in the United States and South Africa. Dr. Kalichman is a recipient of the Distinguished Scientific Award for Early Career Contribution to Psychology in Health from the American Psychological Association and the Distinguished Scientist Award from the Society of Behavioral Medicine. He is the editor of the journal *AIDS and Behavior* and the author of *Denying AIDS: Conspiracy Theories, Pseudoscience, and Human Tragedy.*

Elizabeth A. Klonoff, PhD, is Professor of Psychology at San Diego State University (SDSU) and Professor of Psychiatry at the University of California, San Diego. She serves as the SDSU Codirector of the Joint Doctoral Program in Clinical Psychology. Dr. Klonoff's research focuses on the impact of discrimination and acculturation on health, cancer disparities, and minors' access to tobacco.

Kristin Kuntz, PhD, is Clinical Assistant Professor of Psychiatry at the Ohio State University Wexner Medical Center, where she serves as the Transplant Psychologist of the Comprehensive Transplant Center. Her clinical interests include assisting patients with preparing for organ transplants, helping them adjust to life after transplant, and fostering health behavior change. Dr. Kuntz's research activities involve assessing psychological distress and quality of life in transplant patients and living kidney donors.

Kevin T. Larkin, PhD, ABPP, is Professor of Psychology and Behavioral Medicine and Psychiatry at West Virginia University, where he is Chair of the Department of Psychology. Dr. Larkin's research is in applied psychophysiology, cardiovascular behavioral medicine, and clinical health psychology. He is author of the book *Stress and Hypertension: Examining the Relation between Psychological Stress and High Blood Pressure.*

Elaine A. Leventhal, MD, PhD, is Professor of Medicine Emeritus at Robert Wood Johnson School of Medicine of Rutgers, The State University of New Jersey. She is board certified in Internal and Geriatric Medicine and is a member and former president of the Academy of Behavioral Medicine Research. The many contributions of Dr. Leventhal's clinical expertise to the common-sense model of self-regulation include the design and conduct of studies on the control of distress during childbirth, strategies of conserving resources to minimize distress, and beliefs about sensitivity to medication as a barrier to treatment adherence.

Howard Leventhal, PhD, is Board of Governors Professor of Health Sciences at the Institute for Health at Rutgers, The State University of New Jersey. He is a member of the Institute of Medicine of the National Academy of Sciences, and a recipient of the American Psychological Foundation Life Achievement Award in Psychological Science. He has led in the development of the common-sense model of self-regulation that describes the interplay of cognitive and affective processes involved in both automatic and volitional interpretation of somatic and functional changes from disease and treatment, and the processes involved in the creation of action plans for managing current and future health threats. Dr. Leventhal is committed to multidisciplinary research to develop behavioral science and to influence clinical practice to improve objective health outcomes.

Kenneth L. Lichstein, PhD, CBSM, is Professor of Psychology at the University of Alabama, a past member of the executive board of the Society of Behavioral Sleep Medicine, and the founding editor of *Behavioral Sleep Medicine*. Dr. Lichstein's research interests lie within the area of behavioral sleep medicine, with an emphasis on insomnia in older adults.

Danielle E. McCarthy, PhD, is Associate Professor of Psychology and a member of the Institute for Health, Health Care Policy, and Aging Research at Rutgers, The State University of New Jersey. Her research focuses on identifying malleable, proximal determinants of motivation to smoke cigarettes and targeting these to devise new and improved smoking cessation treatments.

Christina S. McCrae, PhD, CBSM, is Professor in the Department of Health Psychology at the University of Missouri–Columbia. She is past president of the Society of Behavioral Sleep Medicine, a member of the executive board of the American Board of Sleep Medicine, a member of the editorial board of *Behavioral Sleep Medicine*, and former chair of the Insomnia Section of the American Academy of Sleep Medicine. Dr. McCrae's research focuses on sleep and cognition, sleep variability, and insomnia in older adults and medical patients with pain, cancer, or cardiac disease.

Cindy A. McGeary, PhD, ABPP, is Assistant Professor in the Department of Psychiatry at the University of Texas Health Science Center, San Antonio. Dr. McGeary is a former Active Duty

Air Force member and served as the Chief of Training and Research within the largest mental health clinic in the Air Force, where she routinely supervised and trained military psychologists. Dr. McGeary has numerous peer-reviewed articles and book chapters focusing on chronic pain management and occupational burnout.

Donald D. McGeary, PhD, ABPP, is Assistant Professor in the Department of Psychiatry at the University of Texas Health Science Center, San Antonio, and Director of the Health Science Center's Clinical Psychology Internship Program. Dr. McGeary has authored dozens of book chapters and peer-reviewed scientific papers focusing on chronic pain, trauma/resiliency, and telehealth, and is currently on the editorial boards of the *Journal of Applied Biobehavioral Research* and *Pain Practice*. Dr. McGeary helped develop the first integrated behavioral health service in the San Antonio University of Texas Medicine system.

Kate Murray, PhD, is Assistant Professor in the Department of Family and Preventive Medicine at the University of California, San Diego. Her work focuses on using community-based participatory research to address community-identified health and mental health concerns within immigrant and refugee communities.

Howard Newville, PhD, is Associate Research Scientist in the Department of Psychiatry at St. Luke's–Roosevelt Hospital in New York. His research focuses on the treatment of substance abuse in HIV-positive individuals and interventions to improve antiretroviral adherence. He received a National Research Service Award through the National Institute on Drug Abuse to test a behavioral intervention intended to increase antiretroviral adherence and decrease drug use in active substance abusers.

Mary Ellen Olbrisch, PhD, ABPP, is Professor of Psychiatry and Surgery at Virginia Commonwealth University (VCU) and Director of Education and Training in Clinical Health Psychology for the VCU Health System, where she consults to the Weight Loss Surgery Program and serves as the federally designated Living Donor Advocate for the Liver Transplant Program. Dr. Olbrisch has been active in the development of the specialty of clinical health psychology throughout her career. She has served on the American Board of Clinical Health Psychology in various positions since its inception and has been instrumental in developing the standards for competence in the specialty through her work on the Board. Dr. Olbrisch is internationally known for her work in presurgical mental health and behavioral evaluation of patients for organ transplant and bariatric surgery and for exposition of the ethical issues involved in these evaluations.

Jan Passchier, PhD, is Professor in the Psychological Aspects of Somatic Complaints and Academic Director Indonesia at the VU University Amsterdam. His current research focuses on health status and quality of life in Indonesia and the psychological–ethical consequences of participation in medical research.

Lauren M. Penwell-Waines, PhD, is Assistant Professor and Licensed Clinical Psychologist at the Virginia Tech Carilion School of Medicine and Research Institute Department of Family and Community Medicine. Her research interests include stress and health, coping with chronic disease, and integrated care.

Alan L. Peterson, PhD, ABPP (See "About the Editors").

Errol J. Philip, PhD, is Chief Clinical Research Fellow in the Department of Psychiatry and Behavioral Sciences at Memorial Sloan-Kettering Cancer Center. His work spans many issues associated with the late and long-term effects of cancer treatment and diagnosis. He is currently completing a research fellowship with a focus on obesity, diet, and cancer survivorship. Dr. Philip's primary interests include assessing the impact of weight loss on disease biomarkers and quality of life in the context of cancer survivorship.

Lisa M. Schilling, PhD, is a Pediatric Psychologist at Nemours Children's Clinic–Jacksonville in the Division of Psychology and Psychiatry and Assistant Professor of Psychology at the Mayo Clinic College of Medicine. She specializes in the assessment and treatment of children with cancer. Dr. Schilling is involved in research through the Children's Oncology Group and the University of Florida Proton Institute.

Tammy A. Schuler, PhD, is a Clinical Research Fellow in the Department of Psychiatry and Behavioral Sciences at Memorial Sloan-Kettering Cancer Center. Her research interests include development of biobehavioral interventions for couples and families coping with diagnoses of advanced cancers (particularly pancreatic cancer and diagnoses in young adults), longitudinal biobehavioral outcomes following family

involvement in such interventions, and development and psychometric assessment of distress-measurement tools.

Jaclyn A. Shepard, PsyD, is Assistant Professor in the Department of Psychiatry and Neurobehavioral Sciences at the University of Virginia School of Medicine. Her research has focused on psychological and behavioral considerations in the management of chronic illness in pediatric and adult populations, with publications on fear of hypoglycemia and advanced diabetes technology. Dr. Shepard serves as a reviewer for several scientific journals.

Anne-Lise C. Smith, PhD, is completing postdoctoral training at the Massachusetts Mental Health Center and the Brookline Community Mental Health Center. Her research interests involve clinical interventions for anxiety, loss, and trauma.

Merideth D. Smith, PhD, is a clinical psychologist with PsiMed, Inc. in West Virginia. Her research interests focus on functional disability, social support systems, suicide risk, and aging in the prison system.

Todd A. Smitherman, PhD, is Associate Professor in the Department of Psychology at the University of Mississippi. His health psychology research program focuses principally on psychiatric comorbidities in medical conditions such as migraine and chronic pain.

C. Mark Sollars, MS, is Associate Editor at McMahon Publishing Group in New York. Previously he was Research Coordinator at the Montefiore Headache Center, Bronx, New York. He holds graduate degrees in both Counseling and Experimental Psychology, has published on clinical tools used in headache management, and has conducted research on the placebo response.

Karen E. Stewart, PhD, teaches in the Health Psychology Training Program in the Departments of Psychiatry and Gastroenterology at Virginia Commonwealth University Medical Center. Her research and clinical work are focused on the treatment of obesity and disordered eating in adults with medical conditions and the provision of psychological services in medical settings.

Daniel J. Taylor, PhD, CBSM, ABSM, is Associate Professor of Psychology at the University of North Texas and a past member of the executive boards of the Society of Behavioral Sleep Medicine and the American Board of Sleep Medicine. Dr. Taylor is Director of the University's Insomnia Research Laboratory, which focuses on the epidemiology and treatment of insomnia, particularly when comorbid with psychological and medical disorders.

J. Kevin Thompson, PhD, is Professor in the Department of Psychology at the University of South Florida in Tampa. Dr. Thompson's research interests involve the measurement of risk for body image problems and eating disturbances, with a focus on sociocultural factors and interpersonal experiences. He has served on the editorial board of six scientific journals in the areas of psychology and eating disorders. He has written and edited nine books on eating disorders.

Tony Toneatto, PhD, is Associate Professor in the Department of Psychiatry and Director of the Buddhism, Psychology and Mental Health undergraduate program at the University of Toronto.

He has published in the area of substance and gambling addiction treatment.

Brenda B. Toner, PhD, is Full Professor in the Department of Psychiatry and Graduate Coordinator, Institute of Medical Science, Faculty of Medicine, University of Toronto. She was Head of Women's Mental Health in the Department of Psychiatry from 1997 to 2011. Dr. Toner has published over 90 articles and book chapters and has given over 200 presentations on a variety of health-related problems, including eating disorders, anxiety, depression, chronic pelvic pain, chronic fatigue, and irritable bowel syndrome. She is particularly interested in exploring social factors in the lives of women that cut across health and mental health diagnoses, including violence, body dissatisfaction, discrimination, and gender role socialization.

Tovah Yanover, PhD, focuses her research primarily on body image and eating disorders. She has published and presented research at national conferences in these areas.

Contents

PART III. Assessment of Clinical Problems

PART IV. Assessment of Special Populations

PART I

Overview

CHAPTER 1

Introduction to Biopsychosocial Assessment in Clinical Health Psychology

Alan L. Peterson
Jeffrey L. Goodie
Frank Andrasik

Over the past 30 years, clinical health psychology has been one of the fastest growing specialty areas of psychology (Belar & Deardorff, 1995, 2009). A number of terms have been used previously to describe the clinical health psychology specialty area, including psychosomatic medicine (Lipowski, Lipsitt, & Whybrow, 1977), behavioral medicine (Schwartz & Weiss, 1978), behavioral health (Matarazzo, 1980), medical psychology (Prokop & Bradley, 1981), behavioral health psychology (Matarazzo, Weiss, Herd, Miller, & Weiss, 1984), and health psychology (Stone et al., 1987). The term "clinical health psychology" was initially archived by the American Psychological Association in 1997 and is described as the application of "scientific knowledge of the interrelationships among behavioral, emotional, cognitive, social, and biological components in health and disease to the promotion and maintenance of health" (as cited in Belar & Deardorff, 2009, p. 5).

Most specialization training for psychologists comes at the postdoctoral level. Over the past two decades, clinical health psychology has been one of the most popular specialty areas for postdoctoral training. Of the 154 postdoctoral fellowship programs found in an online search of the Association of Psychology Postdoctoral and Internship

Centers directory (Association of Psychology Postdoctoral and Internship Centers [APPIC], 2013), 102 programs (66%) provide specialty training in health psychology.

Another measure of the growth of clinical health psychology is the number of psychologists employed by medical schools. In 1953, a total of 255 psychologists worked at American medical schools (Mensh, 1953). In 2003, a Medical School/Academic Medical Center Psychologists Employment Survey was conducted by the American Psychological Association's Research Office and the Association of Medical School Psychologists' Executive Committee. This survey indicated that the number of psychologists working in academic medical centers had grown to 2,926 (Pate & Kohout, 2004). A more recent survey has not been conducted since 2003, but it has been estimated that the number of psychologists in medical schools continued to increase at a similar rate and reached 4,788 by 2007 (Robiner, Dixon, Miner, & Hong, 2014). Another way to measure the growth of clinical health psychology is by the average number of psychologists at each academic medical center. The average number of psychologists employed by individual academic medical centers has also grown from 2 in the 1950s to 28 in the 1990s (Sheridan, 1999).

A similar rapid growth in clinical health psychologists has occurred in other clinical and research settings. More psychologists are interacting with the medical community to provide clinical services and to conduct research. A plethora of resources have been developed for psychologists to use as references for the assessment and treatment of the most common psychological disorders (e.g., depression, anxiety, couple distress) seen in behavioral health clinics. However, clinical health psychologists are faced with not only addressing traditional behavioral health problems but also understanding how those problems interact with a breadth of medical problems. Clinical health psychologists must work to overcome the mind–body dualism, originally described by Descartes, which continues to be a common way of conceptualizing clinical cases in many medical settings. Rather than attempting to separate contributions of the "mind" versus the "body," which is the goal of many traditional psychological assessments, evidence-based assessments must focus on the interactions among the individual, the disease, and the environment (Belar & Deardorff, 1995, 2009).

The interrelationships of these components are the hallmark feature of the biopsychosocial model. First described by Engel (1977), the biopsychosocial model was initially proposed as a challenge to biomedicine to develop a new medical model for conceptualizing health and illness. Over the past four decades, this model has not only revolutionized the practice of medicine but has also provided the theoretical foundation for clinical health psychology as a specialty area within psychology. A blueprint to address education and training guidelines for the professional practice of psychology in health care settings was recently published by the Health Service Psychology Education Collaborative (2013). This was an interorganizational effort including the American Psychological Association, the Council of Graduate Departments of Psychology, and the Council of Chairs of Training Councils. The blueprint included a statement of core competencies for clinical health psychologists. As highlighted in this blueprint, clinical health psychology may be the one specialty area within psychology that best exemplifies the use of a biopsychosocial approach to assessment and treatment. This chapter provides an overview of biopsychosocial assessment in the field of clinical health psychology.

Domains Included in the Biopsychosocial Model

According to the original definition provided by Engel (1977), the biopsychosocial model refers to biological, psychological, and social domains. Figure 1.1 depicts this basic biopsychosocial model and how biological, psychological, and social factors can influence—and be influenced by—a particular disease, disorder, or illness. For example, cancer can be influenced or caused by a combination of biological, psychological, and social factors. According to the American Cancer Society (2012), cancer is a complex group of diseases with many possible causes, including genetics, lifestyle (e.g., tobacco use, diet, and physical activity), certain types of infections, and environmental exposures to different types of chemicals and radiation. In addition to there being a multitude of potential causes of cancer that can be conceptualized within the domains of the biopsychosocial model, cancer can have an impact on biological, psychological, and social functioning. For example, certain types of cancer can cause pain, weight loss, depression, anxiety, and decreased sexual functioning. The bidirectional influences involved in the biopsychosocial model are important features in the conceptualization of the assessment and treatment of diseases, disorders, and illnesses.

The application of the biopsychosocial model within the field of clinical health psychology, as well as in other disciplines, often includes an expansion of the model beyond the three basic domains. In addition, there is not universal agreement on the specific domains that should be included within an expanded biopsychosocial model. For example, the biological domain can also be referred to or subdivided into physical, physiological, biochemical, nutritional, or genetic domains. The psychological domain is the one most often subdivided by psychologists and can include emotional, affective, cognitive, behavioral, spiritual, and personality domains. The social domain can include environmental, cultural, family, work, and interpersonal domains.

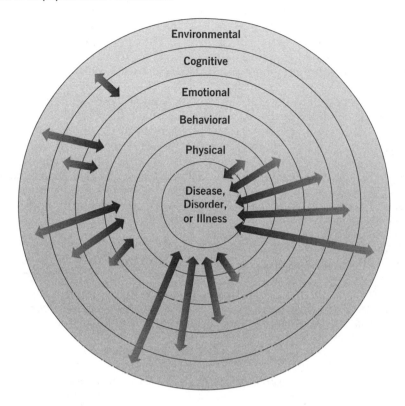

FIGURE 1.1. Domains and bidirectional influences in the expanded biopsychosocial model.

Table 1.1 includes a summary of the primary domains included in the basic as well as expanded versions of the biopsychosocial model. The primary expansion of the model for use by clinical health psychologists is the subdivision of the psychological domain to include behavioral, emotional (or affective), and cognitive domains. For assessments conducted by psychologists, the term "physical

TABLE 1.1. Basic and Expanded Versions of the Biopsychosocial Model

Engle (1977)	American Psychological Association (1997)	Belar & Deardorff (2009)
Biological	Biological	Biological or physical
Psychological	Behavioral Emotional Cognitive	Behavioral Affective Cognitive
Social	Social	Environmental

domain" is a more useful construct than "biological domain." Finally, "environmental factors," as described by Belar and Deardorff (2009), is a preferred domain description over "social" for clinical health psychologists. The environmental domain expands this construct beyond what is ordinarily thought of as "social" to include factors such as the health care system and even climate. These are known to affect some conditions treated by clinical health psychologists, such as Raynaud's disease and systemic sclerosis (Watson, Robb, Belcher, & Belch, 1999).

Evidence-Based Approaches to Biopsychosocial Assessment

The primary goal of evidence-based approaches to biopsychosocial assessment is to identify the unique contributions of multiple domains of possible factors to an individual patient's overall physical and psychological health. As mentioned previously, traditional clinical assessments and case conceptualizations in medical settings have often tried to determine whether an individual patient's medical condition is more psychological or physical. As a result, clinical cases are often conceptualized on a sliding-scale, bimodal continuum anchored on one side with physical factors and the other side with psychological factors (see Figure 1.2). In contrast, the biopsychosocial approach to psychological assessment presumes that there are varying levels of physical, cognitive, emotional, behavioral, and environmental factors that contribute to the overall clinical assessment and conceptualization of every individual case. Rather than trying to determine whether an individual case is more "psychological" or "physical," multiple domains are seen as contributing varying amounts of influence to the overall biopsychosocial conceptualization of an individual case.

The biopsychosocial model has been a critical factor in helping move clinical health psychologists beyond the traditional mind–body dualism approach to the assessment of patients in medical settings. Evidence-based assessment approaches for many diseases, illnesses, and disorders have embraced the biopsychosocial model of clinical assessment. However, much additional work is needed in the development and validation of biopsychosocial assessment instruments and approaches, and it is our hope that the chapters contained in this volume help spur this development.

REFERENCES

American Cancer Society. (2012). *What causes cancer?* Retrieved from *www.cancer.org/Cancer/CancerCauses/index.*

Association of Psychology Postdoctoral and

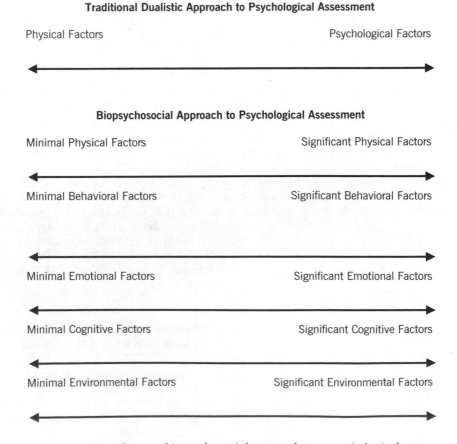

FIGURE 1.2. Traditional versus biopsychosocial approaches to psychological assessment.

Internship Centers (APPIC). (2013). *Postdoctoral directory* [Online directory]. Retrieved from *https://membership.appic.org/directory/search*.

Belar, C. D., & Deardorff, W. W. (1995). *Clinical health psychology in medical settings: A practitioner's guidebook*. Washington, DC: American Psychological Association.

Belar, C. D., & Deardorff, W. W. (2009). *Clinical health psychology in medical settings: A practitioner's guidebook* (2nd ed.). Washington, DC: American Psychological Association.

Engel, G. L. (1977). The need for a new medical model: A challenge for biomedicine. *Science, 196*, 129–136.

Health Service Psychology Education Collaborative. (2013). Professional psychology in health care settings: A blueprint for education and training. *American Psychologist, 68*, 411–426.

Lipowski, Z. J., Lipsitt, D. R., & Whybrow, P. C. (Eds.). (1977). *Psychosomatic medicine: Current trends and clinical applications*. New York: Oxford University Press.

Matarazzo, J. D. (1980). Behavioral health and behavioral medicine: Frontiers for a new health psychology. *American Psychologist, 35*, 807–817.

Matarazzo, J. D., Weiss, S. M., Herd, J. A., Miller, N. E., & Weiss, S. M. (Eds.). (1984). *Behavioral health: A handbook of health enhancement and disease prevention*. New York: Wiley.

Mensh, I. N. (1953). Psychology in medical education. *American Psychologist, 8*, 83–85.

Pate, W. E., II, & Kohout, J. (2004). *Report of the 2003 Medical School/Academic Medical Center Psychologists Employment Survey*. Retrieved from *www.apa.org/workforce/publications/03-amsp/index.aspx*.

Prokop, C., & Bradley, A. A. (1981). *Medical psychology: Contributions to behavioral medicine*. New York: Academic Press.

Robiner, W. N., Dixon, K. E., Miner, J. L., & Hong, B. A. (2014). Psychologists in medical schools and academic medical centers: Over 100 years of growth, influence, and partnership. *American Psychologist, 69*, 230–248.

Schwartz, G. E., & Weiss, S. M. (1978). Yale Conference on Behavioral Medicine: A proposed definition and statement of goals. *Journal of Behavioral Medicine, 1*, 3–12.

Sheridan, E. P. (1999). Psychology's future in medical schools and academic health care centers. *American Psychologist, 54*, 267–271.

Stone, G., Weiss, S., Matarazzo, J., Miller, N., Rodin, J., Belar, C., et al. (1987). *Health psychology: A discipline and a profession*. Chicago: University of Chicago Press.

Watson, H. R., Robb, R., Belcher, G., & Belch, J. J. (1999). Seasonal variation of Raynaud's phenomenon secondary to systemic sclerosis. *Journal of Rheumatology, 26*, 1734–1737.

CHAPTER 2

Fundamentals of Assessment in Clinical Health Psychology

Cynthia D. Belar
William W. Deardorff

The practice of clinical health psychology can probably trace its more recent roots to the biopsychosocial model of illness and health originally proposed by Engel (1977). Briefly, the biopsychosocial model proposes that health and illness are influenced not only by biomedical variables but also by cultural, social, and psychological considerations. Although this concept seems commonplace today, it was somewhat revolutionary at a time when the biomedical model prevailed, including "the notion of the body as a machine, of the disease as a consequence of the breakdown of the machine, and of the doctor's task as repair of the machine" (Engel, 1977, p. 131). Subsequently, Matarazzo's initial definition of health psychology (1980), followed by definitions of clinical health psychology (see Millon, 1982; see also Belar, McIntyre, & Matarazzo, 2003, for a history of health psychology), formed the foundation of a current definition (American Psychological Association):

Clinical health psychology applies scientific knowledge of the interrelationships among behavioral, emotional, cognitive, social and biological components in health and disease to the promotion and maintenance of health; the prevention, treatment and rehabilitation of illness and disability; and the improvement of the health care system. The distinct focus of Clinical Health Psychology is on the physical health problems. The specialty is dedicated to the development of knowledge regarding the interface between behavior and health, and to the delivery of high quality services based on that knowledge to individuals, families and health care systems. (as cited in Belar & Deardorff, 2009, p. 5)

The reader may be wondering why the need for a history lesson. Having knowledge of these historical and definitional issues related to clinical health psychology is critical to understanding the fundamentals of assessment in this area. As can be seen, if one has a good understanding of how clinical health psychology defines itself and its unique realm of practice, then the fundamentals of assessment become clear. As can be derived from the definition, the domains of assessment for the clinical health psychologist must necessarily include physical/biological, affective, cognitive, and behavioral "targets." To make things more interesting (and complicated), these variables or "targets" must be assessed not only relative to the patient but also across various "environments," such as the family, the health care system, and the sociocultural context. Once information is gathered about all of these relevant domains, it must be integrated in a concise and useful format to address the purpose of the assessment and provide answers.

Psychodiagnostic evaluation is a frequent activity of the clinical health psychologist and may serve a number of purposes, such as determining differential diagnosis, guiding a treatment intervention, and planning outcome assessment. One of the unique aspects of clinical health psychology assessment is the integration of the multiple domains of information, as discussed previously. A useful method for approaching the clinical health psychology assessment of any issue is to pose the questions in Table 2.1. The questions can be used to develop the goals of assessment. These were adapted from Belar et al. (2001) relative to the self-assessment of readiness to practice in the area of clinical health psychology. However, they provide an excellent template for building a clinical health psychology assessment approach. The process of clinical health psychology assessment includes determining assessment needs, choosing the appropriate methods of

assessment, gathering information from all the relevant domains, formulating impressions, concisely and efficiently communicating results, and then following through as required.

A Model of Assessment

As evidenced by the many chapters and topics in this volume, clinical health psychology assessment varies widely depending upon a number of factors, including the referral question, patient status, illness/disability issues, the referral source, and the treatment setting. Based on an extension of the biopsychosocial conceptualizations of Engel (1977) and Leigh and Reiser (1980), Belar developed a model for clinical health psychology assessment (Belar, Deardorff, & Kelly, 1987; Belar & Deardorff, 1995, 2009). As can be seen in Table 2.2, this model articulates *targets of assessment* by *domain of information* (biological or physical, affective, cognitive, behavioral) and *unit of assessment* (patient, family, health care system, or sociocultural context). Although by no means exhaustive, each block in the table shows the kinds of information that need to be gathered in an attempt to understand the patient from a biopsychosocial perspective. In addition to current status, each block also has an associated developmental or historical perspective that may be important to fully understanding the problem being assessed. For each block, the clinician should think in terms of assessing current status, changes since onset of the illness or disability, and past history. Also for each block, assessment should focus not only on identification of problems but also on resources and strengths of the patient and his or her environment.

This model is useful for approaching any problem the clinical health psychologist may be confronted with assessing. It ensures that no domain of information is overlooked, facilitates decision making about assessment strategies, assists in the organization of the information obtained, and helps with the formation of intervention strategies. The fact that the model is portrayed as blocks of information should in no way imply a reductionistic focus. The information obtained within each block must be conceptualized as interrelated with all of the

---

TABLE 2.1. Template for Developing the Goals of a Clinical Health Psychology Assessment

1. What are the biological bases of health and disease as related to this problem? How is this related to the biological bases of behavior?

2. What are the cognitive–affective bases of health and disease as related to this problem? How is this related to the cognitive–affective bases of behavior?

3. What are the social bases of health and disease as related to this problem? How are these related to the social bases of behavior?

4. What are the development and individual bases of health and disease as related to this problem? How are these related to the development and individual bases of behavior?

5. What are the interactions among biological, affective, cognitive, social, and developmental components (e.g. psychophysiological aspects)? Do I understand the relationships between this problem and the patient and his or her environment (including family, health care system, and sociocultural environment)?

6. Have I chosen empirically supported clinical assessment methods for these problems, and how might the assessment be affected by information in questions 1–5?

Note. Adapted from Belar et al. (2001, p. 137). Copyright 2001 by the American Psychological Association. Adapted by permission.

TABLE 2.2. Targets of Assessment

Domain of information	Patient	Family	Environment — Health care system	Environment — Sociocultural context
Biological or physical	• Age, sex, race • Physical appearance • Symptoms, health status • Physical examination • Vital signs, lab data • Prescribed medications • Over-the-counter medications • Psychophysiological data • Genetic history and risks • Constitutional factors, disabilities • History of injury, disease surgery, reproduction	• Characteristics of the home setting • Economic resources • Family size • Familial patterning (e.g., headache history) • Other illness in family • Immigration status	• Characteristics of the treatment setting • Characteristics of medical procedures • Availability of prosthetic aids • Accessibility of health care • Gender and cultural disparities in care	• Social services • Financial resources • Social networks • Occupational setting • Health hazards • Exposure to violence, terrorism, war • Global factors (e.g., political, economic)
Affective	• Mood • Affect • Feelings about illness treatment, health care, providers, self, family, jobs, social networks • History of affective disturbance	• Members' feelings about patient, illness, and treatment	• Providers' feelings about patient, illness, and treatment	• Sentiment of culture regarding patient, illness, and treatment
Cognitive	• Cognitive style • Thought content • Intelligence • Education • Knowledge about disease • Health beliefs • Attitudes and expectations regarding illness, treatment, health care, and providers • Perceived meaning of illness • Philosophy of life • Spiritual/religious beliefs	• Knowledge about illness and treatment • Attitudes/expectations about patient, illness	• Providers' knowledge • Providers' attitudes toward patient, illness, and treatment	• Current state of knowledge • Cultural/religious attitudes toward patient and illness
Behavioral	• Activity level/exercise • Interactions with family, friends, providers, and coworkers • Health habits • Health care utilization/history of treatments • Substance abuse • Adherence • Ability to control physical symptoms	• Participation in patient care/caregiving roles • Reinforcement contingencies for health and illness • Family interactions, interpersonal violence • Primary language	• Providers' skills in education and training patients • Reinforcement contingencies for health and illness • Providers' linguistic and cultural competence	• Employment policies • Laws regulating health care practice, disability, provision of care, health habits, accessibility • Customs in symptom reporting and help seeking

Note. Adapted from Belar and Deardorff (2009, pp. 51–53). Copyright 2009 by the American Psychological Association. Adapted by permission.

other compartments. It is noteworthy that this model is consistent with more recent recommendations regarding competencies for *all* psychologists who provide health care services. These competencies are articulated in the Blueprint for Education and Training developed by the Health Service Psychology Education Collaborative (HSPEC; 2013), an interorganizational endeavor including the American Psychological Association, the Council of Graduate Departments of Psychology, and the Council of Chairs of Training Councils.

Patient Targets

Biological Targets

The most basic biological targets include the patient's age, race, sex, and physical appearance. Beyond these obvious variables, other information might include physical examination data, laboratory studies (e.g., blood, urine, imaging), medications, and drug use (current and past). Other important information includes the patient's medical history (e.g., illness, hospitalizations, surgeries), as well as that of his or her family.

Affective Targets

Assessment of affective targets requires developing an understanding of the patient's mood and affect, along with his or her feelings about the illness, treatment, health providers, future, and social support network. Keeping in mind a historical and developmental perspective, it is also important to assess the patient for possible long-term emotional issues (e.g., dysthymia, generalized anxiety) and, as well, his or her response to previous stressors. This will help the clinician more fully understand the patient's current status.

Cognitive Targets

The mental status examination usually forms the core of current cognitive assessment and includes such things as memory, concentration, and intellectual capacity. Further assessment of cognitive function includes the patient's thoughts, beliefs, and attitudes, especially about things related to the purpose of the evaluation (e.g., dis-

ease, disability, health behavior modification). More global cognitive targets include religious beliefs and worldview. All of these factors can help the clinician understand the patient's knowledge about the illness, the perceived meaning of the illness to the patient, the patient's attitudes about medical and other interventions and about health, and the patient's perceived control over physical and psychological symptoms and expectations about outcome.

Behavioral Targets

Behavioral targets include what the patient is doing (action) and the manner in which he or she does it (style). Example of actions include motor behaviors such as facial expression, foot tapping, bracing, body posture, and eye contact. Behavioral styles might include such things as flamboyance, hesitancy, hostility, restlessness, and passivity. Assessment of behavioral targets, including action and style, should give a clinician a good understanding of such things as the patient's level of self-care, health habits, use of the health care system, physician–patient interactions, current and past compliance with treatment regimens, and vocational and avocational pursuits.

Interaction among Patient Targets

It is again important to underscore that, although the targets of assessment are organized as "blocks" or "compartments," they are conceptualized as completely interactive and interrelated. During the assessment, the clinician should always be thinking in terms of how the various findings interrelate. For instance, the mental status examination results (cognitive) may be significantly influenced by biological targets such as medications or by affective targets such as depression. A common example is the assessment of back pain. When the pain is being assessed, the patient might show minimal findings on magnetic resonance imaging (MRI; biological targets), extreme disability, grimacing, and verbalizations of symptoms (behavioral targets), along with depression and anxiety (suffering or affective targets), because he or she thinks the pain is due to a spinal tumor or something that will cause harm (cognitive targets). Integration of these targets of information will guide the multidisciplinary intervention.

Environmental Targets

As suggested in Table 2.2, each of the patient targets must be assessed and understood within the context of the environments within which the patient interacts: the family unit, the health care system, and the sociocultural context (social, work, cultural and ethnic background).

Family Environment

The physical domain of the family environment might include such things as development history, other illnesses in family members, the home setting, and any recent changes in any of these areas. In the affective domain, it is important to understand family members' feelings about the patient, the target of assessment (e.g., illness, health habit change such as smoking cessation or substance abuse), and the treatment rendered. In the cognitive domain, the clinician should assess family members' attitudes, perceptions, and expectations about the patient's condition, treatment, and future. Overall intellectual resources and knowledge about the patient's illness or condition should also be evaluated. Evaluation of the behavioral domain might include such things as how family members act toward the patient, especially in response to "illness behaviors" (e.g., appropriate, nurturing, enabling, punishing, or solicitous actions). Also, any change in the behavior of the family unit, especially as a result of the patient's condition, should be assessed.

Health Care System

Assessment of the physical domain of the health care system might begin with the environment in which the patient is being evaluated or treated (e.g., intensive care unit, rehabilitation hospital, hospice, private practice office, home setting), as this can influence all of the other findings. Special consideration will include privacy issues, prosthetic aids, the degree of sensory stimulation coming from the environment, and the diagnostic tests to which the patient is being subjected. Beyond the physical domain, the clinician must be aware of how the health care staff feels about the patient (affective) and his or her condition. The cognitive domain of the environment includes the staff's knowledge about the patient, the condition being treated, and their expectations for outcome. Unfortunately, medical mistakes are commonplace and often due to a lack of knowledge on the part of health care providers. Assessing the behavior of the health care system requires that the clinician have an understanding of the policies, rules, and regulations that will affect the patient's treatment. This might include such things as staffing patterns, infection control policies, and the discharge planning process. Of particular importance is the behavior of the health care providers toward the patient, especially in complex cases. The patient may be evaluated and treated by myriad specialists, all communicating with and behaving toward the patient in different, and often inconsistent, manners. This situation can be very confusing for the patient and can impede response to treatment.

Sociocultural Environment

The physical aspects of the patient's sociocultural environment include (1) the physical requirements of the occupational setting and (2) the social and financial resources available to the patient. Assessment of the patient's social network, including size, density, proximity, and frequency of contact, is also important. In the affective and cognitive realms of the sociocultural environment, the clinician should understand cultural sentiments, attitudes, and expectations regarding the patient's race, gender, lifestyle, religion, illness, and treatment. Within the behavioral domain, assessment might include such things as employment policies relative to the patient's problem, legislative policies related to health and disability issues, and ethnic customs related to illness, disease, and disability.

Interaction among Patient and Environmental Targets

As discussed previously, and as we emphasize again, the clinician should always be thinking in terms of how the various findings within each "box" interrelate. To extend our example of the patient with back pain: The patient might show minimal findings on MRI (biological); extreme disability, grimacing, and verbalizations of symptoms (behavioral), along with depression and anxiety (suffering or affective), because he or she thinks the pain is due to a spinal tumor or something that will cause harm (cognitive); family members may be angry with him or her due to the disability (family environment) and loss of his or her job (occupational); doctors may not take the time to reassure the patient regarding his or her condition (health care environment); and ethnic customs may influence the patient's expression of depression through increased pain (suffering) rather than directly (cultural environment). If any of these pieces of information were to be missed in the assessment, the treatment plan and intervention would likely be inadequate, with an elevated risk of failure.

Methods and Pitfalls in Assessment

Stemming from the scientist–practitioner model, the clinical health psychologist completing an assessment should consider diverse sources of information and multiple types of data, using a convergent–divergent, hypothesis-testing approach. In making choices about which assessment methods to employ, the clinician will take into consideration a variety of issues, including the purpose of the evaluation, the targets being assessed, the validity of the assessment method relative to the target, and the setting in which the assessment will be completed, as well as feasibility and cost-effectiveness of the assessment approach.

Archival Data

Archival data might include (1) literature reviews about the condition being assessed and (2) the patient's medical records history. In the age of the Internet, completing a literature search relative to the problem being assessed is very efficient. The clinician can rapidly obtain information about the condition being assessed (cause, symptoms, course, prevention, treatment, psychological factors) and recommended assessment methods. Archival data also include the patient's medical history and records (cur-

rent and past). Because most patients tend to be fairly poor historians, these data can be extremely valuable in giving the clinician an accurate picture of previously reported symptoms, what types of treatments have been attempted in the past and the patient's response, and other health care providers' impressions of the patient and problem being assessed.

Pitfalls

Given the ease of access to the Internet, there is really no excuse for a clinician not to avail him- or herself of this information resource. The only pitfall might be getting access to full-text articles rather than just abstracts of articles. For those who have any association with a university, medical school, or hospital (e.g., clinical appointment, staff), full access to the institution's online subscriptions is usually available. For others, consideration might be given to subscribing to an online database such as PsycNET or PsycSCAN. More difficult is obtaining the patient's past medical records, and this might be considered a "pitfall" if not done. Although not always necessary, in complicated cases it is certainly worth the effort. In this age of time-pressured physicians with multiple specialties, each treating a different "part" of the patient's problem, it is not uncommon for important details (either current or historical) to be missed. We cannot count the number of times that the review of medical records has revealed information that the patient did not report during the clinical interview, such as a treatment that has been effective in the past but was not being considered currently, a medication that is being considered but to which the patient had a previous terrible reaction, or significant inconsistencies in the patient's report versus what is documented in the records.

Clinical Interview

The clinical interview is the sine qua non of assessment and the most common form for gathering information. It is generally the initial (and often the only) source of current and historical data across all domains (e.g., physical, affective, cognitive, behavioral) and environments. The interview is also the initial step in forming what may be a working treatment relationship with the patient. The format of the interview will vary depending on the assessment purpose and will range from unstructured to semi-structured to highly structured. The most common elements of the clinical interview include the presenting problem (e.g., symptoms, impact on function), history, psychosocial situation and history, occupational function, and some form of a mental status examination. As is seen throughout this volume, the content and form of the clinical interview will vary greatly depending on the purpose and goal of the overall assessment.

Pitfalls

Probably one of the greatest pitfalls related to the initial clinical interview is the clinician's not establishing the beginnings of a trusting relationship with the patient while also gathering critical information in a timely fashion. Depending on the purpose of the assessment, this can be particularly challenging in clinical health psychology in that patients are often seen within a primarily medical context. Patients can be initially defensive when the "shrink" shows up, especially depending on how the referral was framed by the referral source. This reticence can often be overcome by initially focusing the interview on "medical" issues while also explaining the role of the clinical health psychologist in assessment and treatment.

After a successful initial interview, the patient should have a good understanding of the clinical health psychologist's role in the assessment and treatment of the patient's condition. Also, the patient should feel that he or she was fully "heard" and understood by the clinician while not feeling rushed. On the other hand, the clinician should have obtained enough information necessary to form initial impressions and guide the rest of the assessment, while also engaging the patient in the beginning of the treatment process (as appropriate). The ability to achieve these multifaceted goals, often in less than an hour, is certainly challenging. Developing the interview skills to achieve these goals comes with practice and experience.

Questionnaires

Questionnaires that are clinician-developed and problem-focused can be a very useful and efficient adjunctive method of gathering information. In an outpatient setting, these can often be mailed to the patient prior to the initial evaluation appointment. The use of questionnaires can be a great time saver and often helps to provide more accurate information. For instance, in many of the questionnaires we have developed for various problems, we ask about current and past medications (along with response), past medical treatments, past and current health care providers with contact information, surgical history, and so forth. Patients often cannot provide this information accurately, or at all, when asked as part of the initial evaluation in the office. However, it is often readily available to the patient if he or she has time to collect it as part of completing a questionnaire beforehand. The completed questionnaire that is brought to the initial evaluation can also help guide further information gathering.

Depending on the purpose of the evaluation, questionnaires can also be developed for significant others and health care providers. The form and content of the questionnaire will depend on a variety of factors, including the purpose of the evaluation, the type of treatment intervention, and the patient population. Questionnaires might include a number of different types of inquiry methods, including open-ended and forced-choice surveys, checklists, simple rating scales, or pictorial diagrams (e.g., pain drawings).

Pitfalls

When designing a questionnaire, it is important to keep in mind the person who will be completing it, including such things as educational level, language, and disability issues that might affect the person's ability to complete the assessment. The clinician who designs a 20-page questionnaire written in English at the graduate level of reading comprehension using a 10-point font size will likely be faced with very frustrated patients who, at their initial appointments, bring with them blank questionnaires and an appropriately defensive attitude toward the person who expected them to complete such a task. To carry this hypothetical scenario even further, imagine that the target population is primarily elderly (with possible visual problems) and that Spanish is the predominant primary language.

Diaries

As part of an initial assessment period, patients are often asked to complete diaries of behaviors that are both overt (e.g., pill taking, tics, walking distance, vomiting) and covert (e.g., thoughts, feelings, pain perceptions, blood pressure). These baseline measures are used as part of the initial evaluation to design the intervention and, later, to gauge the effectiveness of the treatment. Diaries can often reveal important information about the frequency, intensity, and duration of targeted behaviors. They also can reveal information about antecedents, consequences, and relationships among internal and external behaviors. Diaries can also be an important source of information to help assess the efficacy of a medical intervention. For instance, when a patient is being considered for a spinal cord stimulator (SCS) implant for pain control, he or she typically undergoes a week-long temporary trial before permanent implantation is considered. In routine practice, the criterion for a "successful" trial and permanent implantation is a 50% or greater reduction in pain. Often, at the end of the week-long trial, the physician will simply ask the patient, "Was your pain reduced by more than half?" Research has demonstrated that memory for pain is notoriously inaccurate and that there can be a significant placebo effect that may influence the patient's assessment of the effectiveness of the trial results (which may lead to permanently implanting an SCS that will not be effective over the long term). To combat these problems and provide better data for decision making, we have patients complete a pain–medication–activity–mood diary for 2 weeks prior to the trial period and during the 1-week trial. These types of data help the physician (and patient) make a better decision about permanent implantation.

Pitfalls

Compliance with completing diaries is probably one of the biggest obstacles to overcome in successfully using this assessment measure. Although the clinician might be tempted to assess myriad variables in the diary, it should be easy to use, nonintrusive, and brief. One of the biggest pitfalls is making the diary too complex and onerous for the patient to complete. Technology is certainly helping with this issue, and the day of the paper-and-pencil diary may be fading. Electronic diary methods are becoming more commonplace (e.g., through smart phones, the Internet), or custom-made devices can be used that require little patient effort to complete the tracking (e.g., of activity during the day, such as "up-time" or pill use).

Psychometrics

Psychometric instruments used in clinical health psychology might be categorized in four general types: broadband—general, broadband—health, narrow focus, and narrow focus—health. Examples of each of these types of instruments can be found in Table 2.3.

The broadband—general measures include those that were not originally designed to assess medical patients or health-related issues. These measures often assess a number of personality, behavioral, or other variables. These assessments were not originally designed to assess medical or health issues, but often normative data for specific populations have been developed to help with generalizability. The Minnesota Multiphasic Personality Inventory–2 (MMPI-2; Butcher et al., 2001) is the most widely used and researched personality inventory. The MMPI-2 was designed to identify psychopathology and personality features; however, it is also one of the most commonly used measures in clinical health psychology for such things as chronic pain, presurgical screening, and other issues. When using broadband—general measures in clinical health psychology practice, the clinician must be well versed in validity, standardization, and interpretation issues to avoid misuse of the test. Example excerpts of three different interpretations of a 1–3/3–1 codetype on the MMPI-2 illustrate this point:

Traditional (often computer generated as part of an interpretative report). Classic conversion symptoms may be present, particularly if scale 2 is considerably lower than scales 1 and 3 (the so called conversion-V pattern). Whereas some tension may be reported, severe anxiety and depression usually are absent. The somatic complaints include headaches, chest pain, back pain, and numbness or tremors in the extremities. Other physical complaints

TABLE 2.3. Examples of Types of Psychometric Instruments Used in Clinical Health Psychology

Broadband—general

- Minnesota Multiphasic Personality Inventory–2 (MMPI-2)
- Personality Assessment Inventory (PAI; Morey, 1991)
- Symptom Checklist-90—Revised (SCL-90-R; Derogatis, 1983)
- Millon Clinical Multiaxial Inventory–III (MCMI-III; Millon, Davis, & Millon, 1997)

Broadband—health

- Millon Behavioral Medicine Diagnostic (MBMD; Millon, Antoni, Millon, Minor, & Grossman, 2001)
- Battery for Health Improvement–2 (BHI-2; Bruns & Disorbio, 2003)
- Sickness Impact Profile (SIP; Bergner, Bobbitt, Carter, & Gilson, 1981)
- Primary Care Evaluation of Mental Disorders (PRIME-MD; Spitzer, Kroenke, & Williams, 1999)
- Health Locus of Control (HLC; Wallston, Wallston, & Devellis, 1978)

Narrow focus—general

- Beck Depression Inventory–II (BDI-II; Beck, Steer, & Brown, 1996)
- Beck Anxiety Inventory (BAI; Beck, Epstein, Brown, & Steer, 1988)
- Posttraumatic Stress Diagnostic Scale (PDS; Foa, 1995)

Narrow focus—health

- Multidimensional Pain Inventory (MPI; Kerns, Turk, & Rudy, 1985)
- Cancer Inventory of Problem Situations (Schag, Heinrich, Aadland, & Ganz, 1990)
- Eating Disorder Inventory—Third Edition (EDI-3; Garner, 2004)

include weakness, fatigue, dizziness, and sleep disturbance. The physical symptoms increase in times of stress, and there is clear secondary gain associated with symptoms. These individuals present themselves as normal, responsible, and without fault. They make excessive use of denial, projection, and rationalization, and they blame others for their difficulties. They tend to be rather immature, egocentric, and selfish. They are insecure and have a strong need for attention, affection, and sympathy. They are very dependent, but they are uncomfortable with the dependency and experience conflict because of it. Although they are outgoing and socially extroverted, their social relationships tend to be shallow and superfi-

cial, and they lack genuine involvement with other people.

Chronic pain. Patients with similar profiles present with a wide variety of vague and diffuse somatic complaints. In these cases, there is often a very low correlation between subjective and objective findings. These patients show pain behaviors and somatic complaints far beyond what would be expected due to nociceptive input and objective findings. These patients show a high readiness to admit pain behaviors, but very little emotional distress associated with their reports of pain and other symptoms (low scale 2). From a positive reinforcement perspective, given the "readiness to emit pain behaviors" there is an increased chance of the patient "using" the pain behaviors to influence his or her environment or of pursuing reinforcing social consequences. From a negative reinforcement perspective, these patients will often use complaints of pain to extricate themselves from stressful situations. Extreme elevations on scales 1 and 3, in conjunction with a nonclinical elevation on scale 2 (depression) suggest that this patient is not uncomfortable in the sick role and may find aspects of it reinforcing. As such, the patient is showing a high readiness to admit pain behaviors, along with multiple somatic complaints, in conjunction with minimal distress regarding these symptoms. (Note: If scale 2 is elevated at or above 1–3, then the patient is expressing distress about being in the sick role or being unhappy and uncomfortable with his or her pain behaviors and, hence, is not as likely to find them reinforcing. This profile suggests less of an influence of environmental contingencies.)

Spine presurgical screening. As discussed by Block, Gatchel, Deardorff, and Guyer (2003, p. 83), elevations on scales 1 and 3 reflect excessive sensitivity to pain rather than the cause of the pain. In other words, in the face of a certain level of nociception, individuals who have high scores on scales 1 and 3 are more likely to experience high pain levels and to be more functionally disabled than those with low scores on these scales. As such, pain sensitivity as assessed by scales 1 and 3 seems to predispose patients towards negative spine surgery results even when the surgery corrects the underlying pathology (Block et al., 2003, p. 84). Individuals with this profile tend to respond very poorly to interventional and invasive pain management techniques aimed at identifying and "fixing" a physical pain generator. The reason they do so poorly is that the other nonphysical factors continue to impact their perception of pain and suffering.

The broadband—health measures are measures that have been specifically developed to assess a number of issues related to health and medical issues, without necessarily focusing on one particular health problem. Examples can be seen in Table 2.3. These tests will often assess psychological and behavioral issues that are intimately related to medical treatment. For instance, the Battery for Health Improvement–2 (BHI-2; Bruns & Disorbio, 2003) is designed "for the psychological assessment of medical patients" and includes scales organized into five domains: validity; physical symptoms; and affective, character, and psychosocial variables. Similarly, the Millon Behavioral Medicine Diagnostic (MBMD; Millon, Antoni, Millon, Minor, & Grossman, 2001) includes domains of response patterns, psychiatric indications, coping styles, stress moderators, treatment prognostics, management guides, and negative health habits. The MBMD now has normative data for general medical patients, patients with chronic pain, and bariatric surgery candidates.

The narrow focus measures include measures that assess a particular psychological issue such as depression, anxiety, suicidality, stress, and coping. Probably two of the most commonly used measures in this category are the Beck Depression Inventory–II (BDI-II; Beck, Steer, & Brown, 1996) and the Beck Anxiety Inventory (BAI; Beck & Steer, 1993). Similar to the MMPI-2, when these measures are used with medical patients, one must be very cautious with interpretation. For instance, the BDI-II is a measure of self-rated depression that contains a number of physical (e.g., weight, sleep, energy) and cognitive (concentration, memory) symptoms, all of which can be differentially affected by depression, pain, some other medical condition, or all of these. Therefore, the clinician should always be aware of the impact of the actual medical problem on the narrow-focus psychological instrument.

The narrow focus—health test is designed to be a brief measure of a specific medical or health condition (see Table 2.3). These tests are valuable for the clinical health psychologist assessing and treating a specific condition. Examples of these tests have been developed for the assessment of chronic pain (often used in conjunction with some of the broad-based measures). For instance, the Multidimensional Pain Inventory (MPI; Kerns, Turk, & Rudy, 1985) includes 13 scales that yield assignment to one of three profiles based on cluster analysis: dysfunctional, interpersonally distressed, and adaptive coper.

Pitfalls

One of the primary pitfalls in clinical health psychological psychometric assessment has already been alluded to: not paying attention to the validity of the test instrument relative to the problem being assessed, along with concomitant interpretation issues. It is always important to keep in mind standardization and basic psychometric issues when using any test on a medical patient population or to address health issues. A second pitfall is not adequately preparing the patient for taking these types of tests, including providing information about the purpose of the test. Problems can really occur when a medical patient is confronted with the types of questions on a broadband—general type of test without any preparation as to why the test is being prescribed. Simple preparation of the patient (e.g., purpose of the test, brief instructions), can avoid problems and generate more useful results.

Observation

Observation is one of the most fundamental methods of assessment for the clinical health psychologist. Observation can be unstructured, such as noting what occurs during the clinical interview or within the assessment setting (e.g., office waiting area, hospital room). It can also be highly structured, such as having the patient complete a specific functional task (e.g., self-administration of insulin, walking down the hallway without assistance). Observations can be made directly by the clinician or by others (family members, health care providers) and might be recorded (video, audio). Highly structured observation is often done in conjunction with research projects, and the results are quantified through the use of validated rating methods for very specific behaviors (e.g., pain behaviors).

Pitfalls

One of the primary pitfalls of observations is the clinician's either ignoring this valuable assessment domain altogether or not integrating (e.g., comparing and contrasting) it with other data sources. We commonly integrate pain behavior observation with that of self-report data in evaluating a patient with chronic pain. For example, we recently evaluated a pain patient who showed significant pain behaviors while walking from the waiting room to the office (limping, using the wall for support, periodic pauses) and during the first 10 minutes of the interview while seated (grimacing, shifting positions, guarding). However, after about 15 minutes into the 2-hour interview, the patient's pain behaviors remitted, his movements became quite fluid, and he remained seated the entire time. In addition, the patient rated his pain "at the time of the interview" at a 9 out of 10 (0–10 scale). Another pitfall is not taking into account observation data relative to the interaction among family members during the evaluation process (when these data are available). This can tell the clinician a lot about what is going on in the naturalistic environment.

Psychophysiological Measures

Psychophysiology refers to the "scientific study by nonsurgical means of the interrelationships between psychological processes and physiological systems in humans" (Cacioppo, Petty, & Marshall-Goodell, 1985, p. 264). Psychophysical measures have become very sophisticated with advancements in technology and include such things as electromyography (EMG; changes in muscle activity), cardiovascular measures (heart rate, beats per minute, heart rate variability, vasomotor activity), skin conductance (galvanic skin response, skin conductance response), electroencephalography (EEG; evoked potentials) and functional magnetic resonance imaging (fMRI). The psychophysiological measures provide assessment and treatment approaches for a variety of conditions, many of which are discussed in this volume. With the advent of sophisticated equipment, psychophysiological treatment approaches (e.g., biofeedback) have been enhanced through such things as what mea-

sures are available to the patient in terms of feedback and how certain stimuli of interest (e.g., desensitization of phobias) can be presented. For example, the technology has gone far beyond the "old days" of having the patient imagine coming close to a snake. Now, through the use of virtual reality technology, the presentation of almost lifelike images is possible and can be controlled by the patient during the treatment process.

Pitfalls

Probably the greatest pitfall in using this approach is a lack of appropriate training on the part of the clinician, along with inadequate treatment interventions, with a disregard for paying attention to generalizing effects outside of the office. Virtually any professional can purchase very sophisticated equipment with little or no advanced training or certification (e.g., EEG biofeedback). The same (unethical) clinician can then begin marketing his or her practice as specializing in the "disorder du jour," such as EEG neurofeedback treatment of attention-deficit/hyperactivity disorder (ADHD) without really having any expertise in that area. In these cases, the patient is often simply "hooked up" to the equipment and told to practice a preprogrammed sequence of tasks. Research has demonstrated that when these approaches are used properly, they can be very powerful interventions. However, the technology can often be very seductive, leading to inappropriate and ineffectual interventions in the actual clinical setting. Secondarily, even when used appropriately in the clinic setting, generalizing treatment results to the naturalistic environment may be an afterthought, if addressed at all.

Understanding the Patient: The Goal Assessment

As discussed by Belar and Deardorff (2009), at the end of the assessment process, the clinician should have an understanding of (1) the patient in his or her physical environment, (2) the patient's relevant strengths and weaknesses, (3) the evidence for psychopathology, (4) the nature of the disease and treatment regimen, and (5) the coping skills being used (p. 79). Upon completion of the assessment and integrating the data, the clinician should be able to answer the following questions (adapted from Moos, 1977, as reprinted in Belar & Deardorff, 2009, p. 79):

1. How is the patient dealing with pain, incapacitation, and other symptoms?
2. How is the patient dealing with the hospital (clinic, hospice, or other) environment and the special treatment procedures?
3. Is the patient developing and maintaining adequate relationships with the health care staff?
4. Is the patient preserving a reasonable emotional balance?
5. Is the patient preserving a satisfactory self-image and maintaining a sense of competence and mastery?
6. Is the patient preserving relationships with family and friends?
7. How is the patient preparing for an uncertain future?

Summary and Conclusions

The purpose of assessment in the practice of clinical health psychology is a complete and thorough understanding of the patient from a biopsychosocial perspective. This is accomplished through assessment of multiple "targets" (patient and environmental) along different "domains" (physical, affective, cognitive, and behavioral). Interaction between each of these areas of evaluation is also taken into account. The methods and tools of assessment available to the clinical health psychologist are vast and will vary depending upon the situation. These include such things as archival data, the clinical interview, questionnaires, psychological testing, and direct observation. Once this comprehensive and multimodal understanding of the patient is established, it can serve a number of purposes, such as differential diagnosis, guiding treatment interventions (both psychological and medical), and planning outcome goals and assessment.

REFERENCES

Beck, A. T., Epstein, N., Brown, G., & Steer, R. A. (1988). An inventory for measuring clini-

cal anxiety: Psychometric properties. *Journal of Consulting and Clinical Psychology, 56,* 893–897.

Beck, A. T., & Steer, R. A. (1993). *Beck Anxiety Inventory manual.* San Antonio, TX: Psychological Corporation.

Beck, A. T., Steer, R. A., & Brown, G. K. (1996). *Manual for the Beck Depression Inventory—II.* San Antonio, TX: Psychological Corporation.

Belar, C., Brown, R. A., Hersch, L. E., Hornyak, L. M., Rozensky, R. H., Sheridan, E. P., et al. (2001). Self-assessment in clinical health psychology: A model for ethical expansion of practice. *Professional Psychology, Research and Practice, 52,* 135–141.

Belar, C. D., & Deardorff, W. W. (1995). *Clinical health psychology in medical settings: A practitioner's guidebook.* Washington, DC: American Psychological Association.

Belar, C. D., & Deardorff, W. W. (2009). *Clinical health psychology in medical settings: A practitioner's guidebook* (2nd ed.). Washington, DC: American Psychological Association.

Belar, C. D., Deardorff, W. W., & Kelly, K. E. (1987). *The practice of clinical health psychology.* New York: Pergamon.

Belar, C. D., McIntyre, T. M., & Matarazzo, J. D. (2003). Health psychology. In I. B. Weiner (Series Ed.) & D. K. Freedheim (Vol. Ed.), *Handbook of psychology: Vol. 1. History of psychology* (pp. 451–464). New York: Wiley.

Bergner, M., Bobbitt, R. A., Carter, W. B., & Gilson, B. S. (1981). The Sickness Impact Profile: Development and final revision of a health status measure. *Medical Care, 19,* 787–806.

Block, A. R., Gatchel, R. J., Deardorff, W. W., & Guyer, R. D. (2003). *The psychology of spine surgery.* Washington, DC: American Psychological Association.

Bruns, D., & Disorbio, J. M. (2003). *Battery for Health Improvement–2.* Minneapolis, MN: Pearson.

Butcher, J. N., Graham, J. R., Ben-Porath, Y. S., Tellegen, A., Dahlstrom, W. G., & Kaemmer, B. (2001). *MMPI-2: Manual for administration, scoring, and interpretation* (rev. ed.). Minneapolis: University of Minnesota Press.

Cacioppo, J. T., Petty, J. N., & Marshall-Goodell, B. (1985). Physical, social, and inferential elements of psychophysiological measurement. In P. Karoly (Ed.), *Measurement strategies in health psychology* (pp. 263–300). New York: Wiley.

Derogatis, L. R. (1983). *SCL-90-R: Administra-

tion, scoring and procedures manual–II. Towson, MD: Clinical Psychometric Research.

Engel, E. L. (1977). The need for a new medical model: A challenge for biomedicine. *Science, 196,* 719–732.

Foa, E. B. (1995). *Posttraumatic Stress Diagnostic Scale manual*. Minneapolis, MN: National Computer Systems.

Garner, D. M. (2004). *Eating Disorder Inventory* (3rd ed.). Lutz, FL: PAR.

Kerns, R. D., Turk, D. C., & Rudy, T. E. (1985). The West Haven–Yale Multidimensional Pain Inventory (WHYMPI). *Pain, 23,* 345–356.

Health Service Psychology Education Collaborative. (2013). Professional psychology in health care services: A blueprint for education and training. *American Psychologist, 68*(6), 411–426.

Leigh, H., & Reiser, M. F. (1980). *Biological, psychological, and social dimensions of medical practice*. New York: Plenum Press.

Matarazzo, J. D. (1980). Behavioral health and behavioral medicine. *American Psychologist, 35,* 807–817.

Millon, T. (1982). On the nature of clinical health psychology. In T. Millon, C. J. Green, & R. B. Meagher (Eds.), *Handbook of clinical health psychology* (pp. 1–27). New York: Plenum Press.

Millon, T., Antoni, M., Millon, C., Minor, S., & Grossman, S. (2001). *Millon Behavioral Medicine Diagnostic*. Bloomington, MN: Pearson Assessments.

Millon, T., Davis, R. D., & Millon, C. (1997). *MCMI-III manual* (2nd ed.). Minneapolis, MN: National Computer Systems.

Moos, R. H. (Ed.). (1977). *Coping with physical illness*. New York: Plenum Press.

Morey, L. C. (1991). *Personality Assessment Inventory: Professional manual*. Tampa, FL: Psychological Assessment Resources.

Schag, C. A., Heinrich, R. L., Aadland, R. L., & Ganz, P. A. (1990). Assessing problems of cancer patients: Psychometric properties of the Cancer Inventory of Problem Situations. *Health Psychology, 9,* 83–102.

Spitzer, R. L., Kroenke, K., & Williams, J. B. W. (1999). Validation and utility of a self-report version of PRIME-MD: The PHQ Primary Care Study. Primary Care Evaluation of Mental Disorders. Patient Health Questionnaire. *Journal of the American Medical Association, 282,* 1737–1744.

Wallston, K. A., Wallston, B. S., & Devellis, R. (1978). Development of Multidimensional Health Locus of Control (MHLC) Scales. *Health Education Monographs, 6,* 160–170.

CHAPTER 3

Medication Adherence

Howard Leventhal
Danielle E. McCarthy
Elaine A. Leventhal
Krysten Williams Bold

The primary objective of our chapter is to present a model of the "common-sense" features of the self-regulatory processes that underlie adherence to treatment across disorders. A central proposition of the common-sense model of health behavior is that two partially correlated processes are involved in treatment adherence and health outcomes: the biological model of disease and treatment and patients' common-sense perceptions and interpretations of their experience of these biological processes. Our second aim is to illustrate ways in which research on medication adherence can illuminate relations between behavior and both soft (quality of life) and hard (onset and/or progression of specific diseases) health outcomes. A third objective is to suggest ways to integrate the common-sense model with cognitive-behavioral theory to generate new effective and efficient interventions to enhance medication adherence and improve health outcomes. We hope to highlight the importance of adherence research, both in practical terms as a way to enhance public health and in theoretical terms as a way to enhance our understanding of the processes that drive health-related behavior.

Medication Adherence: A Gateway for Developing a Comprehensive, Biobehavioral Model

The various proposals for solving the growing health care crisis in the United States (health care consumes 17% of the gross national product; Centers for Medicare and Medicaid Services, 2014; more than 45 million now uninsured; DeNavas-Walt, Proctor, & Smith, 2012) must address the following two facts: (1) approximately 70% of health care dollars are consumed by five chronic conditions (asthma, congestive heart failure, coronary artery disease, diabetes, and depression; Halverson, 2007); (2) cost-effective treatments are available for three of these conditions: asthma, coronary artery disease, and diabetes. Evidence-based practices also exist for depression (Craighead, Craighead, & Ilardi, 1998; Nemeroff & Schatzberg, 1998). In addition, adherence to health recommendations can prevent these chronic conditions. For example, randomized trials provide conclusive evidence that both behavioral lifestyle interventions (changes in diet and physical activities) and medication (metformin) effectively reduce the risk of developing diabetes. In the study by the Diabetes Prevention Program Research Group (2002), 58% fewer of the 1,079 high-risk participants (people showing poor response to a medical test involving blood sugar load) in a lifestyle change intervention developed diabetes over more than 2½ years in comparison with the 1,082 high-risk participants in a standard-care with placebo control condition. The risk-reducing effect of lifestyle change was greater than the reduction achieved by the 1,073 participants (31%) in the medication versus placebo (1,082 participants) arm of the trial (Diabetes Prevention Program Research Group, 2002). A second trial in Finland showed identical short-term effects and a significant lifestyle effect of 48% reduction in diabetes development fully 5 years after the termination of the intervention (Tuomilehto et al., 2001). The reduction in diabetes risk associated with both of these treatments is impressive. It is important to note, however, that such treatments work only when people adhere to them. As Feinstein (1976) pointed out decades ago, a medication that is 100% effective medically will appear less effective in a randomized trial than a medication that is only 75% effective if the perfect medication is taken by only 50% of the participants and the less perfect is taken by 100% of the trial participants. Adherence in chronic conditions requires sustaining behavioral change, whether to lifestyle or medication, over a lifetime.

The picture generated by the diabetes clinical trials contrasts sharply with the evidence for adherence in clinical practice. It has been nearly 40 years since Sackett and Haynes (1976) introduced the one-half-by-one-half-by-one-half rule; half of the population with a disorder such as hypertension is undiagnosed, half of the diagnosed are in treatment, and half of those in treatment are in poor control. The current picture is little better; adherence rates reported in reviews of studies of medication use among patients in treatment hover around 50%; some studies report rates of adherence as low as 20%, others as high as 60%, and some a bit higher (Dunbar-Jacob & Mortimer-Stephens, 2001; Dunbar-Jacob & Schlenk, 2000; Osterberg & Blaschke, 2005; Phillips et al., 2001). The level of adherence is gener-

ally superior for acute, infectious conditions and poorer for chronic conditions (Osterberg & Blaschke, 2005), varies by the population sampled (often related to the catchment for recruitment), and declines over time. For example, patient adherence to beta blockers and angiotensin-converting enzyme (ACE) inhibitors (assessed by pharmacy records for insured patients) following acute myocardial infarction (MI) declined linearly and steadily, settling at 48% after 2 years (Akincigil et al., 2008). It is worth noting that these medications are extremely effective; adherence reduces risk of MI recurrence by 81%, and their use is prescribed by guidelines (Choudhry & Winkelmayer, 2008). Given the known effectiveness of these and other medications—for example, diuretics for hypertension, inhaled corticosteroids for asthma, and so forth—it is reasonable to ask why investigations reporting on the development and testing of innovative, effective, and efficient theory-based interventions to improve adherence for effective treatments are not the main focus of psychological studies examining the relation between behavior and health outcomes.

We view investigations of treatment and/or medication adherence as a gateway to understanding the processes that link a diverse array of antecedent variables to health outcomes across multiple levels of analysis. Adherence is an issue that challenges us to more precisely map the relations among variables that have substantial influence on health-relevant behavior; adherence is at the center of all of the pathways important for behavioral health research. That is, adherence can only be fully understood and explained by examining all of the following influences and levels of analyses: (1) ecological and institutional influences; (2) cultural and sociological influences; (3) interpersonal influences, including interactions with health care providers, family members, and peers; (4) personality traits and individual competencies; and (5) the behavioral biological path defined by research on prolonged and acute stresses as precursors of disease. The data generated in these pathways differ in their value for the development of behavioral theory and interventions, yet all are important pieces of the complex puzzle, as depicted in the conceptual model shown in Figure 3.1.

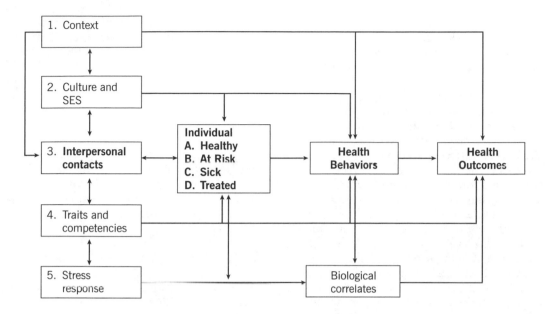

FIGURE 3.1. Hypothesized pathways relating behavior to health. In this organizational framework summarizing behavioral health research, the five classes of causal factors shown at left are thought to influence the health status, behaviors, and outcomes of individuals through various direct and indirect pathways. (1). *Context* refers to the ecological and institutional context in which individuals live. (2). *Culture and socioeconomic status* are factors outside the individual that influence health. (3). *Interpersonal contacts* with health care practitioners, fellow patients, family, and friends are proximal influences on health status and behavior. (4). Psychological *traits*, such as conscientiousness, and *competencies*, such as medication self-efficacy, are another class of hypothesized causal variables influencing health. (5). Physiological, immunological, and emotional *stress responses* make up another well-studied class of health-relevant variables. The central causal pathway showing reciprocal influences between individuals and interpersonal contacts that influence health outcomes through behavior is boldfaced to indicate that this is the focus of the current chapter. Note that many of the other causal pathways also involve indirect effects on health outcomes mediated through health behaviors, which may either promote or jeopardize health.

In this chapter, we focus on interpersonal influences on individual behavior, as this is the area in which the clearest mediating pathways between interventions and positive health outcomes can be articulated and studied. We know relatively little about the mediating pathways that link other, more distal factors to health behavior. Although numerous studies report relationships of regional (e.g., Pickle, Mungiole, & Gillum, 1997), neighborhood (e.g., van Lenthe et al., 2005), and social class (e.g., National Center for Health Statistics, 2011) variables to mortality and rates of chronic illnesses (pathways 1 and 2 in Figure 3.1), few of these studies have examined factors that mediate these relations (Leventhal, Weinman, Leventhal, & Phillips, 2008). For example, we

have not yet explained the high prevalence of chronic diseases and mortality in economically depressed areas by mediators such as exposure to environmental pathogens, risky behaviors (e.g., smoking), healthy behaviors (e.g., exercise), or the beliefs and worries of patients, families, and practitioners that affect access and adherence to care. Surprisingly, perhaps, the picture is not much clearer among studies of the relationship of psychological traits (e.g., depression, Type A behavior, conscientiousness, self-assessment of health) to health outcomes (pathway 4 in Figure 3.1). Although all of these factors predict future illness onset and mortality (e.g., Charles, Gatz, Kato, & Pedersen, 2008), evidence explaining their predictive value is limited. For example, there is no reason to believe that the greater mortality among individuals reporting poor self-ratings of health indicates that poor self-assessments are direct causes of mortality (participants giving self-ratings of poor or fair are 1.5 to 4.0 times more likely to die after controlling for medical and social factors in comparison with those giving very good and excellent ratings; Idler & Benyamini, 1997); there is a difference between a predictive indicator and a causal variable. We know a bit more about the immune-mediated pathways linking stress responses to health outcomes (e.g., Cohen, Doyle, & Skoner, 1999; Glaser, Sheridan, Malarkey, MacCallum, & Kiecolt-Glaser, 2000) and the effects of environmental factors on gene expression (Slavich & Cole, 2013), but the full sequence and the influences that moderate progression through the sequence have not been illuminated. Given the limited understanding of the pathways that link distal influences such as context and culture and personality and stress responses with health-relevant behavior, we believe it makes more sense to focus on the influence of more proximal, interpersonal determinants of health behavior; if studies in pathways 1, 2, 4, and 5 provide less direct evidence regarding the causal factors influencing health behaviors and health than studies in pathway 3, then studies in the latter pathway will provide more evidence for advancing behavioral theory and the implementation of cognitive-behavioral interventions to improve health outcomes.

Studies of adherence and health outcomes (pathway 3) begin with practitioner contact and examine medication adherence for acute conditions and medication and behavioral or lifestyle adherence for chronic conditions (asthma, hypertension, cardiovascular conditions, diabetes, depression). In essence, these are studies of the ways in which a patient's engagement with the health care system influences health behavior and health outcomes. For example, research has examined the ways in which a practitioner frames questions and presents information about diagnosis and how these presentations of treatment affect a patient's recall of treatment advice, disclosure of information, and adherence (Phillips, Leventhal, & Leventhal, 2012). These studies provide a window into the processes that promote or undermine effective use of medical treatments. They also offer the opportunity to build comprehensive models that incorporate ecological, cultural, social, socioeconomic status (SES), and personal factors that may interact with clinical transactions and affect subsequent health behaviors and health outcomes. Research on health care transactions can examine interactions between cultural factors and provider behavior in predicting patient and family views and trust in medical institutions that importantly influence adherence. Such comprehensive models may help us to predict the hard outcomes (e.g., mortality; disease recurrence) of greatest health importance.

A Brief History of Adherence Research

Many investigations of medication adherence conducted during the 1960s and 1970s focused on the relationship of social and personality factors to adherence (for an early review, see Leventhal, Zimmerman, & Gutmann, 1984). Studies of personality traits such as neuroticism and depression and adherence were common during this period (Pugh, 1983); interest in such factors has resurfaced as relationships have been found between adherence and factors such as depression and neuroticism (less adherence: DiMatteo, Lepper, & Croghan, 2000) and conscientiousness (more adherence: Roberts, Walton, & Bogg, 2005). Studies relating personality traits to adherence declined during the 1980s, as these relationships did not offer suggestions for interventions to improve adherence and health outcomes. These studies were also criticized as placing the burden for poor outcomes on the patient, that is, "blaming the patient" (Stimson, 1974). Unfortunately, even the most recent studies fail to conceptualize and describe in detail the perceptions, cognitions, strategies, and tactics involved in planning and specific behaviors that link traits such as conscientiousness to adherence.

The absence of interventions and concerns about blaming patients led clinical investigators to focus on potentially changeable situational factors. Studies reported improvements in adherence through enhanced access to care and improvements in the design and communication of treatment protocols. Access was improved by the creation of work site programs for the treatment of hypertension (Alderman & Schoenbaum, 1975) and community clinics to promote both inoculations and the control of hypertension (Farquhar et al., 1977). Mass media were used for community-wide interventions to reduce risk factors for cardiovascular disease, and competitions were initiated among work sites for reduction of risk factors for cardiovascular disease (Brownell, Cohen, Stunkard, Felix, & Cooley, 1984). Work site clinics improved patient recruitment, but recruitment, retention, and adherence declined over time, leaving the bulk of the nonadherence problem unresolved. Community-wide media interventions had limited efficacy unless backed by intensive cognitive-behavioral treatment of high-risk subgroups (Leventhal, Safer, Cleary, & Gutmann, 1980). Context, however, may enhance the effects of community and nationwide health communication campaigns. For example, community-wide media campaigns promoting family planning proved exceptionally effective when urbanization increased pressure to reduce family size (Rogers et al., 1999), suggesting that contextual factors and interventions may interact to influence health behavior. Such context-by-intervention interactions have not been studied in the medication adherence domain to our knowledge.

Currently, adherence research continues to focus on promoting adherence by improving access to health information and care, making health education materials more accessible and comprehensible (e.g., by attending to the reading level of materials and attempting to address the needs of patients with low health literacy; Chan, Keeler, Schonlau, Rosen, & Mangione-Smith, 2005), and examining provider and system factors affecting health care exchanges and adherence (Phillips et al., 2001). We have yet to explicate the specific causal pathways that link these malleable factors to specific adherence-relevant behaviors or to incorporate the moderating influences of other important factors, such as personality, culture, and context, in adherence research. As such, we have not yet constructed comprehensive models of health behavior such as that depicted in Figure 3.1 that can help us integrate diverse empirical findings and maximize our understanding of the critical determinants of adherence and how to modify them efficiently.

Summary of Empirical Findings

Thousands of small- and large-scale descriptive (cross-sectional and longitudinal) studies and intervention trials of medication adherence related to physical diseases (e.g., HIV/AIDS, asthma, cardiovascular disease, diabetes) and mental disorders (e.g., depression, schizophrenia, smoking cessation) have been published during the 50 and more years of the brief history outlined above. Given the volume and diversity of this literature, it is both impossible and not really useful to attempt a comprehensive literature review. Our reading of existent reviews and specific studies detected six themes that emerge from and have been supported by multiple reviews and specific studies. The themes are as follows.

First, regimen complexity affects adherence for multiple diseases. The more complex the regimen, the less well it is understood, recalled, and followed (Kravitz et al., 1993). More frequent dosage is also associated with worse adherence (see the review by Claxton, Cramer, & Pierce, 2001). Reducing the number of medications is effective for increasing the use of medication for the control of a variety of chronic conditions such as HIV/AIDS, diabetes, and cardiovascular disease (Osterberg & Blaschke, 2005).

Second, adherence declines steadily (often linearly) from the initiation of treatment to later follow-ups; adherence 2 years following initiation may fall to one-half of what it was at time of initiation. This is true for patients initiating treatment after MI (Akincigil et al., 2008), hypertension (see Meyer, Leventhal, & Gutmann, 1985, for inception sample), and type 2 diabetes (Rubin, 2005). Decline in adherence is also apparent for HIV, though usually to a lesser degree than for other chronic conditions (Chesney, 2003).

Third, in addition to documenting the decline in adherence over time, longitudinal studies identify subgroups of patients who vary in adherence patterns over time. Although some patients are stable in adherence (or nonadherence) over time, another common pattern is to engage in episodes of treatment engagement separated by intervals of disengagement and nonadherence. For example, studies have identified patients who initiate and continue to be adherent over long periods of time for bowel disorders (Sewitch et al., 2003) and asthma (Jessop & Rutter, 2003); these patients are likely to remain adherent. It also appears that many patients who have dropped out of treatment return at a later date (Meyer et al., 1985).

Fourth, adherence is typically higher for more life-threatening disorders such as AIDS in comparison with less immediately threatening conditions such as asthma, diabetes, hypertension, and cardiovascular disease. This difference however, appears to reflect the presence and/or proximity of disease-relevant experience. For example, adherence is very high immediately following MI (Akincigil et al., 2008) and high for HIV when disease indicators (e.g., symptoms and viral count) are available on a regular basis (Catz, Kelly, Bogart, Benotsch, & McAuliffe, 2000). As such, the salience or immediacy of health risks seems to promote adherence.

Fifth, medication adherence declines with more adverse symptoms and dysfunctions attributed to treatment. This is true for HIV, diabetes, hypertension, and other chronic conditions (Osterberg & Blaschke, 2005).

Sixth, reviews of interventions to improve medication adherence show modest benefits at best. For example, Kripilani, Yao, and Haynes (2007) found that only 8 of 15 trials achieved better adherence among patients exposed to a combination of information and a behavioral intervention than among patients in information-only conditions (5 trials reported effects on all of the adherence measures taken, 3 trials only on some). Similarly, only 6 of the 10 studies comparing a behavioral intervention alone to information alone showed better adherence for the behavioral intervention. More important, few trials of behavioral interventions showed any effect of the treatments on clinical outcomes. Finally, comparisons of information alone to standard care showed improved adherence in only 4 of 12 trials and no improvement in clinical outcomes for 8 of the 12 trials. Reviews examining the results of larger numbers of studies (using less restrictive rules for inclusion than the Cochrane Reviews), paint a similar picture (Dunbar-Jacob & Mortimer-Stephens, 2001).

Lessons Learned

A number of important lessons emerge from the preceding history and summary of findings. First, the studies relating social factors and personality traits to adherence suffered shortcomings common in epidemiological studies examining predictors of mortality; they typically failed to translate the mechanisms by which social and individual-difference variables relate to the use of medical care and adherence to treatment.

Second, adherence to treatments known to be effective for chronic illness management appears relatively unchanged over most treatment sites for the past 40 and more years. We continue to see that levels of adherence generally hover around 50% and tend to decline over time.

Third, only .03% (38 of 12,106) of published adherence-promoting intervention trials identified in various reference databases met Cochrane criteria (e.g., adequate blinding and controls for confounds for inclusion in the Kripilani et al., 2007, summary of 40 years of randomized trials). Behavioral interventions promoting adherence have not met the stringent criteria set forth for the evaluation of efficacy of medications or psychosocial treatments for other problems.

Fourth, the 38 trials that met Cochrane criteria for evaluation of the effectiveness of interventions for improving adherence and treatment outcome showed that behavioral interventions alone or in combination with informational material were superior to interventions using information alone. However, the effect sizes for measures of adherence were modest, inconsistent across different measures, and less impressive or consistent for clinical outcomes (Kripilani et al., 2007). Thus it is clear that there is still a substantial gap between prescribing a treatment and seeing it enacted, particularly with chronic conditions for which treatment is required for a lifetime.

Fifth, the modest efficacy of the intervention literature contrasts with the much stronger findings of the two best known diabetes prevention trials, suggesting that something is amiss with current approaches to intervention. One might interpret this difference as due to deficiencies in implementation, as few trials have the funds to hire sufficient personnel to devote the time needed to replicate the Diabetes Prevention Program Research Group (2002) diabetes trial that recruited motivated patients and provided 16 contacts with a counselor and numerous phone contacts. Selective recruitment for interventions at this level of intensity is not feasible for most trials and likely impossible to implement in the great majority of health care settings. A second interpretation of the contrast between the diabetes trials and the overall literature is that current interventions are deficient because they are based on theoretical models that fail to capture the processes involved in self-management. This deficit leads to interventions that are complex and expensive and that fail to address and influence the processes underlying self-management.

Sixth, inconsistent findings appear within each of the aforementioned themes, some apparently due to random processes, others to differences in method, and some to differences in implementation that are relevant to behavioral theory. The remainder of our chapter, therefore, discusses a growing body of research that is focused on process; that is, how individual patients and families perceive and interpret illness and treatment; how their perceptions and interpretations are influenced by media and medical communications; and how these processes affect initiation and long-term adherence to treatment. The issue is whether process-oriented work can inform theoretical models that transcend particular places and times and contribute to improvements in practice. The increasing size of the aging population and the high prevalence of chronic illness in that population (National Center for Health Statistics, 2011) are creating pressure for change in the delivery of health care, which may provide a window for process-oriented research that can serve as the basis for effective and efficient clinical interventions.

The Adherence Process

A model describing the processes underlying medication adherence will include behaviors and goals at multiple levels (social, individual) that shift in salience over time. For example, the factors and processes that influence medication adherence may differ during the initiation of a treatment regimen and its maintenance, and different factors may be involved in developing the habits that sustain adherence over decades. Rothman (2000) has suggested that self- and outcome efficacy are critical for initiation of behavior change (e.g., smoking cessation and exercise

adherence following MI), whereas satisfaction is important for subsequent maintenance (Baldwin et al., 2006). Evidence of these effects has been mixed, however (Finch et al., 2005; Linde, Rothman, Baldwin, & Jeffery, 2006). Schwarzer (2008) finds that self-efficacy related to maintenance differs from self-efficacy for achieving recovery from lapses. Although these frameworks are intriguing, they do not provide a theoretical analysis of the components of self-efficacy and therefore do not elucidate the processes involved in the generation of different forms of self-efficacy or satisfaction. These models tend to be descriptive; that is, they are useful for predicting adherence in longitudinal studies and within the intervention arms of experimental studies, but variables that are best predictors typically subsume multiple process variables, only some of which may be optimal targets for future interventions.

Self-Management: The Patient Perspective

Early studies by Ley (1977) and colleagues (Ley, Jain, & Skilbeck, 1976) examined how the organization of information in a clinical encounter affected recall and treatment adherence. For example, recall and adherence were improved when clinicians presented information in discrete categories, such as how the problem was assessed and labeled (diagnosis), what meds if any were needed, how to manage daily behavior, and when to return for follow-up (Leventhal et al., 1984, p. 387). Their studies highlighted the following points: (1) recall of information is essential, as the patient is responsible for implementing treatment (self-management); (2) assimilation and translation of information into behavioral self-management can be conceptualized in an information-processing–problem-solving framework; (3) the clinician is part of the adherence process, and how he or she presents information affects perception, retention, understanding, adherence, and health outcomes; and (4) the patient must translate this information into behavior in his or her home environment. Finally, this entire process takes place in the context of a complex set of interpersonal relationships (practitioner, family, and community) for a particular illness and treatment.

A critical next step in developing a process model for adherence involved the integration of control systems into the clinical context. Miller, Galanter, and Pribram (1960) introduced control-system models to psychology 50 years ago, and these ideas were further elaborated on by Powers (1973). Control models specify start points, that is, a detected discrepancy for beginning action and potential actions and what to monitor to evaluate the efficacy of an action in progressing toward a goal. Such systems send feedback about system functioning (in our case, a symptom such as a sore throat) to a controller (in this case, the patient) to influence choices and behavior (e.g., take prescribed antibiotic) and appraise outcomes (determine whether sore throat improved over 24 hours). Control models were applied to health research in three areas: (1) investigations assessing adherence to recommendations for preventive inoculations and smoking reduction following exposure to fear communications (Leventhal, 1970); (2) preparation of patients to manage noxious medical procedures (Johnson, 1975; Johnson & Leventhal, 1974); and (3) the impact of personality factors, such as optimism about future outcomes, on quality of life and health (Carver et al., 1994; Scheier & Carver, 1987, 1992). From the perspective of the patient, acquiring the self-management skills to adhere to a prescribed treatment (i.e., forming a self-management feedback control) requires mastery of the following processes (see Figure 3.2).

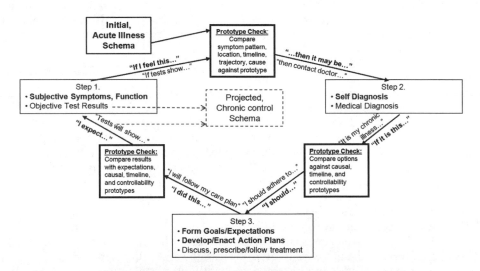

FIGURE 3.2. Common-sense model of patient self-management. According to the common-sense model, individual health behaviors such as medication adherence are influenced by the iterative process depicted in simplified form in this figure. The **bold text** shows the patient's process, whereas the unbolded text illustrates the health care practitioner's parallel process. The cycle begins with a subjective physical symptom or change in functioning or with an objective indicator of illness or dysfunction (e.g., results of a medical test) that is compared with learned prototypes and illness schemas through a prototype check (PC) process. The patient and provider then infer the identity, anticipated timeline, possible consequences, cause, and controllability of the symptoms or change in functioning, as shown in step 2, in which the patient generates a self-diagnosis and may or may not receive a concordant medical diagnosis from providers. This diagnosis then influences the patient's goals and expectations for treatment and shapes behaviors. The patient will continue to monitor changes in symptoms and functioning and compare them with his or her expectations to reactivate the cycle. Repeated cycles influence subsequent ones, as the prototypes and schemas may change with experience or intervention, as shown in the contrast between the bolded initial, acute-illness schema process shown outside the arrows and the projected, chronic control system schema shown inside the arrows that develops over time through collaboration between chronically ill patients and their providers. Through this process, patients and providers can work together to continuously update care goals and maximize adherence and the likelihood of positive health outcomes.

First, the representation, or schema, of an illness must include the perception that the condition, its symptoms, and its consequences can be controlled by treatment. Second, the treatments must make sense in relation to the patient's representation of the illness. Third, the patient must have access to the resources needed to perform self-care and must understand and be competent to perform the specific behaviors. Fourth, the patient needs an action plan to implement behavior in the home environment; chronic illness management does not take place in a clinicians' office. Fifth, the patient needs to evaluate the effects of the treatment; this evaluation requires that the patient know how and when to conduct the evaluation (how and when to check blood pressure and/or blood sugar) and have appropriate expectations as to the meaning and likely value of the evaluation output (e.g., blood pressure norms, desirable blood sugar levels). Sixth, the patient must learn to reconcile inconsistencies between objective evidence and subjective signals (McAndrew, Schneider, Burns, & Leventhal, 2007).

In short, the patient must recognize which cues are valid targets for management and how these cues respond to treatment and must know the time frame in which to observe objective change. Consistency or conflict between the subjective (e.g., feeling better) and objective (e.g., consistent, healthy blood sugar levels) targets for self-management will be critical for adherence. These six steps constitute a control system, a feedback loop for initiation and adherence to treatment, whether the treatment involves medication or lifestyle change.

Two issues need to be addressed about our use of control theory. First, it is important to recognize that factors other than individually controlled feedback systems influence adherence. Adherence can be socially controlled, with the patient on the output side of a social control loop (i.e., an obedient follower of instructions) that bypasses self-regulatory controls for a self-directed pursuit of a health target. For example, in their qualitative study of elderly individuals with congestive heart failure (CHF), Horowitz, Rein, and Leventhal (2004) identified an elderly, cognitively impaired woman who fully adhered to her medication for CHF because her cardiologist son-in-law called

every day to guide her pill taking. Given her limited cognitive-affective competencies, she did not resist being controlled by a valued family member. Patients with CHF who lack effective social control have to monitor breathlessness and swelling of their legs and use these as cues for using diuretic medication or to call for medical assistance. Although response to monitoring is critical for avoiding heart failure and death, as is using ACE inhibitors and beta blockers following MI (Akincigil et al., 2008), patients with CHF in this study did not use medication as prescribed. Something was missing in their self-regulatory systems.

Second, models assuming that action is designed to close a gap between present status and a goal (i.e., negative feedback models) are not the complete self-regulatory system. Goal setting, that is, establishing a next step in a sequence of steps, is intrinsic to self-motivated activity (Locke & Latham, 2002) related to the initiation and maintenance of treatment. This feed-forward process must begin with a choice of a start point that will set the stage for moving to the next goal. Understanding the details of this process will be critical for creating and understanding maintenance of medication adherence and other lasting health behavior change.

Common Sense and Control:
Variables in the Feedback Loops

Feedback and feedforward mechanisms cannot be treated in the abstract if we want to understand how they operate and use them to create interventions. Theory and practice depend on the identification of specific variables affecting the initiation and maintenance of control activities, the responses used for control, the criteria or targets for evaluating effectiveness, and the system involved in signaling next steps. The role of symptoms as initiators of self-regulatory actions, including seeking care and adhering to treatment, has been replicated in numerous studies (Brody & Kleban, 1983; Costa & McCrae, 1980; Stoller, 1998). A study by Cameron, Leventhal, and Leventhal (1993) that monitored spontaneous health care seeking by 111 pairs of elderly individuals provides an excellent example of the power of symptoms in initiating care-seeking behavior. When either member of the pair (members were matched for age, gender, etc.) called for a consultation with his or her primary care physician, he or she and the other member of the pair were interviewed. The data were clear: All (100%) of the participants who called for care reported new symptoms, whereas new symptoms were reported by only 30% of the 111 control participants. A comparison of the symptoms reported by the 111 care seekers and the 33 non-care-seeking but symptomatic matched controls showed that the care seekers were more likely to label their symptoms and describe them as serious and disruptive of daily functioning. The literature is replete with examples of ways in which symptom interpretation affects behavior. For example, chest pain prompts emergency room visits even when this symptom is not related to coronary disease (Aikens, Zvolensky, & Eifert, 2001); symptoms allow patients to recognize that they are suffering from bulimia (Hepworth & Paxton, 2007); patients cut back on or completely stop antiviral medication when symptoms clear (Chesney & Folkman, 1994); and the duration of symptoms is a powerful predictor of the use of health care (Mora, Robitaille, Leventhal, Swigar, & Leventhal, 2002).

In addition, the very same symptoms can be interpreted as benign one day and as threatening the next. For example, ambiguous symptoms, such as fatigue or generalized body aches, do not typically lead to care seeking. Only 18% of a sample of 366 sought health care when experiencing vague symptoms, and the proportion seeking care increased little, if at all, when participants were under a recent life stress (22% sought care). However, 40% of the participants sought care if they experienced vague and/or ambiguous symptoms during a period of relatively prolonged life stress (lasting a month or more; Cameron, Leventhal, & Leventhal, 1995). Thus vague symptoms are interpreted as benign and not requiring care in the presence of acute stress but are interpreted as signs of physical illness and are more likely to prompt care seeking and use of treatment in the context of chronic stress. Life context thus moderates symptom impact on behavior (for an excellent review of symptoms as motivators to care seeking, see Stoller, 1998).

Symptoms also play a significant role in medication adherence; both qualitative (Blumhagen, 1980; Heurtin-Roberts, 1993) and quantitative data show that medication adherence is often symptom-driven. An early study by Meyer et al. (1985) showed a wide gap between what patients believe about the symptom experience of people who are hypertensive and what they believe is true for themselves; 80% of the 50 patients who had been in treatment for elevated blood pressure (and consistent users of care) agreed with the statement that "People *can't* tell when their blood pressure is up"; but when asked, "Do you think you can tell when your blood pressure is up?", 92% said "yes." Of the patients who reported that treatment ameliorated their symptoms, 70% also reported that they were adherent to treatment. Blood pressure readings showed that 62% of those reporting themselves adherent were in good control, in contrast to only 14% of those reporting nonadherence. Thus symptoms prompted sustained adherence when they were assigned meaning: that is, as indicators of effective medication treatment.

Symptom-driven adherence was also visible in a sample of 198 patients hospitalized for severe attacks of asthma; although 80% of these patients agreed that they would definitely or probably have asthma all their lives, 57% also believed they had asthma only when they had symptoms (Halm, Mora, & Leventhal, 2006). Patients who believed that they had asthma only when they had symptoms used their corticosteroid inhaler medication only 45% of the time when they were asymptomatic; this medication is prescribed for daily use when asymptomatic, because it suppresses inflammation. In contrast, those patients who believed they had asthma even when asymptomatic used these inhalers 70% of the time. Thus patients who saw asthma as a series of somewhat unpredictable attacks treated themselves episodically; patients who separated chronic inflammation from symptom episodes were more consistent self-managers. Taken together, these studies suggest that the meaning ascribed to the presence or absence of symptoms influences adherence to medication regimens.

Mapping Symptoms to Prototypes

Symptoms and changes in function, deviations from the underlying image or self-prototype, are the subjective, online cues that are the targets for self-management.

In the common-sense model, the meaning assigned to symptoms is a product of a process in which symptoms are matched and linked to one or another underlying prototype or model of illness. The "meaning" created by this match activates expectations as to how medication will affect both the symptoms and the underlying condition and the interpretation of experienced changes when medication use is initiated, maintained, or discontinued.

The hypothesis that symptoms and functional changes are "mapped" or linked to prototypes is a central assumption of the common-sense model. Indeed, mapping is an active process that is both intrapsychic and interpersonal and familiar to all of us. It involves the actions of a set of prototype checks (PCs). We posit that PCs continually monitor somatic and functional experience, consciously or unconsciously, and compare these experiences with underlying prototypes both of the self and of specific illnesses. There are PCs to assess (1) the *sensory properties* of the somatic display (e.g., aches, dull pressure, sharp pains, throbbing); (2) its *location* (e.g., head, legs, gut, chest); (3) its *timeline* (both felt time and clock time for rate of onset and duration); (4) its *severity*; (5) its *trajectory* (rate of change and whether the change is increasing or worsening, improving, or simply fluctuating); and (6) the *emotional experience* associated with the symptomatic event. PCs will check negative emotions (distress, fatigue, disgust) as signs of harm and positive emotions as signs of benefits. The checks connect or map experience to specific features (receptors or slots; Gobet, 1998) of prototypes both of the self and of specific illnesses. For example, the location and symptom pattern check the *identity* of the prototype (the label and specific properties defining it), and contextual factors, such as stress, injury, ingested food, and so forth, link to the prototype's *causal* feature. Thus sensory properties (pain) and location (head) define a pain as a headache rather than a stomachache, and the antecedent context (long, intense work days; head injury) further defines the condition as a "stress" headache or an injury. Additional signs, for example, visual symptoms, may define it as a migraine. The duration of a symptom (past and expected future) is checked against the prototype's *timeline*. The attribution of swollen legs to aging by

patients with CHF attests to the ease with which practitioners ignore the operation of these simple, common-sense notions (Horowitz et al., 2004).

The prototype's *control* feature creates expectations as to the possible consequences of specific actions; current *distress* and pain are checked against expected pain and distress and with expected changes following action to ameliorate these cues (e.g., taking medication, such as aspirin, will clear a stress headache in an expected time frame; rest will decrease cardiac-induced chest pain). Thus the checks compare and connect experienced changes wrought by action to specific facets of the prototype of the illness and give meaning to symptoms and functional changes experienced prior to and after taking ameliorative action; the experiences also form and enrich the prototypes of the action. The prototypes for chronic illnesses will differ from one another as they reflect the biology that generates disease-specific experience (Hampson, 1997b). The prototypes can also differ between patients with the same chronic condition, and a patient's prototype can change over time. Differences can occur in the number, time frames, disruptiveness and controllability of symptoms, and functional changes associated with the illness label, and these changes will be related to the patient's causal beliefs and anticipated consequences of actions for controlling these events (e.g., if taking medication for CHF does not minimize new symptoms, a patient may call the doctor thinking CHF is getting out of control; Horowitz et al., 2004).

The representation or working model that emerges from the mapping of experience to prototypes includes both cognitive factors that are abstract or conceptual (e.g., labeling a headache a stress headache vs. a headache due to stroke) and cognitive factors that are experience-based and active in recognition. Both levels of cognitive processes define a working model of the condition, but the implication of each level for behavior may differ. For example, the objective duration of a symptom, its clock time, may be far less than its perceived time, and the acceptable time frame for effective control may differ between the two levels. Thus patients often stop treatment when their antibiotics eliminate symptoms, the target for experience, well before the antibiotic has eliminated the underlying bacterial cause of symptoms, the conceptual target (Becker, Drachman, & Kirscht, 1972). As the physiology underlying specific chronic illnesses will differ (e.g., osteoarthritis is symptomatic, whereas hypertension and diabetes are often asymptomatic, except at extremes), their prototypes and the targets and behaviors perceived relevant for self-management will also differ. For example, patients with diabetes perceive a much larger array of negative consequences of their illness and are much more likely to believe their ability to control their illness will improve over time than are people with different disorders, such as depression. For example, patients with diabetes may expect gradual rather than immediate improvement in symptoms (Hampson, 1997a; Hampson, Glasgow, & Toobert, 1990). On the other hand, patients taking antidepressant medications may expect more immediate relief because they experience side effects (e.g., dry mouth) before noticing improvement in depressive symptoms or functioning; as a consequence, they may perceive their medications as ineffective and stop taking them (Keller, Hirschfield, Demyttenaere, & Baldwin, 2002).

Consistency or inconsistency between the behaviors elicited by the conceptualization of an illness and those elicited by its concrete experience can have beneficial or adverse effects for adherence and health outcomes. It is likely that consistency between the concept of heart attack and its somatic expression (angina) can encourage taking beta blockers and ACE inhibitors immediately following acute MI. But as the experience of symptoms and physical dysfunction fade and are replaced by many months of feeling good, the person who had a heart attack may come to believe that heart attacks are acute, curable events and not part of a chronic condition. This experience-based shift in belief may erode the motivation for medication adherence, accounting for the finding that 52% of patients stop taking medication within 2 years of MI (Akincigil et al., 2008). Similarly, lack of symptoms and feelings of wellness are associated with nonadherence to antiviral medication in patients with HIV (Catz et al., 2000). Adherence should be sustained, however, if the concept and the experience are disaggregated; symptomatic attacks may be perceived as episodic

while the underlying condition is viewed as chronic and requiring continued treatment. If patients view treatment as essential to avoid recurrence of attacks and maintenance of vigor and health, rather than as necessary just to ease symptoms and pain, they should be more likely to maintain adherence. Thus the two levels of monitoring and interpretation may have differing or interactive influences on medication adherence. The role of symptoms visible in multiple studies is consistent with the hypothesis that the default mental model for illnesses is for *acute* conditions; the prototype for "acute," episodic illness is consistent with the bulk of life experience for most people, and this should be kept in mind when drafting cognitive-behavioral interventions.

Representations of Actions and Action Plans

Two additional sets of factors are necessary to translate the motivation generated by an illness representation into behavior: the selection of a procedure for self-management and the formation of an action plan. Choice of action is complicated by the simple fact that medically prescribed actions are but one set of elements among a larger set of culturally and socially available procedures for prevention, cure, and/or control of illness threats. Media, family, and friends may encourage a patient to take "alternative" products along with medically prescribed treatments. Because patients appear to use "natural" or other home or culturally, media-, and socially suggested treatments along with their prescribed medications, their use is currently labeled as "complementary" rather than alternative to medication (Barnes, Powell-Griner, McFann, & Nahin, 2004). Unfortunately, self-selected "natural" remedies may be dangerous medically and complementary only in the mind of the user. Cancer patients can put themselves at risk of adverse interactions with medically effective chemotherapy treatments when using herbal or over-the-counter medications to bolster the immune system (Cassileth, 1998). For example, a patient on medication to suppress complications from a coronary valve replacement who takes a supplement to "strengthen" her immune system risks stroke and possible death if the supplements raise levels of vitamin K. Complementary products can, however, be of benefit to adherence. For example, a 50-year-old adult can ensure regular use of his daily antihypertension medication by placing it next to the vitamins he has taken daily for decades.

Representations of Actions

As is the case for illness representations, representations of medications are both abstract and concrete and have substantial effects on adherence. Horne's (1997; Horne, Weinman, & Hankins, 1999) factor analyses of the responses to 18 items made by more than 500 chronically ill patients (with heart disease, asthma, diabetes, or renal disease) yielded four distinct factors. Two factors reflected beliefs about one's own medication: *Specific—Concerns* (e.g., "I sometimes worry about the long-term effects of my medicine"; "I sometimes worry about becoming too dependent on my medicines") and *Specific—Necessity* (e.g., "Without my medicine I would be very ill"; "My medicines protect me from becoming worse"). Two other factors reflected general beliefs about medication: *General—Harm* (e.g., "Medicines do more harm than good") and *General—Overuse* (e.g., "Doctors use too many medicines"; Horne et al., 1999). Differences between necessity and concerns (Necessity scores minus Concerns scores) were significantly correlated with medication adherence in a cross-sectional study of patients with asthma, heart disease, cancer, and renal failure (Horne & Weinman, 1999). The belief that medication is necessary also predicted adherence following MI (Horne & Weinman, 1999). Greater acceptance of highly active antiretroviral therapy (HAART) medications was also found in patients with HIV infection who believed medications necessary and expressed few concerns about their prescribed treatments (Horne, 2003). Groups with high scores for Necessity were more adherent to depression (Aikens, Nau, Klinkman, & Schwenk, 2005) or asthma medication (Menckeberg et al., 2008), regardless of scores on Concerns.

Action Plans

The representations of an illness and medication treatment are insufficient to prompt behavior, however. The formation of explicit action plans is a critical step for the translation of belief systems into behavior (Leventhal, 1970). Plans for the implementation of action identify specific cues for action and a specific set of actions to perform in response to these cues (Gollwitzer, 1999)—for example, check blood sugar 2 hours after eating and take medication if needed. Planning, an executive function, is the most important component of action plans. Planning involves more than the identification of a cue for action and a specific action; it requires that patients review their *behavioral ecology* to identify locations for inserting specific behaviors—for example, "where and how can I (a diabetic) check my blood glucose without being observed and embarrassed while doing it?" The patient rushing to work can easily forget to take her daily antihypertension medication. However, if she always drinks orange juice and/or coffee on rising, it may make sense for her to place the medication near her coffee cup; if she does not always grab a quick bite for breakfast but always brushes her teeth and/or combs her hair, it would be better to place the medication near her hairbrush. Failure to insert actions into the individual's daily schedule increases their burden or "cost" to the patient and increases the risk of nonadherence. The burden to working memory, that is, executive functions, should remain with planning; daily performance should be automatic (Leventhal et al., 2011). Executive skill in planning and automating behavior are critical features of self-efficacy.

There is one significant flaw in the overwhelming evidence for the potency of action plans: Virtually all of the evidence is for the implementation of single actions, such as getting an inoculation for tetanus (Leventhal, Singer, & Jones, 1965) or participating in screening for detection of cancer or other chronic conditions (Hager & Orbell, 2003); there is little evidence of the longer term efficacy of planning (maintenance).

PCs and Dynamic Feedback Loops

Summary scores on the scales assessing beliefs in the *necessity* of medication("Without my medicine I would be very ill"; "My medicines protect me from becoming worse") and the *concerns* about medication("I sometimes worry about the long-term effects of my medicine"; "I sometimes worry about becoming too dependent on my medicines") are based upon personal experience with medication, along with communication about and observations of experience and concerns about medication from others, the media, the Internet, and cultural values. These beliefs activate specific expectations about the meaning of one's experiences when using a medication and shape the individual's appraisals of the effects of the medication and his or her decisions to continue or discontinue its use. For example, the outcome expectancy associated with taking an antihypertensive medication can be a change in symptoms and/or a change in blood pressure reading; if the former is expected and validated, adherence will be high; if not validated, it will be low (Meyer et al., 1985). Patients with HIV who experience multiple, distressing treatment-related symptoms that are perceived as harmful will likely be nonadherent to their HAART regimens, as these symptoms elicit concerns about adverse consequences (Gonzalez et al., 2007). In a qualitative study, 13 of 16 patients with bipolar disorder were intentionally nonadherent to medication when they experienced side effects (Clatworthy, Bowskill, Rank, Parham, & Horne, 2007). The studies suggest that efficacy for self-management is enhanced when the outcomes of volitional and automatic actions are consistent with expectations and reduced when inconsistent.

Anticipated consequences, that is, benefits and concerns, define only one facet of treatment representations. Although they are often implicit rather than explicit, timelines are critical features of medication representations. Timelines are explicit for antibiotics, and many frequently used over-the-counter medications such as aspirin and acetaminophen have stated objective and explicit timelines—for example, they are expected to relieve a stress headache in 20 minutes to an hour and to have effects lasting a few hours. Timelines can be far less clear, however, for many other medications. Patients with Type 2 diabetes should take medication in response to observed changes in blood sugar readings, but unless explicitly instructed, they may be mistaken about the appropriate timing for monitoring. If a patient monitors his or her blood sugar immediately, rather than 2 hours, after eating, before the body

has had time to remove sugars from the bloodstream, he or she may obtain a high reading, take unnecessary medication, and reduce blood sugars to excessively low levels. Similarly, if he or she takes a reading while exercising (blood sugars are elevated during exercise) rather than 2 hours afterward, he or she may conclude incorrectly that exercise is ineffective in lowering blood sugar. Quality of monitoring, rather than mere frequency, appears to be important for behavioral change, for example, adherence to low-fat diets (McAndrew et al., 2011). Patients taking medication to treat eczema expect to experience benefits in days or weeks rather than the 6–7 years it takes to see improvement (Walker, Papadopoulos, Lipton, & Hussein, 2006), which may hinder adherence (Brown, Rehmus, & Kimball, 2006). Temporal factors were evident in the concerns about the long-term consequences of medication expressed by patients with bipolar disorder (Clatworthy et al., 2007). Thus it seems that patients' beliefs regarding the necessity of their medication and concerns about their use are higher-order beliefs that are based on ongoing experience that are checked against underlying, and continually updated, representations of the medication.

Medication beliefs do not operate alone; they are nested under illness representations, and their joint effects are visible in adherence among chronically ill patients. For example, patients who viewed asthma as chronic and believed that medication could control the underlying inflammation, a *coherent* system, were more likely to use preventive medication properly (using inhalers to reduce inflammation, not for relief during attacks) and to intend to adhere in the future (Jessop & Rutter, 2003) than were patients who believed that medication was useful only for relief during attacks. In addition, nonadherent patients in treatment for bipolar disorder believed the condition was not controllable, and some doubted the correctness of their diagnosis (Clatworthy et al., 2007). As a final example, Horne and Weinman (2002) found that patients' chronic timelines and perceived negative consequences of illness were positively related to beliefs in the necessity of treatment that, in turn, predicted medication adherence. Thus patient beliefs about the nature of their conditions and about the treatments prescribed are linked to adherence in important ways. Furthermore, representations of the underlying illness and representations of medication treatment may interact with one another in shaping patients' beliefs regarding the necessity of their medications and their concerns about ongoing use. In addition, prototypes of the self—for example, the belief that one's body is "sensitive" to medication—add yet another source of information to patients' mental models of treatment (Horne et al., 2012). These processes are critical for the development of self-efficacy and appear to influence preferences and selection of behavioral interventions when patients are given treatment choices (Rozanski, Blumenthal, Davidson, Saab, & Kubzansky, 2005).

Linking Inter- and Intrapersonal Processes: The Politics and Affective Processes of Maintenance

The PC process is not exclusively intrapersonal; PCs are the focus of interpersonal communication, as well. Visits to the doctor nearly always involve the exploration of a presenting complaint (visits for inoculations, specific tests, and completion of paperwork may be exceptions). The review of the presenting complaint and the traditional review of systems may open with a friendly query, "How are you?", and move from there to "What's the problem?", "Where is it?", "How does it feel?", "How long has it been going on?", "Did you do something to control it?", "What happened then?", and so on. We hypothesize that this questioning reinforces the patient's belief that PCs—the sensory feel, location, duration, and so forth—are valid tools for diagnosis and for evaluating the efficacy of treatment. The problem is that the informational value of each check depends upon its relationship to an underlying prototype, and the prototypes tested by the patient can be different from those tested by the practitioner. It is critical to note that discussions focused on checks connect an individual's subjective, intrapersonal world to her or his individual personal, interpersonal, or social world. Discussions with practitioners are only part of the picture. The elderly may compare their experiences with peers' symptoms and treatments, discussing how specific medications affect symptoms and function (Brody & Kleban,

1981). The practice is neither confined to the elderly nor strictly between two or more living people, as an endless number of advertisements present testimonials for medication, diets, and other lifestyle behaviors focusing on the experienced benefits of use, including positive feelings, improved function, and the control of specific symptoms. Informal discussion with peers, friends, or family and mass media communications have the potential to influence patient perceptions of the timelines and causes of symptoms and representations of treatment. Social comparison processes embedded in social discourse bring to bear an additional array of check processes involving comparisons based on age, temperament, physical characteristics, and environmental exposures. Once again, we can see that concrete features create mutual sharing and understanding—that is, the concrete links an array of abstract concepts and their associated details.

Representations of Illness and the Self: Feedforward Goal Setting

Our discussion of process has suggested a variety of routes to developing and testing interventions for the initiation and adherence to medication in the short term. Maintenance poses a challenge to any behavioral intervention, regardless of the process model on which it is based. A number of investigators have discussed the changes that take place from the initiation of behavior change to its automatic performance in daily life (Phillips, Leventhal, & Leventhal, 2013; Prochaska & DiClemente, 1984; Rothman, 2000; Schwarzer, 2008). Data related to these models suggest that initiation of change is dependent upon feeling competent to make changes in life patterns (i.e., self-efficacy), whereas maintenance over the short term is dependent upon satisfaction (Rothman, 2000) or maintenance efficacy (Schwarzer, 2008).

What do concepts such as self-efficacy and satisfaction add to the conceptual mix, that is, to the control systems involved in reaching goals? Some (Locke & Latham, 2002) have argued that control models are inappropriate for understanding and intervening in human behavior, as the models are based upon an inflexible device, the thermostat, whereas individuals have shifting goals that change with the accomplishment of prior goals. This depiction of control models as inflexible is incomplete, however. First, feedback models can account for dynamic goals or set points and can provide a clear picture of the processes involved in monitoring movement toward online goals and building self-efficacy. Second, the anticontrol argument fails to recognize the multilevel structure of the feedback system associated with specific prototypes, creating set points (goals) and measuring progress toward them. Most important, controls at the level of executive function are "open" to external and internal inputs, whereas others may be far more closed; for example, intracellular controls involved in gene expression. In the common-sense model, self-efficacy refers to the conceptual and executive processes that compare the present to the past, project future goals and actions, select *start* points for behavioral change, and regulate and shape automatic procedural systems. The specification of this temporal goal sequence is an essential aspect in the creation of a comprehensive script that combines illness and treatment representations with outcome expectations and outcome experience. Thus the feedback control loop involved in current medication use is nested within a conceptual structure specifying a sequence of goals and actions (rather than a static goal); future goals are anticipated once current objectives are met. Creating the sequence of goals and plans for moving from goal to goal, understanding that a start point and procedure can lead to a short-term goal that blocks long-term achievements (e.g., dieting to control blood glucose), are processes that need to be described and understood.

Conceptualizing a condition as chronic poses both opportunities and risks. The opportunities are based upon the function of abstract concepts in linking past and current experience to future goals and plans for goal attainment. Specifically, conceptualizing an illness as chronic creates a framework for future goal setting and action that allows for transitions from initiation through maintenance and development of expertise in self-management. As an example, an elderly individual with type 2 diabetes and elevated hemoglobin A1c (HbA1c in excess of 9.0%) is at high risk of neuropathic complications, including heart disease, blindness, kidney failure, and foot ulceration and amputation. The initial tasks for this patient include adjusting the intake of specific foods, engaging in physical activities that raise and lower blood sugar levels, and regularly monitoring blood glucose with a meter (not by evaluating subjective symptoms that are valid cues for extremely low but not high blood sugar levels). These initial targets are nested, however, under a second, longer term goal for reducing HbA1c; these readings lag the daily blood sugar readings by 3 months or more. As the individual develops skills in management (e.g., "gets the hang of it" and knows how specific foods and activities affect blood sugar levels), fewer daily readings can be used to check the overall quality of management. At this point, the patient is becoming increasingly expert in management using simple heuristics or rules to estimate sugar increases due to food intake and decreases due to physical activity. As these regulatory behaviors occur in a social context, the patient must also manage the interpersonal and economic factors involved in securing and preparing foods, choosing appropriate settings for physical activity, and calling and meeting with clinical practitioners to adjust medication. These actions involve a complex set of goals nested under the abstract conception of diabetes as a chronic illness requiring lifelong management, with a sequence of specific tasks (goals and responses) elaborated in the model's time frame.

The risks involved in holding a chronic model of illness relate to the overlap of its features with the model underlying depressive affect (Abramson, Metalsky, & Alloy, 1989). One challenge, therefore, is to understand the factors that differentiate a chronic functional model from a chronic dysfunctional–depressive model. Although limited in scope, current knowledge suggests that three sets of factors affect the form of chronic illness models: the stability or intelligibility of the biological signals on which the representation is based, the availability of coping responses for controlling illness targets, and the social context. For example, many patients with Type 2 diabetes who have symptoms of peripheral diabetic neuropathy report depressive affect associated with fluctuating pain and loss of sensations in the feet (Vileikyte et al., 2005). The relation between these physical symptoms and depressive affect, with its loss of pleasure in everyday activities, is mediated in part by the fact that these symptoms are episodic and unpredictable, respond poorly to treatment, and disrupt daily activities and one's ability to fulfill social roles. Thus representation of the illness as uncontrollable, along with difficulties in management and disruption of relationships, may contribute to depressive affect in the context of chronic illness models.

A similar set of factors seems to distinguish functional from maladaptive or dysfunctional models guiding self-management for patients with asthma. Unlike patients who hold a functional chronic model, patients who hold an acute model perceive asthma as present only when they are symptomatic and are less likely to monitor their lung function or use preventive medication to control the inflammatory process underlying asthma when they are asymptomatic. In contrast, patients with functional chronic models use peak flow meters and preventive medication as prescribed (Halm et al., 2006). Patients who hold chronic models of asthma may, however, feel frustration and concern about their asthma, worry about becoming addicted to their quick-relief medication (to be used during attacks, not when asymptomatic), and fear that quick-relief medication will not be available when needed. Thus fears that one may be unable to control potentially deadly attacks or become addicted to quick-relief medication appears to be at the heart of inappropriate self-management and reduced quality of life (Ponieman, Wisnivesky, Leventhal, Musumeci-Szabo, & Halm, 2009). The central difficulty for both groups of patients, those with diabetes reporting loss of pleasure in daily life and those with asthma reporting restrictions on activities and reduced quality of life, appears to be inability to successfully manage their illness due either to the uncertain and uncontrollable nature of symptoms and/or to concerns about the medications. Gaps in the conceptual structure of their illness and treatment prototypes, particularly the absence of abstract time frames for identifying risky signs and associated behaviors, underlie deficits in control. In sum, these patients lack self-efficacy, but self-efficacy subsumes and does not identify the specific gaps in the underlying control system.

Cognitive-Behavioral Treatment and the Model of Common-Sense Self-Regulation

The ultimate objective and test of a process model is its utility for designing effective and efficient clinical interventions. Intervention trials for behavioral management of chronic conditions require close attention to at least four different models: (1) the biomedical features of the disease and its treatment; (2) the patients' conceptual and experience-based representation of disease and treatment that underlies ongoing monitoring and response to intervention; (3) a learning model suitable for understanding the acquisition of representations and skills; and (4) a model of an intervention suitable for developing a self-instructional behavioral system for the development of expertise in self-management.

Biomedical Models and Common-Sense Models

Attention to the biomedical model is vitally important for diagnosis and prescribing effective (evidence-based) treatment. The biomedical model is also critical for adherence as it defines the treatment for curing or controlling a disease and associated symptoms and functional changes and provides a rough guide to their anticipated time course. This information needs to be conveyed to the patient and checked against the symptoms and functional changes (prototype checks) the patient uses to assess treatment efficacy. Thus the biomedical model provides a framework for establishing a goal sequence for adherence. To ensure adherence, providers need to identify discrepancies between the biomedically specified control process, targets, responses, and time frames and the self-management control process used by the patient. Attention to patient models of illnesses is likely to be critical to any intervention to promote adherence, as patient beliefs about the controllability of their conditions and the necessity and efficacy of medication are likely some of the most proximal malleable causal factors that influence adherence (Leventhal, Breland, Mora, & Leventhal, 2010; Leventhal, Brissette, & Leventhal, 2003; Leventhal, Dienfenback, & Leventhal, 1992; for hypertension patients, see

Kronish, Leventhal, & Horowitz, 2012; Meyer et al., 1985; for arthritis patients, see Park et al., 1999). For this reason, care providers need to develop expertise in assessing patients' models of their illnesses and available courses of treatment and to help the patient to evaluate these models using both objective information from providers and, perhaps more important, alternative interpretations of the information provided by their own bodies. In this way, the framework provided by the common-sense model suggests an intervention that resembles cognitive-behavioral therapy.

A major task for the members of the health care team, physician, psychologist, nurse, or patient educator is to help patients move from checking subjective cues to objective indicators, to help them learn which cues are valid targets for disease management and which responses close the gaps between current states and targets. For some patients, becoming expert in managing valid biomarkers may require providing them with simple strategies for testing their common-sense models of illness and treatment. For example, this may involve encouraging them to collect more information (e.g., to see how blood sugar readings differ on days the patient does vs. does not take medication as prescribed, checking blood pressure on awakening when blood pressure tends to be high, even after a good night's rest), drawing patients' attention to neglected pieces of information (e.g., helping the patient to remember that he or she reported experiencing foot pain before a recent acute injury, so that current pain cannot be attributed wholly to the injury), or helping patients to consider alternative interpretations of existing data (e.g., to help the patient realize that foot pain may reflect a complication of diabetes rather than an unrelated injury). Disconfirming invalid cues is likely an important part of the learning process.

The instructional value of simple self-conducted "experiments" may prove especially helpful for enhancing adherence and disease control among patients who develop dysfunctional-depressive chronic illness models that resemble the hopelessness that characterizes a subtype of depression (Abramson et al., 1989). In these cases, helping patients to experiment with efforts to control even minor aspects of their ill-

nesses may promote more active adherence, in much the same way that simple behavioral activation seems to prompt improvement in depression (Dimidjian et al., 2006; Jacobson et al., 1996). Both the common-sense model and cognitive-behavioral therapy view patients or clients as lay scientists who may develop somewhat biased or selective ways of interpreting available evidence that limits the repertoire of behavioral responses (Beck, 1987; Beck, Rush, Shaw, & Emery, 1979; Clark, 1999). Perhaps in parallel fashion, then, both models may help individuals to change their behavior by changing their lay-science methods using both behavioral (i.e., experiential) and cognitive (i.e., abstract or conceptual) strategies.

The Executive, Expert Self and Lifelong Self-Management

Although our mission was to focus on medication adherence, we touched upon a range of health-relevant behaviors, including care seeking and use of alternative or complementary treatments. Poorly correlated though they may be (Leventhal, Prochaska, & Hirschman, 1985), these behaviors are involved in the self-management process, and models of health behavior need to account for the situations involved in their initiation and the factors sustaining longer term adherence. Doing this requires understanding and addressing the processes underlying adherence and determining which are merely predictive, which are causal, and which are malleable. The cognitive process that is often most proximal to the initiation and ultimate adherence to these behaviors involves checking changes in symptoms and function against prototypes of the healthy, that is, normal self and prototypes or schemas of frequently experienced acute illnesses. Gathering more information about the development of prototypes and symptom check patterns is a priority for future research.

Effective promotion of lasting behavior change requires greater understanding of how prototypes and the elements defining them change and how to promote this change in the most efficient manner. For example, we are still striving to understand whether cognitive-behavioral therapy truly works by changing the underlying cognitive schemas that lead people with depression to interpret negative events with negative automatic thoughts about the self, the future, and the world (DeRubeis et al., 1990; Hollon & DeRubeis, 2004; Hollon, Stewart, & Strunk, 2006; Strunk, DeRubeis, Chiu, & Alvarez, 2007). The suggestion of the common-sense model that patient prototypes of illnesses are shaped by experience and therefore are flexible and amenable to change is supported by evidence suggesting that, in therapy, patients with depression may let go of beliefs about the causes of their depression that are not relevant to treatment while selectively retaining beliefs that are more closely related to treatment (Leykin, DeRubeis, Shelton, & Amsterdam, 2007). Causal beliefs thus seem to be somewhat flexible. We do not yet know how best to promote change in patient prototypes, but the model suggests that change may be accomplished through both the experiential and conceptual routes. For example, biofeedback training may help patients with asthma learn to detect very subtle changes in lung function that they can track daily in a log to begin to learn through experience that they have asthma even on days on which they do not experience full-fledged asthma attacks (Lehrer et al., 2004). In this way, experience may help alter patients' conceptual models of illness and thereby influence adherence behaviors. Alternatively, cognitive and psychoeducational interventions that seek to correct patients' misapprehensions about the chronic nature of their illness may help some patients with asthma by changing patients' abstract conceptions of their illness, without the need for experiential training. In-depth interviewing with patients with asthma suggests that they are often unaware of the models guiding their self-management behaviors. During interviews, some patients who earlier stated that they used asthma medication only when symptomatic have noted that this must mean that they have asthma only when they are symptomatic. When asked about beliefs about the chronic nature of asthma, one patient noted, "Given what I told you [about using preventer medication only when symptomatic], I guess I must believe that I only have it when I have symptoms." Thus it seems that models underlying self-management behaviors are often implicit

and malleable unless they have been formed over long periods of time and are associated with a variety of "secondary" gains. This hypothesis suggests that intervening to reorganize a patient's common-sense perspective and improving the control of a chronic illness could be a valuable first step in reducing comorbid distress and depression, assuming that the patient perceives a connection between the physical condition and its improvement with the distress symptoms. Behavioral change is more likely to be permanent if action is integrated in a clear conceptual framework and integrated in well-structured daily life patterns.

We need to develop a model of intervention that is informed by the processes that govern adherence and by the ways in which our intervention components alter these processes to promote greater adherence. The model must point to interventions that are effective and efficient and that are usable in practice situations. To arrive at this objective, we must carefully match intervention components to assessments of patient beliefs and contextual factors that may inhibit adherence and evaluate these assessments for efficiency and effectiveness. Strong evidence for treatment effectiveness requires evidence of the pathway through which treatment worked; consistency of outcome is insufficient. The clinical literature is replete with suggestions to examine treatment moderators. For example, the nature of the disease, social context, and culture may shape the prototypes underlying the interpretation of symptoms and functional changes. Our analysis suggests, however, that many moderators can be conceptualized as process variables rather than as static traits. For example, if the incorporation of a behavior such as taking medication into daily life patterns is moderated by conscientiousness, it may make sense to assess the pattern of daily activities to find a slot in which to incorporate medication. Monitoring to locate breaks or inflection points in highly automatic behavioral sequences provides openings for inserting new actions and revising the sequence. This form of monitoring involves more than collecting a series of readings; it creates start points for action. If culture and social context shape prototypes, it may make sense to identify how cultural rules affect the way symptoms are read and the interpretation of symptoms depending on factors such as their pattern, duration, and contingency with environmental events.

As we have suggested throughout the chapter, to help patients learn self-management skills, it is important to first map and then manipulate cognitive and affective factors associated with the development of expertise. The check process provides a unifying theme; PCs (regarding pattern, location, duration, and affect) are involved in mapping experienced symptoms to prototypes, evaluating the efficacy of actions to control health threats, and reshaping views of the self through the executive system. People use function to assess their overall health (Mora, DiBonaventura, Idler, Leventhal, & Leventhal, 2008), and these assessments are powerful predictors of mortality (Idler & Benyamini, 1997). Symptoms and function and estimates of life expectancy reshape the image of self and affect strategies for self-management with advancing age (Baltes & Baltes, 1990). The issue is how best to help the individual use these tools to be more effective in managing a chronic illness while going about daily life. A combination of behavioral strategies and mental tools (what to look for) used in a cognitive–affective framework (prototype) that provides valid feedback should facilitate the change process. Such strategies may be able to be implemented efficiently with the assistance of technology and a team or system approach.

Research in this area is in its infancy, and greater attention to systematic approaches to the development and evaluation of interventions in this area is needed urgently. Considerable flexibility will be needed on the part of the clinician working in a comprehensive framework for assessment and remediation of patient models of illness using psychoeducation and cognitive and behavioral strategies, as needed. The goal is patient control with clinician assistance. The steps to the goal will vary and may include didactic interventions, experimental behavioral (try X and see if you notice Y) exercises, and use of metaphors or analogies (Holyoak & Thagard, 1997). Given that the patient is the arbiter, there may be setbacks from the perspective of the therapist. For example, a patient may be ambivalent about taking medication to manage bipolar swings if he or she values periods of elevated mood (Jamison, 1995) or if the side effects interfere with high-priority activities (e.g., sedation from medications that impair work performance or parenting). The meaning of medication adherence may depend on goals inconsistent with disease control that are important to the patient. The therapist must consider whether the consequences of nonadherence are truly understood (i.e., Are the experiential consequences kept in mind, how it will feel, for how long, and how it will affect other life activities?). We are currently conducting research on provider behavior that suggests that providers vary widely in their attention to and ability to assess patient models of illness and treatment but that the majority of providers do not address this in clinical encounters, even when addressing nonadherence to medication regimens. Given the evidence linking patient representations of illness and treatments to behavior, we suggest that assessing and addressing patient representations may be an important and efficient step toward improving adherence.

Summary

The mechanisms underlying adherence operate in an intrapersonal, interpersonal, and ecological context that influences adherence behaviors through a wide array of not-well-articulated pathways. This is what one would expect from a complex system. The evidence touched upon suggests that interpersonal processes in patient–provider communication are important in facilitating adherence and effective patient management of chronic diseases; a clear opening for cognitive-behavioral interventions. The common-sense self-regulation model provides a framework for developing interventions by advancing our understanding of the array of factors affecting adherence, as it articulates specific, proximal, and malleable processes that influence self-management. This model identifies key sets of factors and processes ranging from matching deviations from prototypes of self to prototypes or schemas of illnesses to schemas of treatments that may or may not make sense relative to the features and perceived causes of illness to the planning process, that is, monitoring behavioral sequences in natural environments to form plans for implementation. This may seem to present an array of variables and processes that would overwhelm research and undermine compliance. The model suggests new approaches to research, such as studying excellent self-managers, to identify the processes underlying the strategies that lead to behavioral expertise. We have reason to believe that work in this area may open new and simpler approaches to the study of adherence and to the improvement of management and ultimately improved, objective health outcomes. Advancing our understanding of the determinants of adherence and our ability to effectively and efficiently promote adherence may depend on our ability to move beyond the identification of predictive factors to a more mechanistic understanding that identifies specific targets and pathways for intervention.

ACKNOWLEDGMENTS

Preparation of this chapter was supported by Grant No. R24-AG023958 from the National Institute on Aging (Howard Leventhal, Principal Investigator).

REFERENCES

Abramson, L. Y., Metalsky, G. I., & Alloy, L. B. (1989). Hopelessness depression: A theory-based subtype of depression. *Psychological Review, 96*, 358–372.

Aikens, J. E., Nau, D. P., Klinkman, M. S., & Schwenk, T. L. (2005). Adherence to maintenance-phase antidepressant medication as a function of patient beliefs about medication. *Annals of Family Medicine, 3*, 23–30.

Aikens, J. E., Zvolensky, M. J., & Eifert, G. H. (2001). Differential fear of cardiopulmonary sensations in emergency room noncardiac chest pain patients. *Journal of Behavioral Medicine, 24*, 155–167.

Akincigil, A., Bowblis, J. R., Levin, C., Jan, S., Patel, M., & Crystal, S. (2008). Long-term adherence to evidence-based secondary prevention therapies after acute myocardial infarction. *Journal of General Internal Medicine, 23*, 115–121.

Alderman, M. H., & Schoenbaum, E. E. (1975). Detection and treatment of hypertension at the work site. *New England Journal of Medicine, 293*, 65–68.

Baldwin, A. S., Rothman, A. J., Hertel, A. W., Linde, J. A., Jeffrey, R. W., Finch, E. A., et al. (2006). Specifying the determinants of the initiation and maintenance of behavior change: An examination of self-efficacy, satisfaction, and smoking cessation. *Health Psychology, 25*, 626–634.

Baltes, P. B., & Baltes, M. M. (1990). *Psychological perspectives on successful aging: The model of selective optimization with compensation.* In P. B. Baltes & M. M. Baltes (Eds.), *Successful aging: Perspectives from the behavioral sciences* (pp. 1–34). New York: Cambridge University Press.

Barnes, P. M., Powell-Griner, E., McFann, K., & Nahin, R. L. (2004, May 27). Complementary and alternative medicine use among adults: United States, 2002. *Advance Data, 343*, 1–19.

Beck, A. T. (1987). Cognitive models of depression. *Journal of Cognitive Psychotherapy, 1*, 5–37.

Beck, A. T., Rush, A. J., Shaw, B. F., & Emery, G. (1979). *Cognitive therapy of depression.* New York: Guilford Press.

Becker, M. H., Drachman, R. H., & Kirscht, J. P. (1972). Predicting mothers' compliance with pediatric medical regimens. *Journal of Pediatrics, 81*, 834–845.

Blumhagen, D. (1980). Hyper-tension: A folk illness with a medical name. *Culture, Medicine, and Psychiatry, 4*, 197–227.

Brody, E. M., & Kleban, M. H. (1981). Physical and mental health symptoms of older people: Who do they tell? *Journal of the American Geriatrics Society, 29*(10), 442–449.

Brody, E. M., & Kleban, M. H. (1983). Day-to-day mental and physical health symptoms of older people: A report on health logs. *Gerontologist, 23*, 75–85.

Brown, K. K., Rehmus, W. E., & Kimball, A. B. (2006). Determining the relative importance of patient motivations for nonadherence to topical corticosteroid therapy in psoriasis. *Journal of the American Academy of Dermatology, 55*(4), 607–613.

Brownell, K. D., Cohen, R. Y., Stunkard, A. J., Felix, M. R., & Cooley, N. B. (1984). Weight loss competitions at the work site: Impact on weight, morale and cost-effectiveness. *American Journal of Public Health, 74*, 1283–1285.

Cameron, L., Leventhal, E. A., & Leventhal, H. (1993). Symptom representations and affect as determinants of care seeking in a community dwelling adult sample population. *Health Psychology, 12,* 171–179.

Cameron, L., Leventhal, E. A., & Leventhal, H. (1995). Seeking medical care in response to symptoms and life stress. *Psychosomatic Medicine, 57,* 37–47.

Carver, C. S., Pozo-Kaderman, C., Harris, S. D., Noriega, V., Scheier, M. F., Robinson, D. S., et al. (1994). Optimism versus pessimism predicts the quality of women's adjustment to early stage breast cancer. *Cancer, 73,* 1213–1220.

Cassileth, B. R. (1998). *The alternative medicine handbook: The complete reference guide to alternative and complementary therapies.* New York: Norton.

Catz, S. L., Kelly, J. A., Bogart, L. M., Benotsch, E. G., & McAuliffe, T. L. (2000). Patterns, correlates, and barriers to medication adherence among persons prescribed new treatments for HIV disease. *Health Psychology, 19,* 124–133.

Centers for Medicare and Medicaid Services. (2014). *National Health Expenditure 2012 highlights.* Retrieved June 12, 2014, from *http://cms.hhs.gov/Research-Statistics-Data-and-Systems/Statistics-Trends-and-Reports/NationalHealthExpendData/Downloads/highlights.pdf.*

Chan, K. S., Keeler, E., Schonlau, M., Rosen, M., & Mangione-Smith, R. (2005). How do ethnicity and primary language spoken at home affect management practices and outcomes in children and adolescents with asthma? *Archives of Pediatric Adolescent Medicine, 159,* 283–289.

Charles, S. T., Gatz, M., Kato, K., & Pedersen, N. L. (2008). Physical health 25 years later: The predictive ability of neuroticism. *Health Psychology, 27,* 369–378.

Chesney, M. (2003). Adherence to HAART regimens. *AIDS Patient Care and STDs, 17,* 169–177.

Chesney, M. A., & Folkman, S. (1994). Psychological impact of HIV disease and implications for intervention. *Psychiatric Clinics of North America, 17*(1), 163–182.

Choudhry, N. K., & Winkelmayer, W. C. (2008). Medication adherence after myocardial infarction: A long way left to go. *Journal of General Internal Medicine, 23,* 216–218.

Clark, D. M. (1999). Anxiety disorders: Why they persist and how to treat them. *Behaviour Research and Therapy, 37,* S5–S27.

Clatworthy, J., Bowskill, R., Rank, T., Parham, R., & Horne, R. (2007). Adherence in medication in bipolar disorder: A qualitative study exploring the role of patients' beliefs about the condition and its treatment. *Bipolar Disorders, 9,* 656–664.

Claxton, A. J., Cramer, J., & Pierce, C. (2001). A systematic review of the associations between dose regimens and medication compliance. *Clinical Therapeutics, 23,* 1296–1310.

Cohen, S., Doyle, W. J., & Skoner, D. P. (1999). Psychological stress, cytokine production, and severity of upper respiratory illness. *Psychosomatic Medicine, 61,* 175–180.

Costa, P. T., & McCrae, R. R. (1980). Somatic complaints in males as a function of age and neuroticism: A longitudinal analysis. *Journal of Behavioral Medicine, 3,* 245–257.

Craighead, W. E., Craighead, L. W. & Ilardi, S. S. (1998). Psychosocial treatments for major depressive disorder. In P. E. Nathan & J. M. Gorman (Eds.), *A guide to treatments that work* (pp. 226–248). New York: Oxford University Press.

DeNavas-Walt, C., Proctor, B. D., & Smith, J. (2012). *Income, poverty, and health insurance coverage in the United States: 2011.* Washington DC: U.S. Government Printing Office. Available at *www.census.gov/prod/2012pubs/p60-243.pdf.*

DeRubeis, R. J., Evans, M. D., Hollon, S. D., Garvey, M. J., Grove, W. M., & Tuason, V. B. (1990). How does cognitive therapy work?: Cognitive change and symptom change in cognitive therapy and pharmacotherapy for depression. *Journal of Consulting and Clinical Psychology, 58,* 862–869.

Diabetes Prevention Program Research Group. (2002). Reduction in the incidence of type 2 diabetes with lifestyle intervention of metformin. *New England Journal of Medicine, 346,* 393–403.

DiMatteo, M. R., Lepper, H. S., & Croghan, T. W. (2000). Depression is a risk factor for noncompliance with medical treatment: Meta-analysis of the effects of anxiety and depression on patient adherence. *Archives of Internal Medicine, 160,* 2101–2107.

Dimidjian, S., Hollon, S. D., Dobson, K. S., Schmaling, K. B., Kohlenberg, R. J., Addis, M. E., et al. (2006). Randomized trial of behavioral activation, cognitive therapy, and antidepressant medication in the acute treatment of adults with major depression. *Journal of Consulting and Clinical Psychology, 74,* 658–670.

Dunbar-Jacob, J., & Mortimer-Stephens, M. K. (2001). Treatment adherence in chronic disease. *Journal of Clinical Epidemiology, 54,* S57–S60.

Dunbar-Jacob, J., & Schlenk, E. (2000). Patient adherence to treatment regimens. In A. Baum, T. A. Revenson, & J. E. Singer (Eds.), *Handbook of health psychology* (pp. 571–580). Mahwah, NJ: Erlbaum.

Farquhar, J. W., Maccoby, N., Wood, P. D., Alexander, J. K., Breitrose, H., Brown, B. W. J., et al. (1977). Community education for cardiovascular health. *Lancet, 1,* 1192–1195.

Feinstein, A. R. (1976). "Compliance bias" and the interpretation of therapeutic trials. In D. L. Sackett & R. B. Haynes (Eds.), *Compliance with therapeutic regimes* (pp. 152–166). Baltimore: Johns Hopkins University Press.

Finch, E. A., Linde, J. A., Jeffrey, R. W., Rothman, A. J., King, C. M., & Levy, R. L. (2005). The effects of outcome expectancies and satisfaction on weight loss and maintenance: Correlational and experimental analyses—a randomized trial. *Health Psychology, 24,* 608–616.

Glaser, R., Sheridan, J., Malarkey, W. B., MacCallum, R. C., & Kiecolt-Glaser, J. K. (2000). Chronic stress modulates the immune response to a pneumococcal pneumonia vaccine. *Psychosomatic Medicine, 62,* 804–807.

Gobet, F. (1998). Expert memory: A comparison of four theories. *Cognition and Emotion, 66,* 115–152.

Gollwitzer, P. M. (1999). Implementation intentions: Strong effects of simple plans. *American Psychologist, 54,* 493–503.

Gonzalez, J. F., Penedo, F. J., Llabre, M. M., Duran, M. H., Antoni, M. H., Schneiderman, N., et al. (2007). Physical symptoms, beliefs about medications, negative mood, and long-term HIV medication adherence. *Annals of Behavioral Medicine, 34,* 46–55.

Hager, M. S., & Orbell, S. (2003). A meta-analytic review of the common-sense model of illness representations. *Psychology and Health, 18,* 141–184.

Halm, E. A., Mora, P., & Leventhal, H. (2006). No symptoms, no asthma: The acute episodic disease belief is associated with poor self-management among inner-city adults with persistent asthma. *Chest, 129,* 573–580.

Halverson, G. (2007). *Health care reform now.* San Francisco: Wiley.

Hampson, S. E. (1997a). Personal models and the management of chronic illness: A comparison of diabetes and osteoarthritis. *European Journal of Personality, 11,* 401–414.

Hampson, S. E. (1997b). Illness representations and the self management of diabetes. In K. J. Petrie & J. A. Weinman (Eds.), *Perception of health and illness: Current research and applications* (pp. 323–347). Amsterdam: Harwood Academic.

Hampson, S. E., Glasgow, R. E., & Toobert, D. J. (1990). Personal models of diabetes and their relations to self-care activities. *Health Psychology, 9,* 632–646.

Hepworth, N., & Paxton, S. J. (2007). Pathways to help-seeking in bulimia nervosa and binge eating problems: A concept mapping approach. *International Journal of Eating Disorders, 40,* 493–504.

Heurtin Roberts, S. (1993). "High-pertension": The uses of a chronic folk illness for personal adaptation. *Social Science and Medicine, 37,* 285–294.

Hollon, S. D., & DeRubeis, R. J. (2004). Effectiveness of treatment for depression. In R. L. Leahy (Ed.), *Contemporary cognitive therapy: Theory, research, and practice* (pp. 45–61). New York: Guilford Press.

Hollon, S. D., Stewart, M. O., & Strunk, D. (2006). Enduring effects for cognitive behavior therapy in the treatment of depression and anxiety. *Annual Review of Psychology, 57,* 285–315.

Holyoak, K. J., & Thagard, P. (1997). The analogical mind. *American Psychologist, 52*(1), 35–44.

Horne, R. (1997). Representations of medication and treatment: Advances in theory and measurement. In K. J. Petrie & J. A. Weinman (Eds.), *Perceptions in health and illness: Current research and applications* (pp. 155–187). London: Harwood Academic Press.

Horne, R. (2003). Treatment perceptions and self-regulation. In L. D. Cameron & H. Leventhal (Eds.), *The self-regulation of health and illness behavior* (pp. 138–154). London: Routledge.

Horne, R., Faasse, K., Cooper, V., Diefenbach, M. A., Leventhal, H., Leventhal, E., et al. (2012). The Perceived Sensitivity to Medicines (PSM) scale: An evaluation of validity and reliability. *British Journal of Health Psychology, 18,* 18–30.

Horne, R., & Weinman, J. (1999). Patients' beliefs about prescribed medicines and their role in adherence to treatment in chronic physical illness. *Journal of Psychosomatic Research, 47*(6), 555–567.

Horne, R., & Weinman, J. (2002). Self-regulation and self-management in asthma: Exploring the role of illness perceptions and treatment beliefs in explaining non-adherence to preventer medication. *Psychology and Health, 17*(1), 17–32.

Horne, R., Weinman, J., & Hankins, M. (1999). The Beliefs about Medicines Questionnaire: The development and evaluation of a new method for assessing the cognitive representation of medication. *Psychology and Health, 14*, 1–24.

Horowitz, C. R., Rein, S. B., & Leventhal, H. (2004). A story of maladies, misconceptions and mishaps: Effective management of heart failure. *Social Science and Medicine, 58*, 631–643.

Idler, E. L., & Benyamini, Y. (1997). Self-rated health and mortality: A review of twenty-seven community studies. *Journal of Health and Social Behavior, 38*, 21–37.

Jacobson, N. S., Dobson, K. S., Truax, P. A., Addis, M. E., Koerner, K., Gollan, J. K., et al. (1996). A component analysis of cognitive-behavioral treatment for depression. *Journal of Consulting and Clinical Psychology, 64*, 295–304.

Jamison, K. R. (1995). *An unquiet mind.* New York: Knopf.

Jessop, D. C., & Rutter, D. R. (2003). Adherence to asthma medication: The role of illness representations. *Psychology and Health, 18*, 595–612.

Johnson, J. E. (1975). Stress reduction through sensation information. In I. L. Sarason & C. D. Spielberger (Eds.), *Stress and anxiety* (pp. 361–373). Washington, DC: Hemisphere.

Johnson, J. E., & Leventhal, H. (1974). Effects of accurate expectations and behavioral instructions on reactions during a noxious medical examination. *Journal of Personality and Social Psychology, 29*, 710–718.

Keller, M. B., Hirschfield, R. M. A., Demyttenaere, K., & Baldwin, D. S. (2002). Optimizing outcomes in depression: Focus on antidepressant compliance. *International Clinical Psychopharmacology, 17*(6), 265–271.

Kravitz, R. L., Hays, R. D., Sherbourne, C. D., DiMatteo, M. R., Rogers, W. H., Ordway, L., et al. (1993). Recall of recommendations and adherence to advice among patients with chronic medical conditions. *Archives of Internal Medicine, 153*, 1869–1878.

Kripilani, S., Yao, X., & Haynes, R. B. (2007). Interventions to enhance medication adherence in chronic medical conditions: A systematic review. *Archives of Internal Medicine, 167*, 540–549.

Kronish, I. M., Leventhal, H., & Horowitz, C. R. (2012). Understanding minority patients' beliefs about hypertension to reduce gaps in communication between patients and clinicians. *Journal of Clinical Hypertension, 14*(1), 38–44.

Lehrer, P. M., Vaschillo, E., Vaschillo, B., Lu, S., Scardella, A., Siddique, M., et al. (2004). Biofeedback treatment for asthma. *Chest, 126*, 352–361.

Leventhal, H. (1970). Findings and theory in the study of fear communications. *Advances in Experimental Social Psychology, 5*, 119–186.

Leventhal, H., Bodnar-Deren, S., Breland, J. Y., Hash-Converse, J., Phillips, L. A., Leventhal, E. A., et al. (2011). Modeling health and illness behavior: The approach of the common-sense model. In A. Baum, T. A. Revenson, & J. Singer (Eds.), *Handbook of health psychology* (pp. 3–36). New York: Psychological Press.

Leventhal, H., Breland, J. Y., Mora, P. A., & Leventhal, E. A. (2010). Lay representations of illness and treatment: A framework for action. In A. Steptoe, K. Freedland, R. Jennings, M. Llabre, S. Manuck, & E. Susman (Eds.), *Handbook of behavioral medicine: Methods and applications* (pp. 137–154). New York: Springer.

Leventhal, H., Brissette, I., & Leventhal, E. A. (2003). The common-sense model of self-regulation of health and illness. In L. D. Cameron & H. Leventhal (Eds.), *The self-regulation of health and illness behaviour* (pp. 42–65). New York: Routledge.

Leventhal, H., Dienfenback, M., & Leventhal, E. A. (1992). Illness cognition: Using common sense to understand treatment adherence and affect cognition interactions. *Cognitive Therapy and Research, 16*, 143–163.

Leventhal, H., Prochaska, T. R., & Hirschman, R. S. (1985). Preventive health behavior across the life span. In J. C. Rosen & L. J. Solomon (Eds.), *Prevention in health psychology* (pp. 191–235). Hanover, NH: University Press of New England.

Leventhal, H., Safer, M., Cleary, P., & Gutmann, M. (1980). Cardiovascular risk modification by community-based programs for life-style change: Comments on the Stanford study. *Journal of Consulting and Clinical Psychology, 48*, 150–158.

Leventhal, H., Singer, R., & Jones, S. (1965).

Effects of fear and specificity of recommendation upon attitudes and behavior. *Journal of Personality and Social Psychology, 2,* 20–29.

Leventhal, H., Weinman, J., Leventhal, E. A., & Phillips, L. A. (2008). Health psychology: The search for pathways between behavior and health. *Annual Review of Psychology, 59,* 477–505.

Leventhal, H., Zimmerman, R., & Gutmann, M. (1984). Compliance: A self regulation perspective. In W. D. Gentry (Ed.), *Handbook of behavioral medicine* (pp. 369–436). New York: Guilford Press.

Ley, P. (1977). Psychological studies of doctor–patient communication. In S. Rachman (Ed.), *Contributions to medical psychology* (pp. 19–42). New York: Pergamon Press.

Ley, P., Jain, V. K., & Skilbeck, C. E. (1976). A method for decreasing patients' medication errors. *Psychological Medicine, 6*(4), 599–601.

Leykin, Y., DeRubeis, R. J., Shelton, R. C., & Amsterdam, J. D. (2007). Changes in patients' beliefs about the causes of their depression following successful treatment. *Cognitive Therapy and Research, 31,* 437–449.

Linde, J. A., Rothman, A. J., Baldwin, A. S., & Jeffery, R. W. (2006). The impact of self-efficacy on behavior change and weight change among overweight participants in a weight loss trial. *Health Psychology, 25,* 282–291.

Locke, E. A., & Latham, G. P. (2002). Building a practically useful theory of goal setting and task motivation: A 35-year odyssey. *American Psychologist, 57*(9), 705–717

McAndrew, L. M., Horowitz, C. R., Lancaster, K. J., Quigley, K. S., Pogach, L. M., Mora, P. A., et al. (2011). Association between self-monitoring of blood glucose and diet among minority patients with diabetes. *Journal of Diabetes, 3,* 147–152.

McAndrew, L., Schneider, S. H., Burns, E., & Leventhal, H. (2007). Does patient blood glucose monitoring improve diabetes control: Always, sometimes, never? A systematic review from the framework of the common-sense model. *Diabetes Educator, 33,* 991–1011.

Menckeberg, T. T., Bouvy, M. L., Bracke, M., Kaptein, A. A., Leufkens, H. G., Raaijmakers, J., et al. (2008). Beliefs about medicine predict refill adherence to inhaled corticosteroids. *Journal of Psychosomatic Research, 64,* 47–54.

Meyer, D., Leventhal, H., & Gutmann, M. (1985). Commonsense models of illness: The example of hypertension. *Health Psychology, 4,* 115–135.

Miller, G. A., Galanter, E. H., & Pribram, K. H. (1960). *Plans and the structure of behavior.* New York: Holt.

Mora, P. A., DiBonaventura, M. D., Idler, E., Leventhal, E. A., & Leventhal, H. (2008). Psychological factors influencing self-assessments of health: Towards an understanding of the mechanisms underlying how people rate their own health. *Annals of Behavioral Medicine, 36,* 292–303.

Mora, P., Robitaille, C., Leventhal, H., Swigar, M., & Leventhal, E. A. (2002). Trait negative affect relates to prior weak symptoms, but not to reports of illness episodes, illness symptoms and care seeking. *Psychosomatic Medicine, 64,* 436–449.

National Center for Health Statistics. (2011). *Health, United States, 2011: With special feature on socioeconomic status and health.* Hyattsville, MD. Available at *www.cdc.gov/nchs/data/hus/hus11.pdf.*

Nemeroff, C. B., & Schatzberg, A. F. (1998). Pharmacological treatment of unipolar depression. In P. E. Nathan & J. M. Gorman (Eds.), *A guide to treatments that work* (pp. 212–225). New York: Oxford University Press.

Osterberg, L., & Blaschke, T. (2005). Adherence to medication. *New England Journal of Medicine, 353,* 487–497.

Park, D. C., Hertzog, C., Leventhal, H., Morrell, R., Leventhal, E., Birchmore, D., et al. (1999). Medication adherence in rheumatoid arthritis patients: Older is wiser. *Journal of the American Geriatrics Society, 47,* 172–183.

Phillips, L. A., Leventhal, H., & Leventhal, E. A. (2012). Physicians' communication of the common-sense self-regulation model results in greater reported adherence than physicians' use of interpersonal skills. *British Journal of Health Psychology, 17,* 244–257.

Phillips, L. A., Leventhal, H., & Leventhal, E. A. (2013). Assessing theoretical predictors of long-term medication adherence: Patients' treatment-related beliefs, experiential feedback, and habit development. *Psychology and Health, 28,* 1135–1151.

Phillips, L. S., Branch, W. T., Cook, C. B., Doyle, J. P., El-Kebbi, I. M., Gallina, D. L., et al. (2001). Clinical inertia. *Annals of Internal Medicine, 135,* 825–834.

Pickle, L. W., Mungiole, M., & Gillum, R. F. (1997). Geographic variation in stroke mortality in blacks and whites in the United States. *Stroke, 28,* 1639.

Ponieman, D., Wisnivesky, J. P., Leventhal, H., Musumeci-Szabo, T. J., & Halm, E. A. (2009). Impact of positive and negative beliefs about inhaled corticosteroids on adherence in inner-city asthmatic patients. *Annals of Allergy, Asthma, and Immunology, 103,* 38–42.

Powers, W. T. (1973). *Behavior: The control of perception.* Chicago: Aldine.

Prochaska, J. O., & DiClemente, C. C. (1984). *The transtheoretical approach: Crossing traditional boundaries of therapy.* Chicago: Dow Jones/Irwin.

Pugh, R. (1983). An association between hostility and poor adherence to treatment in patients suffering from depression. *British Journal of Medical Psychology, 56*(2), 205–208.

Roberts, B. W., Walton, K. E., & Bogg, T. (2005). Conscientiousness and health across the life course. *Review of General Psychology, 9*(2), 156–168.

Rogers, E. M., Vaughan, P. W., Swalehe, R., Rao, N., Svenkerud, P., & Sood, S. (1999). Effects of an entertainment-education radio soap opera on family planning behavior in Tanzania. *Studies in Family Planning, 30,* 193–211.

Rothman, A. J. (2000). Toward a theory-based analysis of behavioral maintenance. *Health Psychology, 19,* 64–69.

Rozanski, A., Blumenthal, J. A., Davidson, K. W., Saab, P. G., & Kubzansky, L. (2005). The epidemiology, pathophysiology, and management of psychosocial risk factors in cardiac practice: The emerging field of behavioral cardiology. *Journal of the American College of Cardiology, 45*(5), 637–651.

Rubin, R. R. (2005). Adherence to pharmacologic therapy in patients with type 2 diabetes mellitus. *American Journal of Medicine, 118* (Suppl. 5A), 27S–34S.

Sackett, D. L., & Haynes, R. B. (1976). *Compliance with therapeutic regimens.* Baltimore: Johns Hopkins University Press.

Scheier, M. F., & Carver, C. S. (1987). Dispositional optimism and physical well-being: The influence of generalized outcome expectancies on health. *Journal of Personality, 55,* 169–210.

Scheier, M. F., & Carver, C. S. (1992). Effects of optimism on psychological and physical well-being: Theoretical overview and empirical update. *Cognitive Therapy and Research, 16,* 201–228.

Schwarzer, R. (2008). Modeling health behavior change: How to predict and modify the adoption and maintenance of health behaviors. *Applied Psychology, 57,* 1–29.

Sewitch, M. J., Abrahamowicz, M., Barkun, A., Bitton, A., Wild, G. E., Cohen, A., et al. (2003). Patient nonadherence to medication in inflammatory bowel disease. *American Journal of Gastroenterology, 98,* 1535–1544.

Slavich, G. M., & Cole, S. W. (2013). The emerging field of human social genomics. *Clinical Psychological Science, 1*(3), 331–348.

Stimson, G. V. (1974). Obeying doctor's orders: A view from the other side. *Social Science and Medicine, 8,* 177–186.

Stoller, E. P. (1998). Dynamics and processes of self-care in old age. In M. Ory & G. DeFriese (Eds.), *Self-care in later life: Research program and policy perspectives* (pp. 24–61). New York: Springer.

Strunk, D. R., DeRubeis, R. J., Chiu, A. W., & Alvarez, J. (2007). Patients' competence in and performance of cognitive therapy skills: Relation to the reduction of relapse risk following treatment for depression. *Journal of Consulting and Clinical Psychology, 75,* 523–530.

Tuomilehto, J., Lindstrom, J., Eriksson, J. G., Valle, T. T., Hamalainen, H., Ilanne-Parikka, P., et al. (2001). Prevention of type 2 diabetes mellitus by changes in lifestyle among subjects with impaired glucose tolerance. *New England Journal of Medicine, 344,* 1343–1350.

van Lenthe, F. J., Borrell, L. N., Costa, G., Diez Roux, A. V., Kaupinnen, T. M., Marinacci, C., et al. (2005). Neighbourhood unemployment and all cause mortality: A comparison of six countries. *Journal of Epidemiology and Community Health, 59,* 231–237.

Vileikyte, L., Leventhal, H., Gonzales, J. S., Peyrot, M., Rubin, R. R., Ulbrecht, J. S., et al. (2005). Diabetic peripheral neuropathy and depressive symptoms: The association revisited. *Diabetes Care, 28,* 2378–2383.

Walker, C., Papadopoulos, L., Lipton, M., & Hussein, M. (2006). The importance of children's illness beliefs: The Children's Illness Perception Questionnaire (CIPQ) as a reliable assessment tool for eczema and asthma. *Psychology, Health and Medicine, 11*(1), 100–107.

PART II

Assessment of Health-Risk Behaviors

CHAPTER 4

Eating Disorders

Susan Himes
Tovah Yanover
J. Kevin Thompson

The field of eating disorders has grown dramatically in the last two decades, and a variety of methods for assessing eating disturbance symptomatology have emerged during this time period (Thompson, 1996, 2004; Thompson & Smolak, 2001). In this chapter, we offer an overview of methods that have received the most empirical evaluation and that appear to offer the best approach for a comprehensive evaluation of the characteristics of eating problems. In the following section, we provide an overview of commonly used, psychometrically sound, and emerging assessment methods for eating disorders. We do not comprehensively review all of the measures that assess domains related to eating disturbance (e.g., body image) or practices central to specific eating disorders (e.g., binge eating disorder [BED], dietary restraint) but focus on the screening and diagnostic methods used for eating disorders. For an in-depth review of body image assessment, see Chapter 2 of *Exacting Beauty* (Thompson, Heinberg, Altabe, & Tantleff-Dunn, 1999); for a review of binge assessment, see Chapter 11 (by Wilson) in *Binge Eating: Nature, Assessment, and Treatment* (Fairburn & Wilson, 1993). For a brief overview of dietary restraint measures, see Chapter 6 (by Anderson and Paulosky) in *The Handbook of Eating Disorders and Obesity* (Thompson, 2004.)

Structured Interviews: The Eating Disorder Examination

The primary interview method utilized for assessing eating disorders is the Eating Disorder Examination (EDE). The EDE (Fairburn & Cooper, 1993) is a semistructured interview created to assess symptoms of anorexia nervosa (AN), bulimia nervosa (BN), and related eating psychopathology. The EDE contains four subscales (Eating Concern, Restraint, Shape Concern, Weight Concern) and two behavioral indices (Overeating, Extreme Methods of Weight Control).

Support for the EDE as a diagnostic and outcome assessment measure is predicated on two arguments. First, the EDE demonstrates excellent psychometric properties, including good interrater reliability (Cooper & Fairburn, 1987; Fairburn & Cooper, 1993), good test–retest reliability (Rizvi, Peterson, Crow, & Agras, 2000), and good internal consistency (Cooper, Cooper, & Fairburn, 1989). Furthermore, the EDE has shown discriminant and concurrent validity (Fairburn & Cooper, 1993). Second, the EDE has substantial empirical support that demonstrates that the measure can differentiate between patients with eating disorders and controls (Cooper et al., 1989) and can differentiate between persons with BN and those with restriction (Cooper et al., 1989; Rosen, Vara, Wendt, & Leitenberg, 1990; Wilson & Smith, 1989). For these reasons, the EDE is considered the gold standard method of eating disorder assessment.

In addition to the psychometric and diagnostic strengths of the EDE structured interview method, the EDE provides a more accurate assessment of binges than self-report measures. Many individuals report a binge when they experience a loss of control and violate their diets without meeting the DSM criteria for consuming a large amount of food (Beglin & Fairburn, 1992; Johnson, Boutelle, Torgrud, Davig, & Turner, 2000; Telch, Pratt, & Niego, 1998). Furthermore, individuals may overestimate their amount of food intake during a given period, reporting a binge when criteria for a large amount of food intake are not met (Anderson, Williamson, Johnson, & Grieve, 1999; Hadigan, Walsh, Lachaussée, & Kissileff, 1992; Schoeller, 1995). Although imperfect because it relies on individuals' self-reported amount of food intake during a perceived binge, the EDE allows the trained interviewer to assess the presence of binge eating, thereby increasing the accuracy for detecting binges (Anderson, Lundgren, Shapiro, & Paulosky, 2004).

The EDE is not without its criticisms, however. The EDE requires interviewer training, the interview may take over an hour to complete, and recent discrepancies between the EDE and other assessment methods have led to questions about its concurrent validity (Anderson & Maloney, 2001; Wilson, 1993). Most frequently, the EDE is used in developing a diagnosis, in assessing treatment outcome, and in conducting research studies (Anderson & Paulosky, 2004; Fairburn & Belgin, 1994). Time constraints limit its use in clinical practice (Anderson & Paulosky, 2004).

The EDE has recently been expanded in two directions; revised versions were created for use with Spanish-speaking populations (S-EDE) and to assess child and adolescent populations with eating disturbance (chEDE). Grilo, Lazano, and Elder (2005) created a Spanish-language version (S-EDE) and assessed a nonclinical sample of monolingual Spanish-speaking women. The S-EDE subscales demonstrate good to excellent test–retest reliability (.67–.90) and interrater reliability (.80–.98); although promising, the new measure has yet to be tested with clinical samples of individuals with AN and BN. In 2012, Grilo and colleagues tested the S-EDE with an overweight and obese binge eating sample and found that the structure of the S-EDE was not supported and that the data better fit a briefer seven-item, three-factor structure that could be utilized instead of the entire measure for binge eating populations (Grilo, Crosby, & White, 2012.) The EDE was modified for use with child and adolescent populations a decade ago (Bryant-Waugh, Cooper, Taylor, & Lask, 1996) and has established psychometric properties (Watkins, Frampton, Lask, & Bryant-Waugh, 2005). The chEDE is considered a simple, age-appropriate version of the EDE, designed for use by children ages 7–14 years. The chEDE demonstrates high interrater reliability (.91–1.0 across subscales), high internal consistency (.80–.91 across subscales), and discriminant validity (Watkins et al., 2005). However, the sample used to test the psychometric properties of the chEDE was small and did not include a specific sample of patients with BN. Although recent additional studies, both internationally (Norway, Germany) and within the United States, have utilized the measure for small samples of children with AN or subjective bulimic episodes, testing with clinical samples of children with eating disorders, including BN, may yield additional support (Frampton, Wisting, Overas, Midtsund, & Lask, 2011; Hilbert et al., 2013; Levine, Ringham, Kalarchian, Wisniewski, & Marcus, 2006).

Self-Report Measures

Screening Measures

Eating Attitudes Test

The most widely used eating disorder screening measure is the Eating Attitudes Test (EAT; Garner & Garfinkel, 1979). After a factor analysis was performed on the original 40-item measure, 26 items that best accounted for variance in the total score were placed into a revised version of the original measure, called the EAT-26 (Garner, Olmstead, Bohr, & Garfinkel, 1982). The EAT-26 is frequently used for eating disorder screenings held in clinics and student counseling centers across the United States during the month of February for Eating Disorders Awareness Week.

The original EAT demonstrates good internal consistency and test–retest reliability (Banasiak, Wertheim, Koerner, & Voudouris, 2001; Carter & Moss, 1984; Garner & Garfinkel, 1979) and good concurrent and discriminant validity (Garner, 1997; Garfinkel & Newman, 2001; Williamson, Anderson, Jackman, & Jackson, 1995). The revised EAT-26 is highly correlated with the original EAT ($r = .98$; Garner et al., 1982), although most psychometric research has been conducted on the original version.

Strengths of the EAT and EAT-26 include its ability to differentiate AN, BN, and BED from controls and to differentiate AN and BN from BED (Garfinkel & Newman, 2001; Williamson et al., 1995). It is a quick, easy method for identifying the presence of eating disturbance. Weaknesses of the EAT include its inability to separate AN from BN (Garfinkel & Newman, 2001; Williamson et al., 1995) and its inability to provide evidence of an eating disorder (Garfinkel & Newman, 2001).

Bulimia Test–R

The original Bulimia Test (BULIT) was created to assess the symptoms of BN (Smith & Thelen, 1984). The BULIT-R is the latest revised version, and it conforms to the diagnostic criteria for BN in DSM-III (Thelen, Farmer, Wonderlich, & Smith, 1991). The two versions of the test are highly correlated ($r = .99$; Thelen et al., 1991). The current BULIT-R is a self-report measure that contains 28 items on a 5-point rating scale.

The psychometric properties of the BULIT-R indicate good internal consistency and test–retest reliability (Thelen et al., 1991) and excellent current, predictive, and discriminant validity (Williamson et al., 1995). More recently, the BULIT-R was found to be reliable and valid for use across ethnic groups (Fernandez, Malcarne, Wilfley, & McQuaid, 2006) and for use with adolescent samples ages 11–18 years (Vincent, McCabe, & Ricciardelli, 1999).

Strengths of the BULIT-R include its ability to discriminate between patients with BN and those with AN and controls, its useful-

ness as a screening tool for BN, and its use as a measure for tracking progress throughout the course of treatment (Anderson & Paulosky, 2004). The primary limitation of the measure is its confinement to use with BN only; it is not recommended for use with AN or BED populations (Anderson & Paulosky, 2004).

Within the last few years, a subset of 23 items from the BULIT-R was extracted to create a new self-report measure for BED, called the Binge Eating Disorder Test (BEDT; Vander Wal, Stein, & Blashill, 2011). The BEDT achieved 100% sensitivity and specificity; however, the sample population was small ($N = 15$) and, although promising, it requires further study.

Eating Disorders Examination–Q

The EDE-Q was created to transcribe the gold standard EDE interview into questionnaire form. The EDE-Q is a 38-item self-report questionnaire; items directly correspond to questions from the structured EDE interview (Beglin & Fairburn, 1994). The EDE-Q was developed to address the need for a brief, easily used questionnaire that would not require the expertise, training, or time to administer that is required by the structured interview EDE (Beglin & Fairburn, 1994). The EDE-Q has gained considerable momentum as a self-report measure of choice in the past decade.

The EDE-Q and EDE were both administered to community and patient samples, and were found to be highly correlated (Beglin & Fairburn, 1994). However, level of agreement across mode of assessment was lower in the domain of binge eating. The EDE-Q derived more frequent reports of binge eating that did not meet clinical criteria for a binge when assessed by interviewers using the EDE. Some studies assessing the differences between the EDE and the EDE-Q have found similar problems with reliability in the domain of binge eating, with EDE-Q reports of more frequent binges (Celio, Wilfley, & Crow, 2004; Wilfley, Schwartz, Spurell, & Fairburn, 1997). However, other studies have found more objective reports of binge eating using the EDE rather than the EDE-Q (Carter, Aime, & Mills, 2001; Grilo, Masheb, & Wilson, 2001; Kalarchian, Wilson, Brolin, & Bradley, 2000). Providing additional nuance, some studies indicate convergence between the EDE and EDE-Q on objective binge eating, with higher rates of overeating obtained by the EDE, and the EDE-Q as less accurate in assessing subjective binge eating (Grilo et al., 2001; Reas, Grilo, & Masheb, 2006). To address difficulties with the EDE-Q, a set of instructions clarifying the definition of binge eating was attached (EDE-Q-I; Celio et al., 2004), which increased agreement with EDE findings. More recently, the EDE-Q has been expanded for use with adolescent populations ages 9–19 years with eating disorders (Binford, le Grange, & Jellar, 2005).

The EDE-Q has been found to have strong psychometric properties, with excellent internal consistency (Peterson, Crosby, & Wonderlich, 2007) and test–retest reliability (Luce & Crowther, 1999), as well as concurrent validity (Beglin & Fairburn, 1994) and acceptable criterion validity (Mond, Hay, & Rodgers, 2004). However, the EDE-Q may have high rates of misclassification in obese binge eaters (Kalarchian et al., 2000).

The EDE-Q can be used as a screening tool or incorporated in the assessment of eating pathology. At this time, there is still concern regarding the EDE-Q's diagnostic capabilities with particular populations; therefore, it should be used in conjunction with other assessment methods (self-monitoring, etc.), and the interviewer should follow up with a brief inquiry to assess whether binge behavior meets clinical criteria for a binge episode. The EDE-Q has similar limitations to other self-report questionnaires, including difficulties with patient recall and retrospective memory.

SCOFF

The SCOFF is a brief self-report questionnaire designed to screen for eating disorders in a primary care population (Morgan, Reid, & Lacey, 1999). The SCOFF consists of five questions that assess some core features of eating disturbance. SCOFF is an acronym that represents key words in assessing features of eating disturbance (making oneself sick, loss of control over eating, one stone loss (weight loss), thoughts of fat, and food dominating life; Cotton, Ball, & Robinson, 2003).

In the early testing of the SCOFF, the questionnaire was provided to adult women primary care patients who were later assessed for an eating disorder using a diagnostic interview. The SCOFF identified patients who met criteria for AN and BN, but did not identify all patients who met criteria for Eating Disorder Not Otherwise Specified (EDNOS; Luck, Morgan, & Reid, 2002). Another study examined the benefits of oral SCOFF assessment versus questionnaire mode assessment; rates of disclosure increased with questionnaire assessment (Perry, Morgan, & Reid, 2002).

Psychometric measurement of a questionnaire with such few items often leads to concerns about compromised reliability; consistent with such concerns, lower internal consistency was found for the SCOFF (r = .47; Siervo, Boschi, & Papa, 2005). Verbal and questionnaire administrations of the SCOFF have high levels of agreement (Perry et al., 2002). However, other studies have found the SCOFF to be less sensitive as a detection tool for identifying eating disorders and EDNOS (Cotton et al., 2003).

In summary, evidence supporting the use of the SCOFF as a screening tool is mixed. Most studies indicate that the use of the screening tool would improve identification and referrals for eating disturbance, although the measure has serious psychometric limitations when compared with other eating disorder screening questionnaires.

Diagnostic Measures

Eating Disorder Inventory–3

The EDI-3 is the latest version of the Eating Disorder Inventory, a 91-item self-report measure that assesses eating disorder symptoms associated with AN, BN, and EDNOS (Garner, 2004). The EDI-3 includes norms from both U.S. and international samples, as well as distinct norms of samples from both adults and adolescents. The EDI-3 includes 12 subscales that assess eating disorder risk (Drive for Thinness, Bulimia, and Body Dissatisfaction) and related psychological constructs associated with the development and maintenance of eating disorders (Low Self-Esteem, Personal Alienation, Interpersonal Insecurity, Interpersonal Alienation, Interoceptive Deficits, Emotional Dysregulation, Perfectionism, Asceticism, and Maturity

Fears). The measure has been widely used and accepted across the field of eating disorders.

The psychometric data supporting the EDI-3 indicate excellent internal consistency, with most scales above .80. Test–retest reliability was reported to be above .90; however, the test–retest measurement was conducted with a small eating disorder sample ($N = 34$). Previous test–retest reliability with the original EDI subscales was shown to be adequate (Crowther, Lilly, Crawford, & Shepard, 1992; Wear & Pratz, 1987). The EDI-3 was administered in conjunction with the EAT-26 and the BULIT-R; there was some support for criterion validity, in particular between the Drive for Thinness (DT) scale and the EAT and the BULIT and the Bulimia (B) scale (Garner, 2004). Overall, there is strong psychometric support for use of the EDI-3.

The original EDI was shown to discriminate between individuals with AN and controls (Garner, Olmstead, & Polivy, 1983) and those with BN and controls (Schoemaker, Verbraak, Breteler, & van der Staak, 1997). The DT, B, and Body Dissatisfaction subscales are most highly correlated with eating pathology (Garner et al., 1983; Hurley, Palmer, & Stretch, 1990).

The EDI-3 is a useful tool for eating disorder assessment and, in conjunction with other data, can be helpful in developing a diagnosis. It is a brief measure, assesses core eating disorder domains, and can be used to measure progress throughout treatment (Anderson et al., 2004).

Eating Disorder Diagnostic Scale

The Eating Disorder Diagnostic Scale (EDDS) is a 22-item, self-report inventory created to diagnose AN, BN, and BED in accordance with DSM-IV criteria (Stice, Telch, & Rizvi, 2000).

The EDDS is a psychometrically sound instrument, with satisfactory test–retest reliability (Stice et al., 2000), high internal consistency reliability (Stice et al., 2000), and good content validity and convergent validity (Stice et al., 2000). More recently, the EDDS was found to have criterion validity with interview-based diagnoses, convergent validity with risk factors for eating pathology, and predictive validity for eating

disturbance onset (Stice, Fisher, & Martinez, 2004). The EDDS has considerable strengths. First, the EDDS is a brief questionnaire that is easily administered. Second, the EDDS assesses and provides a diagnosis for BED in addition to traditionally recognized eating disorders (AN, BN). Third, the EDDS does not use the term "binge" in its scale; this decreases the likelihood of self-reported binge eating that does not meet clinical criteria for a binge episode.

The EDDS is a new measure, and therefore has not yet been widely utilized. However, it is an instrument with excellent psychometric properties and is a very promising diagnostic tool.

Behavioral Assessment of Eating Behaviors

In addition to the self-report and interview methods for the assessment of eating behaviors, more direct methods are also available. These methods offer the opportunity to observe the behavior in action and to collect more detailed information about specific aspects of a given eating episode (e.g., foods and calories consumed, mood, cognitions). Self-report data are, by nature, retrospective. It has been shown that retrospective data do not always match well with data collected in the moment (Shiffman et al., 1997; Stone et al., 1998). The three most common behavioral methods of assessing eating behaviors—test meals, self-monitoring, and ecological momentary assessment—are discussed in this section.

Test Meals

Test meals involve the direct observation of an individual in the process of eating, thereby bypassing some of the pitfalls of self-report data (Anderson & Paulosky, 2004). They also allow the observer to gather information that is not available by any other means, such as eating rate (Anderson & Paulosky, 2004). Despite their usefulness as a data-gathering tool, however, test meals are seldom used (Anderson, 1995; Anderson & Maloney, 2001). Test meals do require a great deal of effort expended to procure and prepare food, as well as time needed to administer the meal. These practical considerations may serve to limit the frequency of their use in regular practice (Anderson & Paulosky, 2004).

Test meals can serve several purposes. During the assessment process, test meals can be used in cases in which denial or minimization of symptoms is suspected. The client is asked to come to the session not having eaten for a prescribed period of time and is then asked to consume a meal of feared or forbidden foods such as sweets, potato chips, or fast food. If the client refuses the test meal, more direct confrontation about symptom denial can follow (Anderson & Paulosky, 2004). Test meals used in this way in laboratory studies have also been shown to elicit binges in self-described binge eaters (e.g., Anderson, Williamson, Johnson, & Grieve, 2001). Williamson (1990) also discusses the usefulness of the test meal for assessing therapy progress. A meal consisting of standard portions from each food group can be given. This method allows for the calculation of the amount of food and calories consumed overall as well as from each of the food groups. The test meal can then be periodically readministered throughout treatment to assess dietary restraint. Change in amount of food and calories consumed acts as an indicator of treatment progress.

Self-Monitoring

Self-monitoring is considered the most common technique for the assessment of eating behaviors (Anderson & Paulosky, 2004). Self-monitoring requires that the individual complete records at each meal or at specific times throughout the day. Self-monitoring allows the assessment of many different factors related to a meal. Self-monitoring can encompass concrete factors such as time of day, amount and type of food consumed, calories consumed, whether the meal was a binge, and whether compensatory behaviors occurred. In addition, self-monitoring can provide data on factors such as location of the meal, time of day, mood and cognitions related to intake, and hunger and satiety (Anderson & Pauloski, 2004). There is no standard set of self-monitoring forms, but several examples are available (e.g., Schlundt, 1995; Williamson, 1990).

Finally, self-monitoring itself can sometimes play a therapeutic role. The act of monitoring may sensitize individuals to their behavior patterns, thus engendering change. Self-monitoring has been associated with behavior change in many populations, including individuals undergoing weight loss treatment (e.g., Foreyt & Goodrick, 1994).

The limitations of self-monitoring data must be kept in mind. Individuals may minimize the severity of symptoms in their records. Food estimation must also be viewed skeptically (Anderson & Paulosky, 2004). Numerous studies have indicated that people are poor estimators of the quantity of food they consume (e.g., Anderson et al., 1999; Zegman, 1984). Inaccurate estimation of food consumed necessarily leads to inaccurate estimation of caloric intake. Caloric estimation also tends to be poor (e.g., Carels, Konrad, & Harper, 2007; Chandon & Wansink, 2007; Stanton & Tips, 1990). Despite these limitations, self-monitoring can provide a great deal of valuable data in the assessment process.

Ecological Momentary Assessment

Ecological momentary assessment (EMA) takes self-monitoring a step further. The individual is asked to keep a diary at specific times of day and to record specific feelings, thoughts, and so forth. They may be signaled to record in their diaries by an electronic signaling device such as a pager, watch, or palmtop computer at specific times of day and/or be asked to record each time a specific event (e.g., eating a feared food) occurs.

In its earliest incarnation, EMA involved paper-and-pencil diaries, which have a number of flaws. Broderick, Schwartz, Shiffman, Hufford, and Stone (2003) placed electronic chips in their paper-and-pencil diaries to detect when they were filled out. Not only did individuals engage in the expected behavior of backfilling the diaries—that is, they filled out the whole day's entries at the end of the day—but they also very frequently forward-filled these diaries, filling out the whole day's entries in the morning. The data do not answer the questions asked when participants back- or forward-fill their diaries. Additionally, a backfilled diary is subject to similar types of biases as other methods of self-report. Furthermore, there has been some suggestion that recall, or at least interview report, may be less accurate than

EMA reporting (le Grange, Gorin, Catkey, & Stone, 2001). At the very least, they suggest different results. le Grange et al. (2001) had women with and without a diagnosis of BED fill out EMA measures of binge eating and found that, using this methodology, both the BED and non-BED groups reported similar levels of binge eating behavior. This finding suggests that individuals may report less accurately in an interview situation than they do when reporting information on a situation in progress. More recently, EMA has come to involve the use of palmtop computers that can time stamp each entry so that the assessor knows when the diary was completed.

Recently, there has been increased interest in the use of EMA as a tool for the assessment of eating behaviors. In addition to the interview study discussed earlier, le Grange, Gorin, Dymek, and Stone (2002) conducted a pilot study to assess the usefulness of EMA as an adjunct to standard cognitive-behavioral therapy (CBT) for BED. No difference was found between the group that used EMA and the standard CBT group. EMA has also proven to be a popular tool for assessing binge precursors and postbinge affect, given that it can assess cognitions and emotions online; there is no need to wait until the individual fills in a self-report measure. For example, Stein et al. (2007) found that hunger and negative mood were elevated before a binge but that negative mood was elevated still further after the binge. Engel et al. (2007) found that anger was predictive of binge eating behavior and that this relationship was moderated by level of impulsivity. Lavender (2013) found that eating disorder behaviors in women with AN or subthreshold AN corresponded to peaks in high levels of anxiety. Furthermore, practices associated with eating behaviors have been identified by EMA. For example, Zunker and colleagues (2011) found that binge eating was more likely to occur on the same day or the following day after food calorie restriction. In contrast, Haedt-Matt (2011) found in a meta-analysis of EMA studies of hunger and binge eating that hunger levels are not excessive prior to binge eating, possibly due to the affective cue component.

There are drawbacks to the use of EMA. If individuals are not compliant with the signals to record or if they neglect to record at a given time, useful data are not obtained from this method of assessment. Research seems to indicate that participants exhibit "good to excellent" compliance with EMA protocols (Engel, Wonderlich, & Crosby, 2005, p. 210). Whether the same compliance rates would be seen in clinical samples remains a question to be answered. Furthermore, it may not be feasible to provide every client with a palmtop computer or electronic signaling device for his or her own use. Despite its drawbacks, however, EMA offers new possibilities for the online assessment of eating behavior beyond the immediate treatment setting.

Summary

A wide variety of methods are available for concurrent and ongoing assessment of eating disturbance symptoms. In Table 4.1, we summarize some of the features of the measures discussed in this chapter.

The specific methods chosen will likely depend on the needs and goals of the assessor and will likely differ depending on the setting, the level of training and expertise, and whether the focus is research or practice.

Overall, we recommend multimethod assessment. The use of different methods to assess eating disturbance (interview, questionnaire, and behavioral monitoring) will allow the assessor to integrate results and to look for convergence from different methods. Multimethod assessment will likely improve diagnostic accuracy and assist in monitoring the patient's eating pathology and treatment progress over time.

REFERENCES

Anderson, A. E. (1995). A standard test meal to assess treatment response in anorexia nervosa patients. *Eating Disorders: Journal of Treatment and Prevention, 3,* 47–55.

Anderson, D. A., Lundgren, J. D., Shapiro, J. R., & Paulosky, C. A. (2004). Assessment of eating disorders: Review and recommendations for clinical use. *Behavior Modification, 28*(6), 763–782.

Anderson, D. A., & Maloney, K. C. (2001). The efficacy of cognitive behavioral therapy on the

TABLE 4.1. Summary of Eating Disorder Screening, Assessment, and Diagnostic Approaches

Purpose	Assessment method	Measure	Author(s)	Description	Psychometric research
Screening	Self-report questionnaire	EAT-26	Garner et al. (1982)	Screening for AN, BN, and BED; 26 items	(psychometrics for original EAT) IC: .79 TR: .84 Validity: content, criterion, construct
	Self-report questionnaire	BULIT-R	Thelen et al. (1991)	Screening for BN; 28 items	IC: .97 TR: .95 Validity: current, predictive, discriminant
	Self-report questionnaire	EDE-Q	Beglin & Fairburn (1994)	Screening and assessment for eating disorders; 38 items	IC: .90 TR: .81–.94 Validity: concurrent, criterion
	Self-report questionnaire	SCOFF	Morgan et al. (1999)	Screening for eating disorders in primary care settings; 5 items	IC: .47
Assessment/ diagnosis	Interview	EDE	Fairburn & Cooper (1993)	Assesses/diagnoses eating disorders; also used as treatment outcome measure; semistructured interview; requires training and approximately 1 hour to complete	IC: .69–1.0 TR: .33–.40 (bulimia episodes); .70–.97 all other scales Validity: discriminant, concurrent
	Self-report questionnaire	EDI-3	Garner (2004)	Assesses eating disorders (AN, BN, EDNOS); measures treatment progress; 91 items	IC: .63–.94 TR: > .90 Validity: criterion
	Self-report questionnaire	EDDS	Stice et al. (2000)	Assesses/diagnoses eating disorders (AN, BN, BED); 22 items	IC: .89 TR: .87 Validity: criterion, predictive, convergent, content
Progress in treatment	Behavioral assessment	Test meals	N/A	Observation of eating a meal; measures rate of eating, consumption of feared foods, assesses presence of binge eating, assesses treatment progress	N/A

(continued)

TABLE 4.1. *(continued)*

Purpose	Assessment method	Measure	Author(s)	Description	Psychometric research
Progress in treatment *(continued)*	Behavioral assessment	Self-monitoring	N/A	Written diary of food intake; measures type and amount of food intake; assesses presence of binge or compensatory behaviors	N/A
	Behavioral assessment	Ecological momentary assessment	Broderick et al. (2003)	Electronic signaling device that requires self-monitoring at specific time points; reduces memory recall biases	N/A

Note. IC, internal consistency; TR, test–retest reliability; N/A, not available.

core symptoms of bulimia nervosa. *Clinical Psychology Review, 21,* 971–988.

Anderson, D. A., & Paulosky, P. A. (2004). Psychological assessment of eating disorders and related features. In J. K. Thompson (Ed.), *Handbook of eating disorders and obesity* (pp. 112–129). Hoboken, NJ: Wiley.

Anderson, D. A., Williamson, D. A., Johnson, W. G., & Grieve, C. O. (1999). Estimation of food intake: Effects of the unit of estimation. *Eating and Weight Disorders, 4,* 6–9.

Anderson, D. A., Williamson, D. A., Johnson, W. G., & Grieve, C. O. (2001). Validity of test meals for determining binge eating. *Eating Behaviors, 2,* 105–112.

Banasiak, S. J., Wertheim, E. H., Koerner, J., & Voudouris, V. J. (2001). Test–retest reliability and internal consistency of a variety of measures of dietary restraint and body concerns in a sample of adolescent girls. *International Journal of Eating Disorders, 29,* 85–89.

Beglin, S. J., & Fairburn, C. G. (1992). What is meant by the term "binge"? *American Journal of Psychiatry, 149,* 123–124.

Beglin, S. J., & Fairburn, C. G. (1994). Assessment of eating disorders: Interview or self-report questionnaire? *International Journal of Eating Disorders, 16*(4), 363–370.

Binford, R. B., le Grange, D., & Jellar, C. C. (2005). Eating Disorders Examination versus Eating Disorders Examination—Questionnaire in adolescents with full and partial-syndrome bulimia nervosa and anorexia nervosa. *International Journal of Eating Disorders, 37*(1), 44–49.

Broderick, J. E., Schwartz, J. E., Shiffman, S.,

Hufford, M. R., & Stone, A. A. (2003). Signaling does not adequately improve dietary compliance. *Annals of Behavioral Medicine, 26,* 139–148.

Bryant-Waugh, R., Cooper, P., Taylor, C., & Lask, B. (1996). The use of the Eating Disorder Examination with children: A pilot study. *International Journal of Eating Disorders, 19*(4), 391–397.

Carels, R. A., Konrad, K., & Harper, J. (2007). Individual differences in food perceptions and calorie estimation: An examination of dieting status, weight, and gender. *Appetite, 49,* 450–458.

Carter, A. C., Aime, A. A., & Mills, J. S. (2001). Assessment of bulimia nervosa: A comparison of interview and self-report questionnaire methods. *International Journal of Eating Disorders, 30*(2), 187–192.

Carter, P. E., & Moss, R. A. (1984). Screening for anorexia and bulimia nervosa in a college population: Problems and limitations. *Addictive Behaviors, 9,* 17–31.

Celio, A. A., Wilfley, D. E., & Crow, S. J. (2004). A comparison of the Binge Eating Scale, Questionnaire for Eating and Weight Patterns–Revised, and Eating Disorder Examination Questionnaire with Instructions with the Eating Disorder Examination in the assessment of binge eating disorder and its symptoms. *International Journal of Eating Disorders, 36*(4), 434–444.

Chandon, P., & Wansink, B. (2007). Is obesity caused by calorie underestimation?: A psychophysical model of meal size estimation. *Journal of Marketing Research, 44,* 84–99.

Cooper, Z., Cooper, P. J., & Fairburn, C. G. (1989). The validity of the Eating Disorder Examination and its subscales. *British Journal of Psychiatry, 154,* 807–812.

Cooper, Z., & Fairburn, C. G. (1987). The Eating Disorders Examination: A semistructured interview for the assessment of the specific psychopathology of eating disorders. *International Journal of Eating Disorders, 6,* 1–8.

Cotton, M., Ball, C., & Robinson, P. (2003). Four simple questions can help screen for eating disorders. *Journal of Internal Medicine, 18*(1), 53–56.

Crowther, J. H., Lilly, R. S., Crawford, P. A., & Shepard, K. L. (1992). The stability of the Eating Disorder Inventory. *International Journal of Eating Disorders, 12,* 97–101.

Engel, S. G., Boseck, J. J., Crosby, R. D., Wonderlich, S. A., Mitchell, J. E., Smyth, J., et al. (2007). The relationship of momentary anger and impulsivity to bulimic behavior. *Behaviour Research and Therapy, 45,* 437–447.

Engel, S. G., Wonderlich, S. A., & Crosby, R. D. (2005). Ecological momentary assessment. In J. E. Mitchell & C. B. Peterson (Eds.), *Assessment of eating disorders* (pp. 203–220). New York: Guilford Press.

Fairburn, C. G., & Belgin, S. J. (1994). Assessment of eating disorders: Interview or self-report questionnaire? *International Journal of Eating Disorders, 16,* 363–370.

Fairburn, C. G., & Cooper, Z. (1993). The Eating Disorder Examination (12th ed.). In C. G. Fairburn & G. T. Wilson (Eds.), *Binge eating: Nature, assessment, and treatment* (pp. 317–360). New York: Guilford Press.

Fairburn, C. G., & Wilson, G. T. (Eds.). (1993). *Binge eating: Nature, assessment, and treatment.* New York: Guilford Press.

Fernandez, S., Malcarne, V. L., Wilfley, D. E., & McQuaid, J. (2006). Factor structure of the Bulimia Test—Revised in college women from four ethnic groups. *Cultural Diversity and Ethnic Minority Psychology, 12*(3), 403–419.

Frampton, I., Wisting, L., Overas, M., Midtsund, M., & Lask, B. (2011). Reliability and validity of the Norwegian translation of the Child Eating Disorder Examination (ChEDE). *Scandinavian Journal of Psychology, 52*(2), 196–199.

Foreyt, J. P., & Goodrick, G. K. (1994). Attributes of successful approaches to weight loss and control. *Applied and Preventative Psychology, 3,* 209–215.

Garfinkel, P. E., & Newman, A. (2001). The

Eating Attitudes Test: Twenty-five years later. *Eating and Weight Disorders, 6,* 1–24.

Garner, D. M. (1997). Psychoeducational principles in treatment. In D. M. Garner & P. E. Garfinkel (Eds.), *Handbook of treatment for eating disorders* (2nd ed., pp. 145–177). New York: Guilford Press.

Garner, D. M. (2004). *Eating Disorder Inventory—3 manual.* Lutz, FL: Psychological Assessment Resources.

Garner, D. M., & Garfinkel, P. E. (1979). The Eating Attitudes Test: An index of the symptoms of anorexia nervosa. *Psychological Medicine, 9,* 273–279.

Garner, D. M., Olmstead, M. P., Bohr, Y., & Garfinkel, P. E. (1982). The Eating Attitudes Test: Psychometric features and clinical correlates. *Psychological Medicine, 12,* 871–878.

Garner, D. M., Olmstead, M. P., & Polivy, J. (1983). Development and validation of a multidimensional eating disorder inventory for anorexia nervosa and bulimia. *International Journal of Eating Disorders, 2,* 15–34.

Grilo, C. M., Crosby, R. D., & White, M. A. (2012). Spanish-language Eating Disorder Examination interview: Factor structure in Latino/as. *Eating Behaviors, 13,* 410–413.

Grilo, C. M., Lazano, C., & Elder, K. A. (2005). Inter-rater and test–retest reliability of the Spanish language version of the Eating Disorder Examination interview: Clinical and research implications. *Journal of Psychiatric Practice, 11*(4), 231–240.

Grilo, C. M., Masheb, R. M., & Wilson, G. T. (2001). A comparison of different methods for assessing the features of eating disorders in patients with binge eating disorder. *Journal of Consulting and Clinical Psychology, 69*(2), 317–322.

Hadigan, C. M., Walsh, B. T., Lachaussée, J. L., & Kissileff, H. R. (1992). 24-hour dietary recall in patients with bulimia nervosa. *International Journal of Eating Disorders, 12,* 107–111.

Haedt-Matt, A. A., & Keel, P. K. (2011). Hunger and binge eating: A meta-analysis of studies using ecological momentary assessment. *International Journal of Eating Disorders, 44*(7), 573–578.

Hilbert, A., Buerger, A., Hartmann, A. S., Spenner, K., Czaja, J., & Warschburger, P. (2013). Psychometric evaluation of the Eating Disorder Examination adapted for children. *European Eating Disorders Review, 21,* 330–339.

Hurley, J. B., Palmer, R. L., & Stretch, D. (1990). The specificity of the Eating Disorders Inventory: A reappraisal. *International Journal of Eating Disorders, 9,* 419–424.

Johnson, W. G., Boutelle, K. N., Torgrud, L., Davig, J. P., & Turner, S. (2000). What is a binge?: The influence of amount, duration, and loss of control criteria on judgments of binge eating. *International Journal of Eating Disorders, 27,* 471–479.

Kalarchian, M. A., Wilson, G. T., Brolin, R. E., & Bradley, L. (2000). Assessment of eating disorders in bariatric surgery candidates: Self-report questionnaire versus interview. *International Journal of Eating Disorders, 28*(4), 465–469.

Lavender, J. M., De Young, K. P., Wonderlich, S. A., Crosby, R. D., Engel, S. G., Mitchell, J. E., et al. (2013). Daily patterns of anxiety in anorexia nervosa: Associations with eating disorder behaviors in the natural environment. *Journal of Abnormal Psychology, 122,* 672–683.

le Grange, D., Gorin, A., Catley, D., & Stone, A. A. (2001). Does momentary assessment detect binge eating in overweight women that is denied at interview? *European Eating Disorders Review, 9,* 309–324.

le Grange, D., Gorin, A., Dymek, M., & Stone, A. (2002). Does ecological momentary assessment improve cognitive behavioral therapy for binge eating disorder?: A pilot study. *European Eating Disorders Review, 10,* 316–328.

Levine, M. D., Ringham, R. M., Kalarchian, M. A., Wisniewski, L., & Marcus, M. D. (2006). Overeating among seriously overweight children seeking treatment: Results of the children's eating disorder examination. *International Journal of Eating Disorders, 39*(2), 135–140.

Luce, K. H., & Crowther, J. H. (1999). The reliability of the Eating Disorder Examination—Self-Report Questionnaire. *International Journal of Eating Disorders, 25*(3), 349–351.

Luck, A. J., Morgan, J. F., & Reid, F. (2002). The SCOFF questionnaire and clinical interview for eating disorders in general practice: Comparative study. *British Medical Journal, 325,* 755–756.

Mond, J. M., Hay, P. J., & Rodgers, B. (2004). Validity of the Eating Disorder Examination Questionnaire (EDE-Q) in screening for eating disorders in community samples. *Behaviour Research and Therapy, 42*(7), 551–567.

Morgan, J., Reid, F., & Lacey, J. H. (1999). The SCOFF questionnaire: Assessment of a new screening tool for eating disorders. *British Medical Journal, 319,* 1467–1468.

Perry, L., Morgan, J., & Reid, F. (2002). Screening for symptoms of eating disorders: Reliability of the SCOFF screening tool with written compared to oral delivery. *International Journal of Eating Disorders, 32*(4), 466–472.

Peterson, C. B., Crosby, R. D., & Wonderlich, S. A. (2007). Psychometric properties of the Eating Disorder Examination—Questionnaire: Factor structure and internal consistency. *International Journal of Eating Disorders, 40*(4), 386–389.

Reas, D. L., Grilo, C. M., & Masheb, R. M. (2006). Reliability of the Eating Disorder Examination—Questionnaire in patients with binge eating disorder. *Behaviour Research and Therapy, 44*(1), 43–51.

Rizvi, S. L., Peterson, C. B., Crow, J. C., & Agras, W. S. (2000). Test–retest reliability of the Eating Disorder Examination. *International Journal of Eating Disorders, 28,* 311–316.

Rosen, J. C., Vara, L., Wendt, S., & Leitenberg, H. (1990). Validity studies of the Eating Disorder Examination. *International Journal of Eating Disorders, 9,* 519–528.

Schoeller, D. A. (1995). Limitations in the assessment of dietary energy intake by self-report. *Metabolism, 44*(Suppl. 2), 18–22.

Schlundt, D. G. (1995). Assessment of specific eating behaviors and eating style. In D. B. Allison (Ed.), *Methods for the assessment and weight-related problems* (pp. 142–302). Newbury Park, CA: Sage.

Schoemaker, C., Verbraak, M., Breteler, R., & van der Staak, C. (1997). The discriminant validity of the Eating Disorder Inventory–2. *British Journal of Clinical Psychology, 36,* 627–629.

Shiffman, S., Hufford, M., Hickcox, M., Paty, J. A., Gnys, M., & Kassel, J. D. (1997). Remember that?: A comparison of real-time versus retrospective recall of smoking lapses. *Journal of Consulting and Clinical Psychology, 65,* 292–300.

Siervo, M., Boschi, V., & Papa, A. (2005). Application of the SCOFF, Eating Attitude Test 26 (EAT 26), and Eating Inventory (TFEQ) questionnaires in young women seeking diet therapy. *Eating and Weight Disorders, 10*(2), 76–82.

Smith, M. C., & Thelen, M. H. (1984.) Development and validation of a test for bulimia.

Journal of Consulting and Clinical Psychology, 52, 863–872.

Stanton, A. L., & Tips, T. A. (1990). Accuracy of calorie estimation by females as a function of eating habits and body mass. *International Journal of Eating Disorders, 9,* 387–393.

Stein, R. I., Kenardy, J., Wiseman, C. V., Dounchis, J. Z., Arnow, B. A., & Wilfley, D. E. (2007). What's driving the binge in binge eating disorder?: A prospective examination of precursors and consequences. *International Journal of Eating Disorders, 40,* 195–203.

Stice, E., Fisher, M., & Martinez, E. (2004). Eating Disorder Diagnostic Scale: Additional evidence of reliability and validity. *Psychological Assessment, 16*(1), 60–71.

Stice, E., Telch, C. F., & Rizvi, S. L. (2000). Development and validation of the Eating Disorder Diagnostic Scale: A brief self-report measure of anorexia, bulimia, and binge eating disorder. *Psychological Assessment, 12,* 123–131.

Stone, A. A., Schwartz, J. E., Neale, J. M., Shiffman, S., Marco, C. A., Hickcox, M., et al. (1998). A comparison of coping assessed by ecological momentary assessment and retrospective recall. *Journal of Personality and Social Psychology, 74,* 1670–1680.

Telch, C. F., Pratt, E. M., & Niego, S. H. (1998). Obese women with binge eating disorder define the term binge. *International Journal of Eating Disorders, 24,* 313–317.

Thelen, M. H., Farmer, J., Wonderlich, S., & Smith, M. (1991). A revision of the bulimia test: The BULIT-R. *Psychological Assessment, 3,* 119–124.

Thompson, J. K. (1996). *Body image, eating disorders and obesity: An integrative guide for assessment and treatment.* Washington, DC: American Psychological Association.

Thompson, J. K. (Ed.). (2004). *Handbook of eating disorders and obesity.* Hoboken, NJ: Wiley.

Thompson, J. K., Heinberg, L. J., Altabe, M., & Tantleff-Dunn, S. (1999). *Exacting beauty: Theory, assessment, and treatment of body image disturbance.* Washington, DC: American Psychological Association.

Thompson, J. K., & Smolak, L. (2001). *Body image, eating disorders, and obesity in youth.* Washington, DC: American Psychological Association.

Vander Wal, J. S., Stein, R. I., & Blashill, A. J. (2011). The EDE-Q, BULIT-R, and BEDT as self-report measures of binge eating disorder. *Eating Behaviors, 12,* 267–271.

Vincent, M. A., McCabe, M. P., & Ricciardelli, L. A. (1999). Factor validity of the Bulimia Test—Revised in adolescent boys and girls. *Behaviour Research and Therapy, 37*(11), 1129–1140.

Watkins, B., Frampton, I., Lask, B., & Bryant-Waugh, R. (2005). Reliability and validity of the child version of the Eating Disorder Examination: A preliminary investigation. *International Journal of Eating Disorders, 38*(2), 183–187.

Wear, R. W., & Pratz, O. (1987). Test–retest reliability for the Eating Disorder Inventory. *International Journal of Eating Disorders, 6,* 767–769.

Wilfley, D. E., Schwartz, M. B., Spurell, E. B., & Fairburn, C. G. (1997). Assessing the specific psychopathology of binge eating disorder patients: Interview or self-report? *Behaviour Research and Therapy, 35*(12), 1151–1159.

Williamson, D. A. (1990). *Assessment of eating disorders: Obesity, anorexia, and bulimia nervosa.* Elmsford, NY: Pergamon Press.

Williamson, D. A., Anderson, D. A., Jackman, L. P., & Jackson, S. R. (1995). Assessment of eating disordered thoughts, feelings, and behaviors. In D. B. Allison (Ed.), *Handbook of assessment methods for eating behaviors and weight-related problems* (pp. 347–386). Newbury Park, CA: Sage.

Wilson, G. T. (1993). Assessment of binge eating. In C. G. Fairburn & G. T. Wilson (Eds.), *Binge eating: Nature, assessment, and treatment* (pp. 227–249). New York: Guilford Press.

Wilson, G. T., & Smith, D. (1989). Assessment of bulimia nervosa: An evaluation of the Eating Disorder Examination. *International Journal of Eating Disorders, 8,* 173–179.

Zegman, M. A. (1984). Errors in food recording and calorie estimation: Clinical and theoretical implications for obesity. *Addictive Behaviors, 9,* 347–350.

Zunker, C., Peterson, C. B., Crosby, R. D., Cao, L., Engel, S. G., Mitchell, J. E., et al. (2011). Ecological momentary assessment of bulimia nervosa: Does dietary restriction predict binge eating? *Behavior Research Therapy, 49,* 714–717.

CHAPTER 5

Tobacco Use

Alan L. Peterson
Antoinette R. Brundige
David Houghton

It is estimated that tobacco use killed 100 million people worldwide during the 20th century (World Health Organization, 2008). According to the U.S. Surgeon General, quitting tobacco is the single most important thing a person can do to improve his or her health (U.S. Department of Health and Human Services, 2004). Of all tobacco products, cigarette smoking is the form of tobacco use with the most significant individual and public health risk. This risk is a result in part of almost a century of mass marketing and production, as well as the relatively inexpensive cost of all tobacco products. The primary emphasis of this chapter is on the assessment of cigarette smoking. However, many of the assessment approaches and measures reviewed in this chapter can easily be adapted to apply to all forms of tobacco use, including smokeless tobacco, chewing tobacco, cigars, bidis, snus, pipe tobacco, and clove cigarettes (Peterson, Vander Weg, & Jaén, 2011).

The American Psychiatric Association's *Diagnostic and Statistical Manual of Mental Disorders* (DSM) and the World Health Organization's *International Classification of Diseases* (ICD) are the most commonly accepted diagnostic systems for classifying disorders related to substance use, including tobacco. The fourth edition, text revision, of DSM (DSM-IV-TR; American Psychiatric Association, 2000) included a diagnostic category for "Nicotine Dependence," but the nomenclature for this category has changed with the release of the fifth edition of DSM (DSM-5; American Psychiatric Association, 2013) and is now termed "tobacco use disorder." The 10th edition of the ICD (ICD-10; World Health Organization, 1992) continues to use "Nicotine Dependence" as a diagnostic category. These terms are both used throughout this chapter to refer to diagnostic criteria. The term "nicotine dependence" may be used as a general descriptor that refers to aspects of both diagnostic categories, as well as to the specific aspects of physical dependence on nicotine. Reference to the ICD-10 diagnostic category of "Nicotine Dependence" is differentiated in this chapter from the more general descriptive term "nicotine dependence" by the use of capitalization when referring to the diagnostic category.

Biopsychosocial Factors in Tobacco Use

The biopsychosocial model (Engel, 1977) is a useful model for the conceptualization of health and illness. It is also useful in the conceptualization of how physical, behavioral, emotional, cognitive, and environmental factors are related to tobacco use and cessation. The biopsychosocial model was adapted by the Tobacco Research Implementation Group (TRIG) into three primary factors related to tobacco use: (1) social, (2) psychological, and (3) biological (TRIG, 1998). TRIG is an interdisciplinary group of scientists representing multiple agencies and institutions, including the National Institutes of Health, academia, and private foundations.

Social Factors

According to TRIG's biopsychosocial model of nicotine addiction, social factors may include culture, environment, socioeconomic status (SES), peer and family modeling, tobacco industry marketing, and media influences. According to the National Cancer Institute (2008) of the National Institutes of Health (NIH), the media were among the most significant social contributors to tobacco use in the 20th century. Cigarettes are one of the most heavily marketed products in the world. Between 1940 and 2005, U.S. cigarette manufacturers spent about $250 billion on cigarette advertising and promotion (National Cancer Institute, 2008). Tobacco advertising has targeted three themes: (1) providing satisfaction (taste, freshness, mildness, etc.), (2) decreasing anxiety about the hazards of smoking, and (3) creating positive associations between smoking and desirable outcomes (independence, social success, sexual attraction, thinness, etc.; National Cancer Institute, 2008). The primary impact of this social marketing has been to recruit new smokers, to expand the market for tobacco products by reinforcing smoking, and to discourage quitting.

Psychological Factors

Psychological factors are perhaps the most complex of all factors related to tobacco use. Psychological factors include comorbid psychological problems, cognitions, emotions, behavioral conditioning, personality, stress, and pleasure that are associated with smoking (Lassner et al., 2000; Ziedonis, Williams, & Smelson, 2003). Tobacco use is a behavior and is subject to the principles of behav-

ioral conditioning and learning. The average smoker consumes about 10,000 cigarettes per year, and each of these events represents an individual conditioning trial. Behavioral factors related to tobacco use include both the relationship between a stimulus and response (classical conditioning) and the relationship between antecedents and consequences (operant conditioning). Antecedents refer to those behavioral factors that occur just prior to each episode of tobacco use. These antecedents become linked to the tobacco use and the consequences that follow and over time become strong triggers for tobacco use. There are strong urges or cravings to use tobacco whenever these antecedents or triggers are present.

Triggers for tobacco use can include the presence of tobacco products themselves (e.g., cigarettes, chew, dip, ashtrays, matches, lighters), as well as behaviors or activities such as drinking coffee, drinking alcohol, finishing a meal, driving a car, and walking out of a building. As stricter environmental tobacco use policies have been imposed (e.g., no smoking in office buildings, restaurants, airplanes), the variety of locations in which people are able to use tobacco has been reduced. In addition, many individuals have imposed their own environmental limitations by opting not to smoke in their cars or inside their homes because of concerns about the impact on future resale of these valuable possessions. As a result, smokers respond to a smaller number of triggers and engage in a larger number of conditioning trials that occur with these triggers. The habit strength or behavioral connection between these environmental events and tobacco use is thus reinforced and becomes more difficult to break.

Behavioral consequences refer to the strong reinforcing properties of nicotine and tobacco that increase the likelihood of future tobacco use. The most obvious consequence is the relief of nicotine withdrawal symptoms (negative reinforcement) that occurs with smoking. However, there are a number of other reinforcing consequences of smoking, which may include increased alertness, social support and networking, and taking a break from work. This complex interaction between stimuli and responses and antecedents and consequences makes quitting tobacco a difficult process.

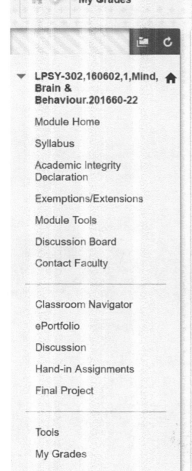

My Grades

| All | Graded | Upcoming | Submitted |

ITEM

Academic Integrity Declaration
Test

Week 01 Discussion Initial Response -- Turnitin
Discussion Initial Response

Week 02 Discussion Follow-on
Discussion Follow-on

Week 2 Hand-in Assignment - FF -- Turnitin
Formative Feedback
View Description

Week 3 Hand-in Assignment - FF -- Turnitin
Formative Feedback

Week 04 Hand-in Assignment Part 1 -- Turnitin
Assignment Part 1

Week 04 Hand-in Assignment Part 2 -- Turnitin
Assignment Part 2

Week 05 Hand-in Assignment -- Turnitin
Individual Assignment (IA)

Week 06 Discussion Initial Response -- Turnitin
Discussion Initial Response

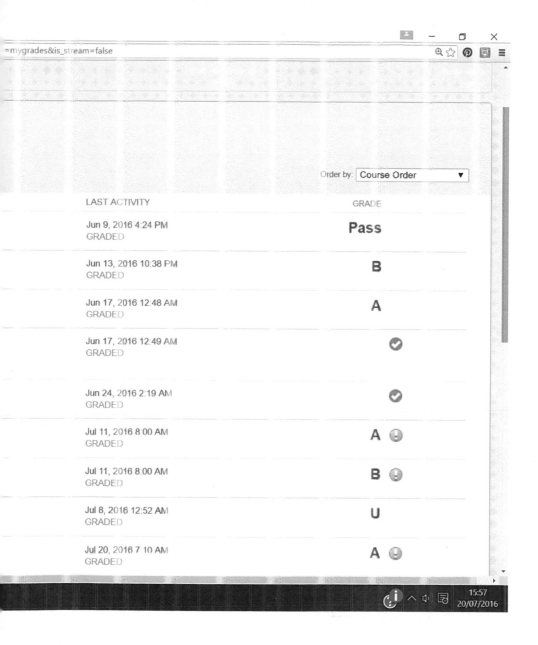

Factors related to stress and stress management also fall under the category of psychological factors, and they are an important link between social and biological factors. Contrary to popular belief, smoking may actually cause stress rather than relieve it. Many people report that smoking helps them manage stress. However, there are many similarities between the symptoms of stress and the symptoms of nicotine withdrawal (Parrott, 1995a, 1995b, 1999). The symptoms of stress include a combination of physical, emotional, and behavioral symptoms. These symptoms are remarkably similar to the symptoms of nicotine withdrawal (Cummings, Giovino, Jaén, & Emrich, 1985; Hughes, 2007). Withdrawal symptoms can begin within about 20–30 minutes after smoking, so individuals need to smoke repeatedly throughout the day in order to maintain a steady dose of nicotine (Teneggi et al., 2002). Therefore, nicotine dependency may actually increase subjective feelings of stress because of these daily fluctuations in blood nicotine levels and the associated levels of subjective stress. What may be perceived as a stress-reducing or relaxing effect after smoking may actually be a reversal of the tension and irritability that develop during nicotine withdrawal.

Another important psychological factor is individuals' beliefs about themselves and their relationship with tobacco. The self-image of a smoker may specifically include smoking as part of who they are ("I'm a smoker"; "Smoking is cool"). Many believe that tobacco helps them perform better at work or at tasks that require significant concentration. They may also have specific thoughts and beliefs about their inability to tolerate nicotine withdrawal symptoms ("I've got to have a smoke"; "There's no way I could quit smoking right now").

Pleasure is another psychological factor related to tobacco use. Many individuals who use tobacco associate it with many of the most pleasurable activities in their lives. Smokeless tobacco users may link it to recreational activities such as playing sports, hunting, fishing, and hanging out with friends. Smokers often link it to drinking alcohol and partying. Smoking after sex is often described as being extremely satisfying and pleasurable. Undoubtedly, combinations of psychological factors are intricately intertwined with tobacco use, and a successful cessation program requires adequately addressing these factors, along with social and biological factors.

Biological Factors

Biological factors in tobacco use include genetics, nutrition, and the physiological dependence or addiction to nicotine that occurs with regular tobacco use (Lerman et al., 1999). Most patients, as well as health care providers, assume that the physical dependence on nicotine is the most significant barrier to successful quitting. However, the physical dependence part of tobacco use may actually be the least difficult part to overcome. The primary reason for this is that once an individual quits all forms of nicotine use (including any nicotine replacement therapy), the physical withdrawal from nicotine dependence peaks during the first week and then lasts for a total of only about 2–4 weeks (Hughes, 2007). Any urges or cravings that occur beyond this point are likely related to behavioral or psychological factors and not physical factors.

Structured Clinical Assessment of Tobacco Use

Effectively addressing issues related to tobacco use begins with a careful assessment. The Clinical Practice Guideline for Treating Tobacco Use and Dependence (Fiore et al., 2008) recommends that every patient presenting to a health care facility be asked if he or she uses tobacco. The most popular brief interview assessment is the "ask" and "assess" portions of the "five A's" approach to tobacco cessation (Andrews, Heath, & Graham-Garcia, 2004; Boyd, 1996; Fiore et al., 2008; Tait et al., 2007). The two assessment questions that make up this approach are "asking" about tobacco use and "assessing" the individual's interest in quitting. The three additional "A's" in the "five A's" approach are focused on cessation and include "advising" the individual to quit tobacco, "assisting" in quitting, and "arranging for follow-up" (Peterson et al., 2011).

The way in which individuals are asked about and assessed on their tobacco use is important. According to the 2007 National

Health Interview Survey (Centers for Disease Control and Prevention, 2008), approximately 80% of all regular smokers use cigarettes on a daily basis, with the remainder being nondaily or intermittent smokers. Simply asking someone whether or not he or she is a "smoker" may not be sufficient, because many nondaily or intermittent smokers do not identify themselves as "smokers." The assessment should focus on patients' self-reported behavior rather than on the way they conceptualize themselves. A good initial assessment question might be, "Do you ever smoke cigarettes, even some of the time?" If the patient positively endorses this initial question, the next steps are to assess the frequency and rate of tobacco use, as well as the level of interest in quitting. The frequency can be assessed by asking, "How often do you smoke?" The rate can be assessed by asking, "About how many cigarettes do you smoke per day (or week or month)?" The assessment of the potential level of interest in quitting can be determined by asking, "Have you thought about quitting tobacco sometime in the near future?" Research has indicated that about two-thirds of all tobacco users indicate that they are interested in quitting in the near future, so asking that question is an important first step (Centers for Disease Control and Prevention, 2002; Hughes, Keely, & Naud, 2004). Knowing how often and how much a patient smokes and his or her interest in quitting provides important information for designing an appropriate cessation intervention. Even if patients indicate that they do not currently use tobacco, it is a good idea to inquire as to whether they have ever used regularly in the past. Because some cigarette smokers remain vulnerable to relapse months or even years after quitting (Fiore et al., 2000), identifying former smokers is important so that supportive messages can be delivered and an intervention can be quickly implemented in the event of a subsequent return to smoking.

Although cigarettes remain the greatest public health threat due to the high prevalence of use and associated health risks, it is also important to inquire about other forms of tobacco use in addition to cigarette smoking. Because of the increasing restrictions on cigarette smoking, many male smokers have started using smokeless tobacco in those settings in which smoking is prohibited. As a result, there appears to be an increasing percentage of dual-use tobacco users (Vander Weg et al., 2008). Therefore, during an initial assessment, patients should also be asked if they ever use any other forms of tobacco, such as chewing tobacco, dip, snuff, snus, cigars, bidis, pipe tobacco, or clove cigarettes (kreteks).

Once tobacco use has been identified, determining whether a patient meets diagnostic criteria for a tobacco-related disorder is often an important consideration. The DSM-5 and ICD-10 are the most commonly accepted diagnostic systems for classifying substance use disorders. Table 5.1 outlines the DSM-5 criteria for tobacco use disorder and Table 5.2 outlines the ICD-10 criteria for Nicotine Dependence.

There are two commonly used approaches to the assessment of tobacco use disorder or Nicotine Dependence: *diagnostic* and *dimensional*. Diagnostic approaches involve determining whether a smoker meets formal diagnostic criteria for tobacco use disorder or Nicotine Dependence. Assessing tobacco use with this approach requires systematically evaluating for the presence or absence of each of the individual symptoms or behaviors included in a given classification system (i.e., DSM-5 or ICD-10) and determining whether an individual meets the necessary diagnostic criteria. This is typically done through a structured or semistructured interview, but it can also be accomplished using self-report checklists. The second is a dimensional approach that is designed to evaluate the degree to which an individual exhibits features believed to be associated with tobacco use disorder or Nicotine Dependence. Unlike an interview approach, which is primarily designed to evaluate the presence or absence of required diagnostic criteria, self-report assessments are geared toward determining a person's level of nicotine dependence based on a continuous scale. The items that make up this type of measure are typically chosen based on empirical associations with smoking or tobacco use characteristics that are believed to be indicative of or related to dependence, such as the heaviness of tobacco use. Frequently used items in dimensional measures of nicotine

TABLE 5.1. DSM-5 Diagnostic Criteria for Tobacco Use Disorder and Tobacco Withdrawal

Tobacco Use Disorder

A. A problematic pattern of tobacco use leading to clinically significant impairment or distress, as manifested by at least two of the following, occurring within a 12-month period:

1. Tobacco is often taken in larger amounts or over a longer period than was intended.

2. There is a persistent desire or unsuccessful efforts to cut down or control tobacco use.

3. A great deal of time is spent in activities necessary to obtain or use tobacco.

4. Craving, or a strong desire or urge to use tobacco.

5. Recurrent tobacco use resulting in a failure to fulfill major role obligations at work, school, or home (e.g., interference with work).

6. Continued tobacco use despite having persistent or recurrent social or interpersonal problems caused or exacerbated by the effects of tobacco (e.g., arguments with others about tobacco use).

7. Important social, occupational, or recreational activities are given up or reduced because of tobacco use.

8. Recurrent tobacco use in situations in which it is physically hazardous (e.g., smoking in bed).

9. Tobacco use is continued despite knowledge of having a persistent or recurrent physical or psychological problem that is likely to have been caused or exacerbated by tobacco.

10. Tolerance, as defined by either of the following:

    a. A need for markedly increased amounts of tobacco to achieve the desired effect.

    b. A markedly diminished effect with continued use of the same amount of tobacco.

11. Withdrawal, as manifested by either of the following:

    a. The characteristic withdrawal syndrome for tobacco (refer to Criteria A and B of the criteria set for tobacco withdrawal).

    b. Tobacco (or a closely related substance, such as nicotine) is taken to relieve or avoid withdrawal symptoms.

Specify if:

In early remission: After full criteria for tobacco use disorder were previously met, none of the criteria for tobacco use disorder have been met for at least 3 months but for less than 12 months (with the exception that Criterion A4, "Craving, or a strong desire or urge to use tobacco," may be met).

In sustained remission: After full criteria for tobacco use disorder were previously met, none of the criteria for tobacco use disorder have been met at any time during a period of 12 months or longer (with the exception that Criterion A4, "Craving, or a strong desire or urge to use tobacco," may be met).

Specify if:

On maintenance therapy: The individual is taking a long-term maintenance medication, such as nicotine replacement medication, and no criteria for tobacco use disorder have been met for that class of medication (except tolerance to, or withdrawal from, the nicotine replacement medication).

In a controlled environment: This additional specifier is used if the individual is in an environment where access to tobacco is restricted.

Coding based on current severity: Note for ICD-10-CM codes: If a tobacco withdrawal or tobacco-induced sleep disorder is also present, do not use the codes below for tobacco use disorder. Instead, the comorbid tobacco use disorder is indicated in the 4th character of the tobacco-induced disorder code (see the coding note for tobacco withdrawal or tobacco-induced sleep disorder). For example, if there is comorbid tobacco-induced sleep disorder and tobacco use disorder, only the tobacco-induced sleep disorder code is given, with the 4th character indicating whether the comorbid tobacco use disorder is moderate or severe: F17.208 for moderate or severe tobacco use disorder with tobacco-induced sleep disorder. It is not permissible to code a comorbid mild tobacco use disorder with a tobacco-induced sleep disorder.

Specify current severity:

305.1 (Z72.0) **Mild:** Presence of 2–3 symptoms.

305.1 (F17.200) **Moderate:** Presence of 4–5 symptoms.

305.1 (F17.200) **Severe:** Presence of 6 or more symptoms.

(continued)

TABLE 5.1. *(continued)*

Tobacco Withdrawal 292.0 (F17.203)

A. Daily use of tobacco for at least several weeks.

B. Abrupt cessation of tobacco use, or reduction in the amount of tobacco used, followed within 24 hours by four (or more) of the following signs or symptoms:
    1. Irritability, frustration, or anger.
    2. Anxiety.
    3. Difficulty concentrating.
    4. Increased appetite.
    5. Restlessness.
    6. Depressed mood.
    7. Insomnia.

C. The signs or symptoms in Criterion B cause clinically significant distress or impairment in social, occupational, or other important areas of functioning.

D. The signs or symptoms are not attributed to another medical condition and are not better explained by another mental disorder, including intoxication or withdrawal from another substance.

Coding note: The ICD-9-CM code is 292.0. The ICD-10-CM code for tobacco withdrawal is F17.203. Note that the ICD-10-CM code indicates the comorbid presence of a moderate or severe tobacco use disorder, reflecting the fact that tobacco withdrawal can only occur in the presence of a moderate or severe tobacco use disorder. It is not permissible to code a comorbid mild tobacco use disorder with tobacco withdrawal.

Note. Reprinted with permission from the *Diagnostic and Statistical Manual of Mental Disorders*, Fifth Edition (Copyright 2013). American Psychiatric Association. All rights reserved.

dependence include the number of cigarettes smoked per day and the amount of time after waking before a person smokes his or her first cigarette in the morning. These items do not assess dependence directly, but they are related to some of its key elements, such as withdrawal symptoms, tolerance, and compulsive smoking. The scores reflect the degree of dependence on nicotine.

As already noted, several measures have been designed to assess whether or not an individual meets the diagnostic criteria for tobacco use disorder according to the DSM-5 or Nicotine Dependence according to the ICD-10. Oftentimes, this process is accomplished informally by simply reviewing each of the individual items with the patient to determine whether he or she meets criteria. Measures that allow the quick and simple assessment of diagnostic criteria and that can be administered in the context of a typical clinical encounter often are preferable to structured diagnostic interviews designed for this purpose. The reason is primarily that the length and time required to administer these instruments, as well as the extensive training required of interviewers, often significantly reduces their utility outside of a research setting.

When patients meet diagnostic criteria for tobacco use disorder or Nicotine Dependence, this diagnosis should be included as an official diagnosis in their medical, dental, or mental health records. In that tobacco use is considered the most significant individual risk factor for morbidity and mortality, it is remarkable how few health care providers list tobacco use disorder or Nicotine Dependence as a clinical diagnosis. One study (Peterson, Hryshko-Mullen, & Cortez, 2003) evaluated how often medical and mental health providers assessed tobacco use and diagnosed tobacco use disorder or Nicotine Dependence when it appeared that the diagnostic criteria were met. The results indicated that the vast majority of medical (87%) and mental health (88%) providers routinely assessed tobacco use. However, only 2% of the mental health records and 7% of the medical records included a diagnosis of tobacco use disorder or Nicotine Dependence for those patients who appeared to meet full diagnostic criteria according to the DSM and ICD.

TABLE 5.2. ICD-10 Diagnostic Criteria for Nicotine Dependence

Three or more of the following manifestations should have occurred together for at least 1 month or, if persisting for periods of less than 1 month, should have occurred together repeatedly within a 12-month period:

1. A strong desire or sense of compulsion to use tobacco;

2. Impaired capacity to control tobacco-taking behavior in terms of its onset, termination, or levels of use, as evidenced by: the substance being often taken in larger amounts or over a longer period than intended; or by a persistent desire or unsuccessful efforts to reduce or control substance use;

3. A physiological withdrawal state when substance use is reduced or ceased, as evidence by characteristic nicotine withdrawal symptoms (see below) or by use of the same (or closely related) substance with the intention of relieving or avoiding withdrawal symptoms.

   A. There must be clear evidence of recent cessation or reduction of substance use after repeated, and usually prolonged and/or high-dose, use of that substance;

   B. Symptoms and signs are compatible with the known features of a withdrawal state from the particular substance or substances (see below):

      Any two of the following signs must be present:

      (1) Craving for tobacco (or other nicotine-containing products)
      (2) Malaise or weakness
      (3) Anxiety
      (4) Dysphoric mood
      (5) Irritability or restlessness
      (6) Insomnia
      (7) Increased appetite
      (8) Increased cough
      (9) Mouth ulceration
      (10) Difficulty in concentrating

   C. Symptoms and signs are not better accounted for by a medical disorder unrelated to substance use, and not better accounted for by another mental or behavioral disorder;

4. Evidence of tolerance to the effects of the substance, such that there is a need for significantly increased amounts of the substance to achieve intoxication or the desired effect, or a markedly diminished effect with continued use of the same amount of the substance;

5. Preoccupation with substance use, as manifested by important alternative pleasures or interests being given up or reduced because of substance use; or a great deal of time spent in activities necessary to obtain, take, or recover from the effects of the substance;

6. Persistent substance use despite clear evidence of harmful consequences, as evidenced by continued use when the individual is actually aware, or may be expected to be aware, of the nature and extent of them.

Note. Adapted and reproduced, with permission of the publisher, from *The ICD-10 Classification of Mental and Behavioural Disorders: Diagnostic Criteria for Research.* Geneva, World Health Organization, 1992. Section F17.3, pp. 8–12, *www.who.int/substance_abuse/terminology/ICD10ResearchDiagnosis.pdf,* retrieved November 20, 2013.

Prior to formulating a treatment plan, it is also important to conduct a clinical interview to assess a patient's history of tobacco use and previous attempts to quit. This information can be useful in identifying individual barriers to a quit attempt and in helping to design an effective treatment approach. The assessment of tobacco use history should include duration of smoking, use of other tobacco products, and prior quit attempts. Providers should determine the number of prior quit attempts, the longest period of abstinence from tobacco, and previous history of nicotine withdrawal symptoms. It can also be helpful to determine the factors that were related to successes and challenges in previous quit attempts. The circumstances in which the individual previously relapsed back into tobacco use and the future high risk of relapse should be assessed. This assessment can be used to plan coping strategies. Finally, it is important to inquire about specific interventions that have been used in prior quit attempts, including both behavioral and pharmacological treatment approaches. This information will help to determine what approaches might be employed in the current quit attempt.

Cigarette smokers are more likely to have one or more psychiatric comorbidities (Breslau, 1995; Degenhardt & Hall, 2001; Pratt & Brody, 2010), which can make quitting more difficult. Therefore, the history of any psychiatric conditions should be assessed and should include any abuse or dependence on other licit and illicit substances of abuse. The presence of certain psychiatric disorders often suggests that a more intensive intervention is indicated and that more frequent contact may be beneficial (Gelenberg, de Leon, Evins, Parks, & Rigotti, 2008; Hitsman, Moss, Montoya, & George, 2009; Ischaki & Gratziou, 2009). In addition, because nicotine withdrawal is often associated with signs such as depressed mood, anxiety or nervousness, irritability, restlessness, and difficulty sleeping, symptoms associated with certain mental health conditions may become exacerbated during the acute withdrawal phase. It is important that the patient understand and prepare for the changes that are likely to occur immediately after quitting smoking. If a patient is experiencing significant levels of acute distress associated with a psychiatric condition, then it may be beneficial to postpone the attempt to quit until the patient's symptoms are better managed. It is also recommended that treatment be coordinated with the provider who is treating the patient's psychiatric condition so that symptoms can be appropriately monitored and any necessary changes in treatment can be rapidly implemented.

One of the most common side effects of successful smoking cessation is weight gain (American Psychiatric Association, 2000; Borrelli, Spring, Niaura, Hitsman, & Papandonatos, 2001). For many people, this weight gain, or the fear of it, is a primary contributor to relapse (Borrelli et al., 2001). On average, the weight gain is relatively modest (about 11.5 pounds for women and 7.5 for men; O'Hara et al., 1998). However, because most people significantly underestimate their current body weight prior to smoking cessation, many individuals believe they have gained about twice as much weight as their actual weight gain after quitting (Peterson, 1999). Therefore, it is highly recommended that patients weigh themselves prior to attempting to quit tobacco to help ensure that they have an accurate assessment of the actual amount of postcessation weight gain.

Self-Report Assessment Measures of Tobacco Use

Numerous self-report measures have been developed to aid in the assessment of tobacco use. This chapter provides a review of 10 of the leading self-report measures for tobacco use (see Table 5.3). In order to be most useful, an instrument should possess the requisite psychometric properties of reliability and validity. Reliable measures of tobacco use will yield similar results when administered at different times, in different settings, and by different clinicians. Valid measures will accurately assess tobacco use disorder or Nicotine Dependence or one of their components (e.g., nicotine withdrawal, tolerance, compulsive use). This is often determined by assessing an instrument's level of association with other accepted measures of tobacco use or biochemical indices of nicotine dependence. Perhaps the most important dimension of validity with regard to the assessment of tobacco use disorder and Nicotine Dependence, however, is predictive validity in determining the likelihood that a person will successfully quit smoking.

Tobacco Use Diary

The most common measure of tobacco use may be a simple self-report tobacco use diary. Although specific psychometric properties of this measure have not been documented, a simple self-report diary can be useful to record the number of cigarettes smoked per day (as well as other forms of tobacco use) prior to initiating smoking cessation. To assist in the assessment of biopsychosocial factors related to smoking, patients can also record the times and locations at which the smoking occurred, as well as factors they believe were associated with each cigarette. These factors might include physical factors, such as nicotine withdrawal symptoms after going several hours without smoking. They might also include behavioral factors, such as linking smoking to driving a car or fin-

TABLE 5.3. Self-Report Measures of Tobacco Use

Name of measure	Description	Estimated time to complete
Tobacco Use Diary	Diary to record the time, location, and number of cigarettes smoked as well as physical, emotional, and behavioral factors related to tobacco use.	< 1 minute
Readiness to Quit Ladder	1–10 hierarchy ladder of statements representing different levels of motivation to quit smoking.	< 1 minute
Heavy Smoking Index	2-item measure for rapid assessment nicotine dependence. Adapted from Fagerström items.	< 1 minute
Fagerström Test for Nicotine Dependence	6-item multiple-choice and yes/no measure of nicotine dependence.	1 minute
Tobacco Dependence Screener	10-item screening assessment of nicotine dependence according to ICD-10 and DSM-IV.	1–2 minutes
Hooked on Nicotine Checklist	10-item yes/no measure of severity of diminished autonomy related to tobacco use.	1–2 minutes
Cigarette Dependence Scale	12-item measure of nicotine dependence closely matched with the DSM-IV and ICD-10 criteria for nicotine dependence.	1–2 minutes
Minnesota Withdrawal Scale—Revised	15-item behavioral rating scale of nicotine withdrawal symptoms.	1–2 minutes
Nicotine Dependence Syndrome Scale	19-item measure including 5 factors relating to nicotine dependence scored on a 5-point Likert scale.	2–3 minutes
Wisconsin Inventory of Smoking Dependence Motives	A 68-item measure of 13 motivational forces and mechanisms that underlie smoking.	10–15 minutes

ishing a meal, or emotional factors such as feeling stressed with the pressures of work. A sample tobacco use diary is included in Figure 5.1.

Readiness to Quit Ladder

It has been suggested that the type of intervention that will be most helpful will depend upon the individuals' level of motivation and readiness to modify their behavior (Niaura & Shadel, 2003). Although several instruments are available to assess readiness to quit smoking, the quickest and most useful include the Contemplation Ladder (Biener & Abrams, 1991) and the newer Readiness to Quit Ladder (Niaura & Shadel, 2003). The Readiness to Quit Ladder (Figure 5.2) takes less than 1 minute to administer and is designed as a hierarchy ladder, including a list of 10 statements representing different

levels of motivation to quit smoking. The hierarchy ranges from 1 to 10, with higher numbers representing greater readiness to quit. Scores of 7 or higher are reported to indicate that the patient is ready for an active intervention. Scores of 6 or below suggest that a motivational intervention may be more appropriate (Abrams et al., 2003).

Heavy Smoking Index

The Heavy Smoking Index (HSI) is another short (< 1 minute to administer) dimensional measure of nicotine dependence that is often useful in a busy clinical setting (Heatherton, Kozlowski, Frecker, Rickert, & Robinson, 1989). The HSI (see Figure 5.3) has most often been used in epidemiological studies, but it can easily be incorporated into clinical settings for the rapid assessment of nicotine dependence. The HSI is composed of two

Time	Location	Triggers		
		Physical	Emotional	Behavioral
Examples: 6:45 A.M.	On back porch	Cravings for nicotine	Feeling tired	Drinking coffee
7:50 A.M.	Driving to work	None	Frustrated with traffic	Being in my car
9:22 A.M.	Smoke break at work	Tightness in neck and shoulder muscles	Feeling stressed	
1.				
2.				
3.				
4.				
5.				
6.				
7.				
8.				
9.				
10.				
11.				
12.				
13.				
14.				
15.				
16.				
17.				
18.				
19.				
20.				
21.				
22.				
23.				
24.				
25.				
26.				
27.				
28.				
29.				
30.				
31.				
32.				
33.				
34.				
35.				

FIGURE 5.1. Tobacco Use Diary

Below are some thoughts that smokers have about quitting. On this ladder, circle the one number that shows what you think about quitting. Please read each sentence carefully before deciding.

10	I have quit smoking, and I never will smoke again.
9	I have quit smoking, but I still worry about slipping back, so I need to keep working on living smoke free.
8	I still smoke, but I have begun to change, like cutting back on the number of cigarettes I smoke. I am ready to set a quit date.
7	I definitely plan to quit smoking within the next 30 days.
6	I definitely plan to quit smoking in the next 6 months.
5	I often think about quitting smoking, but I have no plans to quit.
4	I sometimes think about quitting smoking, but I have no plans to quit.
3	I rarely think about quitting smoking, and I have no plans to quit.
2	I never think about quitting smoking, and I have no plans to quit.
1	I enjoy smoking and have decided not to quit smoking for my lifetime. I have no interest in quitting.

FIGURE 5.2. Readiness to Quit Ladder. From Niaura and Shadel (2003). Copyright 2003 by The Guilford Press. Reprinted by permission.

Items	Response Options	Score
1. How soon after you wake do you smoke your first cigarette?	Within 5 min	3
	6–30 min	2
	31–60 min	1
	After 60 min	0
2. How many cigarettes/day do you smoke?	10 or less	0
	11–20	1
	21–30	2
	31 or more	3

FIGURE 5.3. Heavy Smoking Index. Based on Heatherton, Kozlowski, Frecker, Rickert, and Robinson (1989).

items: (1) the number of cigarettes smoked per day and (2) the time after waking until the first cigarette of the day is smoked. Both of these items are adapted from the Fagerström Test for Nicotine Dependence (FTND; Heatherton, Kozlowski, Frecker, & Fagerström, 1991), and scores on the HSI correlate strongly with total scores on the FTND. The two items have the greatest predictive value in terms of predicting success with quitting smoking.

Fagerström Test for Nicotine Dependence

The FTND is the most commonly used dimensional measure of nicotine dependence (Heatherton et al., 1991). The FTND (see Figure 5.4) was modified from an earlier version of this measure called the Fagerström Tolerance Questionnaire (FTQ; Fagerström, 1978). The FTND is a six-item measure consisting of multiple-choice and yes–no items that patients can complete in about 1 minute. Possible scores range from 0 to 10, with higher scores indicating greater levels of dependence. A score of ≥ 6 is generally taken as indicating high levels of nicotine dependence. The FTND assesses the number of cigarettes smoked per day, the amount of time between first awakening and first cigarette, the frequency of smoking, and the distribution of smoking throughout the day. The FTND also includes items to assess factors such as the tendency to smoke when ill and difficulty in refraining from smoking in situations in which it is not allowed. Initially described as a measure of physical dependence, others have argued that it more specifically assesses aspects of tolerance to the effects of nicotine (Benowitz, 1999) or motivation to remain abstinent in response to the aversiveness of abstinence from tobacco (Piper, McCarthy, & Baker, 2006). Number of cigarettes smoked per day and time until smoking the first cigarette of the day are important physical indicators of dependence that correlate highly with biochemical measures of tobacco use, such as expired-air carbon monoxide levels and salivary cotinine (a metabolite of nicotine), supporting the concurrent validity of the measure. The FTND scales were not intended to assess other important aspects of tobacco use disorder or Nicotine Dependence, such as craving, subjective compulsion to smoke,

Items	Response Options	Score
1. How soon after you wake do you smoke your first cigarette?	Within 5 min	3
	6–30 min	2
	31–60 min	1
	After 60 min	0
2. Do you find it difficult to refrain from smoking in places where it is forbidden, e.g., in a church, at the library, in a cinema, etc.?	Yes	1
	No	0
3. Which cigarette would you hate giving up the most?	The first one in the morning	1
	All others	0
4. How many cigarettes/day do you smoke?	10 or less	0
	11–20	1
	21–30	2
	31 or more	3
5. Do you smoke more frequently during the first hours after waking than during the rest of the day?	Yes	1
	No	0
6. Do you smoke when you are so ill that you are in bed for most of the day?	Yes	1
	No	0

FIGURE 5.4. Fagerström Test for Nicotine Dependence. From Heatherton, Kozlowski, Frecker, and Fagerström (1991). Copyright 1991 by K. O. Fagerström. Reprinted with permission from John Wiley and Sons, publisher, and Karl O. Fagerström, copyright holder.

nicotine withdrawal, behavioral saliency, or behavioral automaticity, which are often regarded as core constructs for dependence (Shiffman, West, & Gilbert, 2004). It also does not include direct assessment of behavioral, cognitive, emotional, or environmental aspects of the biopsychosocial model. However, one question infers emotional association with smoking ("Which cigarette would you hate giving up the most?"), and one question indirectly addresses environmental factors ("Do you find it difficult to refrain from smoking in places where it is forbidden?"). The FTND is most appropri-

ate when assessing patients who are believed to be highly dependent on nicotine. It is not as reliable with those who only demonstrate low dependence, as these patients may tend to score very low and thus may not meet criteria for tobacco use disorder or Nicotine Dependence based on the assessment alone. The limited reliability of the FTND, based on measures of internal consistency, and questionable factor structure are minor limitations of the measure (Piper et al., 2006).

Tobacco Dependence Screener

The Tobacco Dependence Screener (TDS) is a dimensional measure that allows a brief assessment of nicotine dependence (Kawakami, Takatsuka, Inaba, & Shimizu, 1999). The TDS (see Figure 5.5) includes 10 items to screen for Nicotine Dependence or tobacco use disorder according to ICD-10 and DSM-5, and it requires about 1–2 minutes to administer. Smokers are assessed on several symptoms of tobacco use disorder or Nicotine Dependence, such as smoking more than intended, desire to quit smoking, unsuccessful attempts to quit smoking, tobacco craving, withdrawal symptoms, smoking to avoid withdrawal symptoms, and smoking despite serious illness or health problems. The total score is determined by the number of symptoms that are positively endorsed. TDS scores are correlated with other indices of tobacco use, including biochemical measures (e.g., expired-air carbon monoxide levels), cigarettes smoked per day, and years of smoking. The TDS can successfully predict the likelihood of success with smoking cessation. Measures of internal consistency also support the reliability of the TDS.

Hooked on Nicotine Checklist

The Hooked on Nicotine Checklist (HONC; Wellman et al., 2005) is a self-report checklist consisting of 10 items with yes–no responses that requires about 1–2 minutes to complete. The HONC (see Figure 5.6) is scored by counting the number of "yes" responses. It is described as a measure of severity of "diminished autonomy." The number of symptoms a person endorses serves as a measure of the extent to which autonomy has been lost. It is most useful for treatment planning and

Responses are characterized as Yes (1) or No or Not Applicable (0).

1. Have you often had periods or days when you smoked a lot more than you intended to?

2. Have you ever tried to quit or cut down on tobacco and found you could not?

3. Did you crave tobacco after you quit or cut down on it?

4. Did you have any of the following problems when you quit or cut down on tobacco: irritation, nervousness, restlessness, trouble concentrating, headache, drowsiness, upset stomach, heart slowdown, increased appetite or body weight, hand shakes, depression?

5. Did you ever start using tobacco again to keep from having such problems?

6. Have you ever continued to smoke when you had a serious illness that you knew made it unwise to use tobacco?

7. Did you continue to use tobacco after you knew that it caused you health problems?

8. Did you continue to use tobacco after you knew that it caused you mental problems?

9. Have you ever felt like you were dependent on tobacco?

10. Have you ever given up work or social activities so you could use tobacco?

FIGURE 5.5. Tobacco Dependence Screener (TDS). From Kawakami, Takatsuka, Inaba, and Shimizu (1999). Copyright 1999. Reprinted with permission from Elsevier.

outcome management, as it is a good predictor of quitting and long-term usage rates. It addresses all aspects of the biopsychosocial model in direct and inferred ways. Physical dependence is addressed with questions relating to cravings and withdrawal. Behavioral and environmental factors are covered by the question relating to difficulty in not smoking in places in which it is prohibited. Cognitions related to addiction are assessed by asking about the person's subjective need for cigarettes, whether the individual currently smokes because it is difficult to quit, and whether the individual has difficulty concentrating when he or she is without a cigarette. Autonomy and control are important cognitive factors. Emotional factors are addressed in questions asking about irritability, nervousness, and anxiety when not smoking. The HONC can be used with all smokers. It has high internal consistency and is stable over time, with high test–retest reliability. The HONC's ability to predict persistent smoking is a test of its constructive validity as a measure of diminished autonomy, defined as "when the sequelae of tobacco use, either physical or psychological, present a barrier to quitting" (DiFranza et al., 2002, p. 400).

Cigarette Dependence Scale

The Cigarette Dependence Scale (CDS) is another empirically supported self-report measure of nicotine dependence (Etter, Le Houezec, & Perneger, 2003). The CDS is composed of 12 items and was designed to correspond closely with DSM-5 and ICD-10 criteria for tobacco use disorder and Nicotine Dependence, respectively. The CDS also retains features similar to those included in the FTND and can be considered a hybrid approach to assessing elements of both diagnostic and dimensional assessment models. The CDS includes items that measure the compulsion or urge to smoke, withdrawal symptoms, loss of control, the allocation of excessive amounts of time to smoking, neglect of other activities in favor of smoking, and persistence in smoking despite knowledge of the associated health risks. Additional domains assessed by the CDS include average number of cigarettes smoked per day, perceived level of addiction to cigarettes, time until smoking the

	No	Yes
1. Have you ever tried to quit, but couldn't?		
2. Do you smoke *now* because it is really hard to quit?		
3. Have you ever felt like you were addicted to tobacco?		
4. Do you ever have strong cravings to smoke?		
5. Have you ever felt like you really needed a cigarette?		
6. Is it hard to keep from smoking in places where you are not supposed to? When you tried to stop smoking . . . (or, When you haven't used tobacco for a while)?		
7. Did you find it hard to concentrate because you couldn't smoke?		
8. Did you feel more irritable because you couldn't smoke?		
9. Did you feel a strong need or urge to smoke?		
10. Did you feel nervous, restless or anxious because you couldn't smoke?		

FIGURE 5.6. The Hooked on Nicotine Checklist. Adapted from Wellman et al. (2005). Adapted with permission from Oxford University Press.

first cigarette in the morning, and perceived difficulty in quitting smoking. The 12-item CDS takes about 1–2 minutes to administer. A five-item (CDS-5) version of the CDS is also available. Both the CDS and CDS-5 have demonstrated higher levels of internal consistency than has typically been observed for the FTND. In addition, recent evidence suggests that the CDS may possess better construct validity than the FTND, as determined by stronger associations with measures of craving, of self-efficacy to remain abstinent from smoking, and of DSM-5-defined tobacco use disorder (Etter, 2008). Perhaps most important, the CDS (but not the CDS-5) also demonstrated greater ability to predict abstinence after 8 days and after 6 weeks than the FTND. Interestingly, higher scores on the CDS, rather than lower scores, were predictive of abstinence. Etter (2008) has suggested that this may be due to several items correlating with measures of motivation to quit smoking. The items comprising the 5- and 12-item versions of the CDS are presented in Figure 5.7.

Minnesota Withdrawal Scale

The Minnesota Withdrawal Scale (MWS; Hughes & Hatsukami, 1986) is the most widely used measure of nicotine with-

drawal. The MWS takes about 1–2 minutes to administer and includes 15 symptoms associated with the presence and severity of nicotine withdrawal. Severity ratings for each symptom are reported on a scale from 0 (*none*) to 4 (*severe*). Patients should complete the measure for several days prior to their quit attempt and then daily thereafter in order to track changes in withdrawal symptoms accurately over time. It is recommended that the ratings be completed at the end of each day to reflect the patient's overall experiences over the previous 24 hours. The MWS was revised in 2005 (Hughes & Hatsukami, 2005), and a copy of it is included in Figure 5.8.

Nicotine Dependence Syndrome Scale

The Nicotine Dependence Syndrome Scale (NDSS; Shiffman, Waters, & Hickcox, 2004) is a comprehensive measure of nicotine dependence consisting of 19 items scored on a 5-point Likert scale. The NDSS (see Figure 5.9) takes about 2–3 minutes to administer and is useful for both diagnosis and treatment planning. The NDSS can be used as an outcome measure to assess changes in level of dependence across time and smoking status. Development of the scale identified five factors relating to

Questions	Answer	Recoding	Score
* 1. Please rate your addiction to cigarettes on a scale of 0–100, where 0 – I am NOT addicted to cigarettes. 100 = I am extremely addicted to cigarettes.		0–20 = 1 21–40 = 2 41–60 = 3 61–80 = 4 81–100 = 5	
* 2. On average, how many cigarettes do you smoke per day?		0–5 = 1 6–10 = 2 11–20 = 3 21–29 = 4 30+ = 5	
* 3. Usually, how soon after waking up do you smoke your first cigarette? *(Please provide answer in number of minutes.)*		0–5 = 5 6–15 = 4 16–30 = 3 31–60 = 4 61+ = 1	
* 4. For you, quitting smoking would be: *(Enter numerical equivalent in the answer column.)* Impossible = 5 Very difficult = 4 Fairly difficult = 3 Fairly easy = 2 Very easy = 1		No recoding	
Please indicate whether you agree with each of the following statements based on the following scale: *1 = Totally disagree* *2 = Somewhat disagree* *3 = Neither agree nor disagree* *4 = Somewhat agree* *5 = Fully agree*			
* 5. After a few hours without smoking, I feel an irresistible urge to smoke. 1 2 3 4 5		No recoding	
6. The idea of not having any cigarettes causes me stress. 1 2 3 4 5		No recoding	
7. Before going out, I always make sure that I have cigarettes with me. 1 2 3 4 5		No recoding	
8. I am a prisoner of cigarettes. 1 2 3 4 5		No recoding	
9. I smoke too much. 1 2 3 4 5		No recoding	
10. Sometimes I drop everything to go out and buy cigarettes. 1 2 3 4 5		No recoding	
11. I smoke all the time. 1 2 3 4 5		No recoding	
12. I smoke despite the risks to my health. 1 2 3 4 5		No recoding	
CDS-12 Total *(Sum of items 1–12)*			
CDS-5 Total (items marked *) *(Sum of items 1–5)*			

FIGURE 5.7. Cigarette Dependence Scale (CDS). Adapted from Etter, Le Houezec, and Perneger (2003). Copyright 2003 by Nature Publishing Group. Adapted with permission from Macmillan Publishers Ltd.

Please rate yourself for the last 24 hours.

0 = none, 1 = slight, 2 = mild, 3 = moderate, 4 = severe

1. Angry, irritable, frustrated	0	1	2	3	4
2. Anxious, nervous	0	1	2	3	4
3. Depressed mood, sad	0	1	2	3	4
4. Desire or craving to smoke	0	1	2	3	4
5. Difficulty concentrating	0	1	2	3	4
6. Increased appetite, hungry, weight gain	0	1	2	3	4
7. Insomnia, sleep problems, awakening at night	0	1	2	3	4
8. Restless	0	1	2	3	4
9. Impatient	0	1	2	3	4
10. Constipation	0	1	2	3	4
11. Dizziness	0	1	2	3	4
12. Coughing	0	1	2	3	4
13. Dreaming or nightmares	0	1	2	3	4
14. Nausea	0	1	2	3	4
15. Sore throat	0	1	2	3	4

Heart rate _____ bpm

Weight _____ kg

To calculate the total score, sum items 1 through 9. (The first nine items are considered to be well-validated, and should therefore serve as the ones used to determine a total discomfort score. The remaining six items are symptoms that are considered to be possibly related to nicotine withdrawal, but which require additional validation.)

FIGURE 5.8. Minnesota Withdrawal Scale—Revised (MNWS-R). From Hughes and Hatsukami (2005).

dependence, which cover most aspects of the biopsychosocial model.

- *Drive.* "Drive" captures the symptoms of craving, withdrawal, avoidance, and subjective compulsion that are often regarded as core features of addiction.
- *Priority.* "Priority" measures the degree to which smoking comes to be valued over other reinforcers, a concept often described by the discipline of behavioral economics.
- *Tolerance.* "Tolerance" refers to decreased sensitivity to nicotine and/or the escalation of dose needed to overcome such decreases. Tolerance is often considered to be essential for dependence.
- *Stereotypy.* "Stereotypy" refers to the development of rigid or stereotypic patterns of tobacco use, which indicates the behavior's increasing resistance to change.
- *Continuity.* "Continuity" refers to the behavioral momentum, as reflected in its consistency.

Emotional aspects of tobacco use disorder and Nicotine Dependence are not indicated by a specific factor but are addressed by a few individual items within the scale (e.g., "I smoke about the same amount whether I'm relaxed or working, happy or sad, alone or with others, etc."; "The number of cigarettes I smoke per day is often influenced by other factors—how I'm feeling, what I'm doing,

	1 Not at all true	2 Somewhat true	3 Moderately true	4 Very true	5 Extremely true
1 My smoking pattern is very irregular throughout the day. It is not unusual for me to smoke many cigarettes in one hour, then not have another one until hours later.	1 □	2 □	3 □	4 □	5 □
2 My smoking is not much affected by other things. I smoke about the same amount whether I'm relaxed or working, happy or sad, alone or with others, etc.	1 □	2 □	3 □	4 □	5 □
3 Even if traveling a long distance, I'd rather not travel by airplane because I wouldn't be allowed to smoke.	1 □	2 □	3 □	4 □	5 □
4 Sometimes, I decline offers to visit with my non-smoking friends because I know I'll feel uncomfortable if I smoke.	1 □	2 □	3 □	4 □	5 □
5 I tend to avoid restaurants that don't allow smoking, even if I would otherwise enjoy the food.	1 □	2 □	3 □	4 □	5 □
6 I smoke consistently and regularly throughout the day.	1 □	2 □	3 □	4 □	5 □
7 I smoke at different rates in different situations	1 □	2 □	3 □	4 □	5 □
8 Compared to when I first started smoking, I need to smoke a lot more now in order to get what I really want out of it.	1 □	2 □	3 □	4 □	5 □
9 Compared to when I first started smoking, I can smoke much, much more now before I start to feel nauseated or ill.	1 □	2 □	3 □	4 □	5 □
10 After not smoking for a while, I need to smoke in order to keep myself from experiencing any discomfort.	1 □	2 □	3 □	4 □	5 □
11 It's hard to estimate how many cigarettes I smoke per day because the number often changes.	1 □	2 □	3 □	4 □	5 □
12 I feel a sense of control over my smoking. I can "take it or leave it" at any time.	1 □	2 □	3 □	4 □	5 □

(continued)

FIGURE 5.9. The Nicotine Dependence Syndrome Scale. Adapted from Shiffman, Waters, and Hickcox (2004). Adapted with permission from Oxford University Press.

	1 Not at all true	2 Somewhat true	3 Moderately true	4 Very true	5 Extremely true
13 The number of cigarettes I smoke per day is often influenced by other factors—how I'm feeling, what I'm doing, etc.	1 ☐	2 ☐	3 ☐	4 ☐	5 ☐
14 When I'm really craving a cigarette, it feels like I'm in the grip of some unknown force that I cannot control.	1 ☐	2 ☐	3 ☐	4 ☐	5 ☐
15 Since the time when I became a regular smoker, the amount that I smoke has either stayed the same or has decreased somewhat.	1 ☐	2 ☐	3 ☐	4 ☐	5 ☐
16 Whenever I go without a smoke for a few hours, I experience craving.	1 ☐	2 ☐	3 ☐	4 ☐	5 ☐
17 My cigarette smoking is fairly regular throughout the day.	1 ☐	2 ☐	3 ☐	4 ☐	5 ☐
18 After not smoking for a while, I need to smoke to relieve feelings of restlessness and irritability.	1 ☐	2 ☐	3 ☐	4 ☐	5 ☐
19 I smoke about the same amount on weekdays as on weekends.	1 ☐	2 ☐	3 ☐	4 ☐	5 ☐

FIGURE 5.9. *(continued)*

etc."; "After not smoking for a while, I need to smoke to relieve feelings of restlessness and irritability").

The multidimensional classification and comprehensive manner of assessment makes the NDSS widely applicable to different types of smokers. It provides robust discrimination between occasional smokers (often called "chippers") and regular smokers. The NDSS also discriminates levels of intake and dependence within the chippers group, suggesting that the scales are sensitive to individual differences even at the very low end of the dependence continuum. The NDSS has incremental utility, as demonstrated by the subscales, which also serve as independent discriminators, demonstrating the discriminant validity of the subscales. Validity and reliability are higher than that of the FTND, and it can be quite helpful to use the NDSS in conjunction with the FTND, because the measures do not assess exactly the same factors.

Wisconsin Inventory of Smoking Dependence Motives

The Wisconsin Inventory of Smoking Dependence Motives (WISDM-68) is a self-report questionnaire designed to measure the degree of different motivational forces present and mechanisms that underlie smoking (Piper et al., 2004). The WISDM-68 (see Figure 5.10) consists of 68 items (4–7 items per motive) scored on a 7-point Likert scale ranging from 1 (*not true of me at all*) to 7 (*extremely true of me*). The WISDM-68 measures 13 distinct motives related to nicotine dependence. It requires about 10–15 minutes to administer, and it is scored by summing the 13 subscales and the overall total score. It can be useful for treatment planning and provides predictive utility regarding quitting. The WISDM-68 has a reliability coefficient > .90, and the total internal consistency ranged from .97 to .99. The 13 distinct motives related to nico-

Below are a series of statements about cigarette smoking. Please rate your level of agreement for each using the following scale:

1	2	3	4	5	6	7
Not true of me at all						Extremely true of me

1. I enjoy the taste of cigarettes most of the time.   1 2 3 4 5 6 7
2. Smoking keeps me from gaining weight.   1 2 3 4 5 6 7
3. Smoking makes a good mood better.   1 2 3 4 5 6 7
4. If I always smoke in a certain place it is hard to be there and not smoke.   1 2 3 4 5 6 7
5. I often smoke without thinking about it.   1 2 3 4 5 6 7
6. Cigarettes control me.   1 2 3 4 5 6 7
7. Smoking a cigarette improves my mood.   1 2 3 4 5 6 7
8. Smoking makes me feel content.   1 2 3 4 5 6 7
9. I usually want to smoke right after I wake up.   1 2 3 4 5 6 7
10. Very few things give me pleasure each day like cigarettes.   1 2 3 4 5 6 7
11. It's hard to ignore an urge to smoke.   1 2 3 4 5 6 7
12. The flavor of a cigarette is pleasing.   1 2 3 4 5 6 7
13. I smoke when I really need to concentrate.   1 2 3 4 5 6 7
14. I can only go a couple hours between cigarettes.   1 2 3 4 5 6 7
15. I frequently smoke to keep my mind focused.   1 2 3 4 5 6 7
16. I rely upon smoking to control my hunger and eating.   1 2 3 4 5 6 7
17. My life is full of reminders to smoke.   1 2 3 4 5 6 7
18. Smoking helps me feel better in seconds.   1 2 3 4 5 6 7
19. I smoke without deciding to.   1 2 3 4 5 6 7
20. Cigarettes keep me company, like a close friend.   1 2 3 4 5 6 7
21. Few things would be able to replace smoking in my life.   1 2 3 4 5 6 7
22. I'm around smokers much of the time.   1 2 3 4 5 6 7
23. There are particular sights and smells that trigger strong urges to smoke.   1 2 3 4 5 6 7
24. Smoking helps me stay focused.   1 2 3 4 5 6 7
25. Smoking helps me deal with stress.   1 2 3 4 5 6 7
26. I frequently light cigarettes without thinking about it.   1 2 3 4 5 6 7
27. Most of my daily cigarettes taste good.   1 2 3 4 5 6 7
28. Sometimes I feel like cigarettes rule my life.   1 2 3 4 5 6 7
29. I frequently crave cigarettes.   1 2 3 4 5 6 7
30. Most of the people I spend time with are smokers.   1 2 3 4 5 6 7
31. Weight control is a major reason that I smoke.   1 2 3 4 5 6 7
32. I usually feel much better after a cigarette.   1 2 3 4 5 6 7
33. Some of the cigarettes I smoke taste great.   1 2 3 4 5 6 7

(continued)

FIGURE 5.10. The Wisconsin Inventory of Smoking Dependence Motives (WISDM-68). From Piper et al. (2004). Copyright 2004 by the American Psychological Association. Reprinted by permission.

	1	2	3	4	5	6	7
34. I'm really hooked on cigarettes.	1	2	3	4	5	6	7
35. Smoking is the fastest way to reward myself.	1	2	3	4	5	6	7
36. Sometimes I feel like cigarettes are my best friends.	1	2	3	4	5	6	7
37. My urges to smoke keep getting stronger if I don't smoke.	1	2	3	4	5	6	7
38. I would continue smoking, even if it meant I could spend less time on my hobbies and other interests.	1	2	3	4	5	6	7
39. My concentration is improved after smoking a cigarette.	1	2	3	4	5	6	7
40. Seeing someone smoke makes me really want a cigarette.	1	2	3	4	5	6	7
41. I find myself reaching for cigarettes without thinking about it.	1	2	3	4	5	6	7
42. I crave cigarettes at certain times of the day.	1	2	3	4	5	6	7
43. I would feel alone without my cigarettes.	1	2	3	4	5	6	7
44. A lot of my friends and family smoke.	1	2	3	4	5	6	7
45. Smoking brings me a lot of pleasure.	1	2	3	4	5	6	7
46. Cigarettes are about the only things that can give me a lift when I need it.	1	2	3	4	5	6	7
47. Other smokers would consider me a heavy smoker.	1	2	3	4	5	6	7
48. I feel a strong bond with my cigarettes.	1	2	3	4	5	6	7
49. It would take a pretty serious medical problem to make me quit smoking.	1	2	3	4	5	6	7
50. When I haven't been able to smoke for a few hours, the craving gets intolerable.	1	2	3	4	5	6	7
51. When I do certain things I know I'm going to smoke.	1	2	3	4	5	6	7
52. Most of my friends and acquaintances smoke.	1	2	3	4	5	6	7
53. I love the feel of inhaling the smoke into my mouth.	1	2	3	4	5	6	7
54. I smoke within the first 30 minutes of awakening in the morning.	1	2	3	4	5	6	7
55. Sometimes I'm not aware that I'm smoking.	1	2	3	4	5	6	7
56. I'm worried that if I quit smoking I'll gain weight.	1	2	3	4	5	6	7
57. Smoking helps me think better.	1	2	3	4	5	6	7
58. Smoking really helps me feel better if I've been feeling down.	1	2	3	4	5	6	7
59. Some things are very hard to do without smoking.	1	2	3	4	5	6	7
60. Smoking makes me feel good.	1	2	3	4	5	6	7
61. Smoking keeps me from overeating.	1	2	3	4	5	6	7
62. My smoking is out of control.	1	2	3	4	5	6	7
63. I consider myself a heavy smoker.	1	2	3	4	5	6	7
64. Even when I feel good, smoking helps me feel better.	1	2	3	4	5	6	7
65. I reach for cigarettes when I feel irritable.	1	2	3	4	5	6	7
66. I enjoy the sensations of a long, slow exhalation of smoke.	1	2	3	4	5	6	7
67. Giving up cigarettes would be like losing a good friend.	1	2	3	4	5	6	7
68. Smoking is the easiest way to give myself a lift.	1	2	3	4	5	6	7

FIGURE 5.10. *(continued)*

tine dependence that are measured by the WISDM-68 follow (Piper et al., 2004).

- *Affiliative attachment*: strong emotional attachment to smoking and cigarettes.
- *Automaticity*: smoking without awareness or intention.
- *Behavioral choice*: smoking despite constraints on smoking or negative consequences.
- *Cognitive enhancement*: smoking to improve cognitive functioning (e.g., attention).
- *Craving*: smoking in response to craving or experiencing intense and/or frequent urges to smoke.
- *Cue exposure/associative processes*: frequent encounters with nonsocial smoking or a strong perceived link between cue exposure and the desire or tendency to smoke.
- *Loss of control*: based on the notion that once dependence becomes ingrained, the dependent person believes that he or she has lost volitional control over smoking because of any of a variety of factors (e.g., urges, loss of other reinforcers, automaticity).
- *Negative reinforcement*: the tendency or desire to smoke to ameliorate a variety of negative internal states (e.g., dysphoria, stress, withdrawal).
- *Positive reinforcement*: the desire to smoke or experience a "buzz" or a "high" or to enhance an already positive feeling or experience.
- *Social-environmental goals*: social stimuli or contexts that either model or invite smoking.
- *Taste and sensory properties*: the desire or tendency to smoke in order to experience the oral-sensory and/or gustatory effects of smoking.
- *Tolerance*: the principal need of individuals to smoke increasing amounts over time in order to experience the desired effects or the ability to smoke large amounts without acute toxicity.
- *Weight control*: the use of cigarettes to control body weight or appetite.

Biochemical Assessment of Tobacco Use

Although self-report assessment measures of tobacco use have many advantages, such as their low cost, ease of use, and potential for quick scoring and interpretation, there are circumstances in which patients may be motivated to misreport their tobacco use (e.g., during pregnancy or health insurance screenings or in the presence of a smoking-related illness). Objective biochemical measures may have advantages beyond using the number of cigarettes smoked per day for assessing smoking status, tracking changes in cigarette smoking over time, and adjusting the dosage of nicotine replacement therapy (NRT).

Several different biomarkers have been used to quantify levels of tobacco exposure, including nicotine, expired-air carbon monoxide, cotinine, thiocyanate, anabasine, and anatabine. Although nicotine might appear to be the ideal marker for assessing tobacco use and level of exposure, there are actually several properties that significantly limit its utility for this purpose. For example, although plasma nicotine levels obtained during a typical day of smoking correlate well with daily nicotine intake, its short half-life (approximately 2 hours) limit its usefulness for measuring tobacco consumption that has occurred more than 8–12 hours prior to the time of assessment (Society for Research on Nicotine and Tobacco [SRNT] Subcommittee on Biochemical Verification, 2002). The technical difficulties and moderately high expense associated with measuring nicotine levels also detract from its usefulness as a biomarker of tobacco use.

Carbon Monoxide

Expired-air carbon monoxide (CO) is one of the quickest and most easily obtained biomarkers of tobacco smoke exposure. Expired-air CO levels can be readily measured using portable monitors that provide results in a matter of seconds. Levels of 8 to 10 parts per million are the most widely used cutoffs for distinguishing a current smoker from a nonsmoker. However, expired CO does not detect the use of smokeless tobacco products. Consequently, it is possible for an individual to consume high levels of non-smoked forms of tobacco while still testing negative for elevated CO exposure. In addition, due to its relatively short half-life (2–8 hours depending on the activity level of the individual), CO levels may not be noticeably elevated among those who have not recently smoked a cigarette (SRNT Subcommittee on Biochemical Verification, 2002).

Cotinine

Cotinine is the best overall biomarker of tobacco use and cessation (SRNT Subcommittee on Biochemical Verification, 2002). It is a major proximate metabolite of nicotine, with approximately 70–80% of all nicotine absorbed by smokers being subsequently converted to cotinine (Bramer & Kallungal, 2003). Cotinine can be detected in several body fluids, including saliva, blood, and urine. Due to its longer half-life (15–19 hours), cotinine can be detected for several days after tobacco use. Cotinine is also useful for measuring smokeless tobacco use (SRNT Subcommittee on Biochemical Verification, 2002).

Thiocyanate

A metabolite of hydrogen cyanide, thiocyanate is a combustion product that results from the burning of tobacco or certain other materials, such as plastic. The longer half-life of thiocyanate (6–28 days) increases its utility for measuring cigarette smoking over longer periods of time than can be done using nicotine, CO, or cotinine (SRNT Subcommittee on Biochemical Verification, 2002). Considerable time must elapse following cessation for thiocyanate to be useful in determining whether an individual is currently using tobacco. Because thiocyanate is a metabolite of a combustion product, it is also not useful for detecting smokeless tobacco use.

Anabasine and Anatabine

Minor tobacco alkaloids such as anabasine and anatabine, which are present in tobacco products but not in medicinal nicotine products, also have potential for measuring cigarette and other tobacco use, particularly in those using NRT. Urinary levels of both alkaloids have been shown to correlate highly with nicotine intake, with half-lives of approximately 10 hours (anatabine) to 16 hours (anabasine; Jacob, Yu, Shulgin, & Benowitz, 1999). Although the longer half-life and/or greater specificity of these

compounds help to get around some of the previously mentioned limitations associated with CO and cotinine, the added costs and limited number of laboratories that currently provide these assays reduce their utility outside of the context of a research environment, in which they are most commonly used at present.

Selection of Tobacco Use Assessment Measures

Each of the previously described self-report and biochemical measures has clinical utility for assessing tobacco use and nicotine dependence. The choice of measures is best determined based on the goals of the assessment. If the purpose is primarily to formulate a diagnostic impression, then the TDS or a clinical review of DSM-5 and ICD-10 criteria is recommended. However, such measures typically do not provide an adequate index of severity of nicotine dependence across a continuous scale, nor is there good evidence to support their ability to predict severity of withdrawal symptoms or probability of relapse (Piper et al., 2006). The FTND and HSI appear to have somewhat greater utility for predicting the probability of relapse and can be readily administered in a clinical setting. However, the reliabilities of the scales are suboptimal. Furthermore, although the FTND appears to be a good measure of the specific motivational aspects of nicotine dependence related to smoking in order to reduce withdrawal symptoms, it does not address or predict certain components considered to be central to dependence, such as the severity of withdrawal (Piper et al., 2006). The CDS, which combines features of continuous dependence severity scales such as the FTND and those designed to evaluate diagnostic criteria, possesses many of the advantages of both approaches to assessing dependence. The scale's brevity, good reliability, and both construct and predictive validity are additional strengths. Furthermore, recent evidence suggests that it may possess superior psychometric properties to the FTND, although additional confirmatory studies are needed. Because it is a relatively new measure, however, data supporting the extent to which it will prove useful in predicting cessation in different groups of smokers are currently limited (Piper et al., 2006).

In terms of biochemical verification, cotinine is considered the biomarker of choice for assessing tobacco use. Expired-air CO produces rapid results that are not affected by pharmacotherapy use. However, it is limited by a short half-life and the inability to distinguish between elevated CO levels due to tobacco exposure and other sources in the ambient air. Thiocyanate's long half-life makes it possible to assess for tobacco use over much longer periods of time than can be achieved through other biomarkers. Anabasine and anatabine appear to have great utility for measuring tobacco use in general and among patients using NRT specifically. However, despite the potential usefulness of biochemical measures, they have limited utility in most regular clinical practice settings. Therefore, in most instances the verification of self-report with biochemical measures is not worth the additional time and expense incurred.

Summary

Helping patients quit tobacco should be a top priority for all medical, dental, and behavioral health providers. Assessment of tobacco use is the first step in this process. This chapter reviewed a range of tobacco use assessment strategies from a biopsychosocial perspective. As a minimum, providers should assess and document the tobacco use status of every new patient seen in a clinical setting. Asking whether he or she uses tobacco and assessing his or her interest in quitting should be part of this initial assessment. The use of additional structured clinical interviews, self-report assessment measures, and biochemical verification approaches will provide additional information depending on the setting and needs of the clinician or researcher. The majority of patients who quit tobacco do so on their own without any formal intervention by a health care provider (Fiore et al., 1990; Zhu, Melcer, Sun, Rosbrook, & Pierce, 2000). Routine assessment of tobacco use by clinicians may be all that is needed to prompt some patients to quit tobacco all on their own.

REFERENCES

Abrams, D. B., Niaura, R., Brown, R. A., Emmons, K. M., Goldstein, M. G., & Monti, P. M. (2003). *The tobacco dependence treatment handbook*. New York: Guilford Press.

American Psychiatric Association. (2000). *Diagnostic and statistical manual of mental disorders* (4th ed., text rev.). Washington, DC: Author.

American Psychiatric Association. (2013). *Diagnostic and statistical manual of mental disorders* (5th ed.). Arlington, VA: Author.

Andrews, J. O., Heath, J., & Graham-Garcia, J. (2004). Management of tobacco dependence in older adults: Using evidence-based strategies. *Journal of Gerontological Nursing, 30*(12), 13–24. Retrieved from *www.jognonline.com*.

Benowitz, N. L. (1999). Nicotine addiction. *Primary Care: Clinics in Office Practice, 26*, 611–631.

Biener, L., & Abrams, D. B. (1991). The contemplation ladder: Validation of a measure of readiness to consider smoking cessation. *Health Psychology, 10*, 360–365.

Borrelli, B., Spring, B., Niaura, R., Hitsman, B., & Papandonatos, G. (2001). Influences of gender and weight gain on short-term relapse to smoking in a cessation trial. *Journal of Consulting and Clinical Psychology, 69*, 511–515.

Boyd, N. R. (1996). Smoking cessation: A four-step plan to help older patients quit. *Geriatrics, 51*(11), 52–57. Retrieved from *www. modernmedicine.com/modernmedicine/Geriatrics/home/40131*.

Bramer, S. L., & Kallungal, B. A. (2003). Clinical considerations in study designs that use cotinine as a biomarker. *Biomarker, 8*, 187–203.

Breslau, N. (1995). Psychiatric comorbidity of smoking and nicotine dependence. *Behavior Genetics, 25*, 95–101.

Centers for Disease Control and Prevention. (2002). Cigarette smoking among adults—United States, 2001. *Morbidity and Mortality Weekly Report, 51*, 642–645.

Centers for Disease Control and Prevention. (2008). Cigarette smoking among adults—United States, 2007. *Morbidity and Mortality Weekly Report, 57*, 1221–1226.

Cummings, K. M., Giovino, G., Jaén, C. R., & Emrich, L. J. (1985). Reports of smoking withdrawal symptoms over a 21-day period of abstinence. *Addictive Behaviors, 10*, 373–381.

Degenhardt, L., & Hall, W. (2001). The relationship between tobacco use, substance-use disorders and mental health: Results from the National Survey of Mental Health and Well-being. *Nicotine and Tobacco Research, 3*, 225–234.

DiFranza, J. R., Savageau, J. A., Fletcher, K., Ockene, J. K., Rigotti, N. A., McNeill, A. D., et al. (2002). Measuring the loss of autonomy over nicotine use in adolescents: The Development and Assessment of Nicotine Dependence in Youths (DANDY) study. *Archives of Pediatric and Adolescent Medicine, 156,* 397–403.

Engel, G. L. (1977). The need for a new medical model: A challenge for biomedicine. *Science, 196,* 129–136.

Etter, J. F. (2008). Comparing the validity of the Cigarette Dependence Scale and the Fagerström Test for Nicotine Dependence. *Drug and Alcohol Dependence, 95,* 152–159.

Etter, J. F., Le Houezec, J., & Perneger, T. V. (2003). A self-administered questionnaire to measure dependence on cigarettes: The Cigarette Dependence Scale. *Neuropsychopharmacology, 28,* 359–370.

Fagerström, K. O. (1978). Measuring degree of physical dependence to tobacco smoking with reference to individualization of treatment. *Addictive Behaviors, 3,* 235–241.

Fiore, M. C., Bailey W. C., Cohen, S. J., Dorfman, S. F., Fox, B. J., Goldstein, M. G., et al. (2000). *Treating tobacco use and dependence* (AHRQ Publication No. 00-0032.) Rockville, MD: U.S. Department of Health and Human Services, Public Health Service.

Fiore, M. C., Jaén, C. R., Baker, T. B., Bailay, W. C., Benowitz, N. L., Curry, S. J., et al. (2008). *Treating tobacco use and dependence: 2008 update* (AHRQ Publication No. 08-0050-1). Rockville, MD: U.S. Department of Health and Human Services, Public Health Service.

Fiore, M. C., Novotny, T. E., Pierce, J. P., Giovino, G. A., Hatziandreu, E. J., Newcomb, P. A., et al. (1990). Methods used to quit smoking in the United States: Do cessation programs help? *Journal of the American Medical Association, 263,* 2760–2765.

Gelenberg, A. J., de Leon, J., Evins, A. E., Parks, J. J., & Rigotti, N. A. (2008). Smoking cessation in patients with psychiatric disorders. *Primary Care Companion to the Journal of Clinical Psychiatry, 10,* 52–58. Retrieved from *www.psychiatrist.com.*

Heatherton, F. F., Kozlowski, L. T., Frecker, R. C., & Fagerström, K. O. (1991). The Fagerström Test for Nicotine Dependence: A revision of the Nicotine Tolerance Questionnaire. *British Journal of Addiction, 86,* 1119–1127.

Heatherton, F. F., Kozlowski, L. T., Frecker, R. C., Rickert, W., & Robinson, J. (1989). Measuring the heaviness of smoking: Using self-reported time to the first cigarette of the day and number of cigarettes smoked per day. *British Journal of Addiction, 84,* 791–800.

Hitsman, B., Moss, T. G., Montoya, I. D., & George, T. P. (2009). Treatment of tobacco dependence in mental health and addictive disorders. *Canadian Journal of Psychiatry, 54,* 368–378. Retrieved from *http://publications. cpa-apc.org/browse/sections/0.*

Hughes, J. R. (2007). The effects of abstinence from tobacco: Valid symptoms and time course. *Nicotine and Tobacco Research, 9,* 315–327.

Hughes, J. R., & Hatsukami, D. K. (1986). Signs and symptoms of tobacco withdrawal. *Archives of General Psychiatry, 43,* 289–294. Retrieved from *http://archpsyc.ama-assn.org.*

Hughes, J. R., & Hatsukami, D. K. (2005). *Minnesota Withdrawal Scale—Revised.* Retrieved from *www.uvm.edu/~hbpl/?Page=minnesota/ default.html.*

Hughes, J. R., Keely, J., & Naud, S. (2004). Shape of the relapse curve and long-term abstinence among untreated smokers. *Addiction, 99,* 29–38.

Ischaki, E., & Gratziou, C. (2009). Smoking and depression: Is smoking cessation effective? *Therapeutic Advances in Respiratory Disease, 3*(1), 31–38.

Jacob, P., Yu, I., Shulgin, A., & Benowitz, N. (1999). Minor tobacco alkaloids as biomarkers for tobacco use: Comparison of users of cigarettes, smokeless tobacco, cigars and pipes. *American Journal of Public Health, 89,* 731–736.

Kawakami, N., Takatsuka, N., Inaba, S., & Shimizu, H. (1999). Development of a screening questionnaire for tobacco/nicotine dependence according to ICD-10, DSM-III-R, and DSM-IV. *Addictive Behaviors, 24,* 155–166.

Lassner, K., Boyd, J. W., Woolhandler, S., Himmelstein, D. U., McCormick, D., & Bor, D. H. (2000). Smoking and mental illness: A population-based prevalence study. *Journal of the American Medical Association, 284,* 2606–2610.

Lerman, C., Caporaso, N. E., Audrain, J., Main, D., Bowman, E. D., Lockshin, B., et al. (1999).

Evidence suggesting the role of specific genetic factors in cigarette smoking. *Health Psychology, 18*, 14–20.

National Cancer Institute. (2008). *Tobacco control monograph 19: The role of the media in promoting and reducing tobacco use.* Bethesda, MD: U.S. Department of Health and Human Services, National Institutes of Health, National Cancer Institute. Retrieved November 8, 2011, from *www.cancercontrol. cancer.gov/tcrb/monographs/19/index.html.*

Niaura, R., & Shadel, W. G. (2003). Assessment to inform smoking cessation treatment. In D. B. Abrams, R. Niaura, R. A. Brown, K. M. Emmons, M. G. Goldstein, & P. M. Monti (Eds.), *The tobacco treatment handbook: A guide to best practices* (pp. 27–72). New York: Guilford Press.

O'Hara, P., Connett, J. E., Lee, W. W., Nides, M., Murray, R., & Wise, R. (1998). Early and late weight gain following smoking cessation in the Lung Health Study. *American Journal of Epidemiology, 148*, 821–830. Retrieved from *http://aje.oxfordjournals.org.*

Parrott, A. C. (1995a). Smoking cessation leads to reduced stress, but why? *International Journal of the Addictions, 30*, 1509–1516. Retrieved from *www.informaworld.com/ smpp/title~content=t713597302.*

Parrott, A. C. (1995b). Stress modulation over the day in cigarette smokers. *Addiction, 90*, 233–244. Retrieved from *www.addictionjournal.org.*

Parrott, A. C. (1999). Does cigarette smoking cause stress? *American Psychologist, 54*, 817–820.

Peterson, A. L. (1999). Inaccurate estimation of body weight prior to smoking cessation: Implications for quitting and weight gain. *Journal of Applied Biobehavioral Research, 4*, 79–84.

Peterson, A. L., Hryshko-Mullen, A. S., & Cortez, Y. (2003). Assessment and diagnosis of nicotine dependence in mental health settings. *American Journal of Addictions, 12*, 192–197.

Peterson, A. L., Vander Weg, M. W., & Jaén, C. R. (2011). *Advances in psychotherapy— Evidence-based practice* (Vol. 21). *Nicotine and tobacco dependence.* Cambridge, MA: Hogrefe.

Piper, M. E., McCarthy, D. E., & Baker, T. B. (2006). Assessing tobacco dependence: A guide to measure evaluation and selection. *Nicotine and Tobacco Dependence, 8*, 339–351.

Piper, M. E., Piasecki, T. M., Federman, E. B., Bolt, D. M., Smith, S. S., Fiore, M. C., et al. (2004). A multiple motive approach to tobacco dependence: The Wisconsin Inventory of Smoking Dependence Motives (WISDM-68). *Journal of Consulting and Clinical Psychology, 72*, 139–154.

Pratt, L. A., & Brody, D. J. (2010). Depression and smoking in the U.S. household population aged 20 and over, 2005–2008. *National Center for Health Statistics Data Brief, 34*, 1–8. Retrieved from *www.cdc.gov/nchs/data/databriefs/db34.pdf.*

Shiffman, S., Waters. A. J., & Hickcox, M. (2004). The Nicotine Dependence Syndrome Scale: A multidimensional measure of nicotine dependence. *Nicotine and Tobacco Research, 6*, 327–348.

Shiffman, S., West, R., & Gilbert, D. (2004). Recommendation for the assessment of tobacco craving and withdrawal in smoking cessation trials. *Nicotine and Tobacco Research, 6*, 559–614.

Society for Research on Nicotine and Tobacco Subcommittee on Biochemical Verification. (2002). Biochemical verification of tobacco use and cessation. *Nicotine and Tobacco Research, 4*, 149–159.

Tait, R. J., Hulse, G. K., Waterreus, A., Flicker, L., Lautenschlager, N. T., Jamrozik, K., et al. (2007). Effectiveness of a smoking cessation intervention in older adults. *Addiction, 102*, 148–155.

Teneggi, V., Tiffany, S. T., Squassante, L., Milleri, S., Ziviani, L., & Bye, A. (2002). Smokers deprived of cigarettes for 72 h: Effect of nicotine patches on craving and withdrawal. *Psychopharmacology, 164*, 177–187.

Tobacco Research Implementation Group. (1998). *The National Cancer Institute Tobacco Research Implementation Plan: Priorities for tobacco research beyond the year 2000.* Bethesda, MD: U.S. Department of Health and Human Services, National Institutes of Health, National Cancer Institute.

U.S. Department of Health and Human Services. (2004). *The health consequences of smoking: A report of the Surgeon General.* Washington, DC: U.S. Department of Health and Human Services, Centers for Disease Control and Prevention, National Center for Chronic Disease Prevention and Health Promotion, Office on Smoking and Health.

Vander Weg, M. W., Peterson, A. L., Ebbert, J.

E., DeBon, M., Klesges, R. C., & Haddock, C. K. (2008). Prevalence of alternative forms of tobacco use in a population of young adult military recruits. *Addictive Behaviors, 33,* 69–82.

Wellman, R. J., Difranza, J. R., Savageau, J. A., Godiwala, S., Friedman, K., & Hazelton, J. (2005). Measuring adults' loss of autonomy over nicotine use: The Hooked on Nicotine Checklist. *Nicotine and Tobacco Research, 7,* 157–161.

World Health Organization. (1992). *The ICD-10 classification of mental and behavioural disorders: Diagnostic criteria for research.* Geneva, Switzerland: Author.

World Health Organization. (2008). *The WHO report on the global tobacco epidemic, 2008: The MPOWER package.* Geneva, Switzerland: Author. Retrieved from *www.who.int/ tobacco/mpower/mpower_report_full_2008. pdf.*

Zhu, S., Melcer, T., Sun, J., Rosbrook, B., & Pierce, J. P. (2000). Smoking cessation with and without assistance: A population-based analysis. *American Journal of Preventive Medicine, 18,* 305–311.

Ziedonis, D., Williams, J. M., & Smelson, D. (2003). Serious mental illness and tobacco addiction: A model program to address this common but neglected issue. *American Journal of the Medical Sciences, 326,* 223–230. Retrieved from *http://journals.lww.com/ amjmedsci.*

CHAPTER 6

Drug Use and Abuse

Deborah L. Haller
Michelle C. Acosta
Howard Newville
Abigail Herron

In 2010, 8.7% of the U.S. population were found to have current substance use disorders, although only 18% of these (1.6% of the total population) were in treatment. The substance for which the most people sought treatment was alcohol, followed by marijuana (cannabis), pain relievers (opioid analgesics), cocaine, and heroin. Most treatment occurred in self-help groups and drug treatment programs, with less than 30% seen in medical settings (16% in doctors' offices and 11.4% in emergency rooms). Of the 82% of individuals needing but not receiving treatment, 95% did not perceive a need, whereas 3.3% felt they needed treatment but made no effort to obtain it (Center for Behavioral Health Statistics and Quality, 2011). These statistics confirm that there are millions of undiagnosed and untreated substance abusers, most of whom are likewise unaware of having a problem. Highly motivated individuals tend to secure treatment on their own; however, the vast majority either lack problem awareness or are unwilling to change. These individuals are unlikely to come into contact with the drug treatment system, although most will have at least intermittent contact with the larger medical system. "Incidental" medical visits present opportunities to identify and intervene with active drug abusers who otherwise would go undetected and untreated, as they continue to consume a disproportionate share of costly, high-intensity medical services (Kassed, Levit, & Hambrick, 2006–2007).

In recent years, health care providers have begun to screen patients for substance use disorders. SBIRT (Screening, Brief Intervention, and Referral to Treatment), the model being promoted by the federal government, has been implemented in various medical settings, including emergency/trauma centers, primary and specialty care clinics, community health centers, and college health services (*www.samhsa.gov/prevention/SBIRT/index.aspx*). SBIRT differs from traditional psychological assessments in several ways. First, the assessment component is limited to screening, the goal of which is to identify a possible or likely problem. Second, the results of the assessment form the basis of a brief intervention (BI) that typically is delivered during the same session; interventions as simple as personalized feedback and advice to change drug use behavior have been shown to have a positive impact on substance use (Rotgers, Morgenstern, & Walters, 2003). Third, if indicated, referrals are made. Despite its brevity (15–30 minutes), SBIRT has been shown to be an efficacious and cost-effective approach to identifying and intervening with "at risk" drug abusers, including those for whom active drug use could significantly complicate or negatively affect outcomes of other medical problems (e.g., pregnancy, HIV/AIDS, organ transplant). Although SBIRT typically is delivered by medical personnel, there is no reason that psychologists who are interested in conducting substance abuse evaluations should not include it in their "toolboxes." Although SBIRT is conceptualized as a screening and early intervention model, expansion of the assessment and intervention components makes it a viable model for conducting more comprehensive evaluations that incorporate sophisticated psychological tests and evidence-based interventions.

Unfortunately, most psychologists are unfamiliar with the various assessment tools and interventions employed in the drug abuse field. This chapter familiarizes readers with the psychological and biological tools employed in detecting and evaluating the nature and severity of different types of addiction problems in both adults and teens. The psychological measures provide different types of information in order to answer key referral questions pertaining to diagnosis, comorbidity, severity, functional interference due to drug use, and readiness to change drug use behavior. Although the intervention component of the model must remain brief in these "enhanced" interventions, the fact that they will be delivered by experts in behavioral treatment means that they can be more sophisticated—employing norm-based feedback (test results) and various motivational interviewing strategies designed to help patients to recognize that they have a problem with drugs and to accept treatment. Because of their expertise in both assessment and behavioral interventions, psychologists are well positioned to conduct these evaluations.

Epidemiology of Drugs of Abuse

According to the National Survey on Drug Use and Health (Center for Behavioral Health Statistics and Quality, 2011), 22.6 million Americans ages 12 and over (8.9% of the population) reported using illicit drugs during the preceding 30 days (current use). Marijuana (cannabis) was the most frequently used drug (17.4 million); 76.8% of all drug users reported using marijuana, with 60.1% using marijuana exclusively. Furthermore, of the 39.9% (9.0 million) who reported using drugs other than marijuana, only 23.2% did not use marijuana. Although marijuana use is highly prevalent, many people (including health care professionals) minimize its addictive properties. Users can develop mild, moderate, or severe substance use disorders, depending on the number of symptoms they endorse. Physically dependent individuals experience withdrawal symptoms when cessation is abrupt, including tremor, nausea, and sleep disturbances. Other physical sequelae found in heavy users include cognitive dysfunction, respiratory problems, and "amotivational" syndromes. Marijuana also can precipitate delirium, psychosis, and anxiety disorders. Because marijuana is the most used illicit drug, the drug for which the most people seek treatment, and a drug that is highly comorbid with psychiatric disorders, it should be screened for on a routine basis. Most toxicology screens are capable of detecting THC, the active ingredient in marijuana; in addition, cannabis-specific questionnaires (for both adults and teens) are available to assist clinicians in characterizing patients' marijuana use. After marijuana, pharmaceuticals are the next most commonly abused drugs (Center for Behavioral Health Statistics and Quality, 2011). In 2010, 7.0 million Americans reported engaging in "nonmedical" use of pharmaceuticals within the previous 30 days. Nonmedical use is defined as use without a prescription or for nontherapeutic reasons, such as getting high. Pain relievers (opioid analgesics) are the most frequently abused pharmaceuticals, followed by stimulants and sedatives. In 2010, 5.1 million reported using opioid analgesics, up from 4.7 million in 2005. Among those engaged in nonmedical use of opioid analgesics during the 12 months prior to the survey, only 17.3% obtained them from a doctor, whereas 55.0% got them from a friend or relative for free, 11.4% bought them from a friend or relative, 4.8% stole them from a friend or relative, 4.4% obtained them from a drug dealer or a stranger, and 0.4% obtained them via the Internet. Thus less than one-fifth of trafficked opioid analgesics are diverted from the original source (health care providers); rather, they are obtained from friends and family.

The prevalence of drug use varies as a function of demographic characteristics. In 2010, 21.5% of young adults, ages 18–25, reported using illicit drugs within the preceding 30 days. The most frequently used drug was cannabis (18.5%), followed by pharmaceuticals (5.9%), hallucinogens (2.0%), and cocaine (1.5%). Drug use rates were considerably lower for adults over the age of 25 (6.6%): cannabis, 4.8%; pharmaceuticals, 2.2%; and "other" drugs, < 1%. From 2002 to 2010, the percentage of adults ages 50–59 who used illicit drugs doubled (from 2.7 to 5.8%), likely reflecting an aging "baby boomer'" cohort with higher lifetime use rates. In addition to age, gender also is associated with use, with more adult males than females (11.2 vs. 6.8%) reporting previous-30-day use of cannabis (9.1 vs. 4.7%), pharmaceuticals (3.0 vs. 2.5%), and hallucinogens (0.6 vs. 0.3%). Use rates were lower for pregnant (4.4%) than nonpregnant women (10.9%), suggesting that casual users quit after learning they are pregnant. Because of the potential for serious adverse consequences to the fetus, all pregnant women should be screened for all drugs of abuse, including alcohol and tobacco. Regarding adolescents, overall use rates were similar for boys and girls ages 12–17 (9.8 vs. 9.7%); however, boys were more likely to use cannabis (8.3 vs. 6.4%), whereas girls were more likely to use pharmaceuticals (3.7 vs. 2.3%) and opioid analgesics (3.0 vs. 2.0%). Drug use rates also vary by race/ethnicity. Previous-30-day rates were highest for biracial individuals (12.5%), followed by American Indians/Alaskan Natives (12.1%), African Americans (10.7%), European Americans (9.1%), Hispanics (8.1%), Native Hawaiians/Pacific Islanders (5.4%), and Asian Americans (3.5%). A similar pattern was observed among youth ages 12–17: biracial (13.4%), American Indian/Alaska Native (12.7%), Hispanic (11.8%), African American (10.8%), European American (9.7%), Hawaiian/Pacific Islander (4.6%),

and Asian American (4.1%). Risk factors for previous-30-day drug use also include education, employment, and geography. College graduates have the lowest rate (6.3%), and those not graduating from high school the highest rate (10.8%). However, a different pattern was observed for "lifetime" use, with college graduates (52.0%) and those with some college (56.2%) reporting higher rates compared with high school graduates (46.4%) or those not graduating from high school (38.9%). This difference between current and lifetime use likely reflects more experimentation and less frequent use among those with more education. Similarly, fully employed adults had the lowest rate of drug use (8.4%), followed by those employed part time (11.2%); unemployed persons had the highest levels of current drug use (17.5%). Overall, only 65.9% of drug users were employed (either part time or full time). Drug use patterns also vary by geography, being highest in the West (11.0%), followed by the Northeast (9.4%), Midwest (8.2%), and South (7.8%).

Finally, substance abuse is highly prevalent among patients with selected medical conditions or who are being treated in certain settings. For example, although 14% of persons with HIV/AIDS contracted the disease through injection drug use, overall rates of substance abuse are much higher. A study conducted among primary care patients with HIV (Newville & Haller, 2010) revealed that 47% of patients met DSM-IV diagnostic criteria (American Psychiatric Association, 1994) for one or more substance use disorders (8% alcohol only, 22% drugs only, 17% both). Rates of opioid abuse/dependence are higher among patients with pain compared with the general public; furthermore, within pain populations, rates are three to nine times higher among those receiving care in pain management settings (12–34%) than in primary care settings (4%) and may exceed 60% among those with a prior history of illicit drug use (Chabal, Erjavec, Jacobson, Mariano, & Chaney, 1997; Fleming, Balousek, Klessig, Mundt, & Brown, 2007; Hoffman, Olofsson, Salen, & Wickstrom, 1995; Kouyanou, Pither, & Wessely, 1997; Reid et al., 2002; Manchikanti, Fellows, Damron, Pampati, & McManus, 2005).

Comorbidity

National surveys conducted over three decades have found that substance use and psychiatric disorders are highly comorbid. Individuals with mood and anxiety disorders are roughly twice as likely to have a drug use disorder and vice versa. Findings are similar for other psychiatric disorders, including antisocial syndromes (antisocial personality and conduct disorder). There are several possible explanations for this. First, drug abuse can cause symptoms of other mental illnesses; for example, cannabis use increases the risk for psychosis in vulnerable persons. Second, patients with mental illness may use drugs to manage their symptoms. Third, drug dependence and mental illnesses are caused by common factors, including brain deficits and genetic and environmental factors. Relationships among substance use and psychiatric disorders can be complex. For instance, the link between drug abuse and untreated attention-deficit/hyperactivity disorder (ADHD) in youth occurs primarily among those who also have conduct problems (*www.drugabuse.gov/researchreports/comorbidity/whatis.html*).

Psychiatric and substance abuse comorbidity is especially common among certain medical populations. For instance, in a sample of 228 patients with HIV/AIDS (Newville & Haller, 2010), only 22% had no psychiatric or substance use disorder, whereas 30% had psychiatric disorders, 8% substance use disorders, and 40% both psychiatric and substance disorders (based on the University of Michigan version of the Composite International Diagnostic Interview [UM-CIDI]). Among those with both psychiatric and substance use disorders, the most prevalent psychiatric disorders were major depression (91%), panic disorder (35%), dysthymia (34%), and generalized anxiety disorder (32%). Among a cohort of patients with chronic pain and opioid (analgesic) abuse/dependence, 93% qualified for lifetime psychiatric disorders, including depression (85%) and anxiety (61%), with 55% meeting criteria for serious mental illness (e.g., bipolar disorders or recurrent major depression). Two-thirds (67.5%) had a current psychiatric disorder, whereas 37.5% had two or more psychiatric disorders; 22.5% had "double depression." The lifetime comorbidity rate for opioid and other substance use disorders was 52.5%: alcohol (42.5%), cannabis (17.5%), cocaine (10%), sedatives (7.5%), and other drug abuse/dependence (15%), all based on the Structured Clinical Interview for DSM-IV (SCID; Haller & Acosta, 2010). A study testing a behavioral intervention that targeted substance use in patients who were denied organ transplantation due to recent (previous 6 months) drug use produced similar findings, with 53% meeting diagnostic criteria for at least one current non-substance-use psychiatric disorder, based on the Composite International Diagnostic Interview—Short Form (CIDI-SF); this rate increased to 90% when comorbid substance use disorders were included (37% drug and 48% alcohol). Furthermore, based on the Addiction Severity Index (ASI), self-reported substance use among patients who were expected to be abstinent was high: alcohol, 37%; cocaine, 29%; cannabis, 16%; heroin, 5%; and hallucinogens, 3%; 29% reported current polysubstance use (Haller, unpublished data). Medical patients who have psychiatric or drug use disorders should be cross-screened. This includes screening patients with alcohol disorders for drug abuse, and vice versa.

Abuse of Prescribed (Licit) Drugs

"Prescription drug abuse" is an ambiguous term that encompasses misuse of both illicit (nonprescribed) and licit (legally prescribed) pharmaceuticals. Illicit use of pharmaceuticals is a rapidly growing problem in this country, but licit use also may result in addiction for some individuals. Unfortunately, diagnosing an addictive disorder in someone who is using a drug for a legitimate medical purpose is difficult, as our definitions are based on experiences with addicted, rather than medical, populations (Jaffe, 1992; Rinaldi, Steindler, Wilford, & Goodwin, 1988). Under DSM-IV, different sets of diagnostic criteria were used to establish abuse and dependence diagnoses; these were applied to patients taking prescribed medications, even though no studies confirmed their predictive value for this population. In fact, the use of DSM-IV criteria often was inappropriate given that tolerance and dependence (two cardinal features of "dependence" under DSM-IV nomenclature) may have little or no meaning in situations in which patients are being maintained on high-dose opioids for chronic pain. For this reason, providers often focus more on "aberrant drug-taking behaviors" (Table 6.1) that are predictive of abuse of prescribed drugs. Although it is not yet clear how DSM-5 will perform compared with DSM-IV, the fact that only two symptoms (from either the abuse or dependence categories) are needed to get a diagnosis of substance use disorder (mild) likely will produce more diagnoses among medically

ill patients maintained on prescribed medications with abuse liability. If so, then rates of substance use disorders will climb due to changes in diagnostic criteria.

Although most patients take their medications as prescribed, some do not. Epidemiological data (provided earlier) allow insight into which patients may be at increased risk. For instance, an adolescent with ADHD and conduct problems is more likely to engage in drug abuse behaviors than one without conduct disorder. Similarly, individuals with a history of illicit drug use are at risk for engaging in aberrant drug-taking behaviors when prescribed opioids for treatment of pain (Manchikanti et al., 2005; Passik, Kirsh, Donaghy, & Portenoy, 2006). For this reason, at-risk individuals and those with a known history of substance abuse should be carefully evaluated prior to prescribing medications with abuse liability. In some instances, therapy will need to proceed, despite the patient being "at risk." When prescribing drugs with abuse liability to at-risk patients, the following scenarios should be considered: (1) "relapse" (in abstinent patients), including to use of drugs in the same drug class as those previously abused (e.g., opioid analgesics in patients with a history of heroin dependence); (2) "switching" from illicit to licit drugs in the same drug class (e.g., opioids instead of heroin); (3) "supplemental use," wherein patients continue to use other drugs in the same class in combination with prescribed medication (to increase the overall dose); and (4) "mixing" drugs from different drug classes in order to achieve a desired effect (e.g., using prescribed opioids in combination with cocaine, i.e., "speedball") or alcohol. In the absence of any risk factors for drug abuse, some patients may develop "iatrogenic addiction." If the prescribing physician is unaware of these possibilities or ignores telltale signs that a problem exists, he or she may (inadvertently) become the supplier of licit drugs used for illicit purposes. This possibility was brought to light in a *New York Times* cover article (Rosenberg, 2007) titled "When Is a Pain Doctor a Pusher?"

When medical patients abuse prescribed medications, it is important to distinguish true addiction from "pseudoaddiction" (Weissman & Haddox, 1989). Pseudoaddic-

TABLE 6.1. Behaviors That Raise the Suspicion of Addiction or Abuse of Prescribed Drugs

Probably more predictive	Probably less predictive
• Selling prescription drugs	• Aggressive complaining about the need for higher doses
• Prescription forgery	• Drug hoarding during periods of reduced symptoms
• Stealing or "borrowing" drugs from another patient	• Requesting specific drugs
• Injecting oral formulations	• Obtaining prescriptions from multiple providers
• Obtaining prescription drugs from nonmedical sources	• Acquisition of similar drugs from other medical sources
• Concurrent abuse of related illicit drugs	• Unsanctioned dose escalation once or twice
• Multiple dose escalations despite warnings	• Unapproved use of the drug to treat another symptom
• Multiple episodes of lost/stolen prescriptions	• Reporting psychic effects not intended by physician

Note. Adapted from Portenoy (1994) with permission from the International Association for the Study of Pain (IASP). This table may not be reproduced for any other purpose without permission.

tion is characterized by behaviors that resemble addiction (e.g., drug-seeking behavior) that result from undertreatment. Pseudoaddiction is of particular concern for patients receiving opioids because undertreatment of pain provokes drug-seeking behaviors and other aberrant drug-taking behaviors even among those without addiction problems (Schnoll & Weaver, 2003). The treatments for addiction and pseudoaddiction are likely to be different. When undertreated patients (i.e., pseudoaddicts) are given adequate doses of opioid analgesics, their drug-seeking behavior typically subsides; in contrast, those with true addiction may require formal drug treatment and may also need to be tapered off pain medication if unable to adhere. Given the potential adverse consequences of opioid analgesic abuse among patients with pain, it is recommended that candidates for opioid therapy be screened before initiating opioid therapy, as well as after should warning signs emerge. A variety of measures are available to assess for both risk for and current abuse (see Table 6.2).

Medical Marijuana

Some patients use THC (the active ingredient in cannabis) as medicine. In 1985, the Food and Drug Administration (FDA) approved Marinol, a synthetic form of THC, as an antiemetic for use by cancer chemotherapy patients; in 1991, approval also was given for its use as an appetite stimulant for AIDS-related weight loss. In 1999, once it became clear that Marinol was not being diverted for illicit use, it was reclassified from a Schedule II to a Schedule III drug (*www.deadiversion.usdoj.gov/fed_regs/rules/1999/fr0702. htm*), opening the door for "off label" use for other medical indications. Research has confirmed that active cannabis ingredients have therapeutic potential for pain, nausea, anorexia, and ocular pressure. Several cannabinoid-based medications (Marinol and Cesamet) are FDA approved; Sativex, a mixture of plant-derived THC and cannabidiol, formulated as a mouth spray, is approved in Canada and Europe for cancer pain, spasticity, and neuropathic pain in multiple sclerosis. Despite availability of these approved products, many patients prefer to smoke marijuana to address their medical complaints. In 1996, California passed Proposition 215, the "medical marijuana" initiative; currently, smoked marijuana may be used for medical reasons in 16 states and the District of Columbia (*www.drugabuse. gov/tib/marijuana.html*). Although the intent of this act was compassionate, the availability of medical marijuana has led to misuse, abuse, and "self-treatment" of medical conditions for which efficacy has not been proven. Furthermore, in jurisdictions in which medical marijuana is not available, many people use illicit marijuana for medical purposes. Because cannabis is the most abused drug in our society, sanctioned for medical use in many jurisdictions, and used to "self-treat" medical problems in others, it is imperative to screen for use when evaluating medical patients for possible drug abuse problems.

Stimulants

Stimulant drugs such as Adderall, which are prescribed for ADHD, HIV/AIDS, and other legitimate medical conditions, may be misused by the patient and/or diverted for recreational purposes. This problem is more prevalent among young people who have been prescribed stimulants for attention deficit and hyperactivity. Because formal ADHD evaluations may not be conducted prior to making a diagnosis, many prescriptions are written for individuals without clear-cut problems. Accordingly, if a patient with presumptive ADHD is referred for misuse of stimulants, the evaluation should include a formal ADHD evaluation.

Introduction to Drug Abuse Assessment

Medical patients with substance use disorders tend to identify themselves as patients rather than addicts. To decrease resistance during the evaluation, it is important to avoid using pejorative terms such as "addict." If the problem involves misuse of opioid analgesics, for instance, we recommend using the term "medication mismanagement." Treating drug abuse as a medical problem lessens defensiveness and makes patients more amenable to discussing the impact that drug use has on their health. For instance, educating the patient about the impact of cocaine use on hypertension can be helpful. A non-

TABLE 6.2. Psychosocial Measures of Drug Abuse

Test/interview	Population	No. of items	Substances assessed	Diagnosis or severity	Cost/restrictions on use	Languages
Screeners						
Generic self-report questionnaires						
CRAFFT (Car, Relax, Alone, Forget, Friends, Trouble; Knight et al., 1999)	Teens	6	Not drug-specific	Severity	Public domain	English, Chinese, Haitian Creole, French, Japanese, Khmer, Laotian, Portuguese, Spanish, Vietnamese
Drug Abuse Screening Test (DAST; Skinner, 1982)	Adults	10, 20, or 28	Not drug-specific	Severity	Public domain	English
Drug Use Disorders Identification Test (DUDIT; Berman, Bergman, Palmstierna, & Schlyter, 2005)	Adults	11	Not drug-specific	Severity	Public domain	English, Spanish, Swedish
Drug Use Disorders Identification Test—Extended (DUDIT-E; Berman, Palmstierna, Kallmen, & Bergman, 2007)		44				
Drug Use Screening Inventory—Revised (DUSI-R; Tarter, 1990)[a]	Adults and teens	159	Not drug-specific	Severity	$3/paper copy; $495/computer administration and scoring	English, Chinese, Danish, Dutch, Finnish, German, Norwegian, Portuguese, Russian, Spanish, Swedish, Turkish
Global Assessment of Individual Needs Short Screener (GAIN-SS; Dennis, Feeny, & Stevens, 2006)	Adults and teens	23	Not drug-specific	Severity	Copyrighted	English, Spanish
Personal Experiences Inventory (PEI; Winters & Henly, 1989)	Teens	276	Not drug-specific	Severity	Kit—$135	English, Spanish
Personal Experience Screening Questionnaire (PESQ; Winters, 1992)	Teens	40	Not drug-specific	Severity	Kit—$99, $43 for 25 tests	English

(continued)

93

TABLE 6.2. *(continued)*

Test/interview	Population	No. of items	Substances assessed	Diagnosis or severity	Cost/restrictions on use	Languages
Problem-Oriented Screening Inventory for Teenagers (POSIT; Rahdert, 1991)	Teens	139	Not drug-specific	Severity	Public domain	English, Spanish
Substance Abuse Subtle Screening Inventory (SASSI; Lazowski, Miller, Boye, & Miller 1998)[a]	Adults and teens	12 alcohol; 14 drug; 65 general	Not drug-specific	Severity	$125/25 tests	English, Spanish
RAFFT (Relax, Alone, Friends, Family, Trouble; Bastiaens, Francis, & Lewis, 2000; Bastiaens, Riccardi, & Sakhrani, 2002)	Adults and teens	5	Not drug-specific	Severity	Public domain	English, Spanish
			Drug-specific self-report screens			
Benzodiazepine Dependence Self-Report Questionnaire (Bendep-SRQ; Kan, Breteler, Timmermans, van der Ven, & Zitman, 1999)	Adults	Long form: 30 (no attempt to quit); 40 (if attempts to quit)	Benzodiazepines	Severity; problem use; preoccupation; lack of compliance; withdrawal	Public domain	English, Spanish, Dutch, German
Adolescent Cannabis Problems Questionnaire (CPQ-A; Martin, Copeland, Gilmour, Gates, & Swift, 2006)	Teens	Core items: 30; parent: 5; boy-/girlfriend: 5; school: 9; work: 9; total: 58	Cannabis	Severity	Public domain	English, Spanish, French
Cannabis Problems Questionnaire (CPQ; Copeland, Gilmore, Gates, & Swift, 2005)	Adults	22	Cannabis	Severity	Public domain	English, Spanish, French

94

Instrument	Population	Items	Substance	Construct	Cost	Languages
Cannabis Use Disorders Identification Test (CUDIT; Adamson & Sellman, 2003)	Adults	10	Cannabis	Severity; screens for DSM-IV diagnoses	Public domain	English, Spanish
Cannabis Use Disorders Identification Test—Revised (CUDIT-R; Adamson et al., 2010)		8				
Problematic Use of Marijuana (PUM; Okulicz-Kozaryn, 2007)	Adults	8	Cannabis	Severity; IDC-10 harmful use; psychosocial consequences	Public domain	English, Spanish, Portuguese
Cannabis Use Screening Test (CAST; Legleye, Karila, Beck, & Reynaud, 2007)	Adults and teens	6	Cannabis	Severity; psychosocial consequences	Public domain	English, Spanish, German, Chinese, Polish, French
Marijuana Screening Inventory—Experimental Version (MSI-X; Alexander, 2003)	Adults	39	Cannabis	Severity	Public domain	English, Spanish
Severity of Amphetamine Dependence Questionnaire (SAmDQ; Churchill, Burgess, Pead, & Gill, 1993)	Adults	14	Amphetamines	Severity	Public domain	English
Severity of Dependence Scale (SDS general: Gossop et al., 1995; alcohol: Lawrinson, Copeland, Gerber, & Gilmour, 2007; benzodiazepines: de la Cuevas, Sanz, de la Fuente, Padilla, & Berenguer, 2000; cannabis: Martin, Copeland, Gates, & Gilmour, 2006; cocaine: Kaye & Darke, 2002)	Adults and teens	5	Alcohol. amphetamines, benzodiazepines, cannabis, cocaine	Severity	Public domain	English, Spanish, Lithuanian, Czech

(continued)

TABLE 6.2. *(continued)*

Test/interview	Population	No. of items	Substances assessed	Diagnosis or severity	Cost/restrictions on use	Languages
Opioid Risk Tool (ORT; Webster & Webster, 2005)	Adults	5	Prescription opioids	Likelihood of prescription opioid misuse	Copyrighted (use with author's permission)	English
Pain Medication Questionnaire (PMQ; Adams et al., 2004)	Adults	26	Prescription opioids	Severity	Contact author for permission (no mention of cost)	English, Spanish
Prescription Drug Use Questionnaire (PDUQ; Compton, Darakjian, & Miotto, 1998)	Adults	42	Prescription opioids	Severity	Public domain	English, Spanish
Screener and Opioid Assessment for Patients with Pain (SOAPP-V1; Butler, Budman, Fernandez, & Jamison, 2004)	Adults being considered for opioid treatment	5, 14, or 24	Prescription opioids	Likelihood of prescription opioid misuse	Available to registered users at *www.painedu.org*; copyright: *PainEDU@Inflexxion.com*	English, Spanish
Screener and Opioid Assessment for Patients with Pain—Revised (SOAPP-R; Butler, Budman, Fernandez, Fanciullo, & Jamison, 2009)		24				
Current Opioid Misuse Measure (COMM; Butler et al., 2007)	Adults prescribed opioids for chronic pain	17 (original had 40)	Prescription opioids	Adherence to opioid therapy for pain	Available to registered users at *www.painedu.org*; copyright: *PainEDU@Inflexxion.com*	English, Spanish

Embedded drug abuse screens (scales in larger tests)

Test/interview	Population	No. of items	Substances assessed	Diagnosis or severity	Cost/restrictions on use	Languages
Minnesota Multiphasic Personality Inventory (MMPI-2; Butcher, Dahlstrom, Graham, Tellegen, & Kaemmer, 1989)[a]	Adults	567	Not drug-specific	Severity	Scoring kit with 10 test booklets—$700	English, Spanish, French, Hmong

Addiction Potential Scale (APS)
Addiction Admission Scale (AAS)

Instrument	Population	Items	Drug specificity	Type	Cost	Languages
Minnesota Multiphasic Personality Inventory for Adolescents (MMPI-A; Butcher et al., 1992)	Teens	478	Not drug-specific	Severity	Scoring kit with 10 test booklets—$590	English, Spanish
Millon Behavioral Medicine Diagnostic (MBMD; Millon, Antoni, Millon, Meagher, & Grossman, 2001)[a]	Adults	165	Not drug-specific	Severity	Manual—$53 Test booklets—$28.75 per 10 CD—$53.50 Computer software—$89 desktop; $250 networked	English, Spanish, French
Millon Clinical Multiaxial Inventory–III (MCMI-III; Millon, 1994)[a]	Adults	175	Not drug-specific	Severity	Starter kit—$347	English
Alcohol, Smoking and Substance Involvement Screening Test (ASSIST; WHO ASSIST Working Group, 2002)	Adults	8 per substance	NIDA 5, inhalants, sedatives, hallucinogens, other (including tobacco and alcohol)	Severity	Copyrighted; free to use	English, Spanish, Arabic, Farsi, French, German, Hindi, Portuguese, Russian, Ukranian
Comprehensive Adolescent Severity Index for Adolescents (CASI-A; Meyers, McLellan, Jaeger, & Pettinati, 1995)	Teens	Varies	Not drug-specific	Severity	Public domain; training costs $2,000	English, Spanish
Composite International Diagnostic Interview–Substance Abuse Module (CIDI-SAM; Cottler, 2000)[a]	Adults	38	NIDA 5, inhalants, sedatives, club drugs, hallucinogens, caffeine, other	Diagnosis	$35 for paper/pen version, $500 for computerized version	English, Spanish

(continued)

TABLE 6.2. *(continued)*

Test/interview	Population	No. of items	Substances assessed	Diagnosis or severity	Cost/restrictions on use	Languages
University of Michigan Composite International Diagnostic Interview (UM-CIDI; Kessler, 2002)	Adults	Depends on modules administered	All drugs of abuse and alcohol	Substance use and psychiatric disorders (DSM-IV)	Public domain	English, Spanish
MINI-International Neuropsychiatric Interview (MINI and eMINI; Sheehan et al., 1998)[a]	Adults	Depends on modules administered	All drugs of abuse and alcohol	Diagnosis (DSM-IV)	Public domain (paper); $400 for (eMINI)	English, Spanish, French, Chinese
In-depth assessments						
Full interviews						
Addiction Severity Index—5th Edition (ASI; McLellan et al., 1992)[a]	Adults	161	All drugs of abuse and alcohol	Severity of addiction problems and psychosocial consequences	Public domain	English, Spanish, French, Chinese, Arabic, Russian
Addiction Severity Index–Lite (ASI-Lite; McLellan, Cacciola, & Zanis, 1997)	Adults	139	All drugs of abuse and alcohol	Severity of addiction problems and psychosocial consequences	Public domain	English, Spanish, French, Chinese, Arabic, Russian
Teen Addiction Severity Index (T-ASI; Kaminer, Bukstein, & Tarter, 1991)	Teens	154	All drugs of abuse and alcohol	Severity of addiction problems and psychosocial consequences	Public domain	English, Spanish, Russian, Chinese

Instrument	Age	Items	Drugs	Severity/Diagnosis	Cost	Languages
Adolescent Diagnostic Interview (ADI; Winters, Stinchfield, Fulkerson, & Henly, 1993)	Teens	213 (skip patterns when initial question is not endorsed)	Not drug-specific	Severity	Manual—$53; $42 for 5 tests	English, Spanish
Adolescent Drug Abuse Diagnosis (ADAD; Friedman & Utada, 1989)	Teens	150	NIDA 5, sedatives, stimulants, inhalants, hallucinogens, other	Both	Public domain	English, Spanish
Composite International Diagnostic Interview (CIDI; Robins et al., 1988)[a]	Adults and teens	20 major, 59 subquestions	NIDA 5, stimulants, hallucinogens, inhalants, barbiturates, sedatives	Diagnosis	Four-day training session to get the scoring program; costs $1,100	English, Spanish, Chinese, French, Russian
Mini-International Neuropsychiatric Interview (MINI and eMINI; Sheehan et al., 1998) MINI-International Neuropsychiatric Interview (MINI-KID; Sheehan et al., 1998)	Adults and teens	16 modules, 8–10 items each	NIDA 5, stimulants, hallucinogens, inhalants, barbiturates, sedatives, ASP	Diagnosis	Copyrighted; paper versions can be downloaded for free with permission Electronic version available from MOS for unlimited use at $400	English, Spanish, Russian, Chinese, French, Arabic
Structured Clinical Interview for DSM—Axis I Disorders (SCID-I; First, Gibbon, Spitzer, & Williams, 1996)	Adults and teens	226 total (skips sections when the initial question is not endorsed)	NIDA 5, sedatives, stimulants, hallucinogens, other	Diagnosis	Administration booklet—$59 5 scoresheets—$60.50 Purchased together—$101	English, Spanish

Note. More available at *http://pubs.niaaa.nih.gov/publications/Assesing%20Alcohol/factsheets.pdf.* NIDA 5 drugs are cannabinoids, cocaine, amphetamines, opiates, and phencyclidine.
[a]Computerized versions available.

99

judgmental approach is key; if the patient believes the evaluator is likely to be critical of his or her "bad behavior," it is less likely that accurate or complete information will be provided. Treating addiction as a medical problem also unburdens the psychologist, who no longer is in the position of having to confront patients about their bad or illegal behavior. Psychologists who perform the type of evaluations presented in this chapter need not be substance abuse experts, as their roles are limited to identifying drug abuse as a possible problem and assisting patients in making health care decisions—something psychologists do every day. That said, psychologists who lack expertise in addictions may benefit from a "model" for assessing these patients that is consistent with state-of-the-art practice in the drug abuse world. Within this "frame," the administration, scoring, and interpretation of substance abuse measures is only a first step, to be followed by some form of brief intervention and a referral for care if indicated.

SBIRT: A Model for Evaluating Patients for Drug Abuse

SBIRT is a "comprehensive and integrated approach to the delivery of early intervention and treatment services through universal screening for persons with substance use disorders and those at risk" (Babor, McRee, Kassebaum, Grimaldi, & Ahmed, 2007). Research focusing on the individual components of the model has produced valid screening tools, efficacious brief interventions, and valuable insights into implementation. In addition, clinical trials also have produced considerable evidence supporting the model's short-term benefits with regard to drug use and health, although long-term effects are unproven (Babor et al., 2007). The model, designed specifically for use in medical settings, has been successfully implemented in emergency departments, trauma centers, primary care, and specialty medical clinics and, more recently, in community-based health settings, including college counseling centers. Based on efficacy and cost-effectiveness data, the Center for Substance Abuse Treatment (CSAT) now plans to implement SBIRT throughout the entire health care delivery system.

As SBIRT has been more widely disseminated, the scope of the individual components of the model has broadened. Although the screening component originally targeted persons at risk, it now is being used to identify those with more severe addiction problems. Screening evaluations should be used with persons at risk and those who are displaying misuse behavior. Although most patients will screen negative, thus negating the need for steps 2 and 3 of SBIRT, some unknown percentage will screen positive, necessitating BIs and/or referral to drug treatment.

SBIRT should be completed in a single session, allowing 15 minutes per component. Screening tools include both questionnaires and biomarkers. In addition to BIs (i.e., one to two visits to provide information, give advice, and motivate people to change), the model now accommodates brief treatments (i.e., two to six sessions of motivational and/or cognitive-behavioral therapy [CBT] for those at higher risk). Finally, the referral component has grown to include a greater focus on care coordination and integration, which is important because drug treatment programs operate independently from medical services, making it easy for simple referrals to fail, especially in situations in which the patient is ambivalent about change. Based on efficacy and cost-effectiveness data, CSAT plans to implement SBIRT throughout the entire health care delivery system (*www.samhsa.gov/samhsaNewsletter/Volume_17_Number_6/SBIRT.aspxcitation*). Current Procedural Terminology (CPT) codes have been established for commercial insurance carriers, Medicare, and Medicaid. Rates are low, but the amount of time devoted to each component is brief, typically 15–30 minutes; when multiple components of SBIRT are administered, reimbursement is more favorable. Medical psychologists should be aware that primary care and emergency room personnel are being trained to deliver SBIRT. The commitment on the part of the Substance Abuse and Mental Health Services Administration (SAMHSA) to this initiative is evidenced by $3.75 million in grant funding to train medical residents to implement this "evidence-based" approach.

Although the populations being screened using SBIRT have broadened considerably as the model has been disseminated, the assessment component remains minimal in the amount and type of information that may be derived from basic screening tools. This is purposeful by design, as the model was designed to be implemented primarily by medical and other non-mental health staff. At the same time, the entire model holds promise for use by psychologists who are charged with conducting substance abuse consultations in medical settings. In most instances, such evaluations focus mainly on the assessment component, whereas the intervention and referral components are minimal or altogether absent. When working with drug abusers, failure to employ test results to intervene is a wasted opportunity to provide information, increase awareness, address ambivalence regarding substance use, and enhance motivation to change. Psychologists who practice in medical settings may or may not be interested in conducting large-scale screening efforts in at-risk populations using standard SBIRT strategies. However, they may be interested in adopting the overall SBIRT strategy, which has been proven to be efficacious, albeit with an expanded assessment protocol that includes screening tools, structured clinical interviews, and standard psychological tests. To summarize, we are proposing that psychologists use SBIRT as a "conceptual model," with patients receiving either screening or evaluative assessments in combination with brief behavioral interventions and referral as part of a complete evaluation. The intervention component may be as limited as feedback and advice to change drug use behavior or as extensive as a brief treatment using motivational interviewing and/or CBT strategies.

Methods for Evaluating Patients for Drug Abuse Problems

Biomarkers

Primary care providers are mandated to screen for alcohol- and tobacco-related problems (National Guideline Clearinghouse, 2004), though not for drug abuse. In medical settings, screening for drugs of abuse typically is done with the help of biomarkers. Toxicology screens are used in emergency rooms when the visit is drug-related and in specialty clinics serving popu-

lations with high rates of substance abuse. Pregnant women may be screened because the consequences of fetal exposure can be severe. Finally, some pain management programs assess patients prior to initiating opioid therapy in hopes of avoiding problems down the road. Although biomarkers are the "gold standard" for detecting drug use in medical patients, they have a number of limitations that must be recognized. First, most have brief windows of detection (i.e., the amount of time during which a particular drug is detectable in the body). As a consequence, sporadic users and those who are capable of abstaining for several days prior to a scheduled drug test are unlikely to be detected. For standard biological tests such as blood and urine tests to accurately identify drug users, testing must be frequent and random. Table 6.3 shows the windows of detection for various biomarkers. Detection windows are brief for blood and urine, but as long as 90 days for hair and nails. Detection windows vary by drug as well as by test; for example, cocaine is detectable in urine for only 1–3 days, whereas cannabis may be found for several months if use is heavy. Using standard biomarkers means some drugs are more likely to be detected than others, which, in turn, may significantly affect treatment decisions. For instance, findings from a recent study of substance abusers seeking organ transplants showed that hair testing produced twice as many cocaine- and opioid-positive results as urine toxicology or self-report (Haller et al., 2010). Although 6 months of continuous abstinence is required prior to transplantation, standard biomarkers are unable to assess ongoing abstinence; rather, they assess only within the specified window of detection. For this reason, patients who are tested using conventional biomarkers are more likely to go undetected and, therefore, are more likely to have surgery while actively using drugs. Although many psychologists are unfamiliar with biomarkers, those who wish to conduct drug abuse evaluations in medical settings need to understand their benefits and limitations. A positive result is proof of use within the specified window of detection and also may be used to refute a negative self-report; however, it provides no information about whether or not a problem exists and, if so, how severe it may be. Accordingly, biomark-

TABLE 6.3. Biomarkers for Detecting Drug Abuse in Medical Patients

	Urine immunoassay (screen)	Blood (screen)	Hair/nails (screen)	Sweat wipe and patch (screen)	Saliva (screen)	GC/MS (confirmation)
Detectable substances	NIDA 5, benzodiazepines, barbiturates, methadone, buprenorphine, alcohol	NIDA 5*, alcohol	NIDA 5*, benzodiazepines, barbiturates	NIDA 5	NIDA 5, alcohol	Confirmation of urinalysis results; distinguish between members of a class (alprazolam vs. diazepam); synthetic opiates (such as fentanyl, buprenorphine, oxycodone)
Typical cost	$10 per test	Up to $200 per test	$75–100 per test	$35–50 per test	$15–20 per test	$25–30 per test
Window of detection	Drug dependent; 1–3 days (cocaine); weeks if chronic use (cannabis, benzodiazepines)	Minutes to hours; days if chronic use	7–90 days	24 hours for wipe; weeks for patch	1–48 hours	1–3 days; weeks if chronic use
Level of invasiveness	Moderate	High	Moderate	Moderate	Low	Moderate
Point of collection (POC) available?	Yes	No	No	Yes	Yes	No
Timing of results	Minutes (POC); about 24 hours (lab)	24 hours	24–72 hours	Minutes for POC wipe; about a week for patch or confirmatory test results	Minutes for POC; 24–72 hours for confirmatory test	Up to 1 week; dependent on lab used

Advantages					
Inexpensive; onsite results available	Detects acute intoxication; most sensitive method	Provides information about severity of use; unaffected by brief abstinent periods; detects chronic use; directly observable	Easy collection; patch provides prospective information; can be used for monitoring of substance use or abstinence	Can detect drug metabolites; directly observable; easy collection; detects acute intoxication	Highly sensitive and specific; can determine specific drug within a class; provides confirmation of screening results
Disadvantages					
Numerous false positives (over-the-counter medications, codeine products, poppy seeds; ibuprofen for cannabis; decongestants for amphetamines; does not detect acute intoxication	Least commonly used; short window of detection; expensive	Results can be affected by chemical processing of hair, such as dyeing, and melanin content of hair; risk of contamination by passive exposure; does not detect very recent use; requires 90–100 strands of hair	Expensive; variability in amount of sweat production	Very short window of detection; potential contamination by oral, nasal, or inhaled intake	Expensive/long turnaround time for results
Problems in interpretation					
Greatest risk of adulteration		Can be contaminated by passive exposure	Can be contaminated by passive exposure	Can be affected by food or drink; need to refrain from eating, drinking, or smoking for 10 minutes before test	
Qualitative or quantitative results					
Qualitative	Quantitative	Quantitative	Qualitative (POC) and quantitative	Qualitative (POC) and quantitative	Quantitative
Accepted for chain of custody?					
Yes	Yes	Yes	Yes	Yes	Yes

Note. NIDA 5 drugs are cannabinoids, cocaine, amphetamines, opiates (only morphine based, i.e., heroin and codeine), and phencyclidine.

ers should be viewed as "screening tests." Whenever results are positive, a more thorough assessment should be conducted to better characterize the problem.

Questionnaires, Structured Clinical Interviews, and Psychological Tests

Psychosocial evaluations used to assess drug abuse and related constructs include screening questionnaires, structured clinical interviews, and psychological/personality tests. Screening questionnaires can be administered and scored by any health care professional, including a technician. In contrast, structured clinical interviews require diagnostic knowledge; many demand considerable training to administer with fidelity, and some require formal certification. Interviews may be administered and interpreted by any well-trained mental health provider, including psychiatrists, psychologists, and clinical social workers. In contrast, only psychologists may administer and interpret certain psychological tests, as the examiner must be familiar with the psychometric properties of the test, including test construction, validity and reliability, and for which groups norms are available.

Screening Tools

Self-administered drug abuse screening questionnaires are readily available on the Internet. As these are in the "public domain," anyone can use them, including patients who may be questioning whether or not they have a problem. Screening questionnaires tend to be brief, with some having as few as five items. They are easy to score, which makes them ideal for use in situations in which feedback is to be given immediately. However, the type and amount of information produced by screening questionnaires is limited. At best, they reveal the "likelihood" that a problem exists. An example of a screening test for drug abuse is the Drug Abuse Screening Test (DAST; Table 6.2).

Self-Administered Questionnaires

Self-administered questionnaires include those targeting drug abuse (e.g., Substance Abuse Subtle Screening Inventory–3 [SASSI-3]), as well as those designed to assess broader psychopathology (Minnesota Multiphasic Personality Inventory [MMPI-2]) but that contain embedded substance abuse scales (e.g., MMPI-2). Drug-specific tests are longer and more difficult to score; however, they also provide more information. These tests, which are self-administered, can be quite lengthy. In addition, they are more difficult to score and require knowledge of psychometrics to interpret. Personality tests with embedded drug abuse scales may not be designed to detect drug abuse at all. Nevertheless, some have empirically derived scales and subscales that can be useful when considering addiction along with other psychological characteristics. The MMPI-2, for example, has three addiction subscales: the Addiction Potential Scale (APS); the Addiction Acknowledgment Scale (AAS); and the MacAndrew Alcoholism Scale (Mac-R). Unfortunately, with the exception of AAS, these scales have performed poorly in terms of their capacity to predict DSM-IV substance use disorders diagnosed via structured clinical interviews (Clements & Heintz, 2002; Svanum, McGrew, & Erhmann, 1994). The fact that the AAS scale is more sensitive is likely due to the fact that it is a direct measure of substance-related problems, whereas the other two scales are subtle. Thus, whereas a positive AAS likely indicates a problem, a negative APS or Mac-R score should not be viewed as evidence of absence of a problem.

Screening Structured Clinical Interviews

A structured clinical interview is a tool that helps providers and researchers make an accurate diagnosis or qualify the nature of a particular problem with drugs. One of the most popular structured clinical interviews is the SCID, which is capable of providing both lifetime and current (preceding 30 day) diagnoses for all DSM-IV Axis I psychiatric disorders, including alcohol and other substance use disorders. With the introduction of DSM-5, these measures will gradually be phased out. However, updated versions of SCID (both clinician and research versions), based on DSM-5 criteria, currently are being developed.

Structured clinical interviews contain standardized questions to ensure that each patient is interviewed in the same way and that different evaluators will arrive at the same conclusion (i.e., interrater reliability). "Skip patterns" are built into the test so that sections that do not apply may be eliminated from the evaluation to make it shorter and to facilitate making differential diagnoses. Whereas the SCID (all versions) is semistructured, thus allowing evaluators to "probe" when responses are unclear or incomplete, another DSM-IV-based diagnostic interview, the Mini-International Neuropsychiatric Interview (M.I.N.I.), is more proscriptive, giving the evaluator specific phraseology to employ. The M.I.N.I. has the added advantage of having a child/teen version that includes such developmental problems as attachment disorder and conduct disorder. A DSM-5 revision of this measure was recently published. In addition to the full versions of these tests, there also are several screening versions available for use in situations in which the examiner is trying quickly to determine whether someone has a substance use disorder, although these truncated exams also provide limited information that is not drug-specific. Some of these interviews also have computer-administered versions available that allow the examiner to click on criteria during the interview and that generate a printout of which criteria and which diagnoses were met. Additionally, the data are stored in a clinical database that may be used for research or quality improvement purposes. Some of these computer versions may be self-administered, although the evaluator should consider the pros and cons of this type of assessment strategy.

Description of Measures

Measurement selection should be made based on the type of evaluation being conducted (screening vs. comprehensive), the information being sought by the referral source (likely problem, diagnosis, extent of impairment), and the expertise of the psychologist conducting the evaluation. Tables 6.2 and 6.3 provide basic information about psychosocial measures and biomarkers.

Biomarkers

Table 6.3 provides information about biomarkers useful in detecting drug use, including: (1) windows of detection; (2) detectable substances; (3) level of invasiveness; (4) output (qualitative vs. quantitative); (5) costs; (6) availability of point-of-care (POC) test kits; (7) typical time required to obtain results from an outside lab; (8) advantages/disadvantages; and (9) problems in interpretation. If a biomarker is to be used as part of a screening evaluation, the only viable choice is a POC test (i.e., urine or saliva "dipsticks"). POC tests can provide the evaluator with basic information (positive or negative), which can be used for feedback purposes, in less than 5 minutes. POC tests are relatively inexpensive and can be purchased from approved companies with Clinical Laboratory Improvement Amendments (CLIA) waivers that sell direct to customers via the Internet. When using POC tests, the evaluator has the option of selecting various "panels" that screen for different drugs. A limited panel that includes five drugs (e.g., amphetamines, cocaine, benzodiazepines, opioids, and cannabis) can be purchased for about $4. More extensive panels cover as many as 12 drugs and cost about $8 per test. In addition to prepackaged panels, tests for individual drugs can be purchased for a little more than $1. Because biomarkers are easy to use and testing may be billed for using existing CPT codes for drug testing (*www.doh.wa.gov/hsqa/fsl/Documents/LQA_Docs/Waivedtests.pdf*), we recommend use of a POC drug screen along with questionnaires. Although a negative test cannot ensure abstinence (given brief and variable windows of detection), a positive test can refute a negative self-report. If a toxicology screen is positive, the psychologist may request a confirmatory test to determine what drug(s) in a given class have been ingested. A POC test can detect benzodiazepines, but a confirmatory test (employing analytical strategies such as gas chromatography/mass spectrometry [GC/MS]) is needed to differentiate Valium from Xanax or Ambien. POC tests also may be used as part of comprehensive substance abuse evaluations. When used in combination with psychosocial measures, POC tests enhance the overall validity of findings by providing a secondary data source. Other choices also are available, however. Laboratory results typically are available in 1–2 days. Therefore, if the evaluation is expected to occur across several visits, other biomarkers should be considered, as they may provide additional information. Although most biomarkers have windows of detection comparable to those of POC tests, hair and nail testing can detect drug use for up to 90 days and thus is the logical choice when the goal is to evaluate continuous abstinence, such as during pregnancy or while awaiting organ transplant.

Questionnaires and Tests

Appendix 6.1 presents two case examples illustrating measurement selection strategies. When the goal is to screen patients for possible drug use disorders, one may use brief questionnaires and/or POC drug tests. Questionnaires are self-administered and cost-effective and have relatively long windows of detection; some measure current status, whereas others inquire about the previous 30 days or 12 months. Like POC drug tests, results are immediately available for feedback purposes during the screening session. Some screening questionnaires are "generic" (non-drug-specific); others are drug-specific. The type of screening questionnaire that should be selected depends on the purpose of screening, as well as the population. For example, any drug use during pregnancy can result in adverse consequences for both mother and child; therefore, a generic screen is most appropriate for use in obstetrics clinics (e.g., the Drug Use Disorders Identification Test [DUDIT] or the DAST). In contrast, pain providers may wish to assess an individual's risk for opioid abuse before initiating opioid therapy; in this instance, the goal would be better met by using a screening tool designed specifically for this purpose (e.g., the Screener and Opioid Assessment for Patients with Pain—Revised [SOAPP-R]). Table 6.2 provides a comprehensive list of measures used to evaluate for drug abuse. These are grouped by type (questionnaire, interview, etc.), population (adult, teen, both), length, substances assessed, and output (diagnosis vs. severity, cost/availability, languages and availability of computerized versions).

Screening tests vary in the type and amount of information they provide. The DUDIT and the Cannabis Use Disorders Identification Test (CUDIT-R), patterned after the Alcohol Use Disorders Identification Test (AUDIT), employ cut scores that correspond to problem severity. Many of the items map onto both DSM-IV and DSM-5 criteria, making it possible to obtain a presumptive diagnosis in some instances. Other screening tests employ standard scores that make it possible for the patient's scores to be directly compared with those of normative samples (e.g., the SASSI). This type of information can be extremely helpful during a feedback session. Some screens assess for alcohol and drug-related problems (e.g., the SASSI), yet still lack specificity. Instruments that assess for both alcohol and drug abuse are particularly useful, because these problems are highly comorbid. However, in instances in which a generic screen is positive, additional testing is needed to define the drug problem. In general practice, we recommend starting with a broad screen. If this is positive, it can be useful to simply ask the patient what drugs he or she has used and then select follow-up screens accordingly. For instance, if the DAST is positive and the patient acknowledges marijuana use, the next step might be to administer the CUDIT-R. If it is unclear how many or what drugs are being used, the next step might be a screening interview such as the Alcohol, Smoking and Substance Involvement Screening Test (ASSIST), which was developed for the World Health Organization (WHO). The ASSIST was developed to detect substance use and related problems in primary and general medical care settings and therefore is ideal for psychologists in medical settings (*www.who.int/substance_abuse/activities/assist/en/index.html*). There may be situations in which a particular drug is of concern. In these instances, a drug-specific screen may be sufficient to answer the referral question. For example, if a pain provider is concerned that a patient with chronic pain who is being treated with opioid analgesics may be abusing prescribed medication, then the Prescription Drug Use Questionnaire (PDUQ) may be an appropriate prescreen. If the patient screens positive, a structured clinical interview may be administered to confirm an opioid use disorder. This "stepped" approach to evaluation is similar to that employed with other medical conditions, with additional tests ordered only when routine tests are abnormal.

Comprehensive substance abuse evaluations focus on: (1) diagnosis, (2) severity, (3) comorbidity, and (4) functional interference secondary to drug abuse. To make a DSM-based diagnosis, a structured clinical interview is the best option. Most diagnostic interviews are lengthy and difficult to administer, score, and interpret. Extensive training (even certification) may be required. Many of these interviews (e.g., SCID) began life as research instruments, although clinician-friendly versions now are available for some (e.g., SCID-CV). The M.I.N.I. and M.I.N.I.-Kid are easier to administer and score than SCID; additionally, a computer-administered version is available that can be self- or interviewer-administered; this instrument also is being updated for DSM-5 but is not yet commercially available; accordingly, clinicians and researchers continue to utilize the existing versions. The M.I.N.I. tests cover all drugs of abuse, including hallucinogens, inhalants, and steroids, but the examiner may "unselect" modules that are not appropriate. Because these interviews cover all DSM-based diagnoses, they are an excellent means of ascertaining both psychiatric and substance use comorbidity. Although psychologists who work in research settings are quite familiar with these measures and some savvy clinical psychologists have begun incorporating them into their test batteries, they remain underused by psychologists, but they definitely should be considered for this type of evaluation. The most widely used substance abuse measure is the Addiction Severity Index (ASI), which also is an interview. The ASI is not a diagnostic tool but rather measures problem severity for alcohol and drugs and five other areas of functioning affected by substance use: medical, psychiatric, family/social, employment, and legal. Norms also are available for many subgroups of substance abusers to allow comparisons.

Substance abuse severity (as opposed to presence/absence of diagnosis) typically is measured via questionnaires. Whereas diagnostic tests are categorical (yes–no), most severity measures are continuous. Severity measures are particularly advantageous when reevaluation is planned, as improvement (or lack thereof) can be shown. Self-report severity measures include drug abuse tests such as the SASSI and the Drug Use Screening Inventory—Revised (DUSI-R) for adults and the Personal Experiences Inventory (PEI) for teens. Some traditional psychological tests, such as MMPI-2, have "embedded" drug abuse scales. Because these tests were designed for other purposes and the items rarely correspond to actual drug use behaviors, elevations on these scales should not be considered firm evidence of a drug abuse problem. However, an elevated score should trigger a more focused substance abuse evaluation. Most severity instruments are self-report. An important exception is the ASI, a biopsychosocial measure that assesses problem severity in seven domains: alcohol, drug, medical, psychiatric, family/social, legal, and employment.

Personalized Feedback as a Universal Intervention

"Practice guidelines" for psychiatric consultations in medical settings (Bronheim et al., 1998) describe a consultation process that is far removed from the patient. Nowhere in the document does it mention that patients should: (1) receive direct feedback regarding the test results, (2) receive brief interventions to educate or motivate change, or (3) be part of the decision-making process, so far as referral is concerned. Failure to provide face-to-face feedback to anyone who tests positive for a drug use disorder should be seen as a lost opportunity. Feedback can help patients to understand the implications of drug use on their health and can motivate them to change their drug use behavior or enter treatment. Because feedback is both hard to deliver and hard to hear, we recommend using a motivational approach when sharing results of substance abuse evaluations with patients. Motivational interviewing (MI) is "a client-centered, directive method for enhancing intrinsic motivation to change by exploring and resolving ambivalence" (Miller & Rollnick, 2002, p. 25). MI uses an empathic, nonjudgmental, nonconfrontational style that assumes that patients have mixed feelings about their drug use and that ambivalence is normal. A patient may realize that his or her drug use is problematic but continue to use because he or she is obtaining some benefit from using (e.g., improved sleep, decreased stress). It is the clinician's job to help patients weigh the pros and cons of continued drug use. The goal of an MI intervention is to decrease resistance to change as evidenced through "change talk" (i.e., when a patient begins to express the need to make a change). MI is compatible with the transtheoretical model (Miller & Rollnick, 2002) in which patients progress through stages of change, beginning with precontemplation (not recognizing the need for change) through contemplation (thinking about making a change), preparation (preparing to make a change), action (changing), and maintenance (consistently making better choices). The clinician's goal is to increase the patient's intrinsic motivation to change and, once motivated to change, to assist him or her in identifying and overcoming barriers to change. By comparing patients' assessment results with those of the general population, clinicians can illustrate the severity of the problem without appearing overly critical. Provision of information about the impact of drug use on comorbid medical conditions is especially helpful. For example, a patient may not be aware that his or her cocaine use is responsible for high blood pressure and renal problems. Providing factual, nonjudgmental information on the short- and long-term consequences of drug use may help patients to decide to make a change. In fact, many individuals become aware that their drug use is problematic only once they receive feedback. For those who already are aware that their drug use is problematic (i.e., are in the contemplation stage) but who continue to use anyway, a frank discussion of the consequences of use, along with advice to reduce drug use, may assist them in changing their behavior. For some patients, providing brief feedback and advising them to change may not be effective because their problem severity is too great. In these cases, patients should be provided with feedback, advised to change, and referred for formal drug treatment.

There may be a tendency to refer all drug abusers to treatment, although this may not be necessary, and many patients simply will not go. The following guidelines will assist the psychologist in deciding when and where to refer. Patients with severe drug problems likely will require specialty care. This includes individuals who require a medically supervised taper or opioid replacement therapy (i.e., methadone or buprenorphine) or who need intensive treatment due to comorbid psychiatric conditions. Patients with "abuse" diagnoses may be able to be handled in the medical clinic, whereas those with "dependence" may require a higher level of care. Some medications to treat addiction problems can be prescribed through the medical clinic if the clinic has providers who are willing to do this. If not, patients requiring such medications as buprenorphine and naltrexone will need to be referred to addiction specialists. Patients who abuse cannabis or prescription drugs may be able to be managed in the medical clinic; in contrast, injection drug users and those using illicit drugs such as heroin, cocaine, and methamphetamine may require a higher level of surveillance than can be provided in medical clinics. Due to increased psychosocial severity among users of street drugs, ancillary services (e.g., housing, HIV-related) may be required that are not available in general medical settings. Opioid analgesic abusers who require opioids to manage chronic pain may be able to be managed in the medical system; however, modifications to clinic and prescribing practices and procedures to enhance opioid adherence likely will be required (Schnoll & Weaver, 2003). In such instances, the expertise and willingness of medical staff must be taken into consideration. Patients may wish to be treated in one or the other setting; however, staff may not be able to provide the needed services or support. In this instance, patients also will need to be referred.

Sample Feedback Session

Prior to delivering "personalized feedback" to a patient, the clinician should ask permission. Agreeing to listen to information is an initial step in the change process. Once the feedback session is concluded, it can be helpful to assess importance, confidence, and readiness to change drug use behavior using "readiness rulers" (*www.ncbi.nlm.nih.gov/books/NBK64975*). Finally, options for treatment should be discussed, if indicated. Following is a transcript from a feedback session conducted with a patient who was denied a heart transplant due to marijuana use:

CLINICIAN: I would like to share your test results with you if that's OK? Perhaps the information will help you put things in perspective so you can decide what steps you want to take.

PATIENT: I can't believe I can't get a transplant because of marijuana . . . what's the big deal anyway? I already gave up alcohol and I need something for my nerves.

CLINICIAN: You have a difficult choice to make. You don't want to quit smoking, but you can't get a new heart until you've been drug-free for 6 months.

PATIENT: I already gave up cigarettes and alcohol. I only smoke weed once in a while and I don't think it's doing me any harm.

CLINICIAN: You've already made some changes and you don't see smoking marijuana as a problem except that if you continue to smoke you can't qualify for a transplant. You have a big decision to make. Why don't we review your test results and discuss your options. Sound OK?

PATIENT: I feel I'm being forced to do something I don't want to do. What choice do I really have? Without the surgery I know I'm going to die . . .

CLINICIAN: What you decide to do is totally up to you. No one can make you quit. Quitting can be difficult, but you can do it if you really want to, and we are here to help you.

Anyway, the tests you took confirm that you quit cigarettes and alcohol, just like you said. That's great! On the other hand, you have marijuana in your system, and your test results say you qualify for "problem use." You're smoking three to four times per week and staying stoned for three to four hours at a time. You sometimes smoke more than you plan to, and you've blown off responsibilities because you were high. Your family is complaining . . . they're really frightened for you. The biggest thing is that you can't get surgery and yet you continue to use anyway. Aside from helping you manage your anxiety . . . what else is marijuana doing for you?

PATIENT: All of my friends smoke. They know I'm not supposed to, so now they avoid me. My wife is upset because she thinks I'm going to die . . . she says its suicide. After the doctor told me I needed a heart transplant, I started having panic attacks. Marijuana just takes the edge off. If I stop, can you give me something for the anxiety?

CLINICIAN: Anxiety is normal for someone who's facing what you're facing. If you decide to quit, we can discuss other ways of dealing with anxiety, including medication and counseling. You also should know that marijuana can actually make anxiety worse. You think it's helping you, but maybe it's not.

So, given what we have been talking about . . . that smoking weed is keeping you from getting a new heart, possibly causing anxiety and upsetting your family, how IMPORTANT is it for you to quit on a scale of 1 to 10, with 1 being "not at all important" and 10 being "extremely important" . . . ?

PATIENT: I guess it's a 10 when you say it that way . . .

CLINICIAN: So it's EXTREMELY IMPORTANT for you to quit smoking. You need a new heart. You don't want to die. I can see why it is so important for you to stop using. On that same scale of 1 to 10, can you tell me how CONFIDENT you are that you can quit, just like you did with cigarettes and alcohol?

PATIENT: It's going to be harder than alcohol because it's the last thing . . . maybe a 4 or 5. Maybe I can do it if I get something else for anxiety.

CLINICIAN: So it's extremely important for you to quit, but you think it's going to be pretty hard and you're not so sure you can do it. Any thoughts about what might make it easier?

PATIENT: Maybe it won't be as bad as I think. I need to focus on getting the surgery and staying alive.

CLINICIAN: You know it's going to be hard to quit, but now you're thinking maybe you can do it if you just stay focused on getting the surgery and staying alive. So, on the same 1 to 10 scale, how READY are you to give it a try?

PATIENT: If I have to wait six months to get the surgery, I guess I better get started.

The only thing I am thinking about is the anxiety. Can you give me something for the anxiety?

CLINICIAN: I can have the doctor talk to you about your medication options if you like. What about someone to talk to about all of this? Having a transplant is very stressful. There also are lifestyle changes to discuss, including medications to prevent rejection of your new heart and how to keep yourself healthy. Many people find it helps to talk to someone. We also have a group for transplant patients at this hospital. Is this something you might be interested in?

PATIENT: I'd rather do this on my own. I gave up cigarettes and alcohol, so why not pot? Can I call you if I run into trouble?

CLINICIAN: Sure. Here's my card in case you run into difficulty or change your mind about counseling. I think you've made the right decision . . . to try to save your life. Remember, since you can't be listed until you have six months' abstinence, the sooner you get started, the better.

In this vignette, the patient went from being overtly resistant about having to give up marijuana in order to get a heart transplant (despite the potentially devastating consequences of failing to do so) to expressing the importance of quitting and evidencing increased self-efficacy within the feedback session. The patient did not accept the recommendation for counseling but is interested in receiving medication for anxiety and did request a phone number from the examiner. The patient moved from the precontemplation to the contemplation stage of change during the session and now appears ready to take the next step, which would put him in preparation. This is an excellent outcome for a brief 15-minute feedback session.

Conclusions

Psychologists have an important role to play in evaluating medical patients for substance use disorders. Despite their lack of familiarity with the models and measures employed with this population, they should be able to develop competency in this area by adhering to a proven intervention model (SBIRT) and

through use of valid and reliable tests/measures designed specifically for this purpose. Substance abuse evaluations differ from other psychological evaluations in several important ways. First, there is emphasis on screening at-risk populations, such as pregnant women and individuals with HIV/AIDS or chronic pain or who are pursuing organ transplantation. The goal of screening and early intervention is to identify patients earlier in the disease process, before any medical sequelae become severe. This approach has significant public health implications. For instance, a May 2009 *New York Times* article reported that government spending related to substance abuse had reached $468 billion, with $207.2 billion going toward direct health care costs (e.g., cirrhosis, overdoses) versus $8.8 billion for prevention, drug treatment, and research (*www. nytimes.com/2009/05/28/us/28addiction. html*).

Second, the drug abuse field has produced an efficacious and cost-effective model for assessing and treating drug abusers: SBIRT. Over the years, this three-component model has expanded to include more comprehensive assessments, a greater variety of behavioral interventions, and more systems-conscious referral strategies. Given the success of SBIRT and the government's commitment to implementing the model throughout the U.S. health care system, it makes sense for psychologists, who have expertise in both assessment and brief behavioral interventions, to be "early adopters."

A third way in which substance abuse evaluations differ from other psychological evaluations involves the supplemental use of biomarkers. When evaluating patients for drug abuse problems, the use of biomarkers is strongly recommended, either as a frontline screening technique or as a means of confirming or disputing a negative self-report. Because some patients have strong incentives to deny or minimize their use of substances in situations in which a false-negative finding may have dire consequences, use of multiple methods of detection, administered sequentially, is recommended. For instance, a positive POC toxicology screen for marijuana conducted in a specialty medical clinic could be followed by the CUDIT-R to determine quantity, frequency of use, and problem severity. If both tests are positive, then a structured clinical interview should be administered to determine a diagnosis, to identify comorbid psychiatric and substance use disorders that may be complicating the patient's presentation (e.g., cannabis-induced psychotic symptoms), and/or to determine the impact of drug use on psychosocial functioning. Although some psychologists may be uncomfortable with the idea of using biomarkers, they are easy to obtain, inexpensive, and accurate (within designated windows of detection). Furthermore, because results are immediately available when POC tests are used, the findings can be incorporated into personalized feedback at the end of the evaluation component of SBIRT.

A fourth difference between substance abuse evaluations and other psychological assessments pertains to instrumentation. Many substance abuse tests are self-administered questionnaires designed to detect and gauge the severity of drug abuse problems. Some of these tests are simple to administer, score, and interpret, whereas others are more sophisticated, requiring manuals and interpretation guides with reference norms. Some psychological tests, developed to assess for broad psychopathology (e.g., MMPI-2), have substance abuse scales that can provide helpful information; however, as these tests were not designed to assess for drug abuse, they should not be used in isolation. Still, patients who are administered the MMPI-2 and who score high on the addiction subscales should be assessed further, using addiction-specific tests. Because diagnosis is critical in determining the course of treatment for drug abusers, these evaluations emphasize diagnosis more than personality characteristics and symptom severity. This shift in focus (from psychological characteristics to psychiatric diagnosis) is necessary to distinguish substance-induced and withdrawal-related syndromes from primary mood, anxiety, and psychotic disorders. For instance, cocaine withdrawal may produce symptoms consistent with major depression, but the course of symptoms is only 7–10 days. Therefore, it is critical to determine the temporal relationship between drug use, cessation, and onset of depressive symptoms, as there is no specific treatment for cocaine withdrawal. Many psychologists have basic familiarity

with the DSM criteria but are less aware of specific criteria and strategies for making a differential diagnosis when substance abuse is present. Thus a working knowledge of DSM generally is insufficient to confirm or distinguish a primary from a secondary substance use disorder or to rule out a mood or psychotic disorder that is secondary to drug use. For this reason, we strongly recommend that evaluators become fully trained in at least one diagnostic interview, such as SCID or M.I.N.I. For those who do not have the time, energy, and/or desire to participate in a formal training process, M.I.N.I. is an excellent option, as it is more structured, with built-in skip patterns, and is available in an automated version with a one-time charge for unlimited use.

Finally, adherence to the SBIRT model demands that testing psychologists conduct brief substance abuse interventions and make referrals to drug treatment as indicated. This process departs from the Practice Guidelines for Psychiatric Consultation in the General Medical Setting (Bronheim et al., 1998), but it is more appropriate to this population, whose contact with the medical system may be sporadic and who are prone to denial and minimization of their drug use. Because the focus of this chapter is on assessment, we have not gone into depth regarding these other components. However, the types of interventions that are being used are quite familiar to health psychologists, including personalized feedback, information about the relationship between drug use and health, and various MI and CBT exercises designed to decrease resistance and enhance motivation to change. In contrast, making appropriate referrals to drug treatment programs may be challenging for someone for whom substance abuse is not a focus. Some hospitals have in-house treatment programs that may serve as universal referral sources. In the absence of this resource, however, it is recommended that the testing psychologist develop a consultative relationship with an addiction expert who can provide assistance.

In this chapter, we have attempted to provide psychologists with a "road map" for conducting competent substance abuse evaluations in medical populations. To accomplish this task, we have introduced an evidence-based evaluation–early intervention model (SBIRT) designed for use in medical populations. A growing literature shows that this model is effective when applied both to at-risk individuals and to those with serious drug abuse problems being treated in emergency departments and trauma centers, primary care and specialty medical clinics, and community-based health clinics. Given SBIRT's strong track record and trajectory, it makes sense for medical psychologists to familiarize themselves with this approach and to consider adopting it as their platform for conducting this type of evaluation. In addition to promoting SBIRT as an overall framework for evaluating substance abusers, we have recommended a "stepped" evaluation process (screening, followed by more in-depth assessments) to keep assessment burden at a minimum. Finally, we have provided guidance regarding specific tests, including both biomarkers and psychosocial measures. We appreciate that biomarkers may be unfamiliar to many psychologists. However, these can be especially helpful when evaluating patients for drug use disorders and thus need to be incorporated into the psychologist's toolbox if possible. All of the tests we are recommending are valid and reliable, with sound psychometric properties. As with any other psychological tests, the evaluator will need to familiarize him- or herself with the instrument's psychometric properties and manuals. In contrast, our suggestion that medical/health psychologists make greater use of diagnostic interviews may necessitate additional training. Diagnostic evaluations are a critical component of comprehensive substance abuse evaluations because it is essential to determine primary versus secondary disorders and to rule out substance-induced and withdrawal-related syndromes. It thus is critical that psychologists not focus exclusively on substance abuse; rather, they must consider drug use disorders within the larger context of psychopathology. For psychologists who are new to substance abuse evaluations, we would suggest beginning with simple screening evaluations before progressing to more complex assessments. Perhaps this is as far as you will get; however, those who become interested in the complex interplay between substance abuse and other types of psychopathology hopefully will view these assessments as an interesting challenge.

REFERENCES

Adams, L. L., Gatchel, R. J., Robinson, R. C., Polatin, P., Gajraj, N., Deschner, M., et al. (2004). Development of a self-report screening instrument for assessing potential opioid medication misuse in chronic pain patients. *Journal of Pain and Symptom Management, 27,* 440–459.

Adamson, S. J., Kay-Lambkin, F. J., Baker, A. L., Lewin, T. J., Thornton, L., Kelly B. J., et al. (2010). An improved brief measure of cannabis misuse: The Cannabis Use Disorders Identification Test—Revised (CUDIT-R). *Drug and Alcohol Dependence, 110,* 137–143.

Adamson, S. J., & Sellman, J. D. (2003). A prototype screening instrument for cannabis use disorder: The Cannabis Use Disorders Identification Test (CUDIT) in an alcohol-dependent clinical sample. *Drug and Alcohol Review, 22,* 309–315.

Alexander, D. (2003). Clinical pilot experiences using the Marijuana Screening Inventory (MSI-X): Screening guidelines and case illustrations. *Journal of Social Work Practice in the Addictions, 3,* 29–51.

American Psychiatric Association. (1994). *Diagnostic and statistical manual of mental disorders* (4th ed.). Washington, DC: Author.

Babor, T. F., McRee, B. G., Kassebaum, P. A., Grimaldi, P. L., & Ahmed, K. (2007). Screening, brief intervention and referral to treatment (SBIRT): Toward a public health approach to the management of substance abuse. *Substance Abuse, 28,* 7–30.

Bastiaens, L., Francis, G., & Lewis, K. (2000). The RAFFT as a screening tool for adolescent substance use disorders. *American Journal on Addictions, 9,* 10–16.

Bastiaens, L., Riccardi, K., & Sakhrani, D. (2002). The RAFFT as a screening tool for adult substance use disorders. *American Journal of Drug and Alcohol Abuse, 28,* 681–691.

Berman, A. H., Bergman, H., Palmstierna, T., & Schlyter, F. (2005). Evaluation of the Drug Use Disorders Identification Test (DUDIT) in criminal justice and detoxification settings in a Swedish population sample. *European Addiction Research, 11,* 22–31.

Berman, A. H., Palmstierna, T., Kallmen, H., & Bergman, H. (2007). The self-report Drug Use Disorders Identification Test—Extended (DUDIT-E): Reliability, validity, and motivational index. *Journal of Substance Abuse Treatment, 32,* 357–369.

Bronheim, H. E., Fulop, G., Kunkel, E. J., Muskin, P. R., Schindler, B. A., Yates, Y. R., et al. (1998). Practice guidelines for psychiatric consultation in the general medical setting. *Psychosomatics, 39*(4), S8–S30.

Butcher, J. N., Dahlstrom, W. G., Graham, J. R., Tellegen, A., & Kaemmer, B. (1989). *Minnesota Multiphasic Personality Inventory (MMPI-2).* Minneapolis: University of Minnesota Press.

Butcher, J. N., Williams, C. L., Graham, J. R., Archer, R., Tellegen, A., Ben-Porath, Y. S., et al. (1992). *Minnesota Multiphasic Personality Inventory—Adolescent (MMPI-A): Manual for administration, scoring, and interpretation.* Minneapolis: University of Minnesota Press.

Butler, S. F., Budman, S. H., Fernandez, K. C., Fanciullo, G. J., & Jamison, R. N. (2009). Cross-validation of a screener to predict opioid misuse in chronic pain patients (SOAPP-R). *Journal of Addiction Medicine, 3,* 66–73.

Butler, S. F., Budman, S. H., Fernandez, K. C., Houle, B., Benoit, C., Katz, N., et al. (2007). Development and validation of the Current Opioid Misuse Measure. *Pain, 130,* 144–156.

Butler, S. F., Budman, S. H., Fernandez, K., & Jamison, R. N. (2004). Validation of a screener and opioid assessment measure for patients with chronic pain. *Pain, 112,* 65–75.

Center for Behavioral Health Statistics and Quality. (2011). *Results from the 2010 National Survey on Drug Use and Health: Summary of National Findings* (NSDUH Series H-41, HHS Publication No. SMA 11-4658). Rockville, MD: Substance Abuse and Mental Health Services Administration.

Chabal, C., Erjavec, M. K., Jacobson, L., Mariano, A., & Chaney, E. (1997). Prescription opiate abuse in chronic pain patients: Clinical criteria, incidence, and predictors. *Clinical Journal of Pain, 13*(2), 150–155.

Churchill, A. C., Burgess, P. M., Pead, J., & Gill, T. (1993). Measurement of the severity of amphetamine dependence. *Addiction, 88,* 1335–1340.

Clements, R., & Heintz, J. M. (2002). Diagnostic accuracy and factor structure of the AAS and APS scales of the MMPI-2. *Journal of Personality Assessment, 79*(3), 564–582.

Compton, P., Darakjian, J., & Miotto, K. (1998). Screening for addiction in patients with chronic pain and "problematic" substance use: Evaluation of a pilot assessment tool. *Journal of Pain and Symptom Management, 16*(6), 355–363.

Copeland, J., Gilmore, S., Gates, P., & Swift, W. (2005). The Cannabis Problems Questionnaire: Factor, structure, reliability and validity. *Drug and Alcohol Dependence, 80,* 313–319.

Cottler, L. B. (2000). *Composite International Diagnostic Interview—Substance Abuse Module (SAM).* St. Louis, MO: Washington University School of Medicine, Department of Psychiatry.

de la Cuevas, C., Sanz, E. J., de la Fuente, J. A., Padilla, J., & Berenguer, J. C. (2000). The Severity of Dependence Scale (SDS) as screening for benzodiazepine dependence: SDS validation study. *Addiction, 95,* 245–250.

Dennis, M. L., Feeny, T., & Stevens, L. H. (2006). *Global Appraisal of Individual Needs Short Screener (GAIN-SS): Administration and scoring manual for the GAIN-SS Version 2.0.1.* Bloomington, IL: Chestnut Health Systems.

First, M. B., Gibbon, M., Spitzer, R. L., & Williams, J. B. W. (1996). *User's guide for the Structured Clinical Interview for DSM-IV Disorders, Research Version* (SCID-I, Version 2.0). New York: Biometrics Research.

Fleming, M. F., Balousek, S. L., Klessig, C. L., Mundt, M. P., & Brown, D. P. (2007). Substance use disorders in a primary care sample receiving daily opioid therapy. *Pain, 8*(7), 573–582.

Friedman, A. S., & Utada, A. (1989). A method for diagnosis and planning the treatment of adolescent drug abusers: The Adolescent Drug Abuse Diagnosis (ADAD). *Journal of Drug Education, 19,* 285–312.

Gossop, M., Darke, S., Griffith, P., Hando, J., Powis, B., Hall, W., et al. (1995). The Severity of Dependence Scale (SDS): Psychometric properties of the SDS in English and Australian samples of heroin, cocaine and amphetamine users. *Addiction, 90,* 607–614.

Haller, D. L., & Acosta, M. C. (2010). Characteristics of pain patients with opioid-use disorders. *Psychosomatics, 51,* 257–266.

Haller, D. L., Acosta, M. C., Lewis, D., Miles, D. R., Schiano, T., Shapiro, P. A., et al. (2010). Hair analysis versus conventional methods of drug testing in substance abusers seeking organ transplantation. *American Journal of Transplantation, 10,* 1305–1311.

Hoffman, N. G., Olofsson, O., Salen, B., & Wickstrom, L. (1995). Prevalence of abuse and dependency in chronic pain patients. *International Journal of Addictions, 30,* 919–927.

Jaffe, J. H. (1992). Current concepts of addiction. In C. P. O'Brien & J. H. Jaffe (Eds.), *Addictive states* (pp. 1–21). New York: Raven Press.

Kaminer, Y., Bukstein, O., & Tarter, R. E. (1991). The Teen-Addiction Severity Index: Rationale and reliability. *International Journal of Addictions, 26*(2), 219–226.

Kan, C. C., Breteler, M. H. M., Timmermans, E. A. Y., van der Ven, A. H. G. S., & Zitman, F. G. (1999). Scalability, reliability, and validity of the Benzodiazepine Dependence Self-Report Questionnaire in outpatient benzodiazepine users. *Comprehensive Psychiatry, 40,* 283–291.

Kassed, C. A., Levit, K. R., & Hambrick, M. M. (2006–2007). *Hospitalizations related to drug abuse, 2005* (Statistical Brief No. 39). Rockville, MD: Agency for Health Care Policy and Research.

Kaye, S., & Darke, S. (2002). Determining a diagnostic cut-off on the Severity of Dependence Scale (SDS) for cocaine dependence. *Addiction, 97,* 727–731.

Kessler, R. C. (2002). *National Comorbidity Survey 1990–1992.* Ann Arbor, MI: Interuniversity Consortium for Political and Social Research. Available at *www.hcp.med.harvard.edu/ncs/ftpdir/Baseline%20NCS.pdf.*

Knight, J. R., Shrier, L. A., Bravender, T. D., Farrell, M., Vander Bilt, J., & Shaffer, H. J. (1999). A new brief screen for adolescent substance abuse. *Archives of Pediatrics and Adolescent Medicine, 153*(6), 591–596.

Kouyanou, K., Pither, C. E., & Wessely, S. (1997). Medication misuse, abuse and dependence in chronic pain patients. *Journal of Psychosomatic Research, 43,* 497–504.

Lawrinson, P., Copeland, J., Gerber, S., & Gilmour, S. (2007). Determining a cut-off on the Severity of Dependence Scale (SDS) for alcohol dependence. *Addictive Behaviors, 32,* 1474–1479.

Lazowski, L. E., Miller, F. G., Boye, M. W., & Miller, G. A. (1998). Efficacy of the Substance Abuse Subtle Screening Inventory—3 (SASSI-3) in identifying substance dependence disorders in clinical settings. *Journal of Personality Assessment, 71*(1), 114–128.

Legleye, S., Karila, L., Beck, F., & Reynaud, M. (2007). Validation of the CAST, a general population Cannabis Abuse Screening Test. *Journal of Substance Use, 12,* 233–242.

Manchikanti, L., Fellows, B., Damron, K. S., Pampati, V., & McManus, C. D. (2005). Prevalence of illicit drug among individuals with chronic pain in the Commonwealth of Kentucky: An evaluation of patterns and trends. *Journal of the Kentucky Medical Association, 103*(2), 55–62.

Martin, G., Copeland, J., Gates, P., & Gilmour, S. (2006). The Severity of Dependence Scale (SDS) in an adolescent population of cannabis users: Reliability, validity and diagnostic cut-off. *Drug and Alcohol Dependence, 83,* 90–93.

Martin, G., Copeland, J., Gilmour, S., Gates, P., & Swift, W. (2006). The Adolescent Cannabis Problems Questionnaire (CPQ-A): Psychometric properties. *Addictive Behaviors, 31*(12), 2238–2248.

McLellan, A. T., Cacciola, J. S., & Zanis, D. (1997). *The Addiction Severity Index— "Lite" (ASI-"Lite").* Philadelphia: Center for the Studies of Addiction, University of Pennsylvania/Philadelphia VA Medical Center.

McLellan, A. T., Kushner, H., Metzger, D., Peters, R., Smith, I., Grissom, G., et al. (1992). The fifth edition of the Addiction Severity Index. *Journal of Substance Abuse Treatment, 9,* 199–213.

Meyers, K., McLellan, A. T., Jaeger, J. L., & Pettinati, H. M. (1995). The development of the Comprehensive Addiction Severity Index for Adolescents (CASI-A): An interview for assessing multiple problems of adolescents. *Journal of Substance Abuse Treatment, 12,* 181–193.

Miller, W. R., & Rollnick, S. (2002). *Motivational interviewing: Preparing people for change* (2nd ed.). New York: Guilford Press.

Millon, T. (1994). *MCMI-III manual.* Minneapolis, MN: National Computer Systems.

Millon, T., Antoni, M., Millon, C., Meagher, S., & Grossman, S. (2001) *Millon Behavioral Medicine Diagnostic.* Minneapolis, MN: NCS Assessments.

National Guideline Clearinghouse. (2004). Screening and behavioral counseling interventions in primary care to reduce alcohol misuse: Recommendation statement. *Annals of Internal Medicine, 140*(7), 554–556.

Newville, H., & Haller, D. L. (2010). Psychopathology and transmission risk behaviors in patients with HIV/AIDS. *AIDS Care, 22*(10), 1259–1268.

Okulicz-Kozaryn, K. (2007). Evaluation of psychometric properties of the *problematic use of marijuana* (PUM) for adolescents. *Progress of Psychiatry and Neurology, 16,* 105–111.

Passik, S. D., Kirsh, K. L., Donaghy, K. B., & Portenoy, R. K. (2006). Pain and aberrant drug-related behaviors in medically ill patients with and without histories of substance abuse. *Clinical Journal of Pain, 22*(2), 173–181.

Portenoy, R. K. (1994) Opioid therapy for chronic nonmalignant pain: Current status. In H. L. Fields & J. C. Liebeskind (Eds.), *Progress in pain research and management* (Vol. 1, pp. 247–287). Seattle, WA: IASP Press.

Rahdert, E. (Ed.). (1991). *Adolescent Assessment/Referral System manual.* Washington, DC: National Institute on Drug Abuse.

Reid, M. C., Engles-Horton, L. L., Weber, M. B., Kerns, R. D., Rogers, E. L., & O'Connor, P. G. (2002). Use of opioid medications for chronic noncancer pain syndromes in primary care. *Journal of General Internal Medicine, 17*(3), 173–179.

Rinaldi, R. C., Steindler, E. M., Wilford, B. B., & Goodwin, D. (1988). Clarification and standardization of substance abuse terminology. *Journal of the American Medical Association, 259,* 555–557.

Robins, L. N., Wing, J., Wittchen, H. U., Helzer, J. E., Babor, T. F., Burke, J., et al. (1988). The Composite International Diagnostic Interview: An epidemiologic instrument suitable for use in conjunction with different diagnostic systems and in different cultures. *Archives of General Psychiatry, 45,* 1069–1077.

Rosenberg, T. (2007, June 17). When is a pain doctor a pusher? *The New York Times.* Retrieved from *http://www.nytimes.com.*

Rotgers, F., Morgenstern, J., & Walters, S. T. (Eds.). (2003). *Treating substance abuse: Theory and technique* (2nd ed.). New York: Guilford Press.

Schnoll, S. H., & Weaver, M. F. (2003). Pain and addiction. *American Journal on Addictions, 12*(Suppl. 2), S27–S35.

Sheehan, D. V., Lecrubier, Y., Sheehan, K. H., Amorim, P., Janavs, J., Weiller, E., et al. (1998). The Mini-International Neuropsychiatric Interview (M.I.N.I.): The development and validation of a structured diagnostic psychiatric interview for DSM-IV and ICD-10. *Journal of Clinical Psychiatry, 59,* 22–33.

Skinner, H. A. (1982). The Drug Abuse Screening Test. *Addictive Behaviors, 7,* 363–367.

Svanum, S., McGrew, J., & Erhmann, L. (1994). Validity of the substance abuse scales of MMPI-2 in a college student sample. *Journal of Personality Assessment, 62*(3), 427–439.

Tarter, R. (1990). Evaluation and treatment of adolescent substance abuse: A decision tree method. *American Journal of Drug and Alcohol Abuse, 16,* 1–46.

Webster, L. R., & Webster, R. M. (2005). Predicting aberrant behaviors in opioid-treated patients: Preliminary validation of the Opioid Risk Tool. *Pain Medicine, 6,* 432–442.

Weissman, D. E., & Haddox, J. D. (1989). Opioid pseudo-addiction: An iatrogenic syndrome. *Pain, 36,* 363–366.

WHO ASSIST Working Group. (2002). The Alcohol, Smoking and Substance Involvement Screening Test (ASSIST): Development, reliability and feasibility. *Addiction, 97,* 1183–1194.

Winters, K. C. (1992). Development of an adolescent substance abuse screening questionnaire. *Addictive Behaviors, 17,* 479–490.

Winters, K. C., & Henly, G. A. (1989). *Personal Experience Inventory (PEI) test and manual.* Los Angeles: Western Psychological Services.

Winters, K. C., Stinchfield, R. D., Fulkerson, J., & Henly, G. A. (1993). Measuring alcohol and cannabis use disorders in an adolescent clinical sample. *Psychology of Addictive Behaviors, 7,* 185–196.

APPENDIX 6.1. Measurement Selection Examples

Case 1: Adolescent with ADHD Referred by Pediatrician

Background Information

The patient is a 13-year-old European American male referred for evaluation of a possible substance use disorder by his pediatrician, who has been treating him for ADHD for the past 4 years. During the past 6 months, his grades have fallen from B's to D's. He has skipped school and missed curfew on multiple occasions. He also was caught stealing money from his mother's purse. He has been withdrawn at home and has begun hanging out with a different peer group. Concerned about possible drug abuse, the pediatrician administered the CRAFFT, which was positive (score ≥ 2), prompting referral to the psychologist. On the CRAFFT, the patient admitted to drinking and smoking marijuana but denied using any other drugs.

Assessment Strategy

Results of CRAFFT indicate the patient should be assessed for alcohol and cannabis (at a minimum). Although the 58-item Cannabis Problems Questionnaire (CPQ-A) could be used to gauge the severity of cannabis-related problems, the fact that alcohol and conduct problems also are present suggests that the 270-item Personal Experience Inventory (PEI-A) would be a better choice. The PEI-A is not a diagnostic test, but it does provide information about problem severity for multiple drugs, other problematic behaviors, and risk factors that can be used for treatment planning purposes. The normative group was composed of teens in drug treatment. The PEI-A includes the following scales: (1) substance use problem severity (10 scales); (2) treatment receptiveness (1 scale); (3) substance use frequency/onset (20 items); (4) personal risk factors (8 scales); (5) environmental risk factors (3 scales); (6) problem screens (10 screens); and (7) validity indices (5 scales).

Case 2: HIV-Positive Inpatient with History of Opioid, Cocaine and Cannabis Abuse

Background Information

The patient is a 37-year-old African American male admitted to a medical unit for treatment of pneumocystis pneumonia; this is his third admission in a year for AIDS-related illnesses. He has a history of intravenous heroin and cocaine use. He also smokes cannabis and cigarettes (half a pack per day), and binge drinks. He is noncompliant with HIV care and last attended drug treatment (methadone clinic) 5 years ago. He is unstably housed but has disability income. Because of his drug use history, the attending physician requested a substance abuse/psychiatric evaluation to confirm his current status and assist with linkage to care.

Assessment Strategy

If the patient recently was admitted (past 48 hours) to the hospital, a broad toxicology screen should be ordered. Because he is known to have multiple drug use disorders, screening tests are not appropriate in this case. Rather, a diagnostic interview (e.g., MINI or SCID) is needed to clarify diagnoses (lifetime/current, severity). In addition, the ASI could be used to determine psychosocial functioning in seven domains: (1) medical; (2) family/social; (3) employment; (4) legal; (5) alcohol; (6) drug; and (7) psychiatric. Norms are available for HIV-positive patients and various drug groups, including heroin addicts. Finally, because the patient is out of care (for both HIV and drug abuse), it would be helpful to administer a measure of treatment motivation/readiness (e.g., University of Rhode Island Change Assessment [URICA]). Findings from these three assessments should be adequate to determine what type of drug treatment is appropriate (e.g., residential, methadone maintenance) and what motivation interventions may facilitate linkage to care.

CHAPTER 7

Alcohol Use

Tony Toneatto
Mekhala Gunaratne

Population surveys indicate that alcohol consumption ranks second in prevalence to caffeine use (American Psychiatric Association, 2000). Up to 44% of the adult U.S. population reported having consumed at least 12 alcoholic drinks within the past year (Dawson, Grant, Chou, & Pickering, 1995). It is not surprising that up to 7.4% of the U.S. population met current diagnostic criteria for either alcohol dependence or abuse. The National Longitudinal Alcohol Epidemiologic Survey (Grant, 1997) reported that the lifetime prevalence of alcohol dependence approximates 13%. For heavy drinkers, the damage inflicted by alcohol abuse on the economy, the life of the abuser, and his or her family, friends, and society as a whole is staggering (e.g., Klatsky, 2010). In 1998, economic costs of alcohol problems were estimated to be close to $200 billion (U.S. Department of Health and Human Services, 2000).

In DSM-5 (American Psychiatric Association, 2013), alcohol use disorder is only 1 of 10 alcohol-related psychiatric diagnoses.[1] The biopsychosocial assessment of each of these disorders is beyond the scope of this chapter. Many of these disorders lack well-validated assessment tools and may rely only on the expertise of a clinician with considerable experience within the whole range of alcohol-induced psychopathology. Consequently, the focus of this chapter is limited to the biopsychosocial assessment of alcohol abuse and dependence disorders for which numerous evaluative instruments have already been developed and carefully validated.

Assessment and evaluation are the foundation for prudent decisions regarding the

---

[1]These include but are not limited to alcohol intoxication delirium, alcohol withdrawal delirium, alcohol-induced psychotic disorder, alcohol-induced bipolar disorder, alcohol-induced depressive disorder, alcohol-induced anxiety disorder, alcohol-induced sleep disorder, alcohol-induced sexual dysfunction, and alcohol-induced major or mild neurocognitive disorder.

treatment of alcohol problems. A comprehensive assessment can effectively guide the selection of the most efficient treatments that correspond with the specific needs of the individual and provide feedback about their clinical efficacy. Because alcohol problems have multifactorial etiologies and a diverse set of conditions and variables that contribute to their onset, a multivariate assessment of alcohol misuse is often indicated to fully characterize the disorder (Capuzzi & Stauffer, 2008). However, this is not always possible or desirable. For example, in primary care or in outpatient settings treatments may be very brief and may neither require nor justify a comprehensive assessment (e.g., Bradley, Kivlahan & Williams, 2009). In many cases, tools required to assess alcohol misuse may be expensive to use, may require specialized training, or may need to be administered only by qualified professionals. Thus the assessment tools discussed in this chapter should simply be considered as options to choose from in response to the specific needs of the client and the clinical setting.

A biopsychosocial assessment will assist in the identification, description, and quantification of the biological, cognitive, affective, behavioral, social, and environmental factors associated with hazardous alcohol use. With this valuable information, the selection of the most appropriate interventions—whether focused on the individual (e.g., psychopharmacological, cognitive), the environment (e.g., behavioral) or the person–environment interaction (e.g., social, interpersonal interventions)—can be made. In addition to providing a comprehensive evaluation of the alcohol problem that facilitates an empirically based intervention approach, assessment should also be capable of measuring changes that occur as a result of treatment.

Piazza (2002) has identified reliability, validity, specificity, sensitivity, and cost efficiency as characteristics of acceptable assessment instruments. At the minimum, any tool adopted to evaluate alcohol use disorders must possess both reliability and validity. The former includes primarily test–retest reliability (i.e., the temporal stability of the score) and interrater reliability (i.e., scores obtained by one clinician should easily be replicated by another clinician). The lat-

ter should encompass both construct validity (i.e., the assessment instrument actually assesses the biopsychosocial process) and predictive validity (i.e., one may confidently rely on the test scores to determine prognosis). Tarter (2005) has indicated that incremental validity should also characterize the assessment instrument. That is, the administration of each test should provide information that is above and beyond what causal or informal assessments would obtain. For example, there is little value in assessing behavioral risks for alcohol abuse if the individual has already articulated them. Thus the skillful application of an efficient assessment protocol should yield clinically useful data that would otherwise be too complex or subtle to observe in less formal evaluations.

As is demonstrated in this chapter, the reliability and internal consistency of scales measuring alcohol problem severity have been documented extensively in clinical and general population samples. Their concurrent and convergent validity have been established in comparisons with other severity scales and/or measures of alcohol dependence, alcohol consumption patterns and biomarkers, psychological functioning and social adjustment, and treatment goals and progress (Devos-Comby & Lange, 2008; Donovan et al., 2006; Thomas & McCambridge, 2008).

Screening, Assessment, and Diagnosis

The evaluation of alcohol misuse can be classified according to screening, assessment, and diagnostic instruments. Screening instruments are mainly used to inform the clinician whether the alcohol consumption of an individual is clinically significant. These methods tend to be brief and can be administered by individuals with limited clinical experience. However, they do not yield a diagnosis or extensive information about the alcohol concern. Ideally, screening instruments identify individuals who have an alcohol problem (when results indicate high true positive rates) and rule out those who do not have the problem (when results indicate high true negative rates). Sensitivity, or true positive, and specificity, or true negative, results that accurately reflect the individual's true condition (i.e., the screening instrument should confirm that an individual with an alcohol problem does in fact have one and vice versa) should be maximized. At the same time, the probability of encountering false negative and false positive results should be minimized in order to avoid inaccurate conclusions (i.e., that an alcohol problem exists when it actually does not and vice versa).

Conceptually, there are two models for alcohol screening: (1) disease detection and (2) risk reduction. Whereas earlier screening instruments that focused on disease detection sought to identify individuals with clear evidence of an alcohol misuse disorder, more recent instruments have been designed to detect hazardous drinking patterns with the goal of risk reduction in mind (e.g., Mundt, Zakletskaia, & Fleming, 2009). Such instruments identify individuals with modifiable behavioral risk factors who are not currently experiencing an alcohol problem (Rubinsky, Kivlahan, Volk, Maynard, & Bradley, 2010).

Alcohol assessments are more labor intensive than the screening process and intend to provide additional information into the nature of the alcohol problem to help render a diagnosis. For the past quarter century, alcohol assessment has been strongly influenced by the dependence syndrome delineated by Griffith Edwards and colleagues (1976). The dependency syndrome includes the following elements: (1) specific cognitive, behavioral, and physiological symptoms related to a common addictive process; (2) distribution of symptoms along a severity dimension; and (3) independence of dependence symptoms from the negative consequences of alcohol use. Because assessments are central to effective treatment planning and thus include a referral process for further assessment, a comprehensive evaluation of the impact of alcohol misuse on the individual's life, as well as any characteristics that may affect the person's response to treatment, is essential.

Although assessment and screening are usually conducted by paraprofessionals or can even be done by the patient him- or herself, the determination of a diagnosis typically requires a clinician possessing an advanced degree and considerable clinical experience with the disorder. Diagnosis is the process by which the individual with an alcohol problem exhibits a prescribed set of symptoms that are believed to meet criteria for a psychiatric disorder. DSM-5 (American Psychiatric Association, 2013) represents the latest version of these criteria and provides a consistent means for communication within clinical and research settings. From a historical perspective, the evolution of DSM demonstrates that specific components of diagnosis can vary over time.

The vast majority of information gathered during screening, assessment, and diagnosis is based largely on self-report. An issue that is often raised when evaluating alcohol problems is reliability of self-report. For a variety of reasons, such self-report has often been considered to depict inaccurate representations of an individual's behavior. However, empirical research has demonstrated that an alcohol misuser's self-report is valid and can be relied upon when obtained under the following conditions (Sobell & Sobell, 2003): complete sobriety during the assessment; assurance of confidentiality; freedom to self-report any drinking; unambiguous questioning; accurate definition of amounts of alcohol; use of memory aids; assumption of heavy drinking to encourage honest disclosure; nonjudgmental attitude when discrepancies become apparent; distinction between irregular alcohol consumption and normal drinking patterns (Sobell & Sobell, 2003; Room, 2000).

Screening

No single instrument comprehensively assesses all aspects of alcohol use problems. Some focus on quantity or frequency, whereas others may emphasize severity and patterns of use. The Michigan Alcoholism Screening Test (MAST; Selzer, 1971) in its original formulation is an easy-to-administer test containing 25 true–false items (some of which are weighted more heavily than others) used to measure severity of alcohol use. A score of 5 or 6 is considered to indicate probable alcohol dependence, and a score of 7 or greater is considered to represent alcohol dependence. Reliance on a single score assumes that the MAST's items represent a single latent variable (Thurber & Snow, 2001), although some critics suggest that there are multiple facets within the MAST (e.g., Parsons, Wallbrown, & Myers, 1994). Though often considered the gold standard of screening instruments, its transparency has rendered it vulnerable to criticisms. Opponents suggest that the MAST reflects the intention of an individual to admit to an alcohol problem (Martin, Liepman, & Young, 1990). Several brief versions of the original MAST have also been developed, such as the B-MAST (Pokorny, Miller, & Kaplan, 1972).

The Alcohol Use Disorders Identification Test (AUDIT; Saunders, Aasland, Babor, de la Fuente, & Grant, 1993) was developed by the World Health Organization (Hodgson et al., 2003). Requiring approximately 3 minutes to administer, the AUDIT consists of 10 items assessing quantity and frequency of alcohol use, hazardous drinking, intoxication, and alcohol-related negative consequences. In a review of relevant literature (Fielling, Reid, & O'Connor, 2000; Reinert & Allen, 2007), the recommended AUDIT cutoff score of 8 yielded a sensitivity and specificity score between .80 and .95. Fielling et al. (2000) concluded that the AUDIT is best suited to detect milder alcohol problems instead of alcohol abuse or dependence. The AUDIT has been as good as or superior to other screening measures such as the CAGE, MAST, or Alcohol Dependence Scale (ADS) in identifying problem drinkers (Barry & Fleming, 1993). Other screens related to the AUDIT have been produced, such as the Fast Alcohol Screening Test (FAST) and AUDIT-C. The FAST consists of four questions derived from the original AUDIT (Hodgson et al., 2003). It can be administered in as little as a few seconds and is ideal for medical settings. The sensitivity and specificity of the FAST range from .89 to .95 and .84 to .90, respectively, and correlates highly with the full AUDIT. The AUDIT-C uses the first three AUDIT questions and maintains high sensitivity and specificity (e.g., Bush, Kivlahan, McDonell, Fihn, & Bradley, 1998). It appears to be more efficacious in screening hazardous drinking than alcohol use or dependence. Strengths of the AUDIT include its ability to screen using a continuum of severity, to distinguish preceding-year and lifetime use, to evaluate each symptom on a continuum rather than a yes-or-no basis, and to assess hazardous consumption.

Very brief screening instruments have been developed to detect alcohol problems. The CAGE (Ewing, 1984), originally designed for primary care physicians, is best at detecting alcohol dependence. It asks the following four questions: (1) Have you ever wanted to Cut back or stop drinking? (2) Have you ever felt Annoyed or angry after someone commented on your drinking? (3) Have there been instances when you've felt Guilty about or regretted outcomes that were a result of drinking? (4) Have you ever used alcohol to help you get started in the morning to steady your nerves (Eye-opener)? The cutoff score for an alcohol problem is two positive answers. The CAGE's diagnostic accuracy ranges between 40 and 95% (Sokol, Martier, & Ager, 1989) and sensitivity ranges between 60 and 95% (O'Connor & Schottenfeld, 1998). As initially designed, the CAGE does not differentiate between lifetime and current alcohol problems and could potentially classify an individual in remission as having an alcohol problem (a 50% false-positive rate has been reported by Fleming, 1993). The CAGE appears to be transparent and as a result is subject to manipulation.

The T-ACE (Chang, 2001), specifically developed to assess alcohol risk among pregnant women, consists of four items related to Tolerance, Annoyance, efforts to Cut down, and an Eye-opener drink, thus resembling the CAGE. Typically, a score of 2 reflects at-risk alcohol consumption. Among African American women, cutoff points of 1, 2, and 3 produced sensitivity coefficients of .83, .70, and .45, respectively, and specificity coefficients of .75, .85 and .97, respectively (Russell et al., 1994). In a more diverse ethnic group, the sensitivity and specificity for risky drinking were reported to be .92 and .38, respectively.

The TWEAK (Cherpitel, 1999), derived from the MAST, CAGE, and T-ACE, is similarly brief and consists of five items that particularly aid in screening alcohol misuse among women, especially those who are pregnant. Scored on a 7-point scale, the TWEAK items include the assessment of Tolerance (How many drinks can you hold, or how many drinks does it take to get high?), Worry (Have close friends or relatives worried about your drinking?), Eye-Opener (Do you sometimes take a drink in the morning to wake up?), **Amnesia** (Has a friend or family member ever told you things you said or did while you were drinking that you could not remember?), **K** (Cut; do you sometimes feel the need to cut down on your drinking?). The cutoff score for an alcohol problem is three positive answers. Cutoff points of 1, 2, and 3 produced sensitivity estimates of .87, .79, and .59, respectively, and specificity ratings of .72, .83, and .94, respectively (Russell et al., 1994). A review by Bradley, Boyd-Wickizer, Powell, & Burman (1998) concluded that the TWEAK was the best instrument for identifying alcohol dependence among women. However, an opposing view by Cherpitel (1997) suggests that the TWEAK is more sensitive at detecting alcohol problems in men than in women.

The Rapid Alcohol Problem Screen (RAPS) consists of five items derived from the TWEAK, MAST, CAGE, and AUDIT that effectively identify emergency room patients who abuse or depend on alcohol (Cherpitel, 1995). A 4-item version of this instrument (RAPS4) had a sensitivity of 93% for alcohol dependence but a sensitivity of 55% for hazardous drinking (Cherpitel, 2000).

Likely the briefest screen for hazardous drinking has been developed by Vinson, Kruse, and Seale (2007), who have defined two questions based on (1) recurrent drinking in hazardous situations and (2) consuming more alcohol than intended. A high degree of specificity and sensitivity was reported in a variety of diverse samples.

Smith, Herrmann, and Bartlett (2011) conducted a qualitative content analysis of several brief alcohol screen inventories, including the AUDIT, CAGE, brief MAST, and TWEAK. They identified six major themes or core constructs in the assessment of alcohol dependence and abuse: consequences, consumption, emotions, eye-opener, perceptions, and risks.

Assessment

The Addiction Severity Index (ASI; McLellan, Luborsky, Woody, & O'Brien, 1980) has been used to assess alcohol severity, in addition to several other domains related to addiction, such as medical history, legal records, psychiatric status, family history, employment background, and social functioning. A valued aspect of the ASI is its utility in treatment planning and its availability in the public domain. Though computerized and online versions of the ASI are available, it is typically administered during an oral interview that lasts approximately 1 hour. Both the client and assessor produce ratings of severity, ranging from "no problem" to "severe" problem, during the previous 30 days. The psychometric properties of the ASI have generally been supportive (e.g., Butler et al., 2001; Rist, Glockner-Rist, & Demmel, 2009; Donovan et al., 2006), although a review by Makela (2004) concluded that acceptable internal consistency coefficients were not established for all of the composite scores.

The Comprehensive Drinker Profile (CDP; Miller & Marlatt, 1984) evaluates several areas related to alcohol, such as drinking history and patterns, reasons for drinking, expectancies, and self-efficacy. The administration of the CDP requires approximately 2 hours. A similar instrument is the Alcohol Use Inventory (AUI; Horn, Wanberg, & Foster, 1987), which consists of 228 items that measure the multivariate aspects of alcohol use problems and which focuses primarily on the motivational aspects of alcohol use, including benefits of drinking, drinking styles, consequences, and admitting to an alcohol problem. The AUI can also be administered in groups.

The Drinker Inventory of Consequences (DrInC; Miller, Tonigan, & Longabaugh, 1995) assesses, over the lifetime and in recent months, alcohol-related negative effects of drinking. Specifically, the effects of heavy alcohol consumption on physical health, social obligations, impaired control, and inter- and intrapersonal consequences are evaluated. A 15-item shorter version of the DrInC, the Short Inventory of Problems (SIP; Feinn, Tennen, & Kranzler, 2003), has been found to be psychometrically robust. Recently, the 27-item Addiction Severity Assessment Tool (ASAT; Butler et al., 2006) has been developed to multidimensionally assess the effect of alcohol misuse on daily functioning, social relations, mood states, severity, and self-efficacy. Intended to be used with individuals seeking treatment, its advantages over instruments such as the ASI are its brevity and use as a self-report instrument. It can also be used to measure effects of treatment. Preliminary psychometric properties of the ASAT are encouraging (Butler et al., 2006).

Although most assessment instruments are rational (i.e., they contain items that are transparent), there has been effort to develop less transparent measures to minimize the possibility of response manipulation. The Minnesota Multiphasic Personality Inventory (MMPI-2) has generated a subscale, the MacAndrew Alcoholism Scale—Revised (Mac-R), constructed using the criterion-keying method (Graham, 2000). The Mac-R, consisting of 49 items, is used to distinguish those with alcohol addiction from those without alcohol dependence. A score of 28 or more is associated with alcohol abuse. Butcher, Dahlstrom, Graham, Tellegen, and Kaemmer (1989) found internal consistency estimates of .56 for men and .45 for women. Higher coefficients were reported by Laux, Newman, and Brown (2004) in outpatients (alpha = 0.88) and by Laux, Salyers, and Kotova (2005) in a college sample (alpha = 0.82). One valued aspect of the Mac-R is its assessment of personality characteristics often associated with alcohol misuse, such as impulsivity, sensation seeking, and impaired judgment. In addition, the Mac-R understood within the MMPI validity scales has the added advantage of identifying individuals who may be motivated to hide or minimize their addictive behavior. As the Mac-R screens for substance use, additional assessment would be required to determine which substance was actually producing the elevated score. A review of the Mac-R by Miller, Shields, Campfield, Wallace, and Weiss (2007) concluded that the Mac-R produces generally unreliable scores (~ .47) and suggested relying on more direct measures such as the CAGE, AUDIT, and MAST instead. Miller et al. (2007) also failed to discriminate types of substance abusers and thus did not necessarily detect alcohol use problems.

The Addiction Acknowledgement Scale (AAS), another MMPI-2 subscale, consists of 13 items that measure substance abuse (Graham, 2000). T-scores above 60 indicate acknowledgement of substance abuse. However, because the items are transparent, it may also indicate efforts to hide substance abuse. Reviews of the psychometric properties of the AAS compared with the Mac-R generally show it to be a superior subscale of the MMPI substance abuse scales.

The Substance Abuse Subtle Screening Inventory-3 (SASSI-3; Lazowski, Miller, Boye, & Miller, 1998), another empirically developed measure, consists of 67 true–false questions unrelated to substance use but established to discriminate individuals with a substance use disorder from those without one. These items comprise eight empirically established subscales measuring causes, consequences, and correlates of substance use, the clients' admission of abuse-related difficulties, and defensiveness. Some evidence suggests that the SASSI-3 has excellent internal consistency for face-valid scales (Laux, Perera-Diltz, Smirnoff, & Salyers, 2005) and was superior to the CAGE, MAST, and Mac-R in 1-week test–retest reliability and internal consistency (Laux, Salyers, & Kotova, 2005). Swartz (1998) concluded that the SASSI-3 effectively discriminated severe and moderate dependence.

The Clinical Institute Withdrawal Assessment for Alcohol—Revised (CIWA-Ar; Sullivan, Sykora, Schneiderman, Naranjo, & Sellers, 1989) assesses vital signs and 10 symptoms of withdrawal, such as nausea, vomiting, agitation, headache, anxiety, tremor, and sensory disturbances. The CIWA-Ar can be useful in making treatment decisions and can be administered by a wide range of clinical staff.

Diagnosis

Structured clinical interviews have been the most commonly used approaches to the diagnostic assessment of alcohol use disorders. This approach to diagnostic assessment is also useful when other psychiatric disorders are concurrently present with the alcohol misuse and the determination of a primary alcohol use disorder is necessary. The Structured Clinical Interview for DSM-IV Axis I Disorders, Patient Edition, version 2.0 (SCID-I/P; First, Spitzer, Gibbon, & Williams, 1996) is among the most commonly used semistructured instruments that permit the interviewer to probe for additional information. Its modular nature allows the interview to be shortened to diagnose only those disorders of interest. It is important that the interviewer be a skilled professional, as it requires sound clinical judgment. A self-administered computer screen version of the SCID, as well as a computer-assisted interview, is also available for use (First, Gibbon, Williams, Spitzer, & MHS Staff, 2001).

The Schedule for Affective Disorders and Schizophrenia (SADS; Spitzer, Endicott, & Robins, 1975) is semistructured, thus requiring a high degree of clinical skill to administer and interpret the results. The Diagnostic Interview Schedule (DIS; Robins et al., 2000) can be administered by paraprofessionals without clinical training, because it is fully structured. A computerized version of the DIS (CDIS-IV) yields only lifetime diagnoses.

The Psychiatric Research Interview for Substance and Mental Disorders (PRISM) is similar to the SCID and must also be administered by skilled clinicians. Its main use is to improve the diagnosis of Axis I disorders in substance abusing populations (Hasin, Trautman, & Endicott, 1998).

The Schedule for Clinical Assessment in Neuropsychiatry (SCAN; Wing et al., 1990) resembles the SCID in being semistructured and requiring administration by trained professionals. Lifetime and current diagnoses consistent with DSM-IV and ICD-10 nosologies are produced. Cottler and colleagues (1997) reported strong psychometric properties for the SCAN.

The MMPI-2, although not yielding a diagnosis, can provide an overview of the severity of psychopathology that can be important in treatment planning. In addition, the MMPI-2 provides information on the test-taking attitude of the respondent (either the under- or overreporting of symptoms) through the interpretation of the validity scales.

Severity of alcohol dependence is not an element of the DSM-5 diagnostic system. However, several measures of dependence are available that can provide this continuum of severity. The Alcohol Dependence Scale (ADS; Skinner & Allen, 1982) consists of 25 items measuring alcohol withdrawal, lack of control, compulsivity, and tolerance within the past year. It can be administered using computer, paper-and-pencil, and online methods (Miller et al., 2002; Murphy & MacKillop, 2011). Doyle and Donovan (2009) identified a three-factor structure

that constitutes the ADS: loss of behavioral control and heavy drinking, obsessive–compulsive drinking style, and psychoperceptual and psychophysical withdrawal. The Severity of Alcohol Dependence Questionnaire (SADQ; Stockwell, Murphy, & Hodgson, 1983) consists of 20 items emphasizing withdrawal, craving, and heavy consumption within the previous 30 days.

Treatment-Related Assessment

Alcohol Consumption

Quantity–frequency (QF) measures of alcohol consumption pertain to the average amount of alcohol consumed (usually expressed in standard drinks) on the average frequency of drinking days (usually expressed in days per week or month; Sobell & Sobell, 2003). Typically, separate estimates for wine, beer, and spirits are obtained. QF measures allow estimates of number of drinking days over a period of time and total amount of alcohol consumed. Because QF measures do not usually gather information about heavy drinking days (i.e., emphasizing the average instead), they may underestimate alcohol consumption.

Heavy drinking days are assessed in Midanik's Graduated Frequency (GF; Midanik, 1994), which measures alcohol consumption at different levels (i.e., 1–2 drinks, 3–4 drinks, up to 12 or more drinks). The GF yields more accurate information on drinking patterns and eliminates the need to determine the average amount of drinks consumed. When it is desirable to obtain information regarding drinking patterns over a lengthy period of time, such as an individual's lifetime, the Lifetime Drinking History (LDH; Skinner & Sheu, 1982) is useful. The LDH identifies distinct phases in an individual's drinking history, assesses QF within each phase, and specifies maximum drinking days. One of the more extensively evaluated measures of alcohol consumption, the Alcohol Timeline Followback (TLFB; Sobell & Sobell, 2000), assesses any psychoactive substance using a calendar that encompasses the past 30, 60, 90, or even 360 days. Abstinent days and the amount of alcohol consumed on drinking days are recorded. The TLFB is valuable when patterns of drinking, variability in drinking, or accurate amounts of consumption and frequency are desirable. The TLFB is available in paper-and-pencil, interview, and computerized versions.

Readiness to Change

The variability in motivational status on the preparedness to make changes in alcohol consumption has long been recognized (Miller & Rollnick, 2002). Prochaska and DiClemente's (1986) well-known conceptual framework has identified several stages that may characterize an individual's readiness to change (i.e., precontemplation, contemplation, determination, action, maintenance, and relapse) and has been immensely influential throughout the addiction treatment field. Several self-report measures of readiness to change alcohol behavior have been developed and can provide important information on the most appropriate form of clinical intervention.

The 28-item University of Rhode Island Change Assessment (URICA; DiClemente & Hughes, 1990) measures four stages of change in alcohol treatment seekers: precontemplation, contemplation, action, and maintenance. A readiness score, calculated by subtracting the precontemplation score from the sum of the other three scores, strongly predicted treatment outcome in Project MATCH (Project MATCH Research Group, 1997).

The 39-item Stages of Change Readiness and Treatment Eagerness Scale (SOCRATES; Miller & Tonigan, 1996) measures all of the stages of change except relapse. The Readiness to Change Questionnaire (RTCQ; Rollnick, Heather, Gold, & Hall, 1992) uses 12 items to measure the following three stages: precontemplation, contemplation, and action. It was originally intended to assess readiness to change in heavy drinkers presented in medical settings. The RTCQ-TV (Heather, Luce, Peck, Dunbar, & James, 1999) is a 15-item version of the RTCQ suitable for assessing readiness to change in treatment-seeking hazardous drinkers.

Reasons for Drinking

Most empirically based treatments for alcohol misuse assist the individual to develop more effective coping skills in the presence of potent triggers for heavy drinking. Among the most widely used instruments to assess such triggers is the Inventory of Drinking Situations (IDS; Annis, Graham, & Davis, 1987). The original version consisted of 100 items reflecting Marlatt's (Marlatt & Gordon, 1985) categories of high-risk situations: pleasant emotions, negative emotional states, interpersonal conflict, physical discomfort, testing personal control, social pressure to drink, pleasant social situations, urges, and temptations. A profile depicting the drinker's risk for drinking heavily when exposed to these situations can be produced. However, a much briefer, 42-item version of the IDS (IDS-42; Isenhart, 1993) has been developed and is psychometrically equivalent to the IDS.

The Reasons for Drinking Questionnaire (RFDQ; Zywiak, Connors, Maisto, & Westerberg, 1996) requires the individual to rate the importance of 16 reasons, related to Marlatt's categories, in the relapse to alcohol use. The RFDQ possesses positive psychometric support (Zywiak et al., 1996).

Self-Efficacy

Self-efficacy theory conceptualizes the likelihood to relapse as a result of the individual's confidence in his or her ability to cope with high-risk alcohol situations. Alcohol treatments often incorporate efforts to increase such confidence with adequate training in cognitive and behavioral coping skills. Several questionnaires have been developed to measure self-efficacy among alcohol misusers, such as the Situational Confidence Questionnaire (SCQ-39; Annis & Graham, 1988). It measures self-efficacy in response to the same eight categories of high-risk situations defined by Marlatt and Gordon (1985). Greater self-efficacy (as measured on a continuum from 0 to 100%) in the ability to resist the urge to drink in these situations has been associated with superior treatment outcomes up to a year posttreatment (Greenfield et al., 2000). DiClemente, Carbonari, Montgomery, and Hughes (1994) have developed the Alcohol Abstinence Self-Efficacy Scale (AASE) that assesses the degree of temptation and confidence to resist drinks in the face of 20 high-risk drinking situations. A briefer version of the SCQ, the

Brief SCQ (BSCQ), consists of eight items, each representing one of the eight subscales (Breslin, Sobell, Sobell, & Agrawal, 2000).

Coping Skills

Assessment of coping skills is an important component of treatment planning given the centrality of such skills in the effective management of alcohol consumption emphasized in cognitive-behavioral therapies. The 36-item Coping Behaviours Inventory (CBI; Litman, Stapleton, Oppenheim, & Peleg, 1983) measures the effort to avoid relapse. It consists of four factors: seeking social support, negative thinking, positive thinking, and avoidance/distraction. The Coping Response Inventory (CRI; Moos, 1992) measures approach coping (e.g., logical analysis, positive reappraisal) and avoidance coping (e.g., cognitive avoidance, emotional discharge) responses when faced with high-risk situations for drinking.

Alcohol Expectancies

Drinking behavior may be influenced by expectations that the drinker may have based on the reinforcing and punishing consequences of alcohol consumption. Treatment interventions often attempt to alter alcohol expectancies in order to modify those that may facilitate abusive drinking. The Alcohol Expectancy Questionnaire (AEQ; Brown, Goldman, Inn, & Anderson, 1980) evaluates six positive expectancies of alcohol consumption: global positive expectancy, improved sexual performance, social/physical pleasure, social assertiveness, tension reduction, and increased power/aggression. The Drinking Expectancy Questionnaire (DEQ; Young & Knight, 1989) measures both negative and positive alcohol expectancies, and the Negative Alcohol Expectancy Questionnaire (NAEQ; Jones & McMahon, 1994) focuses exclusively on the assessment of expectancies of alcohol-related negative consequences. Spada and Wells (2008) have focused on alcohol-related metacognitions, beliefs about alcohol-related cognitive processes. Two metacognitive measures have been developed, the Positive Alcohol Metacognitions Scale (PAMS) and the Negative Alcohol Metacognitions Scale (NAMS). Both instruments were characterized by good classification accuracy, reliability and validity.

Cravings and Urges

Given the central role that urges and cravings to drink have in the conceptualization of hazardous drinking and in treatment interventions, several instruments have been developed to assess this construct. The Yale–Brown Obsessive–Compulsive Scale—Heavy Drinkers (YBOCS-HD; Modell, Glaser, Mountz, Schmaltz, & Cyr, 1992) is composed of 10 items measuring obsessional thinking patterns and compulsive behaviors related to hazardous drinking. The Alcohol Urge Questionnaire (AUQ; Bohn, Krahn, & Staehler, 1995) is a brief, 8-item questionnaire measuring current urge to drink (i.e., current desire for alcohol, positive expectancies, difficulty resisting alcohol). The Alcohol Craving Questionnaire (ACQ; Singleton, 1996) is composed of 47 items that measure current craving for alcohol and consist of four factors: emotionality, purposefulness, compulsivity, and expectancy (Singleton & Gorelick, 1998).

Psychiatric Comorbidity

Given the compelling evidence of the presence of psychiatric disorders among alcohol misusers, it is important to accurately diagnose the presence of concurrent psychopathology. Epidemiological studies (e.g., Kessler et al., 1997; Grant, 1995) report very high lifetime rates (> 75%) of psychiatric pathology among those with alcohol dependence. Rates among clinical populations are also elevated, especially among those with mood, anxiety, and personality disorders. For example, marked comorbidity between alcohol use and anxiety disorders in both clinical and community populations have been repeatedly demonstrated (e.g., Grant et al., 2004; Kessler et al., 1994; Kushner, Abrams, & Borchardt, 2000; Thomas & McCambridge, 2008), with some evidence suggesting that concurrent alcohol use and anxiety disorders predict poorer alcohol treatment outcomes and greater likelihood of relapse (e.g., Burns, Teesson, & O'Neill, 2005; Driessen et al., 2001; Willinger et al., 2002). Because concurrent psychiatric disorders may affect the course of treatment, it is important to accurately measure such symptoms in addition to rendering a psychiatric diagnosis.

The Beck Depression Inventory (BDI-II; Beck, Steer, & Brown, 1996) and the Beck Anxiety Inventory (BAI; Beck, Epstein, Brown, & Steer, 1988) are commonly used self-report questionnaires measuring depression and anxiety. Other self-report scales, such as the Symptom Checklist 90—Revised (SCL-90-R; Derogatis, 1983), can be rapidly administered and provide a profile along nine dimensions of psychopathology. Briefer versions of this instrument, such as the Brief Symptom Inventory (BSI; Derogatis & Melisaratos, 1983), measures psychopathology along the same nine dimensions found in the SCL-90-R. The BSI-18 (Derogatis, 2000), which concentrates on depression, anxiety, and somatoform symptoms, can rapidly assess concurrent psychopathology when a diagnosis is not essential or possible (e.g., when skilled assessors are unavailable).

Alcohol Biomarkers

When the validity of self-report is questioned or when corroborative information is required, it is useful to consider obtaining biological markers to indicate alcohol consumption. Although ethanol can be detected in urine, saliva, and blood or on the breath, the elimination of alcohol from the blood within 6–8 hours makes it impractical to conclude that alcohol consumption has occurred. The inclusion of biochemical measures can assist in adopting a convergent validity approach to assessment. The use of a breath analyzer is a simple way of detecting the presence of recent drinking and an important consideration in assessing the validity of self-report. Also, because very tolerant individuals may not exhibit obvious evidence that they have been drinking and thus escape clinical judgment, the use of biochemical approaches can be informative and revealing (Sobell, Toneatto, & Sobell, 1994).

Urine tests can provide evidence of alcohol use both qualitatively (i.e., type of substance) and quantitatively (i.e., amount consumed when the substance's half-life is known) but may not be as informative or accurate

regarding when alcohol was ingested (Dilts, Gendel, & Williams, 1996).

Several tests are useful for detecting the presence of heavy drinking. Serum gamma-glutamyltransferase (GGT) has long been considered an effective test (sensitivity 50%, specificity 80%) for early liver problems. GGT levels typically begin to rise after several weeks of heavy alcohol consumption and then return to normal within 4–6 weeks of abstinence. Because elevated GGT levels can be caused by several medical conditions, false positives are likely. Erythrocyte mean corpuscular volume (MCV), triglycerides, serum alkaline phosphates, serum bilirubin, and uric acid have all been used as biomarkers.

Recently, carbohydrate-deficient transferring (CDT) has been shown to increase in response to several weeks of daily alcohol consumption of at least five drinks and to normalize within 2 weeks of abstinence (Allen & Anthenelli, 2003). CDT elevations can also be due to other medical conditions, but overall, CDT, though more expensive, is more accurate than GGT or other liver function tests (Litten, Allen, & Fertig, 1995).

Generally, using a combination of markers is recommended due to an individual's variability in responsiveness to heavy drinking. The utility of biomarkers is to monitor drinking status of drinkers during treatment, to provide feedback, and to enhance motivation (Allen, Sillanaukee, Strid, & Litten, 2003).

Conclusions

The alcohol assessment field has matured sufficiently to make available a wide variety of assessment instruments to meet the needs of a population as diverse as alcohol abusers. Because individuals with alcohol problems can appear in a wide variety of clinical settings (e.g., hospital emergency rooms, physician offices, outpatient clinics, and specialized addiction clinics) and meet with a variety of professionals (e.g., psychiatrists, physicians, counselors, social workers, nurses), there may be a variety of practical limitations in the time and expertise available to conduct an assessment. Fortunately, with the abundance of instruments available, the most appropriate assessment tool can be selected to screen, assess, and diagnose alcohol problems and obtain data most relevant to treatment planning. This chapter has described some of the more established assessment instruments to assist clinicians in their approach toward conducting an assessment that meets their needs, the needs of their clients, and those of the setting in which treatment services take place.

REFERENCES

Allen, J. P., & Anthenelli, R. M. (2003). Getting to the bottom of problem drinking: The case for routine screening. *Journal of Family Practice, 2*(6). Available at *www.currentpsychiatry. com/the-publication/past-issue-single-view/ getting-to-the-bottom-of-problem-drinking- the-case-for-routine-screening/70bb0fa422be f4ce5e73d8b735ef651a.html*.

Allen, J. P., Sillanaukee, P., Strid, N., & Litten, R. Z. (2003). Biomarkers of heavy drinking. In J. P. Allen & V. B. Wilson (Eds.), *Assessing alcohol problems: A guide for clinicians and researchers* (2nd ed., pp. 37–53). Rockville, MD: U.S. Department of Health and Human Services, National Institute on Alcohol Abuse and Alcoholism.

American Psychiatric Association. (2000). *Diagnostic and statistical manual of mental disorders* (4th ed., text rev.). Washington, DC: Author.

American Psychiatric Association. (2013). *Diagnostic and statistical manual of mental disorders* (5th ed.). Arlington, VA: Author.

Annis, H. M., & Graham, J. M. (1988). *Situational Confidence Questionnaire (SCQ 39): User's guide.* Toronto, Ontario, Canada: Addiction Research Foundation.

Annis, H. M., Graham, J. M., & Davis, C. S. (1987). *Inventory of Drinking Situations (IDS) user's guide.* Toronto, Ontario, Canada: Addiction Research Foundation.

Barry, K. L., & Fleming, M. F. (1993). The Alcohol Use Disorders Identification test (AUDIT) and the SMAST-13: Predictive validity in a rural primary care sample. *Alcohol and Alcoholism, 28,* 33–42.

Beck, A. T., Epstein, N., Brown, G., & Steer, R. (1988). An inventory for measuring clinical anxiety: Psychometric properties. *Journal of Consulting and Clinical Psychology, 56,* 893–897.

Beck, A. T., Steer, R. A., & Brown, G. K. (1996). *Beck Depression Inventory–II.* San Antonio, TX: Psychological Corporation.

Bohn, M. J., Krahn, D. D., & Staehler, R. A. (1995). Development and initial validation of a measure of drinking urges in abstinent alcoholics. *Alcoholism: Clinical and Experimental Research, 19,* 600–606.

Bradley, K. A., Boyd-Wickizer, J., Powell, S. H., & Burman, M. L. (1998). Alcohol screening questionnaires in women: A critical review. *Journal of the American Medical Association, 280,* 166–171.

Bradley, K. A., Kivlahan, D. R., & Williams, E. C. (2009). Brief approaches to alcohol screening: Practical alternatives for primary care. *Journal of General Internal Medicine, 24,* 881–883.

Breslin, F. C., Sobell, L. C., Sobell, M. B., & Agrawal, S. (2000). A comparison of a brief and long version of the Situational Confidence Questionnaire. *Behaviour Research and Therapy, 38,* 1211–1220.

Brown, S. A., Goldman, M. S., Inn, A., & Anderson, L. (1980). Expectations of reinforcement from alcohol: Their domain and relation to drinking patterns. *Journal of Consulting and Clinical Psychology, 48,* 419–426.

Burns, L., Teesson, M., & O'Neill, K. (2005). The impact of comorbid anxiety and depression on alcohol treatment outcomes. *Addiction, 100,* 787–796.

Bush, K. R., Kivlahan, D. R., McDonell, M. B., Fihn, S. D., & Bradley, K. A. (1998). The AUDIT alcohol consumption questions (AUDIT-C): An effective brief screening test for problem drinking. *Archives of Internal Medicine, 158,* 1789–1795.

Butcher, J. N., Dahlstrom, W. G., Graham, J. R., Tellegen, A., & Kaemmer, B. (1989). *Minnesota Multiphasic Personality Inventory—2 (MMPI-2): Manual for administration, scoring, and interpretation, revised.* Minneapolis: University of Minnesota Press.

Butler, S. F., Budman, S. H., Goldman, R. J., Newman, F. L., Beckley, K. E., Trottier, D., et al. (2001). Initial validation of a computer-administered Addiction Severity Index: The ASI-MV. *Psychology of Addictive Behaviors, 15,* 4–12.

Butler, S. F., Budman, S. H., McGee, M. D., Davis, M. S., Cornelli, R., & Morey, L. (2006). Addiction Severity Assessment Tool: Development of a self-report measure for clients in substance abuse treatment. *Drug and Alcohol Dependence, 80,* 349–360.

Capuzzi, D., & Stauffer, M. D. (2008). *Foundations of addictions counseling.* Boston: Pearson Education.

Chang, G. (2001). Alcohol-screening instruments for pregnant women. *Alcohol Research and Health, 25,* 204–209.

Cherpitel, C. J. (1995). Screening for alcohol problems in the emergency room: A rapid alcohol problems screen. *Drug and Alcohol Dependence, 40,* 133–137.

Cherpitel, C. J. (1997). Brief screening for alcohol problems. *Alcohol Health and Research World, 21,* 348–351.

Cherpitel, C. J. (1999). Screening for alcohol problems in the U.S. general population: A comparison of the CAGE and TWEAK by gender, ethnicity, and service utilization. *Journal of Studies on Alcohol, 60,* 112–121.

Cherpitel, C. J. (2000). A brief screening instrument for problem drinking in the emergency room: The RAPS4. *Journal of Studies on Alcohol, 61,* 447–449.

Cottler, L. B., Grant, B. F., Blaine, J., Mavreas, V., Pull, C., Hasin, D., et al. (1997). Concordance of DSM-IV alcohol and drug use disorder criteria and diagnoses as measured by AUDADIS-ADR, CIDI and SCAN. *Drug and Alcohol Dependence, 47,* 195–205.

Dawson, D. A., Grant, B. F., Chou, S. P., & Pickering, R. P. (1995). Subgroup variation in U.S. drinking patterns: Results of the 1992 National Longitudinal Alcohol Epidemiologic Survey. *Journal of Substance Abuse, 7,* 331–344.

Derogatis, L. R. (1983). *SCL-90-R: Administration, scoring and procedures manual–II* (Revision). Towson, MD: Clinical Psychometric Research.

Derogatis, L. R. (2000). *BSI-18: Administration, scoring and procedures manual.* Minneapolis, MN: National Computer Systems.

Derogatis, L. R., & Melisaratos, N. (1983). The Brief Symptom Inventory: An introductory report. *Psychological Medicine, 13,* 595–605.

Devos-Comby, L., & Lange, J. E. (2008). Standardized measures of alcohol-related problems: A review of their use among college students. *Psychology of Addictive Behaviors, 22,* 349–361.

DiClemente, C. C., Carbonari, J. P., Montgomery, R. P. G., & Hughes, S. O. (1994). The Alcohol Abstinence Self-Efficacy Scale. *Journal of Studies on Alcohol, 55,* 141–148.

DiClemente, C. C., & Hughes, S. O. (1990). Stages of change profiles in outpatient alcoholism treatment. *Journal of Substance Abuse, 2,* 217–235.

Dilts, S. L., Gendel, M. H., & Williams, M. (1996). False positives in urine monitoring of substance abusers: The importance of clinical context. *American Journal on Addictions, 5,* 66–68.

Donovan, D. M., Kivlahan, D. R., Doyle, S. R., Longabaugh, R., & Greenfield, S. (2006). Concurrent validity of the Alcohol Use Disorders Identification Test (AUDIT) and AUDIT zones in defining levels of severity in the COMBINE study. *Addiction, 101,* 1696–1704.

Doyle, S. R., & Donovan, D. M. (2009). A validation study of the Alcohol Dependence Scale. *Journal of Studies on Alcohol, 70,* 689–699.

Driessen, M., Meier, S., Hill, A., Wetterling, T., Lange, W., & Junghanns, K. (2001). The course of anxiety, depression and drinking behaviours after completed detoxification in alcoholics with and without comorbid anxiety and depressive disorder. *Alcohol and Alcoholism, 36,* 249–255.

Edwards, G., & Gross, M. M. (1976). Alcohol dependence: Provisional description of a clinical syndrome. *British Medical Journal, 1,* 1058–1061.

Ewing, J. (1984). Detecting alcoholism: The CAGE questions. *Journal of the American Medical Association, 252,* 1905–1907.

Feinn, R., Tennen, H., & Kranzler, H. R. (2003). Psychometric properties of the short index of problems as a measure of recent alcohol-related problems. *Alcoholism: Clinical and Experimental Research, 27,* 1436–1441.

Fielling, D. A., Reid, M. C., & O'Connor, P. G. (2000). Screening for alcohol problems in primary care: A systematic review. *Archives of Internal Medicine, 160,* 1977–1989.

First, M. B., Gibbon, M., Williams, J. B. W., Spitzer, R. L. & the MHS Staff. (2001). *SCID Screen Patient Questionnaire (SSPQ) and SCID Screen Patient Questionnaire—Extended (SSPQ-X): Computer programs for Windows software manual.* Toronto, Ontario: Canada: Multi-Health Systems/American Psychiatric Press.

First, M. B., Spitzer, R. L., Gibbon, M., & Williams, J. B. W. (1996). *Structured Clinical Interview for DSM-IV Axis I Disorders— Patient Edition (SCID-I/P, Version 2.0).* New York: New York State Psychiatric Institute Biometrics Research Department.

Fleming, M. F. (1993). Screening and brief intervention for alcohol disorders. *Journal of Family Practice, 37*, 231–234.

Graham, J. R. (2000). *MMPI-2: Assessing personality and psychopathology* (3rd ed.) New York: Oxford University Press.

Grant, B. F. (1995). The DSM-IV field trial for substance use disorders: Major results. *Drug and Alcohol Dependence, 38*, 71–75.

Grant, B. F. (1997). Prevalence and correlates of alcohol use and DSM-IV alcohol dependence in the United States: Results of the National Longitudinal Alcohol Epidemiologic Survey. *Journal of Studies on Alcohol, 58*, 464–473.

Grant, B. F., Stinson, F. S., Dawson, D. A., Chou, P., Dufour, M. C., Compton, W., et al. (2004). Prevalence and co-occurrence of substance use disorders and independent mood and anxiety disorders. *Archives of General Psychiatry, 61*, 807–816.

Greenfield, S. F., Hufford, M. R., Vagge, L. M., Muenz, L. R., Costello, M. E., & Weiss, R. D., (2000). The relationship of self-efficacy expectancies to relapse among alcohol-dependent men and women: A prospective study. *Journal of Studies on Alcohol, 61*, 345–351.

Hasin, D., Trautman, K., & Endicott, J. (1998). Psychiatric Research Interview for Substance and Mental Disorders: Phenomenologically based diagnosis in patients who abuse alcohol or drugs. *Psychopharmacology Bulletin, 34*, 3–8.

Heather, N., Luce, A., Peck, D., Dunbar, B., & James, I. (1999). The development of a treatment version of the Readiness to Change Questionnaire. *Addiction Research, 7*, 63–68.

Hodgson, R. J., John, B., Abassi, T., Hodgson, R. C., Waller, S., Thom, B., et al. (2003). Fast screening for alcohol misuse. *Addictive Behaviors, 28*, 1453–1463.

Horn, J. L., Wanberg, K. W., & Foster, F. M. (1987). *Guide to the Alcohol Use Inventory*. Minneapolis, MN: National Computer Systems.

Isenhart, C. E. (1993). Psychometric evaluation of a short form of the Inventory of Drinking Situations. *Journal of Studies on Alcohol, 54*, 345–349.

Jones, B. T., & McMahon, J. (1994). Negative and positive alcohol expectancies and predictors of abstinence after discharge from a residential treatment program: A one-month and three-month follow-up study in men. *Journal of Studies on Alcohol, 55*, 543–548.

Kessler, R. C., Crum, R. M., Warner, L. A., Nelson, C. B., Schulenberg, J., & Anthony, J. C. (1997). Lifetime co-occurrence of DSM-III-R alcohol abuse and dependence with other psychiatric disorders in the National Comorbidity Survey. *Archives of General Psychiatry, 54*, 313–321.

Kessler, R. C., McGonagle, K. A., Zhao, S., Nelson, C. B., Hughes, M., Eshleman, S., et al. (1994). Lifetime and 12-month prevalence of DSM-III-R psychiatric disorders in the United States: Results from the National Comorbidity Survey. *Archives of General Psychiatry, 51*, 8–19.

Klatsky, A. L. (2010). Alcohol and cardiovascular health. *Physiology and Behavior, 100*, 76–81.

Kushner, M. G., Abrams, K., & Borchardt, C. (2000). The relationship between anxiety disorders and alcohol use disorders: A review of major perspectives and findings. *Clinical Psychology Review, 20*, 149–171.

Laux, J. M., Newman, I., & Brown, R. (2004). The Michigan Alcoholism Screening Test (MAST): A psychometric investigation. *Measurement and Evaluation in Counseling and Development, 36*, 209–225.

Laux, J. M., Perera-Diltz, D., Smirnoff, J., & Salyers, K. M. (2005). The SASSI-3 Face-Valid Other Drug Scale: A psychometric investigation. *Journal of Addictions and Offender Counseling, 26*, 15–23.

Laux, J. M., Salyers, K. M., & Kotova, E. (2005). A psychometric evaluation of the SASSI-3 in a college sample. *Journal of College Counseling, 8*, 41–51.

Lazowski, L. E., Miller, F. G., Boye, M. W., & Miller, G. A. (1998). Efficacy of the Substance Abuse Subtle Screening Inventory-3 (SASSI-3) in identifying substance dependence disorders in clinical settings. *Journal of Personality Assessment, 71*, 114–128.

Litman, G. K., Stapleton, J., Oppenheim, A. N., & Peleg, M. (1983). An instrument for measuring coping behaviors in hospitalized alcoholics: Implications for relapse prevention treatment. *British Journal of Addictions, 78*, 269–276.

Litten, R. Z., Allen, J. P., & Fertig, J. B. (1995). Gamma-glutamyltranspeptidase and carbohydrate deficient transferrin: Alternative measures of excessive alcohol consumption. *Alcoholism: Clinical and Experimental Research, 19*, 1541–1546.

Makela, K. (2004). Studies of the reliability and validity of the Addiction Severity Index. *Addiction, 99*, 411–418.

Marlatt, G. A., & Gordon, J. R. (Eds.). (1985). *Relapse prevention*. New York: Guilford Press.

Martin, C. S., Liepman, M. R., & Young, C. M. (1990). The Michigan Alcoholism Screening Test: False positive in a college student population. *Alcoholism: Clinical and Experimental Research, 14,* 853–855.

McLellan, A. T., Luborsky, L., Woody, G. E., & O'Brien, C. P. (1980). An improved diagnostic evaluation instrument for substance abuse patients: The Addiction Severity Index. *Journal of Nervous and Mental Disease, 168,* 26–33.

Midanik, L. T. (1994). Comparing usual quantity/frequency and graduated frequency scales to assess yearly alcohol consumption: Results from the 1990 U.S. National Alcohol Survey. *Addiction, 89,* 407–412.

Miller, C. S., Shields, A. L., Campfield, D., Wallace, K. A., & Weiss, R. D. (2007). Substance use scales of the MMPI: An exploration of score reliability via meta-analysis. *Educational and Psychological Measurement, 67,* 1052–1065.

Miller, E. T., Neal, D. J., Roberts, L. J., Baer, J. S., Cressler, S. O., Metrik, J., et al. (2002). Test–retest reliability of alcohol measures: Is there a difference between Internet-based assessment and traditional methods? *Psychology of Addictive Behaviors, 16,* 56–63.

Miller, W. R., & Marlatt, G. A. (1984). *Manual for the Comprehensive Drinker Profile*. Odessa, FL: Psychological Assessment Resources.

Miller, W. R., & Rollnick, S. (2002). *Motivational interviewing: Preparing people for change* (2nd ed.). New York: Guilford Press.

Miller, W. R., & Tonigan, J. S. (1996). Assessing drinkers' motivations for change: The Stages of Change Readiness and Treatment Eagerness Scale (SOCRATES). *Psychology of Addictive Behaviors, 10,* 81–89.

Miller, W. R., Tonigan, J. S., & Longabaugh, R. (1995). *The Drinker Inventory of Consequences (DrInC): An instrument for assessing adverse consequences of alcohol abuse* (Project MATCH Monograph Series, Vol. 4, NIH Publication No. 95-3911). Rockville, MD: National Institute on Alcohol Abuse and Alcoholism.

Modell, J. G., Glaser, F. B., Mountz, J. M., Schmaltz, S., & Cyr, L. (1992). Obsessive and compulsive characteristics of alcohol abuse and dependence: Quantification by a newly developed questionnaire. *Alcoholism: Clinical and Experimental Research, 16,* 144–150.

Moos, R. H. (1992). *Coping Response Inventory: Adult form manual*. Palo Alto, CA: Stanford University Center for Health Care Evaluation and Department of Veterans Affairs Medical Centers.

Mundt, M. P., Zakletskaia, L. I., & Fleming, M. F. (2009). Extreme college drinking and alcohol-related injury risk. *Alcoholism: Clinical and Experimental Research, 33,* 1532–1538.

Murphy, C. M., & MacKillop, J. (2011). Factor structure validation of the Alcohol Dependence Scale in a heavy drinking college sample. *Journal of Psychopathology and Behavioral Assessment, 33,* 523–530.

O'Connor, P. G., & Schottenfeld, R. S. (1998). Patients with alcohol problems. *New England Journal of Medicine, 338,* 592–602.

Parsons, K. J., Wallbrown, F. H., & Myers, R. W. (1994). Michigan Alcoholism Screening Test: Evidence supporting general as well as specific factors. *Educational and Psychological Measurement, 54,* 530–536.

Piazza, N. J. (2002). Screening for alcohol and other substance use disorders. In R. S. Weiner (Ed.), *Pain management: A practical guide for clinicians* (3rd ed., pp. 825–832). Boca Raton, FL: CRC Press.

Pokorny, A. D., Miller, B. A., & Kaplan, H. B. (1972). The Brief MAST: A shortened version of the Michigan Alcoholism Screening Test. *American Journal of Psychiatry, 129,* 342–345.

Prochaska, J. O., & DiClemente, C. C. (1986). Toward a comprehensive model of change. In W. R. Miller & N. Heather (Eds.), *Treating addictive behaviors: Processes of change* (pp. 3–27). New York: Plenum Press.

Project MATCH Research Group. (1997). Matching alcoholism treatments to client heterogeneity: Project MATCH post-treatment drinking outcomes. *Journal of Studies on Alcohol, 58,* 7–29.

Reinert, D. F., & Allen, J. P. (2007). The Alcohol Use Disorders Identification Test: An update of research findings. *Alcoholism: Clinical and Experimental Research, 31,* 185–199.

Rist, F., Glockner-Rist, A., & Demmel, R. (2009). The Alcohol Use Disorders Identification Test revisited: Establishing its structure using nonlinear factor analysis and identifying subgroups of respondents using latent class factor analysis. *Drug and Alcohol Dependence, 100,* 71–82.

Robins, L. N., Cottler, L. B., Bucholz, K. K., Compton, W. M., North, C. S., & Rourke, K. M. (2000). *Diagnostic Interview Schedule for the DSM-IV (DIS-IV).* St. Louis, MO: Washington University School of Medicine.

Rollnick, S., Heather, N., Gold, R., & Hall, W. (1992). Development of a short "Readiness to Change Questionnaire" for use in brief, opportunistic interventions among excessive drinkers. *British Journal of Addiction, 87,* 743–754.

Room, R. (2000). Measuring drinking patterns: The experience of the last half century. *Journal of Substance Abuse, 12,* 23–31.

Rubinsky, A. D., Kivlahan, D. R., Volk, R. J., Maynard, C., & Bradley, K. A. (2010). Estimating risk of alcohol dependence using alcohol screening scores. *Drug and Alcohol Dependence, 108,* 29–36.

Russell, M., Martier, S. S., Sokol, R. J., Mudar, P., Bottoms, S., Jacobson, S., et al. (1994). Screening for pregnancy risk-drinking. *Alcoholism: Clinical and Experimental Research, 18,* 1156–1161.

Saunders, J. B., Aasland, O. G., Babor, T. F., de la Fuente, J. R., & Grant, M. (1993). Development of the Alcohol Use Disorders Identification Test (AUDIT): WHO collaborative project on early detection of persons with harmful alcohol consumption: II. *Addiction, 88,* 791–804.

Selzer, M. (1971). The Michigan Alcoholism Screening Test: The quest for a new diagnostic instrument. *American Journal of Psychiatry, 127,* 1653–1658.

Singleton, E. G. (1996). Alcohol Craving Questionnaire (ACQ-NOW). *Alcohol and Alcoholism, 32,* 344.

Singleton, E. G., & Gorelick, D. A. (1998). Mechanisms of alcohol craving and their clinical implications. In M. Galanter (Ed.), *Recent developments in alcoholism: Vol. 14. The consequences of alcoholism* (pp. 177–195). New York: Plenum Press.

Skinner, H. A., & Allen, B. A. (1982). Alcohol dependence syndrome: Measurement and validation. *Journal of Abnormal Psychology, 91,* 199–209.

Skinner, H. A., & Sheu, W. J. (1982). Reliability of alcohol use indices: The Lifetime Drinking History and the MAST. *Journal of Studies on Alcohol, 43,* 1157–1170.

Smith, S. D., Herrmann, E. V., & Bartlett, K. A. (2011). A content analysis of brief alcohol screening inventories. *Counseling Outcome Research and Evaluation, 2,* 37–58.

Sobell, L. C., & Sobell, M. B. (2000). Alcohol Timeline Followback (TLFB). In American Psychiatric Association (Ed.), *Handbook of psychiatric measures* (pp. 477–479). Washington, DC: American Psychiatric Association.

Sobell, L. C., & Sobell, M. B. (2003). Alcohol consumption measures. In J. P. Allen & V. Wilson (Eds.), *Assessing alcohol problems: A guide for clinicians and researchers* (rev. ed.). Rockville, MD: U.S. Department of Health and Human Services, National Institute on Alcohol Abuse and Alcoholism.

Sobell, L. C., Toneatto, T., & Sobell, M. B. (1994). Behavioral assessment and treatment planning for alcohol, tobacco, and other drug problems: Current status with an emphasis on clinical applications. *Behavior Therapy, 25,* 533–580.

Sokol, R. J., Martier, S. S., & Ager, J. W. (1989). The T-ACE questions: Practical prenatal detection of risk-drinking. *American Journal of Obstetrics and Gynecology, 160,* 863–870.

Spada, M. M., & Wells, A. (2008). Metacognitive beliefs about alcohol use: Development and validation of two self-report scales. *Addictive Behaviors, 33,* 515–527.

Spitzer, R. L., Endicott, J., & Robins, E. (1975). Clinical criteria for psychiatric diagnosis and DSM-III. *American Journal of Psychiatry, 132,* 1187–1192.

Stockwell, T., Murphy, D., & Hodgson, R. (1983). The Severity of Alcohol Dependence Questionnaire: Its use, reliability, and validity. *British Journal of Addiction, 78*(2), 145–155.

Sullivan, J. T., Sykora, K., Schneiderman, J., Naranjo, C. A., & Sellers, E. M. (1989). Assessment of alcohol withdrawal: The revised Clinical Institute Withdrawal Assessment for Alcohol scale (CIWA-Ar). *British Journal of Addiction, 84,* 1353–1357.

Swartz, J. A. (1998). Adapting and using the Substance Abuse Subtle Screening Inventory—2 with criminal justice offenders. *Criminal Justice and Behaviors, 25,* 344–365.

Tarter, R. E. (2005). Psychological evaluation of substance use disorder in adolescents and adults. In R. J. Frances, S. I. Miller, & A. H. Mack (Eds.), *Clinical textbook of addictive disorders* (3rd ed., pp. 37–62). New York: Guilford Press.

Thomas, B. A., & McCambridge, J. (2008). Comparative psychometric study of a range of hazardous drinking measures administered online in a youth population. *Drug and Alcohol Dependence, 96*, 121–127.

Thurber, S., & Snow, M. (2001). Item characteristics of the Michigan Alcoholism Screening Test. *Journal of Clinical Psychology, 57*, 139–144.

U.S. Department of Health and Human Services. (2000). *10th Special Report to Congress on Alcohol and Health*. Rockville, MD: Author.

Vinson, D. C., Kruse, R. L., & Seale, J. P. (2007). Simplifying alcohol assessment: Two questions to identify alcohol use disorders. *Alcoholism: Clinical and Experimental Research, 31*, 1392–1398.

Willinger, U., Lenzinger, E., Hornik, K., Fischer, G., Schonbeck, G., Aschauer, H. N., et al. (2002). Anxiety as a predictor of relapse in detoxified alcohol-dependent patients. *Alcohol and Alcoholism, 37*, 609–612.

Wing, J. K., Babor, T., Brugha, T., Burke, J., Cooper, J. E., Giel, R., et al. (1990). SCAN: Schedule for Clinical Assessment in Neuropsychiatry. *Archives of General Psychiatry, 47*, 589–593.

Young, R. M., & Knight, R. G. (1989). The Drinking Expectancy Questionnaire: A revised measure of alcohol-related beliefs. *Journal of Psychopathology and Behavioral Assessment, 11*, 99–112.

Zywiak, W. H., Connors, G. J., Maisto, S. A., & Westerberg, V. S. (1996). Relapse research and the Reasons for Drinking Questionnaire: A factor analysis of Marlatt's relapse taxonomy. *Addiction, 91*(Suppl.), 121–130.

CHAPTER 8

Social Support

Merideth D. Smith
Amy Fiske

Social support is an important factor in understanding the onset, progression, and outcomes of physical health problems. It is a multifaceted construct that can provide a better conceptualization of a patient's potential resources and risks for both physical and mental health outcomes. The individual facets of social support may have differential associations with health outcomes. This chapter outlines the components of social support, the relation between these components of social support and physical health, and measures that can be used to assess social support in a patient population. We begin by reviewing the following five components of support: the structure of the support, amount of support received, the perception of the support, reciprocity in the relationship, and negative interactions.

Five Components of Social Support

One facet that has received considerable attention and that can be objectively measured is the structural component of social support. This component includes characteristics such as the size of the network (i.e., the number of supports), the types of inter-actions within that network, the physical proximity to the members of the network, and the frequency of contact with network members (Berkman, Glass, Brissette, & Seeman, 2000). Measuring an individual's social network may also provide information regarding how isolated an individual is from other people (Thoits, 1992).

Another important facet of social support is the amount of support received from others (Cohen & Wills, 1985). This can be measured by examining the specific function that the received support serves (Oxman & Berkman, 1990). Functions can be emotional (e.g., providing comfort or a listening ear), instrumental/tangible (e.g., providing transportation or assistance), or informational (e.g., providing advice; Cohen & Wills, 1985; Oxman & Berkman, 1990). Received support is often provided or sought in response to a stressor (Uchino, 2009). The amount of support received from others can have a differential impact on patients depending upon the function of the support. Whereas the receipt of emotional support is associated with positive health outcomes, informational or tangible support can be inversely associated with health outcomes (Uchino, 2004). For example, for patients recovering from a stroke, emotional support was significantly correlated with increased functioning at a 6-month follow-up, whereas instrumental support was found to be associated with increased functioning only when provided in moderate amounts (Glass & Maddox, 1992). Individuals who require larger amounts of support may be experiencing a more severe illness and would have little improvement in functioning regardless of the support received. The differential impact of instrumental support may also be explained by the quality of support received—poor quality support would not result in improvements in functioning. Alternatively, receiving high levels of instrumental support may threaten the individual's self-esteem or sense of independence (Uchino, 2004).

Perceived social support is the appraisal of the availability and adequacy of support (Oxman & Berkman, 1990). Perceived social support takes into account whether the support received meets the needs of the patient and whether that support is available when needed (Cohen & Wills, 1985). The literature suggests that the perceived quality of support may be a more valuable component of support to assess than the amount of support received or the structure of the support network when predicting psychological and physical health outcomes (Penninx, Kriegsman, van Eijk, Boeke, & Deeg, 1996). Surprisingly, the amount of support received from others is only moderately related to the perception of availability and quality of support received from others (Haber, Cohen, Lucas, & Baltes, 2007). Several factors may influence how one perceives the support received. For example, the perception of support may be influenced by enduring predispositions, such as personality factors or a cognitive schema developed over the life span that an individual uses to explain social interactions (Uchino, 2009). Individuals reporting poor quality or poor availability of support may have a more negative outlook, which influences how the support is perceived (Kitamura et al., 2002). The association between support received and the perception of that support may also be influenced by the amount of support the care receiver gives back to the social network. In a community sample of older adults, individuals who reported giving support to their families were more likely to report a better perception of the support received from others (Krause, 1999).

The construct of social exchanges takes into consideration the reciprocal nature of social interactions, that is, the relation between support received and support given to others. This concept of reciprocity has come out of the work evaluating the theory of equity (Liang, Krause, & Bennett, 2001; Walster, Berscheid, & Walster, 1973). Reciprocity is the social norm dictating that within a relationship both members engage in a balance of providing and receiving support, so both members maximize the benefits derived from the relationship (Walster et al., 1973). The theory of equity predicts that deviations from this balance will cause distress to the individual who *over*benefits (receives more support than she or he gives) and to the individual who *under*benefits (provides more support than she or he receives). The provision of support to others is related to both the perceived quality of support received and the amount of support received (Dunkel-Schetter & Skokan, 1990; Krause, 1999).

Finally, negative social interactions (negative support) can have a dramatic impact on health and functioning and may reduce the beneficial effects of positive social interactions (Uchino, 2006). Negative support can include isolation from others, interactions that increase distress or negative emotions, support that is overwhelming, support that threatens a person's independence, or interactions that lead to feelings of burdensomeness, that is, feeling burdened by the other individual (Cohen, 2004). Additionally, members of the social network can have a negative influence on others and may promote unhealthy behaviors such as smoking (Burg & Seeman, 1994).

Loneliness, although related, is distinct from the constructs discussed above. Defined as an unpleasant emotional state associated with perceived deficits in social relationships, loneliness is more closely aligned with perceived support than with social isolation (Hawkley et al., 2008). Loneliness is not typically assessed by social support instruments, but well-validated measures are available (e.g., the revised UCLA Loneliness Scale; Russell, Peplau, & Cutrona, 1980).

Social Support and Health Outcomes

There is an abundance of literature suggesting that structural, received, and perceived social support are related to lower mortality rates across diseases (see Penninx et al., 1996, and Uchino, 2004, for reviews). Additionally, both providing support to others and volunteering are related to lower mortality rates (Brown, Nesse, Vinokur, & Smith, 2003; Oman, Thoresen, & McMahon, 1999). An extensive body of literature has examined the impact of social support on the cardiovascular system and, to a lesser extent, on immune and endocrine system functioning.

Structural, received, and perceived quality of support have been linked to cardiovascular disease. A review by Lett et al. (2005) found increased risk for onset of coronary heart disease and mortality in patients with coronary heart disease with smaller network size, less social support received from others, and lower perceived quality and availability of support. Negative social interactions were associated with poor health at discharge in patients hospitalized due to strokes (Stephens, Kinney, Norris, & Ritchie, 1987). Additionally, there is evidence that relates social supports to lower blood pressure, decreased heart rate during a stressor task, faster recovery of systolic blood pressure after a stressor, lower ambulatory blood pressure, and slower progression of plaque buildup (Grant, Hamer, & Steptoe, 2009; Uchino, 2006, 2009).

Structural support, received emotional support, and perceived social support are related to increased natural killer cell activity, indicating improved immune system functioning (Uchino, 2006; Uchino, Cacioppo, & Kiecolt-Glaser, 1996). Further, in men with HIV, poor perceived availability of social support was related to an increased deterioration of the immune system over a 5-year period compared with men with HIV with good perceived availability of support (Theorell, Blomkvist, Jonsson, & Schulman, 1995). Negative interactions may also be related to suppressed immune functions. Negative social interactions in animal studies resulted in increased susceptibility to viruses (DeVries, Glasper, & Detillion, 2003). Social support can also affect the functioning of the endocrine system. In response to stressors, the presence of support or perceived availability of support is related to a decrease in the release of stress hormones such as cortisol and catecholamines (Uchino, 2006). The perceived strength of a partner's support was related to increased oxytocin levels after physical contact with that partner (Grewen, Girdler, Amico, & Light, 2005).

Process Models of Social Support

There are several models to describe the process by which social support influences physical health. The models addressed in this chapter include the direct-effects model, including the social control model; a model that posits alteration of acute stressors; and a model that involves improved psychological health. The social convoy model places the process within a developmental context. The direct-effects model suggests that social support may directly influence health through the type of support received or through social influence (Cohen, 1988). A patient might receive health-related information or financial help that promotes better health and maintains healthy behaviors (Croyle & Hunt, 1991; O'Reilly & Thomas, 1989). Additionally, social support can have a direct effect on health through the mechanism of social control. Members of the social network can exert social influence on the individual by encouraging the individual to engage in positive health behaviors (Cohen, 1988; Uchino, 2004). Attempts at social control were more associated with health-enhancing behaviors, such as exercise, compared with the association between social control and risky health behaviors (Lewis & Rook, 1999).

Social support may also affect health by altering the experience of acute stressors. Positive social interactions may directly affect an individual's reaction to stress by changing how an individual perceives a stressful situation (Thoits, 1992). Social support may also increase an individual's sense of well-being, decrease the amount of daily stress, and subsequently decrease the number of major life stressors (Russell & Cutrona, 1991). The physiological reaction to the stressor can also be influenced, as social support decreases the fight-or-flight and stress response (Berkman et al., 2000; Cohen, 1988; Lepore, 1998; Uchino, 2009).

Social support may affect physical health by altering psychological factors that are associated with improved health. For example, support may improve an individual's self-efficacy (or confidence in the ability to perform an activity), level of self-esteem, psychological health, or positive emotions (Cohen, 1988). Additionally, social support may serve as a means for the regulation of emotion. The socioemotional selectivity theory posits that individuals who have a time-limited perspective (as may be the case in individuals with terminal illness) will invest their resources and remaining time in maintaining the relationships that provide positive support and decrease negative interactions (Carstensen, Isaacowitz, & Charles, 1999). By focusing on increasing positive interactions and decreasing negative interactions, an individual can increase positive experiences and positive emotions. Positive emotions can have a beneficial impact on health (see review by Pressman & Cohen, 2005).

Regardless of the mechanisms through which social support may influence health outcomes, it is important to consider stability and change in social factors over the life span. The social convey model (Kahn & Antonucci, 1980) suggests that individuals are surrounded by a relatively stable social network, the composition of which reflects both personal and situational variables. Consistent with this model, the composition of social networks—particularly among the closest members of the network—appears to be relatively stable over time, although network size declines in late life (Antonucci, Akiyama, & Takahashi, 2004).

Thus social support is an important factor to consider when assessing an individual who is experiencing physical and mental health problems. Information about the resources available to the patient, the patient's perception of those resources, and potential sources of stress can be important in treatment planning. The assessment of social support can include an overview of the available support resources (structural components), the support currently received, the perception of support availability and quality, the perception of reciprocity, and negative interac-

tions. This assessment can be accomplished through an unstructured clinical interview or through the measures described in the next section. The following sections review measures that assess the five components of social support (structural, amount received, perception of support, reciprocity, and negative social interactions). Psychometric information is included in Table 8.1.

Structural Components of Social Support

Structural aspects of social support include, on the one hand, the number of social ties and frequency of contact with them (conceptualized as social integration vs. isolation) and, on the other hand, the systemic characteristics of the social network itself, such as network density and stability (Berkman et al., 2000). Understanding of the individual's social network provides the clinician with information about the person's context, including potential resources that may aid in treatment.

Social integration is often measured by asking about intimate partners, whether the person lives alone or with others, participation in community organizations, and frequency of social contacts. These questions can be incorporated into an unstructured clinical interview or assessed as part of a more formal social network analysis. Aspects of the network structure that can be evaluated include network size, density (the extent to which network members interact with one another), multiplexity (the extent to which network members fulfill more than one function), physical proximity of network members, and temporal stability. Following are commonly used measures of the structural aspect of social support. Measures of social integration are discussed first, followed by measures that provide more extensive analyses of social network characteristics.

The Social Network Index (SNI; Berkman & Syme, 1979) is used specifically to compile an inventory of social network members in each of four categories. The respondent is asked about marital status, number of close relatives and friends, church participation, and participation in other organizations. The number of contacts, weighted by the relative importance of the relationship, is used to categorize the network on a 4-point scale from fewest to most connections. Evidence of reliability was not located (nor is internal consistency relevant for measures of this sort). Evidence of construct validity can be found in the strong relation with mortality (Berkman & Syme, 1979). Originally developed for use in epidemiological research, the measure was validated using large representative samples.

Several measures assess both social integration variables and aspects of received or perceived support. A widely used measure of this sort is the 10-item Lubben Social Network Scale (LSNS; Lubben, 1988). Developed specifically for use with older adults, questions assess the number of family members or friends seen at least once a month (on a 0–5 scale ranging from none to 9 or more), as well as the perceived closeness of the relationships. Low scores on the LSNS have been associated with a wide range of health outcomes, including mortality, all-cause hospitalization, physical health problems, depression, and poor health practices (Lubben et al., 2006). The measure has been translated into numerous languages (e.g., Chinese, German, Japanese, Korean, Spanish). An abbreviated, 6-item version (LSNS-6; Lubben et al., 2006) has demonstrated similar psychometric properties to the full-length scale, including acceptable internal consistency and correlation with various social and health indicators (e.g., self-rated health, limitations in activities of daily living). Subscales assessing support from family and non-kin sources have demonstrated convergent and discriminant validity.

The Duke Social Support Index (DSSI; Koenig et al., 1993; Landerman, George, Campbell, & Blazer, 1989) assesses the nature of the social ties and frequency of contact, as well as support received and satisfaction with that support. The original DSSI includes 35 items that factor into five subscales: Social Network, Social Interaction (e.g., number of times in past week the person spent time with someone he or she is not living with), Subjective Support, Instrumental Support, and Other Items. A 23-item version includes only the Social Interaction, Subjective Support, and Instrumental Support subscales (Koenig et al., 1993). An 11-item version (Koenig et al., 1993) or a 10-item subset (Powers, Goodger, & Byles,

2004) includes only the Social Interaction and Subjective Support factors. Thus the appropriate version of the DSSI depends on the type of social support one wishes to measure. The Social Network subscale is only weakly related to mental or physical health outcomes, whereas the Social Interaction, Subjective Support, and Instrumental Support subscales are associated with a variety of health outcomes (Koenig et al., 1993). The Subjective Support subscale has demonstrated good internal consistency, whereas only moderate internal consistency has been demonstrated for the Social Interaction subscale (Koenig et al., 1993; Powers et al., 2004). Reliability was not reported by the authors for the other subscales.

The Norbeck Social Support Questionnaire (NSSQ; Norbeck, Lindsey, & Carrieri, 1981) is a self-report measure of the function of support (affect, affirmation, and aid), size of the network, stability of the network, the availability of support, frequency of contact, and loss of important social relationships within the past year. Respondents are asked to identify up to 20 significant relationships and the type of relationship (i.e., family, friend). For each item, respondents are asked to rate the network members listed as significant relationships using a 5-point Likert-type scale, ranging from *not at all* to *a great deal*. The items load onto three factors: Aid, Affect, and Affirmation (Gigliotti, 2002). All items had good test–retest reliability over a 1-week period in a sample of graduate students. Items of support received were highly correlated. Items measuring the network structure were also highly correlated. The measures of numbers of relationships lost and quality of those lost relationships were moderately correlated. The NSSQ had convergent validity with other measures of social integration and affection (Norbeck, Lindsey, & Carrieri, 1983). This measure had similar internal reliability in a population of patients receiving care in a psychiatric unit (Byers & Mullis, 1987).

Numerous measures include only one or several questions about social integration but primarily evaluate other aspects of social support. These measures are discussed in the relevant sections.

The most comprehensive method of assessing the structure of an individual's social network is a formal network analysis, derived

TABLE 8.1. Summary of Social Support Measures

Measure	Description	No. of items	Validity	Internal reliability	Test–retest reliability
			Structural: Social integration/isolation		
Social Network Index (SNI; Berkman & Syme, 1979)	Assesses frequency of contact within four categories: marital status, number of close relatives and friends, church participation, other organizations.				
Lubben Social Network Scale (LSNS; Lubben, 1988); short form (LSNS-6; Lubben & Gironda, 2000; Lubben et al., 2006)	Screens for social isolation. Assesses frequency of contact and perceived availability of support from family, friends, and confidants; helping others; living arrangements. Developed for older adults. Short form includes only Family and Friend subscales.	Two versions: 10-item, 6-item	Short form correlates with mortality, all-cause hospitalization, physical health, depression, health behaviors.	*10-item:* alpha = 0.70 *6-item:* Total score: alpha = 0.83 Family: alpha = 0.84–0.89 Non-kin: alpha = 0.80–0.82	
Duke Social Support Index (DSSI; Landerman et al., 1989; Koenig et al., 1993)	Assesses social network, social interaction, subjective support, instrumental support, other items; 23-item version omits network, other items; 11-item version omits instrumental support.	Three versions: 35-item, 25-item, 11-item	*Short forms:* Subjective Support subscale inversely related to mental distress, use of health services.	*23-item:* Subjective support: alpha = 0.71–0.81 *11-item:* Subjective Support alpha = 0.80 Social Interaction alpha = 0.58 10-item total alpha = 0.76 (Powers et al., 2004)	
Norbeck Social Support Questionnaire (NSSQ; Norbeck et al., 1981)	Assesses network size, stability, availability, frequency of contact, losses within past year.	9 items per network member (up to 20 members)		alpha = 0.69–0.98	r = .85–.92

Measure	Description	No. items	Validity	Reliability	Test–retest
Social Network List (SNL; Hirsch, 1979, 1980; adapted by Stokes, 1983)	Identifies up to 20 social network members; assesses supports received over past 14 days (Stokes: month) in 5 domains: cognitive guidance, social reinforcement, tangible assistance, emotional support, socializing; measure yields network size and density, number of confidants, percent relatives.		Structural: Social network analysis Network size correlates with SSQ number of supports.		Over 4 weeks: total network size r =.45; satisfaction r = .16; family size, r = .49; friend size, r = .54 (Bass & Stein, 1997)
Hierarchical Mapping Technique (Antonucci & Israel, 1986; Antonucci, 1986)	Semistructured interview; concentric circles are presented in which respondent places at least 10 network members who provide or receive support (confiding; reassurance; respect; sick care; talk when upset, nervous, or depressed; and talk about health).		Received support Veridicality (correspondence with network member report) = 49–54% for specific types of support, 79% for any support; veridicality is highest for spouses and when respondent feels close to network member.		
Arizona Social Support Interview Schedule (ASSIS; Barrera, 1980)	Structured interview; assesses available support and actual support received in the last month (material aid, physical assistance, intimate interaction, guidance, feedback, positive social interaction); administration: 15–20 minutes.	6 × 2-part questions	Convergent validity with ISSB (available and conflicted network size).	Satisfaction, alpha = 0.33 Support need, alpha = 0.52	Received support: r = .88 Conflicted support: r = .54 Satisfaction: r = .69 Support need: r = .80
Inventory of Socially Supportive Behaviors (ISSB; Barrera et al., 1981)	Questionnaire; assesses frequency of supportive behaviors received in past month: directive guidance (advice); nondirective guidance (emotional support); positive social interaction; tangible assistance.	40	Convergent validity with ASSIS available support, actual support, network size and Moos's Family Environment Scale, Cohesion subscale.	alpha = 0.93–0.94	r = .88 (2 days)

(continued)

TABLE 8.1. *(continued)*

Measure	Description	No. of items	Validity	Internal reliability	Test-retest reliability
			Perceived social support		
Social Support Questionnaire (Sarason, Levine, Basham, & Sarason, 1983)	Assesses network size and satisfaction with support received.	Two versions: 27-item, 6-item	Related to anxiety, depression, hostility, neuroticism, loneliness, and social skills. Converges with other measures of social support.	*27-item:* Network factor: alpha = 0.97; Satisfaction factor: alpha = 0.94; *6-item:* In 3 samples: alphas ranged from 0.90–0.93 for both factors.	*27 item:* Network factor: $r = .90$ Satisfaction factor: $r = .83$
Social Relationship Scale (McFarlane, 1981)	Network size, helpfulness of the support received, and reciprocity in the areas of work, money/finances, home/family, personal/social, personal health, and problems in society.			Helpfulness scales: Work alpha = 0.94; money, alpha = 0.54; home, alpha = 0.84; health, alpha = 0.60; personal, alpha = 0.94; and society alpha = 0.72	Number of people in the network: median across categories $r = .91$ (.62–.99) Helpfulness: median across categories $r = .78$ (.54–.94)
Perceived Social Support—Family/ Friends (Procidano & Heller, 1983)	Measures the satisfaction with support received from family and friends.	40	Related to worry, anxiety, and social alienation.	Friends factor: alpha = 0.88; Family factor alpha = 0.90.	Total PSS $r = .83$
Interpersonal Support Evaluation List (Cohen & Hoberman, 1983; Cohen et al., 1985)	Measures the perceived availability of material aid, belonging, self-esteem, appraisal support. Two versions: Student version and General Population version.	Two versions: Student version: 48 items; General version: 40 items	Converges with other measures of perceived social support. Related to positive life events and depressive symptoms. Moderates the relation between negative life events and physical symptoms. Related to physical health symptoms.	*Student version:* Total score: alpha = 0.77; tangible: alpha = 0.71; belonging: alpha = 0.75; self-esteem: alpha = 0.60; appraisal: alpha = 0.77 *General version:* tangible: alpha = 0.73–0.82; belonging: alpha = 0.73–0.78; self-esteem: alpha = 0.62–0.73; appraisal: alpha = 0.76–0.82	*Student version* Total score: $r = .87$; tangible: $r = .80$; belonging: $r = .82$; self-esteem: $r = .71$; appraisal: $r = .87$ *General version:* Total score: $r = .70$; tangible: $r = .69$; belonging: $r = .65$; self-esteem: $r = .68$; appraisal: $r = .69$
Family Relationship Index (Holahan & Moos, 1982)	Measures the satisfaction with family in the areas of cohesion, expressiveness, and conflict.	27	Related to physical symptoms and depressive symptoms across men and women.	alpha = 0.89	

Measure	Description	Number of items	Validity	Reliability (alpha)	Correlations (r)
Social Support Appraisals (Vaux, 1986)	Measures perception of feeling loved, esteemed, and involved with support network. Has three factors: Friends, Family, and Other Individuals.	23	Convergent with other measures of perceived social support and depressive symptoms.	Family: alpha = 0.90; Friends: alpha = 0.81; Other Individuals: alpha = 0.84	
Multidimensional Scale of Perceived Social Support (Zimet, Dahlem, Zimet, & Farley, 1988)	Measures adequacy of support from family, friends, and significant others.	12	Related to depressive and anxiety symptoms.	Total scale: alpha = 0.88, test–retest: .85; Family: alpha = 0.91, test–retest: .85; Friends: alpha = 0.87, test–retest: .75; Significant others: alpha = 0.85, test–retest: .72	Total scale: $r = .85$; Family: $r = .85$; Friends: $r = .75$; Significant others: $r = .72$
Positive and Negative Social Exchanges (Newsom et al., 2005)	Measures the satisfaction with positive interactions across 4 areas (informational support, instrumental support, emotional support, companionship) and the level of bother experienced with negative interactions across 4 areas (unwanted advice/intrusion, failure to provide help, unsympathetic/insensitive behavior, and rejection/neglect).	24	Related to distress and well-being.	Positive appraisal: alpha = 0.68; Negative appraisal: alpha = 0.75	
MOS–Social Support Survey (Sherbourne & Stewart, 1991)	Measures the perceived availability of support across areas: tangible support, affectionate support, emotional/informational support, and positive interactions.	Three versions: 18-item, 12-item, 4-item		*18-item* tangible: alpha = 0.92; affection: alpha = 0.91; positive social interactions: alpha = 0.91; emotional/informational: alpha = 0.96 *12-item* Total score: alpha = 0.94 *4-item* Total score: alpha = 0.83	*18-item* tangible: $r = .74$; affection: $r = .76$; positive social interactions: $r = .72$; emotional/informational: $r = .72$; total score: $r = .78$

(continued)

TABLE 8.1. *(continued)*

Measure	Description	No. of items	Validity	Internal reliability	Test–retest reliability
Interview Schedule for Social Interaction (ISSI; Henderson et al., 1980; Eklund et al., 2007; Undén & Orth-Gomér, 1989)	Measures the Availability of Attachment (AVAT), the perceived Adequacy of the Attachment (ADAT), the Availability of Social Integration (AVSI), and the perceived Adequacy of the Social Integration (ADSI).	Two versions: 52-item; 30-item	Related to psychological health, trustfulness, smoking behaviors, and physical symptoms.	*52-item version:* AVAT: alpha = 0.67; ADAT: alpha = 0.81; AVSI: alpha = 0.71; ADSI: alpha = 0.79 *30-item version:* AVAT: alpha = 0.74; ADAT: alpha = 0.63; AVSI: alpha = 0.66; ADSI: alpha = 0.76	*52-item version:* AVAT: $r = .76$; ADAT: $r = .79$; AVSI: $r = .75$; ADSI: $r = .75$
Social Support Network Inventory (SSNI; Flaherty et al., 1983)	Measures availability of support, emotional help, practical support, and reciprocity within the respondent's five most important relationships.	11	Convergent validity with clinician ratings of support in depressed patients ($r = .68$). Related to depressive symptoms and social adjustment.	Total score: Kuder–Richardson–20 alpha = 0.821; availability of support: Kuder–Richardson–20, alpha = 0.76; practical help: Kuder–Richardson–20, alpha = 0.84; emotional support: Kuder–Richardson–20, alpha = 0.90; event-related support: Kuder–Richardson–20, alpha = 0.84; reciprocity scales: Kuder–Richardson–20, alpha = 0.81	$r = .87$
			Reciprocity		
Hatfield Global Measure (Hatfield, Walster, & Berscheid, 1978)	Measures perceived exchange of support in marital relationship.	1			

Instrument	Description	No. of items	Related constructs	Internal consistency	Test–retest reliability
Traupmann–Utne–Hatfield Scale (Traupmann, Utne, & Hatfield, 1981)	Measures the perception of benefits derived from intimate partners (output) and benefits given to intimate partner (input) across personal, emotional, and day-to-day situations. Also measures opportunities lost or gained in marriage.	44	Equitable relationships related to satisfaction with relationship and mood.	Total input scale: alpha = 0.90; Total output scale: alpha = 0.87	
Interpersonal Relationship Index (Tilden, Nelson, & May, 1990)	Measures beliefs and behaviors across support, reciprocity, and conflict domains within relationships.	39	Related to physical health. Conflict scale related to social desirability.	Support: alpha = 0.92; Reciprocity: alpha = 0.83; Conflict: alpha = 0.81	Support: $r = .91$; Reciprocity: $r = .84$; Conflict: $r = .81$
Social Support Scale (Krause & Markides, 1990)	Measures support provided to others across emotional, tangible, and informational domains.	13	Related to self-esteem, negative affect.	Emotional support: alpha = 0.83; Tangible support: alpha = 0.63; Informational support: alpha = 0.84	
Negative social interactions					
Test of Negative Social Exchange (Ruehlman & Karoly, 1991)	Measures interactions across four domains: hostility/impatience, insensitivity, interference, and ridicule.	18	Related with social desirability, depressive symptoms, and anxiety symptoms.	Hostility/impatience: alpha = 0.83; Insensitivity: alpha = 0.82; Interference: alpha = 0.75; Ridicule: alpha = 0.70	Hostility/impatience: $r = .80$; Insensitivity: $r = .72$; Interference: $r = .65$; Ridicule: $r = .7$
Zarit Burden Interview (Bédard, Molloy, Squire, Dubois, Lever, & O'Donnell, 2001; Zarit, Reever, & Bach-Peterson, 1980)	Measures the perceived level of personal strain and role strain in caregivers.	12		Total score: alpha = 0.88; Personal strain: alpha = 0.89; Role strain: alpha = 0.77	

from the anthropological research tradition. In this approach, the object is to evaluate aspects of the network as a system rather than aspects of the individual. This approach is represented by the Network Analysis Profile (Sokolovsky & Cohen, 1981). Developed for research with community-dwelling psychiatric populations, in whom self-report of social networks was found to be problematic at times, this method involves interviews with the individual, as well as confirmation with collateral sources. Three dimensions are assessed, including network member attributes (e.g., age, sex, occupation), linkage attributes (i.e., the types of interactions between the individual and each network member), and network attributes (including interconnections between network members and fluctuations in the network over time). The authors report high interrater reliability (.83–.92). A drawback of this method is the length of time required to train interviewers (8–10 hours) and to administer the profile (2 hours on average, with a range from 30 minutes to 6 hours).

A more economical method of assessing network attributes is the Social Network List (SNL; Hirsch, 1979, 1980; adapted and described by Stokes, 1983). The SNL involves asking an individual to identify up to 20 members of the social network with whom the individual has had contact within the last month. For each relationship, the interviewer queries whether the person is a relative, whether the person is considered a confidant, and with which other network members that person has contact at least monthly. Scores provided by the measure include network size, number of confidants, percentage of relatives, and density (actual relationships among network members as a proportion of possible relationships). The measure also assesses the nature of the support received in the domains of cognitive guidance, social reinforcement, tangible assistance, emotional support, and socializing. The measure was validated using samples composed primarily of undergraduate students (Hirsch, 1979, 1980; Stokes, 1983). We were unable to obtain reliability information for this measure.

As can be seen, there are numerous measures available for use in compiling a comprehensive picture of a person's social world. Because the comprehensive assessment of social network variables (e.g., network density, proximity, multiplexity) can be time-consuming, it may be feasible only in exceptional cases, whereas the assessment of social integration variables (number of social ties and frequency of contacts) would be warranted on a routine basis. Any analysis of social networks, however, only provides information about the structure of an individual's social relationships.

Received Support

In addition to understanding the structure of an individual's social network, it can be useful to evaluate the nature and quantity of support the individual actually receives. As noted earlier, the relation between received support and health outcomes varies by type of support received, current stressful life events, and the personality of the care receiver (Sarason & Sarason, 1994; Uchino, 2004), so any assessment of received support should differentiate by type, such as emotional support, instrumental/tangible support, or informational support (Cohen, 1988; Oxman & Berkman, 1990). Further, the assessment of received support should be placed in the context of recent life events and personality factors of the individual receiving the support. Both interview and self-report methods of assessing received support have been developed. Although these methods both rely on an individual's report of support received, evidence suggests that received support can be reliably measured, perhaps reflecting the more behavioral nature of the construct, in contrast with the more subjective construct of perceived support (Haber et al., 2007).

Antonucci and colleagues (Antonucci, 1986; Antonucci & Israel, 1986) have developed a comprehensive interview method for evaluating support received, consistent with the social convoy model of support (Kahn & Antonucci, 1980). The interviewer begins by drawing three concentric circles, representing differential levels of closeness to the respondent, and eliciting at least 10 network members that the respondent locates within one of the circles. Respondents are asked to indicate which network members provide each of six functions (and to whom each type of support is provided by the respondent): confidences, reassurance, respect, sick care, talk when upset, nervous, or depressed, and talk about health. On average, the agreement between respondent and network member report for specific type of support was 49–54%, and for receipt or provision of any support was 79%. Agreement was highest among spouses and lowest among friends and was correlated with feelings of closeness. Originally developed for use with adults and older adults, this method has been adapted for use with children as young as 6 years old (Levitt, Guacci-Franco, & Levitt, 1993). This approach yields comprehensive information about social integration, as well as received support.

The Arizona Social Support Interview Schedule (ASSIS; Barrera, 1980) provides a more delimited method of assessing provided support. This structured interview evaluates actual support received, as well as available support, conflicted support, and satisfaction with the support within the past 6 months in the following categories: material aid, physical assistance, intimate interaction, guidance, feedback, and positive social interaction. Additionally, the ASSIS measures whether the individual would have liked more support and whether he or she received the support needed. Both support received and conflicted support were stable over a 2-day period in an undergraduate population. The Support Satisfaction scale was stable but did not have good internal reliability. The Support Need scale was stable over 2 days and had poor internal reliability. The interview requires 15–20 minutes to administer.

The most widely used self-report assessment of received support is the Inventory of Socially Supportive Behaviors (ISSB; Barrera, Sandler, & Ramsay, 1981). The respondent rates the frequency of occurrence in the past month (1 = *not at all*, 5 = *about every day*) of 40 potentially supportive behaviors. Factors assessed include directive guidance (advice); nondirective guidance (emotional support); positive social interaction; and tangible assistance. Internal consistency is good, as is test–retest reliability over 2-day and 1-month intervals (Barrera et al., 1981; Barrera & Ainlay, 1983). Convergent validity with the ASSIS and other measures of social support has been established (Barrera et al., 1981).

As noted earlier, several measures assess received support, as well as other aspects of social support. The DSSI (Landerman et al., 1989), discussed earlier, measures received support, in addition to social integration variables. The more extensive measures of social network characteristics discussed previously, the SNL (Hirsch, 1979, 1980; adapted and described by Stokes, 1983) and the Network Analysis Profile (Sokolovsky & Cohen, 1981) also incorporate detailed evaluations of support received.

Perception of Support

Perceived social support is an individual's appraisal of the support received from formal and informal sources and whether it meets the needs of the individual, is available when needed, and is desired (Cohen & Wills, 1985). The perception of support quality is an important construct in predicting physical and psychological health (Penninx et al., 1996). Clinical assessments and the available measures of perceived social support often include questions designed to assess the perceived availability of the support, the quality of the support received, and whether the support received is desired. Several measures described previously include an assessment of perceived support (see LSNS, DSSI, and ASSIS). Following is a brief discussion of self-report and interviewer-administered measures that assess the perceived quality and availability of support.

The Social Support Questionnaire (SSQ; Sarason, Levine, Basham, & Sarason, 1983; Sarason, Sarason, Shearin, & Pierce, 1987) is one of the more widely used measures of perceived quality of support received. There are two versions of the SSQ, a 27-item and a 6-item version. Respondents are asked to list people who provide support in the manner described in each item and to indicate whether they are satisfied with that support. In the SSQ, both the satisfaction factor and the network size factor had stable test–retest reliability in a population of college students (Sarason et al., 1983). Additionally, both factors had good internal reliability in the 27-item SSQ. The 6-item version had similar internal reliability to the full version within three samples of college students for both factors (Sarason et al., 1987). High satisfaction with support was significantly related to less anxiety, depression, hostility, and neuroticism in women, but only to less depression in men (Sarason et al., 1983). Neither the report of network size nor satisfaction with support was related to social desirability. The 6-item version of the SSQ had similar correlations with anxiety, depression, and social desirability to the 27-item version of the SSQ (Sarason et al., 1987).

The Social Relationship Scale (SRS: McFarlane, 1981) is an interviewer-administered measure used to assess several components of social relationships. This measure assesses the network size, the helpfulness of support received, and whether the respondent reciprocates that support. The respondent is asked to list initials and type of relationship of individuals who have provided support in the areas of work, money/finances, home/family, personal/social, personal health, and problems in society. The respondent rates the support from each member on a 7-point Likert-type scale representing the level of helpfulness and indicates which relationships are reciprocal. Psychometrics were established in undergraduate students. The network size had good test–retest reliability in each area. The helpfulness of support received in the areas of work, money, home, health, personal life, and society were stable over a 1-week period. Responses were not influenced by a tendency to respond in a socially desirable manner.

The Perceived Social Support scale (Procidano & Heller, 1983) assesses the perception of satisfaction with the support received from friends (PSS-Fr) and support received from family (PSS-Fa). The PSS is a 40-item measure with three response options (*yes, no,* or *don't know*). In a sample of undergraduate students, the test–retest reliability of the PSS measure was stable over a 1-month period. Both factors had good internal reliability. The Friends and Family scales were related to measures of worry, anxiety, and social alienation. The Family scale was related to depressive symptoms. Positive mood induction did not influence the reporting of satisfaction of support from family or friends. Induction of a negative mood resulted in lower reports of satisfaction with friends. This implies that satisfaction with support is influenced by a negative

mood state, whereby individuals presenting with depression or negative affect may report poor quality of support. A 20-item abbreviated version of the PSS has similar internal reliability in a sample of caregivers for individuals with Alzheimer's disease (PSS-Family: alpha = 0.89; PSS-Friends: alpha = 0.90; Wilks, 2009). In three different samples of individuals seeking treatment for alcohol addiction, a 7-item version of the PSS-Family scale had internal reliability ranging from alpha = 0.76 to .82, and the 7-item PSS-Friend scale had internal reliability ranging from alpha = 0.84 to 0.91 (Rice & Longabaugh, 1996). The 7-item subscales also demonstrated good test–retest reliability (PSS-Family: r = .94; PSS-Friends: r = .88).

The Family Relationship Index (FRI: Holahan & Moos, 1982) is a 27-item measure derived from the Family Environment Scale to assess the quality of relationships within a family across three domains: cohesion, expressiveness, and conflict. The FRI has good internal consistency in a sample of community-dwelling adults. This measure has also been found to be related to psychosomatic and depressive symptoms in both men and women.

The Interpersonal Support Evaluation List (ISEL: Cohen & Hoberman, 1983; Cohen, Mermelstein, Kamarck, & Hoberman, 1985) is a 48-item measure that assesses the perceived availability of material aid (tangible), people with whom the interviewee can engage in activities (belonging), people with whom the respondent can make positive self-comparisons (self-esteem), and people with whom the interviewee can talk (appraisal). This scale uses a 4-point Likert-type scale ranging from *definitely false* to *definitely true*. The internal reliability of the total score was good, and the internal reliability for each factor was adequate in both an undergraduate student sample and five samples of adults in the community. The ISEL is related to experiencing more positive events and fewer depressive symptoms (Cohen, McGowan, Fooskas, & Rose, 1984). In the community adult sample, the ISEL was related to psychological symptoms and physical symptoms (Cohen et al., 1985).

The Social Support Appraisals (SSA; Vaux, 1986) scale measures the perception of feeling loved, esteemed, and involved with family, friends, and other individuals. The SSA has 23 items that use a 4-point Likert-type scale, wherein response choices range from *strongly agree* to *strongly disagree*. In a sample of college students, the internal reliability for the three factors (family, friends, and other individuals) was good. In a sample of community members (age range 12–85), the internal reliability for the Family, Friends, and Other Individuals factors was also good and similar to the alpha levels in the college sample. The SSA is related to other measures of perception of social support, including the PSS, FRI, and SSQ. The perceived quality of support from friends, family, and others was inversely related to depressive symptoms in both the community and undergraduate samples.

The Multidimensional Scale of Perceived Social Support (MSPSS; Zimet, Dahlem, Zimet, & Farley, 1988) is a 12-item measure that assesses the adequacy of support received from family, friends, and significant others. This measure uses a 7-point Likert-type scale that ranges from *very strongly disagree* to *very strongly agree*. The internal reliability of the total scale and the factor scales was good in a sample of undergraduate students. This measure is stable over a period of 2–3 months. The MSPSS is inversely related to depressive symptoms and anxiety symptoms. Additionally, this measure demonstrates good psychometric qualities in African American adolescents, psychiatric patients, and Arab American adolescents and women (Aroian, Templin, & Ramaswamy, 2010; Canty-Mitchell & Zimet, 2000; Cecil, Stanley, Carrion, & Swann, 1995; Ramaswamy, Aroian, & Templin, 2009).

The Positive and Negative Social Exchanges (PANSE; Newsom, Rook, Nishishiba, Sorkin, & Mahan, 2005) scale is a measure of both positive and negative interactions and the appraisal of quality for each type of interaction. Twenty-four items assess positive and negative interactions across eight areas (informational support, instrumental support, emotional support, companionship, unwanted advice/intrusion, failure to provide help, unsympathetic or insensitive behavior, and rejection/neglect). Satisfaction is assessed using 12 items with a 4-point Likert-type scale that ranges from *not at all satisfied* to *very satisfied*. Nega-

tive appraisal is measured with 12 items by asking the interviewee how bothered he or she was by each type of negative interaction. These items are rated on a 4-point Likert-type scale ranging from *not at all bothered* to *very bothered*. The positive appraisal scale had adequate internal reliability, and the negative appraisal had good internal reliability in a sample of older adults. Both positive and negative appraisals of support were related to distress and well-being.

The Medical Outcomes Study Social Support Survey (MOS-SSS; Sherbourne & Stewart, 1991) is an 18-item measure that assesses the perceived availability of support in four areas: tangible support, affectionate support, emotional/informational support, and positive social interactions. The items are rated on a 5-point Likert-type scale ranging from *none of the time* to *all of the time*. The total score and four factors have good internal reliability in a sample of adults. The measure was stable over 1 year in a sample of chronically ill adults. Two abbreviated versions of the MOS-SSS, with 12 items and 4 items, respectively, have also been developed (Gjesfjeld, Greeno, & Kim, 2008). Both the 12-item and 4-item MOS-SSS demonstrated good internal reliability in a sample of adult women.

The Interview Schedule for Social Interactions (ISSI; Henderson, Duncan-Jones, Byrne, & Scott, 1980) is a 52-item measure of both structural components of support and the perception of support. The factors measured in the ISSI include the Availability of Attachment (AVAT), the perceived Adequacy of the Attachment (ADAT), the Availability of Social Integration (AVSI), and the perceived Adequacy of the Social Integration (ADSI). The ISSI was originally conceived as an interview that lasted approximately 45 minutes. These factors had adequate internal reliability and remained stable over a 4-, 8-, and 12-month period in a sample of community adults. The AVAT, ADAT, AVSI, and ADSI were moderately correlated with neuroticism. This measure was designed using a general population sample. An abbreviated questionnaire version of the ISSI (30 items) was assessed using a Swedish population of men at risk for ischemic heart disease and individuals with mental illness (Eklund, Bengtsson-Tops, & Lindstedt, 2007; Undén & Orth-Gomér, 1989). In the sample of

Swedish men, the internal reliability was adequate (Undén & Orth-Gomér, 1989). The ISSI factors were related to psychological health, trustfulness, smoking behaviors, and physical symptoms. In the study utilizing three samples of patients with mental illness, the abbreviated ISSI had only two factors that were similar to the 52-item measure (AVSI and ADSI). The AVAT and ADAT were not stable factors in the abbreviated ISSI, which suggests that those factors may not be reliable in this version of the ISSI (Eklund et al., 2007).

The Social Support Network Inventory (SSNI; Flaherty, Gaviria, & Pathak, 1983) is an 11-item measure that assesses availability of support, practical help, emotional support, and reciprocity within the individual's five most important relationships. The internal reliability of the availability of support, practical help, emotional support, event-related support, and reciprocity scales was good in a mixed sample of undergraduate students and adults in an urban neighborhood and adults in a religious community. The test–retest reliability was high over a 2-week period. A factor analysis of the 11 items identified two factors: Perceived Support (availability, emotional, practical, and reciprocity) and Support Received in Response to a Stressor (event-related support). Higher SSNI scores were related to lower depressive symptoms and better social adjustment.

Reciprocity and Support Provided

The need to understand both sides of social interactions has often been overlooked, but both providing and receiving support appear to have beneficial effects for physical health (Brown et al., 2003). Additionally, measures that assess the provision of support to another individual are measures of reciprocity, or the balance of support given and received (Walster et al., 1973). Development of measures to assess support given to others in a variety of relationships is needed. As mentioned in previous sections, the SRS and the social convoy model measure developed by Antonucci and Israel (1986) measured reciprocity (Antonucci & Israel, 1986; McFarlane, 1981). To assess for reciprocity and support-giving behaviors within rela-

tionships, available measures assess the individual's perception of balance between support given and received, which also could include an assessment of the individual's perception of being burdened by others or being a burden to others. Additionally, the support-giving behaviors may be important to assess, including the support provided to the social network, as well as support the individual gives to the community through volunteer work. In this section we review reciprocity and support-giving measures that are currently used in the literature.

The Hatfield Global Measure (Hatfield, Walster, & Berscheid, 1978) is a single self-report item that assesses the individual's perception of give-and-take in an intimate relationship. The participant has six response options, ranging from "My partner is doing a lot more for me than I am doing for him/her" to "My partner is doing a lot less for me than I am doing for him/her." This item is a face-valid measure of perceived equity in the marital relationship. The Hatfield item is often combined with the Traupmann–Utne–Hatfield Scale (Traupmann, Petersen, Utne, & Hatfield, 1981). This measure consists of 44 items that evaluate the perception of benefits derived from intimate partners (output) and benefits given to intimate partners (input) across personal, emotional, and day-to-day situations. This measure also assesses opportunities lost or gained in marriage. The measure uses an 8-point Likert-type scale ranging from *extremely positive* to *extremely negative*. The internal reliabilities for the input and output scales were good in a sample of opposite-sex married or dating community adults. Within this sample, this measure was also related to relationship satisfaction and mood.

The Interpersonal Relationship Index (IPRI; Tilden, Nelson, & May, 1990) is a 39-item measure that assesses support received, reciprocity, and conflict within relationships. The IPRI assesses beliefs, for which it uses a 5-point Likert-type scale with response options ranging from *strongly disagree* to *strongly agree,* and behaviors, for which it uses a 5-point Likert-type scale with response options ranging from *very often* to *never.* The support, reciprocity, and conflict factors had good internal reliability in a mixed sample of college students and adults in the community experiencing significant life stressors (homelessness, individuals with chronic illness, and pregnancy). These three factors were stable over a 2-week period. The conflict scale was correlated with social desirability. Additional studies utilizing this measure have found significant relationships between the support received and reciprocity factors in predicting health outcomes (Tilden, Hirsch, & Nelson, 1994).

Krause and Markides (1990) developed a 13-item measure of support-providing behaviors using a sample of adults ages 65 years and older. It assesses the frequency of three types of support provided to others (emotional, tangible, and informational). Participants are asked to rate how often they provide each type of support; response choices range from *never* to *very often*. These scales had good internal consistency in a sample of older adults.

Negative Interactions

Historically, negative social interactions have not been as frequently assessed in the research addressing the relation between social support and health (Rook, 1992). However, the importance of this construct in understanding the impact of social interactions on health has been demonstrated, and it is becoming a more frequently assessed support factor. Continued research on measures designed to assess negative interactions is still needed. Clinical interviews may include an assessment of interactions that are perceived as causing negative emotions or stress. Additionally, interactions may be negative if they are perceived as being a burden or if they challenge the individual's perception of his or her identity or social role. Several measures described in previous sections include factors related to negative interactions, such as the ASSIS, IPRI, FRI, and the PANSE. The next two measures discussed specifically assess different forms of negative social interactions.

The Test of Negative Social Exchange (TENSE; Ruehlman & Karoly, 1991) is an 18-item self-report measure that assesses interactions in four areas: hostility/impatience, insensitivity, interference, and ridicule. A 5-point Likert-type scale is used with a response range of *not at all* to *about every day*. The four factors had good internal reliability in a sample of college students. Test–retest reliability was also good across each factor. This measure was moderately correlated with social desirability. The TENSE was related to increased reports of depressive symptoms and anxiety symptoms. (The TENSE can be purchased through Psychological Assessments and Training, LLC.)

One setting in which negative social interactions have been examined is among caregivers. Although caregiver burden is not equivalent to negative interactions, it is an important component of social interactions that may be producing negative outcomes for individuals providing care to others. The shortened Zarit Burden Interview is one example of an efficient measure of the level of perceived burden on the caregiver (Bédard et al., 2001; Zarit, Reever, & Bach-Peterson, 1980). This measure assesses level of personal strain and the level of role strain using a 5-point Likert-type scale. Internal reliability for the total score and the two factors was good in a sample of caregivers for older adults with cognitive impairment.

Conclusions

Social support is a multifaceted construct that can be useful in understanding the health of patients. Social support encompasses the structural characteristics of a social network, the amount and type of support received from that network, the perception of quality and availability of that support, the reciprocity within relationships, and negative social interactions. It is important to be cognizant of the type of support component being measured, as each facet has a different influence on physical and psychological health. The assessment of social support can include an unstructured interview or any of the measures described herein. Further, additional constructs that are not traditionally included in the literature investigating social support, such as reciprocity, negative support, and loneliness, can provide valuable information in a clinical setting. Awareness of the support resources, the perception of the support, and possible negative interactions can help a clinician in conceptualizing the patient's strengths and areas of risks and may aid in treatment planning.

REFERENCES

Antonucci, T. C. (1986). Hierarchical mapping technique. *Generations: Journal of the American Society on Aging, 10*(4), 10–12.

Antonucci, T. C., Akiyama, H., & Takahashi, K. (2004). Attachment and close relationships across the life span. *Attachment and Human Development, 6*, 353–370.

Antonucci, T. C., & Israel, B. A. (1986). Veridicality of social support: A comparison of principal and network members' responses. *Journal of Consulting and Clinical Psychology, 54*, 432–437.

Aroian, K., Templin, T. N., & Ramaswamy, V. (2010). Adaptation and psychometric evaluation of the Multidimensional Scale of Perceived Social Support for Arab immigrant women. *Health Care for Women International, 31*(2), 153–169.

Barrera, M., Jr. (1980). A method for the assessment of social support networks in community survey research. *Connection, 3*, 8–13.

Barrera, M., Jr., & Ainlay, S. L. (1983). The structure of social support: A conceptual and empirical analysis. *Journal of Community Psychology, 11*(2), 133–143.

Barrera, M., Jr. Sandler, I., & Ramsay, T. (1981). Preliminary development of a scale of social support: Studies on college students. *American Journal of Community Psychology, 9*(4), 435–447.

Bass, L. A., & Stein, C. H. (1997). Comparing the structure and stability of network ties using the Social Support Questionnaire and the Social Network List. *Journal of Social and Personal Relationships, 14*(1), 123–132.

Bédard, M., Molloy, D., Squire, L., Dubois, S., Lever, J., & O'Donnell, M. (2001). The Zarit Burden Interview: A new short version and screening version. *Gerontologist, 41*(5), 652–657.

Berkman, L. F., Glass, T., Brissette, I., & Seeman, T. E. (2000). From social integration to health: Durkheim in the new millennium. *Social Science and Medicine, 51*(6), 843–857.

Berkman, L. F., & Syme, S. L. (1979). Social networks, host resistance, and mortality: A nine-year follow-up study of Alameda County residents. *American Journal of Epidemiology, 109*, 186–204.

Brown, S., Nesse, R., Vinokur, A., & Smith, D. (2003). Providing social support may be more beneficial than receiving it: Results from a prospective study of mortality. *Psychological Science, 14*(4), 320–327.

Burg, M. B., & Seeman, T. E. (1994). Families and health: The negative side of social ties. *Annals of Behavioral Medicine, 16*(2), 109–115.

Byers, P. H., & Mullis, M. R. (1987). Reliability and validity of the Norbeck Social Support Questionnaire in psychiatric inpatients. *Educational and Psychological Measurement, 47*, 445–448.

Canty-Mitchell, J., & Zimet, G. D. (2000). Psychometric properties of the Multidimensional Scale of Perceived Social Support in urban adolescents. *American Journal of Community Psychology, 28*(3), 391–400.

Carstensen, L. T., Isaacowitz, D. M., & Charles, S. T. (1999). Taking time seriously: A theory of socioemotional selectivity. *American Psychologist, 54*(3), 165–181.

Cecil, H., Stanley, M. A., Carrion, P. G., & Swann, A. (1995). Psychometric properties of the MSPSS and NOS in psychiatric outpatients. *Journal of Clinical Psychology, 51*(5), 593–602.

Cohen, L., McGowan, J., Fooskas, S., & Rose, S. (1984). Positive life events and social support and the relationship between life stress and psychological disorder. *American Journal of Community Psychology, 12*(5), 567–587.

Cohen, S. (1988). Psychosocial models of the role of social support in the etiology of physical disease. *Health Psychology, 7*(3), 269–297.

Cohen, S. (2004). Social relationships and health. *American Psychologist, 59*(8), 676–684.

Cohen, S., & Hoberman, H. M. (1983). Positive events and social supports as buffers of life change stress. *Journal of Applied Social Psychology, 13*(2), 99–125.

Cohen, S., Mermelstein, R., Kamarck, T., & Hoberman, H. M. (1985). Measuring the functional components of social support. In I. G. Sarason & B. R. Sarason (Eds.), *Social support: Theory, research, and applications* (pp. 73–94). The Hague, Netherlands: Martinus Nijhoff.

Cohen, S., & Wills, T. (1985). Stress, social support, and the buffering hypothesis. *Psychological Bulletin, 98*(2), 310–357.

Croyle, R., & Hunt, J. (1991). Coping with health threat: Social influence processes in reactions to medical test results. *Journal of Personality and Social Psychology, 60*(3), 382–389.

DeVries, A., Glasper, E., & Detillion, C. (2003). Social modulation of stress responses. *Physiology and Behavior, 79*(3), 399–407.

Dunkel-Schetter, C., & Skokan, L. (1990). Determinants of social support provision in personal relationships. *Journal of Social and Personal Relationships, 7*(4), 437–450.

Eklund, M., Bengtsson-Tops, A., & Lindstedt, H. (2007). Construct and discriminant validity and dimensionality of the Interview Schedule for Social Interaction (ISSI) in three psychiatric samples. *Nordic Journal of Psychiatry, 61*(3), 182–188.

Flaherty, J., Gaviria, F., & Pathak, D. (1983). The measurement of social support: The Social Support Network Inventory. *Comprehensive Psychiatry, 24*(6), 521–529.

Gigliotti, E. (2002). A confirmation of the factor structure of the Norbeck Social Support Questionnaire. *Nursing Research, 51*(5), 276–284.

Gjesfjeld, C., Greeno, C., & Kim, K. (2008). A confirmatory factor analysis of an abbreviated social support instrument: The MOS-SSS. *Research on Social Work Practice, 18*(3), 231–237.

Glass, T., & Maddox, G. (1992). The quality and quantity of social support: Stroke recovery as psycho-social transition. *Social Science and Medicine, 34*(11), 1249–1261.

Grant, N., Hamer, M., & Steptoe, A. (2009). Social isolation and stress-related cardiovascular, lipid, and cortisol responses. *Annals of Behavioral Medicine, 37*(1), 29–37.

Grewen, K., Girdler, S., Amico, J., & Light, K. (2005). Effects of partner support on resting oxytocin, cortisol, norepinephrine, and blood pressure before and after warm partner contact. *Psychosomatic Medicine, 67*(4), 531–538.

Haber, M., Cohen, J., Lucas, T., & Baltes, B. (2007). The relationship between self-reported received and perceived social support: A meta-analytic review. *American Journal of Community Psychology, 39*(1), 133–144.

Hatfield, E., Walster, G. W., & Berscheid, E. (1978). *Equity: Theory and research*. Boston: Allyn & Bacon.

Hawkley, L. C., Hughes, M. E., Waite, L. J., Masi, C. M., Thisted, R. A., & Cacioppo, J. T. (2008). From social structural factors to perceptions of relationship quality and loneliness: The Chicago Health, Aging, and Social Relations Study. *Journal of Gerontology: Social Sciences, 63B*, S375–S384.

Henderson, S., Duncan-Jones, P., Byrne, D., & Scott, R. (1980). Measuring social relationships: The Interview Schedule for Social Interaction. *Psychological Medicine, 10*(4), 723–734.

Hirsch, B. J. (1979). Psychological dimensions of social networks: A multimethod analysis. *American Journal of Community Psychology, 7*, 263–277.

Hirsch, B. J. (1980). Natural support systems and coping with major life changes. *American Journal of Community Psychology, 8*(2), 159–172.

Holahan, C., & Moos, R. (1982). Social support and adjustment: Predictive benefits of social climate indices. *American Journal of Community Psychology, 10*(4), 403–415.

Kahn, R. L., & Antonucci, T. C. (1980). Convoys over the life course: Attachment roles and social support. In P. B. Baltes & O. G. Brim (Eds.), *Life-span development and behavior* (pp. 253–286). New York: Academic Press.

Kitamura, T., Watanabe, K., Takara, N., Hiyama, K., Yasumiya, R., & Fujihara, S. (2002). Precedents of perceived social support: Personality, early life experiences and gender. *Psychiatry and Clinical Neurosciences, 56*(2), 169–176.

Koenig, H. G., Westlund, R. E., George, L. K., Hughes, D. C., Blazer, D. G., & Hybels, C. (1993). Abbreviating the Duke Social Support Index for use in chronically ill elderly individuals. *Psychosomatics, 34*, 61–69.

Krause, N. (1999). Assessing change in social support during late life. *Research on Aging, 21*(4), 539–569.

Krause, N., & Markides, K. (1990). Measuring social support among older adults. *International Journal of Aging and Human Development, 30*(1), 37–53.

Landerman, R., George, L. K., Campbell, R. T., & Blazer, D. G. (1989). Alternative models of the stress buffering hypothesis. *American Journal of Community Psychology, 17*, 625–642.

Lepore, S. (1998). Problems and prospects for the social support–reactivity hypothesis. *Annals of Behavioral Medicine, 20*(4), 257–269.

Lett, H., Blumenthal, J., Babyak, M., Strauman, T., Robins, C., & Sherwood, A. (2005). Social support and coronary heart disease: Epidemiologic evidence and implications for treatment. *Psychosomatic Medicine, 67*(6), 869–878.

Levitt, M. J., Guacci-Franco, N., & Levitt, J. L. (1993). Convoys of social support in childhood and early adolescence: Structure and function. *Developmental Psychology, 29*, 811–818.

Lewis, M., & Rook, K. (1999). Social control in personal relationships: Impact on health behaviors and psychological distress. *Health Psychology, 18*(1), 63–71.

Liang, J., Krause, N., & Bennett, J. (2001). Social exchange and well-being: Is giving better than receiving? *Psychology and Aging, 16*(3), 511–523.

Lubben, J. E. (1988). Assessing social networks among elderly populations. *Family and Community Health, 11,* 42–52.

Lubben, J. E., Blozik, E., Gillmann, G., Iliffe, S., von Renteln Kruse, W., Beck, J. C., et al. (2006). Performance of an abbreviated version of the Lubben Social Network Scale among three European community-dwelling older adult populations. *Gerontologist, 46,* 503–513.

Lubben, J. E., & Gironda, M. W. (2000). Social support networks. In D. Osterweil, K. Brummel-Smith, & J. C. Beck (Eds.), *Comprehensive geriatric assessment* (pp. 121–137). New York: McGraw-Hill.

McFarlane, A. (1981). Methodological issues in developing a scale to measure social support. *Schizophrenia Bulletin, 7*(1), 90–100.

Newsom, J., Rook, K., Nishishiba, M., Sorkin, D., & Mahan, T. (2005). Understanding the relative importance of positive and negative social exchanges: Examining specific domains and appraisals. *Journals of Gerontology: Series B. Psychological Sciences and Social Sciences, 60*(6), P304–P312.

Norbeck, J. S., Lindsey, A. M., & Carrieri, V. L. (1981). The development of an instrument to measure social support. *Nursing Research, 30,* 264–269.

Norbeck, J. S., Lindsey, A. M., & Carrieri, V. L. (1983). Further development of the Norbeck Social Support Questionnaire: Normative data and validity testing. *Nursing Research, 32,* 4–9.

Oman, D., Thoresen, C., & McMahon, K. (1999). Volunteerism and mortality among the community-dwelling elderly. *Journal of Health Psychology, 4*(3), 301–316.

O'Reilly, P., & Thomas, H. (1989). Role of support networks in maintenance of improved cardiovascular health status. *Social Science and Medicine, 28*(3), 249–260.

Oxman, T., & Berkman, L. (1990). Assessment of social relationships in elderly patients. *International Journal of Psychiatry in Medicine, 20*(1), 65–84.

Penninx, B., Kriegsman, D., van Eijk, J., Boeke, A., & Deeg, D. (1996). Differential effect of social support on the course of chronic disease: A criteria-based literature study. *Families, Systems, and Health, 14*(2), 223–244.

Powers, J. R., Goodger, B., & Byles, J. E. (2004). Assessment of the abbreviated Duke Social Support Index in a cohort of older Australian women. *Australasian Journal on Aging, 23,* 71–76.

Pressman, S., & Cohen, S. (2005). Does positive affect influence health? *Psychological Bulletin, 131*(6), 925–971.

Procidano, M., & Heller, K. (1983). Measures of perceived social support from friends and from family: Three validation studies. *American Journal of Community Psychology, 11*(1), 1–24.

Ramaswamy, V., Aroian, K. J., & Templin, T. (2009). Adaptation and psychometric evaluation of the Multidimensional Scale of Perceived Social Support for Arab American adolescents. *American Journal of Community Psychology, 43*(1–2), 49–56.

Rice, C., & Longabaugh, R. (1996). Measuring general social support in alcoholic patients: Short forms for perceived social support. *Psychology of Addictive Behaviors, 10*(2), 104–114.

Rook, K. (1992). Detrimental aspects of social relationships: Taking stock of an emerging literature. In H. O. F. Veiel & U. Baumann (Eds.), *The meaning and measurement of social support* (pp. 157–169). Washington, DC: Hemisphere.

Ruehlman, L., & Karoly, P. (1991). With a little flak from my friends: Development and preliminary validation of the Test of Negative Social Exchange (TENSE). *Psychological Assessment, 3*(1), 97–104.

Russell, D., & Cutrona, C. E. (1991). Social support, stress, and depressive symptoms among the elderly: Test of a process model. *Psychology and Aging, 6*(2), 190–201.

Russell, D., Peplau, L. A., & Cutrona, C. E. (1980). The revised UCLA Loneliness Scale: Concurrent and discriminant validity evidence. *Journal of Personality and Social Psychology, 39,* 472–480.

Sarason, I. G., Levine, H. M., Basham, R. R., & Sarason, B. R. (1983). Assessing social support: The Social Support Questionnaire. *Journal of Personality and Social Psychology, 44*(1), 127–139.

Sarason, B. R., & Sarason, I. G. (1994). Assessment of social support. In S. A. Shumaker & S. M. Czajkowski (Eds.), *Social support and car-*

diovascular disease (pp. 41–63). New York: Plenum Press.

Sarason, I. G., Sarason, B. R., Shearin, E. N., & Pierce, G. R. (1987). A brief measure of social support: Practical and theoretical implications. *Journal of Social and Personal Relationships, 4*(4), 497–510.

Sherbourne, C., & Stewart, A. (1991). The MOS social support survey. *Social Science and Medicine, 32*(6), 705–714.

Sokolovsky, J., & Cohen, C. I. (1981). Toward a resolution of methodological dilemmas in network mapping. *Schizophrenia Bulletin, 7,* 109–116.

Stephens, M., Kinney, J., Norris, V., & Ritchie, S. (1987). Social networks as assets and liabilities in recovery from stroke by geriatric patients. *Psychology and Aging, 2*(2), 125–129.

Stokes, J. P. (1983). Predicting satisfaction with social support from social network structure. *American Journal of Community Psychology, 11,* 141–152.

Theorell, T., Blomkvist, V., Jonsson, H., & Schulman, S. (1995). Social support and the development of immune function in human immunodeficiency virus infection. *Psychosomatic Medicine, 57*(1), 32–36.

Thoits, P. (1992). Social support functions and network structures: A supplemental view. In H. O. F. Veiel & U. Baumann (Eds.), *The meaning and measurement of social support* (pp. 57–62). Washington, DC: Hemisphere.

Tilden, V., Hirsch, A., & Nelson, C. (1994). The Interpersonal Relationship Inventory: Continued psychometric evaluation. *Journal of Nursing Measurement, 2*(1), 63–78.

Tilden, V., Nelson, C., & May, B. (1990). The IPR Inventory: Development and psychometric characteristics. *Nursing Research, 39*(6), 337–343.

Traupmann, J., Petersen, R., Utne, M., & Hatfield, E. (1981). Measuring equity in intimate relations. *Applied Psychological Measurement, 5*(4), 467–480.

Uchino, B. (2004). *Social support and physical health: Understanding the health consequences of relationships.* New Haven, CT: Yale University Press.

Uchino, B. (2006). Social support and health: A review of physiological processes potentially underlying links to disease outcomes. *Journal of Behavioral Medicine, 29*(4), 377–387.

Uchino, B. (2009). Understanding the links between social support and physical health: A life-span perspective with emphasis on the separability of perceived and received support. *Perspectives on Psychological Science, 4*(3), 236–255.

Uchino, B., Cacioppo, J., & Kiecolt-Glaser, J. (1996). The relationship between social support and physiological processes: A review with emphasis on underlying mechanisms and implications for health. *Psychological Bulletin, 119*(3), 488–531.

Undén, A., & Orth-Gomér, K. (1989). Development of a social support instrument for use in population surveys. *Social Science and Medicine, 29*(12), 1387–1392.

Vaux, A. (1986). The Social Support Appraisals (SS-A) scale: Studies of reliability and validity. *American Journal of Community Psychology, 14*(2), 195–219.

Walster, E., Berscheid, E., & Walster, G. (1973). New directions in equity research. *Journal of Personality and Social Psychology, 25*(2), 151–176.

Wilks, S. E. (2009). Support for Alzheimer's caregivers: Psychometric evaluation of familial and friend support measures. *Research on Social Work Practice, 19*(6), 722–729.

Zarit, S. H., Reever, K. E., & Bach-Peterson, J. (1980). Relatives of the impaired elderly: Correlates of feeling of burden. *Gerontologist, 20*(6), 649–655.

Zimet, G. D., Dahlem, N. W., Zimet, S. G., & Farley, G. K. (1988). The Multidimensional Scale of Perceived Social Support. *Journal of Personality Assessment, 52*(1), 30–41.

CHAPTER 9

Coping

Lauren M. Penwell-Waines
Kevin T. Larkin
Jeffrey L. Goodie

Individual differences exist in how people respond to stress, with some experiencing extreme stress responses and others merely becoming annoyed in response to identical stressful events. Although there are myriad individual-difference characteristics known to influence the magnitude of these stress responses (e.g., genetic factors, engagement in health behaviors), a significant source of variance in explaining the magnitude of one's stress response focuses on an individual's coping skills. Perhaps one of the most well-known definitions of coping was provided by Lazarus and Folkman (1984), who described coping as the "constantly changing cognitive and behavioral efforts to manage specific external and/or internal demands that are appraised as taxing or exceeding the resources of the person" (p. 141). Note that this definition refers to both covert and overt coping behaviors and that appraisal serves as a central component of their model. According to this perspective, having a solid repertoire of coping skills not only assists individuals in responding to demands appraised as exceeding one's resources but also reduces the probability of making this type of appraisal in the first place. Inherent in this definition is the biopsychosocial model, which provides a template for understanding the complexities of stress and coping. According to the biopsychosocial model, what individuals think and do (psychological factors) in response to environmental stressors (social environmental factors) determines the magnitude of their physical and emotional response, which in turn influences health status (biological factors). Measuring how people cope with the demands, stressors, and unpleasant (or pleasant) events in their lives has long been a hallmark of clinical health psychology.

Although clinical health psychologists agree that measurement of coping is important for understanding how stress leads to physical disease and for working with individual patients in health care environments, disagreement exists regarding how coping should be assessed. Folkman and Moskowitz (2004) described three significant sources of debate regarding the assessment of coping, including differing opinions regarding which instrument for measuring coping should be used, differing nomenclatures used to define the underlying conceptual model of coping, and differing positions regarding the efficacy of employing specific coping strategies for reducing the impact of or preventing disease consequences. Across recognized methods of assessing coping, there are significant inconsistencies in how the thoughts, behaviors, and emotions associated with coping are categorized. Schwarzer and Schwarzer (1996), in their review of measures of coping, acknowledged that many researchers relied on two basic dimensions of coping, which were labeled as (1) instrumental/attentive/vigilant/confrontative or (2) avoidant/palliative/emotional. However, the assessment of coping can be more complex due to the multiple dimensions of coping that can be measured. Skinner, Edge, Altman, and Sherwood (2003) identified at least 15 different "higher-order distinctions" among types of coping. Others have focused on conceptualizing coping as higher-order categories, including problem-focused versus emotion-focused coping, approach versus avoidance coping, primary control versus secondary control, assimilation versus accommodation, social versus solitary coping, effortful versus involuntary coping, receiving good news versus bad news, as well as approximately 400 other labels that have been identified to name different aspects of coping (Skinner et al., 2003). Of these, the dimensions of coping that have been studied with the most fervor are dispositional versus situational coping, approach–avoidance paradigms (including monitoring and blunting styles), and emotion-focused versus problem-focused coping.

Dispositional versus Situational Conceptualizations of Coping

Some researchers have approached coping as a stable disposition and suggested that individuals tend to use similar coping strategies across multiple situations (e.g., Carver, Scheier, & Weintraub, 1989; Terry, 1994). Dispositional measures of coping typically ask respondents to describe how they generally cope with stress. Alternatively, they may be asked how they coped with a recent stressor, and inferences are made from these responses to describe how an individual generally copes. Ptacek, Pierce, and Thompson (2006) argued that, although trait coping measures may not be able to predict a single instance of coping behavior, they do have the potential to describe consistent coping patterns over time, as Schoen, Altmaier, and Tallman (2007) observed in patients undergoing bone marrow transplantation.

Schwarzer and Schwarzer (1996) suggested that measures of dispositional coping should be studied intensively, as their potential for predicting adaptive outcomes could provide useful information both for scientists examining the role of coping in serious medical illnesses and for patients directly confronting these diseases.

In contrast, situation-specific approaches to coping examine how a person actually responds to an identified stressor, considering cognitive, affective, behavioral, and perhaps physiological responses. Numerous studies have provided evidence that measures of coping are not very stable and change over time, suggesting that measuring current, situation-specific coping strategies may be a more prudent approach (e.g., Danhauer, Crawford, Farmer, & Avis, 2009; Nolen-Hoeksema & Larson, 1999). Using ecological momentary assessment (EMA) methods (i.e., by which the respondent endorses coping responses immediately following engagement with a stressor), Schwartz, Neale, Marco, Shiffman, and Stone (1999) found that measures of dispositional coping were poor predictors of coping methods actually used in specific stressful situations encountered throughout daily life. Taking an extreme position, Steed (1998) suggested that situation-specific coping measures should always be used. Additionally, because some dispositional measures of coping present respondents with scenarios and instructions to respond "as if" the situations were actually occurring, test stimuli may not be personally relevant to respondents, and less valid inferences regarding typical coping styles would be made (Bijttebier, Vertommen, & Vander Steene, 2001).

Although situation-specific coping measures have some advantages over dispositional measures, they are difficult to use in daily life without the use of EMAs. Additionally, because real life is not standardized across individuals, one can never be sure whether responses obtained from situation-specific measures are a reflection of actual coping behaviors or are related to the unique stressors persons encounter throughout daily life. Schwarzer and Schwarzer (1996) concluded that it was important to state clearly the purpose for assessing coping prior to deciding whether to use dispositional or situational coping measurement strategies. For example, empirical questions pertaining to how different individuals cope with a specific stressor or how individuals cope with a stressor at different time points may lead to selecting certain types of assessment methods. Using this approach, both dispositional and situation-specific methods are important but aim to address different empirical or clinical questions.

Approach–Avoidance Coping

The approach–avoidance paradigm represents a style of dispositional coping that ranges from tendencies to confront the source of stress directly to avoiding stressful stimuli altogether (Ptacek et al., 2006; Roth & Cohen, 1986). Reminiscent of the literature on repression–sensitization (see Bell & Byrne, 1978), approach versus avoidance styles of coping have long been recognized as distinctive strategies for responding to various forms of environmental stress. For example, Roth and Cohen (1986) noted support for using avoidance strategies to cope with uncontrollable stressors and using approach strategies for coping with controllable, solvable stressors. In health care settings, one such application of this dimension of coping has distinguished monitoring and blunting styles of information processing (Miller, 1987). Monitoring involves seeking out information related to a diagnosis or health concern, whereas blunting is characterized by avoiding information or distracting oneself from information presented (Miller & Mangan, 1983). Although monitoring appears to be an active coping approach and blunting an avoidant coping approach, Myers and Derakshan (2000) reported a negative relation between monitoring and active coping, indicating that an exact correspondence between the constructs was lacking. Nevertheless, the dimensions share some conceptual similarity.

Efficacy of active versus avoidant strategies for coping with health-related problems appears to differ depending upon the duration of the health problem being investigated. In several studies, it has been shown that approach-oriented coping strategies were associated with less distress than avoidance-oriented strategies (e.g., Geirdal & Dahl, 2008; Penedo et al., 2003) and

that avoidant coping may be more adaptive for responding to short-term stressors and approach strategies better for responding to long-term stressors (Suls & Fletcher, 1985). However, in the case of chronic health-related coping, there is some consensus that monitoring is associated with poorer behavioral health than blunting (Constant et al., 2005; Miller & Mangan, 1983; Tercyak et al., 2001; Voss, Kolling, & Heidenreich, 2006). In contrast, use of avoidance coping strategies has been shown to be problematic regarding adherence to some types of treatments, including treatment for cystic fibrosis (Abbott, 2003). In support of these seemingly contradictory findings, Lazarus and Folkman (1984) argued that one cannot make broad conclusions about a coping style as being wholly positive or negative because the context of the coping behavior is a critical factor. Barnoy, Bar-Tal, and Zisser (2006), in their study of coping among cancer patients, reported that congruence of coping and information-gathering styles between patients and members of their support systems is also important for better psychological adjustment.

Emotion-Focused versus Problem-Focused Coping

One of the most commonly used distinctions discussed in the coping literature is between emotion- and problem-focused coping. Emotion-focused coping generally involves cognitive attempts to decrease emotional distress (Lazarus & Folkman, 1984). Problem-focused coping, in contrast, involves cognitive and overt behavioral efforts to modify the stressor or the impact of the stressor on the individual. Baker and Berenbaum (2007) described the relations between problem- and emotion-focused coping and several other variables. In their study, people who used problem-focused coping reported more negative affect than those who used emotion-focused coping, but people who attended to their emotions reported more physical symptoms on a measure of subjective health than problem-focused copers. Additionally, emotion-focused strategies were utilized more often to cope with interpersonal stressors, and problem-focused strategies were utilized more often to cope with achievement-oriented stressors. In another study, the use of emotion-focused coping before a stressor was associated with higher negative affect and problem-focused coping with lesser negative affect (Sideridis, 2006). In response to a stressor task, however, a combination of emotion-focused and problem-focused coping strategies was associated with the lowest negative affect and heart rate reactivity (Sideridis, 2006). In a study of children coping with cancer (Sorgen & Manne, 2002), additional evidence regarding the importance of matching coping strategy with the type of situation being confronted was reported. Children tended to use problem-focused strategies in situations perceived as more controllable but emotion-focused strategies in situations perceived as being less controllable, and children who matched coping responses to the context the best reported the least distress (Sorgen & Manne, 2002). Similar to the approach–avoidance distinction, it appears important to consider the context in which coping occurs, as well as other psychosocial and demographic variables of the individual, in making a determination regarding optimal coping strategies.

Given the lack of coherence that exists among conceptualizations of coping, it is not surprising that a wide range of measures has been devised to assess coping, none of which serves as a universally adopted measure. Researchers and clinicians then are faced with the daunting task of selecting appropriate methods for assessing coping in patients dealing with a variety of health problems or other stressors in their lives. There are as many instruments to measure coping as there are conceptualizations of it, with the format of measures ranging from paper-and-pencil tests to clinical interviews to think-aloud procedures (e.g., Heiden, Larkin, & Knowlton, 1991). Keeping in mind the conceptual issues raised in the previous pages, the remaining portion of this chapter provides an overview of the existing measures of coping that make up the current state of this literature.

Measures of Coping

Numerous measures have been developed over the years that measure coping, most of which rely on retrospective reporting of how individuals think and what they do in response to various stressors. Given the centrality of cognitive appraisal in the model of stress outlined by Lazurus and Folkman (1984) and the importance of covert mental activity involved in problem-focused and emotion-focused coping, self-report strategies for assessment have been the primary method used for measuring coping. Although some coping strategies involve observable phenomena (e.g., making use of social support, engaging in substance use) and would be amenable to other behavioral assessment strategies, the vast majority of behavior that occurs during coping is internal, cognitive activity. Although we may eventually be able to isolate neural activity associated with various types of coping through cortical imaging, this assessment strategy is currently not used. Based on these limitations, the descriptions of the various assessment strategies that follow all rely on accurate self-reporting of the process of coping, a strategy unfortunately known to be influenced by respondent demand characteristics and imprecise recollection.

Presentation of measures is organized using the various dimensions discussed on the preceding pages. Instruments typically conceptualized as dispositional measures are presented first, followed by instruments typically conceptualized as more situational in nature, including those aimed at coping with specific medical problems. The dimensions of approach versus avoidance and emotion-focused versus problem-focused coping are considered when relevant. This information also appears in Tables 9.1 and 9.2 for easy reference.

Dispositional Measures

Ways of Coping Checklist and Ways of Coping Questionnaire

In an initial attempt to measure the various aspects of coping, Folkman and Lazurus (1980) developed the Ways of Coping Checklist. Although devised as a situational measure of coping (i.e., participants were asked to respond with a specific stressor in mind), inferences regarding respondents' scores are typically made to describe whether they use problem-focused or emotion-focused coping strategies with a range of stressful events.

TABLE 9.1. Dispositional Measures of Coping

Measure	Citation	No. of items	Test–retest reliability coefficients	Internal consistency reliability coefficients	Dimensions			
					EF	PF	AP	AV
COPE and	Carver et al. (1989)	60	.42–.89	.45–.92			X	X
Brief COPE	Carver (1997)	28		.50–.90			X	X
Coping Inventory for Stressful Situations (CISS)	Endler & Parker (1990a)	48	.51–.73	.75–.90	X	X		X
Frankfurt Monitoring Blunting Scale (FMBS)	Voss et al. (2006)	8	NR	.70–.79			X	X
Mainz Coping Inventory (MCI)	Krohne, Egloff, et al. (2000)	8	.70–.84	.75–.82			X	X
Miller Behavioral Style Scale (MBSS)	Miller (1987)	8	.72–.75	.69–.79			X	X
Ways of Coping Questionnaire (WCQ)	Folkman & Lazarus (1985)	66	.25–.47	.61–.79	X	X		

Note. NR, not reported; EF, emotion-focused coping; PF, problem-focused coping; AP, approach coping; AV, avoidance coping.

TABLE 9.2. Situation-Specific Measures of Coping

Measure	Citation	No. of items	Test–retest reliability coefficients	Internal consistency reliability coefficients	Dimensions			
					EF	PF	AP	AV
Respondent-identified stress								
Billings & Moos Coping Checklist	Billings & Moos (1984)	19	.59–.71	.41–.66	X	X	X	X
COPE	Carver et al. (1989)	60	.42–.89	.45–.92			X	X
Coping Strategies Inventory (CSInv) and	Tobin et al. (1989)	75	.67–.83	.71–.94	X	X		X
CSInv–Short Form	Addison, et al. (2007)	15		.58–.72	X	X		X
Coping Strategy Indicator (CSI)	Amirkhan (1990)	33	.77–.86	.83–.92		X		X
Ways of Coping Questionnaire (WCQ)	Folkman & Lazarus (1985)	66	.25–.47	.61–.79	X	X		
Coping with pain								
Chronic Pain Acceptance Questionnaire (CPAQ)	McCracken et al. (2004)	20	NR	.78–.82			X	X
Chronic Pain Coping Inventory (CPCI)	Jensen et al. (1995)	65	.66–.90	.70–.93			X	X

(continued)

TABLE 9.2. *(continued)*

Measure	Citation	No. of items	Test–retest reliability coefficients	Internal consistency reliability coefficients	EF	PF	AP	AV
Coping Strategies Questionnaire–R (CSQ-R)	Riley & Robinson (1999)	27	.60–.90	.65–.86				
Vanderbilt Pain Management Inventory (VPMI)	Brown & Nicassio (1987)	18	.65–.69	.71–.82			X	X
Coping with cancer								
Mental Adjustment to Cancer (MAC)	Watson et al. (1988)	40	.38–.65	.65–.84				
Revised Ways of Coping—Cancer Version (WCQ-CA)	Dunkel-Schetter et al. (1992)	52	NR	NR			X	X
Coping with other medical conditions								
Coping Questionnaire for Coronary Patients	Maes & Bruggemans (1990)	NR	NR	.78–.87			X	X
Coping Questionnaire for Asthmatic Patients	Maes & Schlosser (1987)	93	NR	.63–.84	X	X	X	X
Coping with Surgical Stress (CoSS)	Krohne, de Bruin, et al. (2000)	27	NR	.55–.79			X	X
Jalowiec Coping Scale (JCS)	Jalowiec et al. (1984)	60	.79–.86	.85	X	X		
Medical Coping Models Questionnaire (MCMQ)	Feifel et al. (1987)	19	NR	.66–.70			X	X
Threatening Medical Situations Inventory (TMSI)	Van Zuuren et al. (1996)	24	.82	>.70			X	X

Note. NR, not reported; EF, emotion-focused coping; PF, problem-focused coping; AP, approach coping; AV, avoidance coping.

The Ways of Coping Questionnaire (WCQ) was created by modifying the Ways of Coping Checklist, as there were concerns about the psychometric properties of the original measure (Folkman & Lazarus, 1985; see Table 9.1 for additional information). Factor analyses have yielded an eight-factor solution, including Confrontive Coping, Distancing, Self-Controlling, Seeking Social Support, Accepting Responsibility, Escape-Avoidance, Planful Problem Solving, and Positive Reappraisal, although other ways of grouping the subscales are possible (Schwarzer & Schwarzer, 1996). Thus the WCQ was expanded to measure dimensions beyond the emotion-focused–problem-focused dichotomy presented in the initial version of the instrument. The WCQ continues to be used and has been shown to predict differences in appraisal of illness severity among patients with chronic fatigue syndrome (Walker, Lindner, & Noonan, 2009) and distress among caregivers for individuals with traumatic brain injuries (Davis et al., 2009).

*Coping Orientations to Problems
Experienced and Brief Coping Orientations
to Problems Experienced*

The Coping Orientations to Problems Experienced (COPE; Carver et al., 1989), constructed as a dispositional measure of coping, instructs individuals to respond according to what they "generally do and feel" in response to stressful events. However, it has also been shown to provide valid measures of situational coping by asking individuals to report how they responded to a specific, self-identified stressor (Carver et al., 1989). The 15-factor structure, confirmed by Clark, Bormann, Cropanzano, and James (1995), includes Active Coping, Planning, Suppression of Competing Activities, Restraint Coping, Seeking Instrumental Support, Seeking Emotional Social Support, Positive Reinterpretation, Acceptance, Denial, Turning to Religion, Focus on and Venting of Emotions, Behavioral Disengagement, Mental Disengagement, Humor, and Substance Use. However, other researchers have described different factor structures (Eisengart et al., 2006; Zuckerman & Gagne, 2003). The subscales also can be grouped into an Avoidant and an Active coping factor (Kershaw et al., 2008).

An abbreviated form of the COPE, known as the Brief COPE, contains fewer items and only measures 14 subscales (Carver, 1997). Compared to the original COPE, two scales were omitted (i.e., Restraint Coping and Suppression of Competing Activities), three scales were modified, and one scale (i.e., Self-Blame) was added (Carver, 1997). Factor analysis and reliability analysis suggested that the Brief COPE and the COPE exhibited similar psychometric characteristics. The Brief COPE has been used with a variety of patient populations, including those with breast cancer (Kershaw, Northouse, Kritpracha, Schafenacker, & Mood, 2004), head and neck cancer (Harrington, McGurk, & Llewellyn, 2008), heart failure (Klein, Turvey, & Pies, 2007), and multiple sclerosis (Sinclair & Scroggie, 2005). Forms of approach coping (Seeking Social Support and Problem Engagement) measured via the COPE have also been shown to be related to lower daily cortisol levels (O'Donnell, Badrick, Kumari, & Steptoe, 2008).

Coping Inventory for Stressful Situations

Developed by Endler and Parker (1990a, 1990b), the Coping Inventory for Stressful Situations (CISS) is a three-factor (i.e., Task-Oriented, Emotion-Oriented, and Avoidance-Oriented) measure of coping based on a situation × disposition model of psychological assessment. Items that make up the Task-Oriented factor resemble problem-focused coping, and items that make up the Emotion-Oriented factor resemble emotion-focused coping. The factor structure was confirmed by factor analysis, and the scales were found to have high levels of internal consistency among samples of college students, adults, adolescents, and psychiatric patients (Endler & Parker, 1994). Factor structure of these items is fairly consistent across all of these samples as well.

Mainz Coping Inventory

The Mainz Coping Inventory (MCI) was developed to distinguish between Vigilance (i.e., orienting toward a threatening situation) and Cognitive Avoidance (i.e., orienting away from a threatening situation), representing a measure of coping from the approach–avoidance paradigm. The MCI includes eight stressful scenarios, including ego-threatening and physically threatening situations. Respondents rate the degree to which they would use Vigilant and Cognitive-Avoidant strategies in response to these scenarios (Krohne, Egloff, et al., 2000). Schwarzer and Schwarzer (1996) argue that, although the two-factor solution is strong and is supported for use in regard to physically threatening stimuli, it is limited in its scope of measuring coping responses to the range of stimuli people encounter in their daily lives.

Miller Behavioral Style Scale

The Miller Behavioral Style Scale (MBSS; Miller, 1987) was designed to measure how individuals process information using the monitoring–blunting dichotomization. Four threatening scenarios are depicted, followed by items assessing whether individuals prefer to seek out information about stressors (i.e., monitors) or avoid seeking information about stressors (i.e., blunters). The initial validation of the MBSS was conducted using the scale to predict responses of students exposed to aversive laboratory situations (e.g., threat of electric shock and a cognitive stressor). The two-factor (Monitoring, Blunting) structure of the MBSS was confirmed by Muris and Schouten (1994) in a sample of students, and a shortened version of the instrument has been developed (Steptoe, 1989). The MBSS has been used in numerous studies to predict health outcomes, including cancer rehabilitation (Petersson et al., 2002), insomnia (Voss, Kolling, & Heidenreich, 2006), and HIV-testing (Warburton, Fishman, & Perry, 1997).

Frankfurt Monitoring Blunting Scale

The Frankfurt Monitoring Blunting Scale (FMBS; Voss, Muller, & Schermelleh-Engel, 2006) extends the MBSS by adding scenarios of controllable situations to the uncontrollable threatening scenarios from the MBSS. This was an important development because, as the authors noted, an individual's tendency to engage in monitoring or blunting may be influenced by the perceived controllability of the situation portrayed. Using the FMBS, monitoring and blunting scores were computed separately for the distinct types of situations to categorize individuals as "rigid" or "adaptive" copers. Whereas rigid copers were hypothesized to maintain their coping styles regardless of the situation, adaptive copers were hypothesized to alter coping styles in response to different types of situations. However, results from the initial trial showed that only 5% of the sample were classified as adaptive copers, and the majority of individuals reported using a monitoring coping style regardless of controllability of the situation.

Situation-Specific Measures

Situation-specific measures of coping often resemble the paper-and-pencil format seen among dispositional measures of coping. In fact, both the WCQ and the COPE have been used as situation-specific measures of coping by simply altering the instructions to the respondent (Carver et al., 1989; Folkman & Lazarus, 1980). Development of

these types of instruments involves either (1) requesting respondents to consider a recent stressful situation or event they encountered and complete the questionnaire with that situation or event in mind, or (2) selecting items that are pertinent to a common situation or event that all respondents are encountering. The former approach requires a broad and general set of response options that could easily be applied to the plethora of situations or events respondents report. In this regard, items on these instruments often resemble items on the dispositional measures discussed previously. The latter approach enables the test developer to consider response options specific to the situation or event on which the instrument is centered. Although specific assessment instruments could be theoretically devised for any stressful situation or event (e.g., the Athletic Coping Skills Inventory; Smith, Schutz, Smoll, & Ptacek, 1995), only those pertinent to coping with medical illnesses or conditions are included here. Details regarding studies employing situation-specific measures of coping are depicted in Table 9.2.

Coping with Respondent-Identified Stressors

Billings and Moos Coping Checklist. The Billings and Moos Coping Checklist was developed to assess how individuals coped with a self-identified crisis (Billings & Moos, 1981). Five subscales were initially reported: Active Behavioral, Active Cognitive, Avoidant Coping, Problem-Focused Coping, and Emotion-Focused Coping. However, Oxlad, Miller-Lewis, and Wade (2004) found that the original Billings and Moos Coping Checklist exhibited only four factors, measuring Positive Reappraisal, Social Support Seeking, Avoidance, and Information Seeking Coping Strategies. Furthermore, internal consistency and test–retest reliability estimates were only low to moderate among university students and patients awaiting coronary artery bypass graft surgery. The authors revised the measure so that individuals rated the frequency with which they used each of the coping options in response to a recent stressor. According to the authors, the revised version assesses three factors: Appraisal-Focused Coping, Problem-Focused Coping, and Emotion-Focused Coping.

Coping Strategy Indicator. Similar to the Billing and Moos Coping Checklist, the Coping Strategy Indicator (CSI; Amirkhan, 1990) instructs respondents to describe a stressful situation and indicate to what degree they used each of three coping strategies: Problem Solving, Seeking Social Support, and Avoidance Coping. Clark et al. (1995) confirmed the three-factor model and found the scales of the CSI to have high internal consistency and adequate convergent and discriminant validity.

Coping Strategies Inventory and Coping Strategies Inventory Short Form. The original Coping Strategies Inventory (CSInv), typically abbreviated CSI in the literature, was developed by Tobin, Holroyd, Reynolds, and Wigul (1989). Respondents describe a stressful event and use a five-item Likert response format to indicate the degree to which they used a coping strategy. The CSInv includes 72 items with eight primary factors, including Problem Solving, Cognitive Restructuring, Express Emotions, Social Support, Problem Avoidance, Wishful Thinking, Self-Criticism, and Social Withdrawal (Tobin et al., 1989). A Spanish translation has been shown to have a similar factor structure to its English counterpart (Cano García, Rodríguez Franco, & García Martínez, 2007). The CSInv Short Form (CSInv-SF), developed by Addison and colleagues (2007), includes 15 items forming four primary factors: Problem-Focused Engagement, Problem-Focused Disengagement, Emotion-Focused Engagement, and Emotion-Focused Disengagement.

Coping with Specific Medical Diseases or Conditions

Sachs (1991) noted the importance that coping can have on disease outcomes, conferring either a buffer against the physical and psychological stress associated with disease processes or an enhanced stress response that interferes with optimal recovery. Thus the context of a person's health status has led to the development of several situation-specific measures of coping with specific medical conditions. Although there has been a significant amount of research examining relations between stress, coping, and disease outcomes, the results of these studies have been inconclusive. In cancer research, for example, relations between coping and medical outcomes are known to be influenced by type of cancer, stage of cancer, presence of medical complications, demographic variables, personality variables, or any number of other factors (e.g., Baider et al., 2003). As such, it is probably not that surprising that measures of dispositional coping yield very little new information in predicting treatment outcome. In these cases, it may be advantageous to develop measures of coping response that tap into domains of coping unique to the specific medical disease or condition. For one medical condition, adaptive coping that promotes optimal treatment outcomes may involve bed rest, whereas adaptive coping for another condition may involve adopting an active lifestyle incorporating daily exercise. Over the past decade, researchers have developed and validated several assessment instruments designed to assess coping specific to medical procedures and chronic health conditions. These disease-specific instruments are typically characterized by several features: (1) consideration of the subjective experience of disease prognosis in comparison to the magnitude of the emotional reaction an individual is experiencing, (2) assessment of how an individual engages in long-term problem solving with respect to the disease, (3) acknowledgement of the variety of coping strategies that could be used and the personal factors that influence which ones are chosen, (4) consideration of the context in which the illness and the coping are occurring, and (5) the ability of the assessment process to be iterative (Maes, Leventhal, & de Ridder, 1996).

Coping with Chronic Pain

Several instruments have been developed to measure how individuals deal with chronic pain on a daily basis. This is probably not surprising, given the enormity of this medical condition both in terms of reduced quality of life and increased health care costs. Many of these instruments have employed the classification of coping into active or passive strategies (i.e., the approach–avoidance paradigm). How a patient with chronic pain perceives or appraises his or her experience of pain appears to influence choice of coping strategy, so that appraisals of threat lead to passive coping and appraisals of pain as a challenge lead to active coping. Studies have demonstrated that passive coping indeed is associated with greater pain and impairment (e.g., Ramirez-Maestre, Esteve, & Lopez, 2008). Researchers have also suggested that acceptance-based active coping strategies are more valuable for measuring treatment-related improvements in chronic pain (e.g., McCracken & Eccleston, 2006).

Coping Strategies Questionnaire—Revised

The Coping Strategies Questionnaire (CSQ; Rosenstiel & Keefe, 1983) comprises six subscales measuring cognitive strategies and two subscales measuring behavioral strategies for coping with pain. Coping strategy subscales include Diverting Attention, Reinterpreting Pain Sensations, Coping Self-Statements, Ignoring Pain Sensations, Praying or Hoping, Catastrophizing, Increasing Activity Level, and Increasing Pain Behavior. As studies on the original CSQ suggested problems with scale psychometrics and stability of its factor structure, Riley and Robinson (1997) revised the scale, known as the CSQ-R. Their analysis revealed three factors: Cognitive Coping and Suppression, Helplessness, and Diverting Attention and Praying. Harland and Georgieff (2003) also developed a shorter version of the CSQ called the CSQ24, which contains only four factors: Catastrophizing, Diversion, Cognitive Coping, and Reinterpreting. Although factor structures across various versions of this instrument were generally consistent, they did not parallel the standard dichotomies of active–avoidant coping or problem-focused–emotion-focused coping. Despite this limitation, elements of standard coping style dichotomies are evidenced within the observed factor analytic structures of the CSQ and CSQ24. Coping strategies using the CSQ-R have been described for patients with cancer pain (Utne et al., 2009), arthritic pain (Park, 1994), chronic low back pain (Rosenstiel & Keefe, 1983), and spinal cord lesions (Elfstrom, Ryden, Kreuter, Taft, & Sullivan, 2005).

Chronic Pain Coping Inventory. The Chronic Pain Coping Inventory (CPCI; Jensen, Turner, Romano, & Strom, 1995) assesses a wide range of coping strategies typically employed by chronic pain patients, some of which are generally encouraged by health professionals (termed "wellness-focused") and others that are not viewed positively ("illness-focused"). As such, it can be conceptualized as a measure of mal-adaptive versus adaptive coping, with items on the illness-focused scale reflecting passive coping approaches and items on the wellness-focused scale reflecting active coping approaches (Jensen et al., 1995). Subscales from the CPCI include Professional Service Utilization, Medication Usage, Asking for Assistance, Seeking Information, Seeking Social Support, Ignoring Pain, Reinterpreting Pain Sensations, Counter-Stimulation, Guarding, Resting, Relaxation, Task Persistence, Stretching, Exercising, and Coping Self-Statements. In general, greater use of the wellness-focused strategies has been shown to be negatively associated with psychological distress and pain ratings, and illness-focused coping shares a positive relation with poorer outcomes (Jensen et al., 1995). An 18-item Brief CPI (BCPI; McCracken, Eccleston, & Bell, 2005) also has been developed and validated.

Vanderbilt Pain Management Inventory. The Vanderbilt Pain Management Inventory (VPMI; Brown & Nicassio, 1987) was developed to assess active versus passive coping strategies among chronic pain patients. Active coping strategies have been shown to be correlated with less pain, depression, and functional impairment, whereas passive coping strategies showed the opposite relation.

Chronic Pain Acceptance Questionnaire. Integrating the importance of the attitude of acceptance into current interventions for chronic pain conditions, McCracken and colleagues devised the Chronic Pain Acceptance Questionnaire (CPAQ), a two-factor measure of coping with chronic pain; the factors are Activity Engagement (AE) and Pain Willingness (PW; McCracken, Vowles, & Eccleston, 2004; Vowles, McCracken, McLeod, & Eccleston, 2008). Additionally, Vowles and colleagues (2008) reported that these two dimensions formed three response types: high AE/high PW, high AE/low PW, and low AE/low PW. These response types were found to be predictive of pain-related outcomes; for example, the low AE/low PW type was associated with more pain, depression, anxiety, and disability than other types. Although this instrument only measures a few specific types of coping with pain, the response types appear to have value in predicting important clinical outcomes.

Coping with Cancer

Research on coping with cancer has revealed a strong association between patient perception of illness and coping strategies (Koehler, Koeningsmann, & Frommer, 2009). In brief, two specific coping strategies have emerged as being associated with positive treatment outcomes: those used to obtain control and those used to raise hope (Koehler et al., 2009). As with medical coping, Koehler and colleagues (2009) proposed that coping with cancer should be assessed as an iterative process, examining how coping strategies and their relative effectiveness change over the course of the illness.

Mental Adjustment to Cancer. The Mental Adjustment to Cancer (MAC; Watson et al., 1988) was developed based on previous research that indicated that several main types of coping were used among cancer patients: Fighting Spirit, Fatalistic (or Stoic) Acceptance, Hopelessness/Helplessness, Anxious Preoccupation, and Avoidance (Watson et al., 1988). The subscales correlated in the expected directions with measures of anxiety and depression. Cultural and age differences in coping using the MAC have been described, including differing factor structures (Baider et al., 2003; Costa-Requena & Gil, 2009). Using a large sample of cancer patients, factor analytic results yielded two broad factors: Positive Adjustment and Negative Adjustment (Watson & Homewood, 2008). As expected, Negative Adjustment was correlated with anxiety and depression.

Revised WCQ—Cancer Version. Based upon the structure of the WCQ, the WCQ—Cancer Version (WCQ-CA) was developed to assess how cancer patients cope across several important domains: Cognitive Escape-Avoidance, Behavioral Escape-Avoidance, Seek and Use Social Support, Focus on the

Positive, and Distancing (Dunkel-Schetter, Feinstein, Taylor & Falke, 1992). These strategies can be assessed regardless of cancer stage or type and current treatment status. When assessing how women with breast cancer coped with specific stressors, results indicated that those with the best adjustment exhibited variation in coping style in response to the type of stressor they were confronting (Manuel et al., 2007).

Other Medical Coping Measures

Coping with Surgical Stress Scale. The Coping with Surgical Stress Scale (CoSS) was developed to assess styles of presurgical coping that may influence postoperative functioning (Krohne, de Bruin, El-Giamal, & Schmukle, 2000). Subscales on the CoSS measure are Rumination, Optimism and Trust, Turning to Social and Religious Resources, Threat Avoidance, and Information Seeking. Thus at least some items on the instrument measure the approach–avoidance dimension of coping. Various relations have been observed between the subscales and measures of trait anxiety, surgical anxiety, and postoperative adjustment (Krohne, de Bruin, et al., 2000).

Threatening Medical Situations Inventory. The Threatening Medical Situations Inventory (TMSI) is a measure of monitoring versus blunting specific to medical situations (Van Zuuren, de Groot, Mulder, & Muris, 1996). Individuals are presented with four medical threat scenarios and asked to report how they would respond, choosing among the monitoring and blunting options listed. Convergent validity for the TMSI has been reported, comparing it favorably with the MBSS in a community sample (Wakefield, Homewood, Mahmut, Taylor, & Meiser, 2007). Additionally, blunting, as measured by the TMSI, has been shown to be negatively related to anxiety among a sample of individuals undergoing genetic testing for cancer risk (Wakefield et al., 2007).

Medical Coping Models Questionnaire. The Medical Coping Models Questionnaire (MCMQ) was designed to facilitate the assessment of coping with a variety of health-related stressors (Feifel, Strack, & Nagy, 1987). Rodrigue, Jackson, and Perri

(2000) noted that the MCMQ was preferable to other medical coping measures, as it strikes a balance between being specific enough to capture coping with illness, but not just one illness in particular. The scale is composed of three subscales: Confrontation, Avoidance, and Acceptance-Resignation. In a study of patients with HIV/AIDS, the latter two subscales were associated with greater psychological distress (Sun, Zhang, & Fu, 2007). The three-factor structure has been confirmed in a sample of transplant patients, in which the Acceptance-Resignation and Avoidance subscales were also found to be correlated with poorer psychological functioning (Rodrigue et al., 2000). However, another factor analysis indicated the presence of a fourth subscale among cancer patients that was named Nondominant (Shapiro, Rodrigue, Boggs, & Robinson, 1994).

Coping Questionnaire for Coronary Patients. Using the approach–avoidance paradigm, the Coping Questionnaire for Coronary Patients was developed to assess how individuals respond to worry about cardiac events or the actual experience of them (Maes & Bruggemans, 1990). The coping strategies are considered within three contexts: medical, psychological, and social.

Coping Questionnaire for Asthmatic Patients. Patients with asthma cope with two features of the disease: knowing they have a chronic disease and having acute asthma attacks. The Coping Questionnaire for Asthmatic Patients was constructed with two distinct subscales: Asthma Coping State Scale and Asthma Coping Trait Scale. Scores on the coping subscales have been shown to predict patients' well-being and the number of days they missed work due to asthma, but were not able to predict number of hospital admissions for asthma conditions or amount of asthma medications taken in a given day (Maes & Schlosser, 1987).

Jalowiec Coping Scale. The Jalowiec Coping Scale (JCS) was designed specifically for use by emergency room patients and patients with hypertension (Jalowiec, Murphy, & Powers, 1984). The 40 coping strategies that make up this measure can be categorized into problem-focused or emotion-focused coping strategies. However, factor analysis yielded a four-factor solution that classifies coping strategies as Problem-Focused, Palliative, Pessimistic, and Support-Related. Other factor analyses have yielded different factor structures, including subscale clusters named Confrontive, Evasive, Optimistic, Fatalistic, Emotive, Palliative, Supportive, and Self-Reliant. Neither factor structure was supported among a sample of coronary patients (Ulvik et al., 2008). Willoughby, Kee, Demi, and Parker (2000) also reported psychometric problems with some of the subscales of the JCS, but other subscales were successful in predicting adjustment outcomes on the Psychosocial Adjustment to Illness Scale.

Think-Aloud Methods of Assessment

Questionnaire measures of coping depend upon respondents accurately reporting their coping responses that occurred days, weeks, or even years earlier. This is particularly true for assessing dispositional measures of coping that require respondents to synthesize lifetimes of coping responses into a single questionnaire. Situation-specific assessment instruments are influenced to a lesser extent by this limitation, as long as the measure is completed immediately following the stressful situation or event or as it is actually occurring. Presumably, most of the measures devised for coping with medical conditions are obtained while the patient is experiencing the condition, making these measures less susceptible to delayed recall problems.

Another strategy for assessing coping *in vivo* involves training respondents to report their thought processes verbally while engaging in a stressful situation, a method known as the think-aloud procedure. This procedure enables covert activity to be accessed and recorded in real time while coping is occurring. This method, however, is not without its problems. For example, it is unknown to what extent thinking aloud actually influences the content of thinking that typically occurs during coping. In this regard, this measurement strategy might interfere or alter the content of the cognitive appraisals that actually occur when confronting a stressful situation. Furthermore, most stressful situations that are encountered in laboratory stress manipulations and certainly in daily life require cognitive activity that would be seriously disrupted if think-aloud procedures were implemented. Think-aloud procedures can be used effectively to access thought content during relatively passive stress manipulations such as being exposed to pain (Heiden et al., 1991) but are less helpful in accessing thought content during active stress manipulations such as engaging in mental tasks or interpersonal tasks.

Ecological Momentary Assessment of Coping

Using the technological advances in portable data collection equipment, strategies for accessing information regarding coping responses immediately following stressful situations or encounters that occur in real life are now possible. In these studies (e.g., Schwartz et al., 1999) handheld computer devices are programmed to prompt respondents to answer brief questions regarding levels of stress encountered and their associated coping responses. These approaches have a substantial advantage over questionnaire approaches in obtaining information within moments of stressful encounters. Additionally, because data are gathered using ambulatory devices, the generalizability of results from these studies to coping during real-life situations is enhanced. EMAs have been used to measure coping responses among smokers, adding support for the use of EMA as a valid tool to measure coping (O'Connell et al., 1998). However, there remains relatively little research published describing the use of EMA for measuring coping.

Summary and Conclusions

Despite the years of development and progression, some researchers have suggested that existing coping measures continue to be psychometrically inadequate (Parker & Endler, 2006). Paradoxically, as the research literature expands, there seems to be less clarity about the best ways to measure coping. Schwarzer and Schwarzer (1996) argue that the development and empirical construction of the scales themselves are less important than how they are used. They have proposed adopting multiple time points for assessing coping and causal modeling for validation.

Additionally, they echo the sentiment that EMA strategies may provide the best tool for representing the range of an individual's actual coping behaviors. However, not all researchers have access to such instrumentation, nor will all clinical health psychologists have access to these devices should they desire to assess coping in a clinical setting. In this regard, it appears that both researchers and clinicians in clinical health psychology must strike a balance between assessing general coping skills and gathering information about coping with a designated specific stressor. Information about patterns of coping both over time and in concrete situations also appears to be of interest, with preference given to assessments of actual, real-time coping. Although there are many instruments that measure coping in a dichotomous fashion (i.e., monitoring–blunting; emotion-focused vs. problem-focused coping), it has become increasingly clear that conceptualizing the range of coping strategies along a continuum yields important information. Folkman and Moskowitz (2004) identified several new directions for future research on coping, including:

1. A focus on proactive coping (i.e., how people cope prior to an event to decrease the impact of future stressors).
2. The dual-process model of coping (i.e., "oscillating between loss and future orientations, between approach and avoidant coping, and between positive and negative reappraisals"; Folkman & Moskowitz, 2004, p. 758).
3. Social aspects of coping, religious coping (Pargament, Koenig, & Perez, 2000).
4. New directions for emotional coping and emotion regulation.

Perhaps taking advantage of the multitude of instruments available and sampling from the different conceptualizations of coping can provide a well-rounded glimpse of one's coping styles. More important than style, however, is determining the effectiveness of an individual's coping strategies. Inquiries regarding coping should include a regular assessment of how well the strategies are working to reduce the anxiety and distress associated with confronting various life stressors. This is where clinicians will be able to offer interventions to best serve the needs of their patients.

REFERENCES

Abbott, J. (2003). Coping with cystic fibrosis. *Journal of the Royal Society of Medicine, 96,* 42–50.

Addison, C., Campbell-Jenkins, B., Sarpong, D., Kibler, J., Singh, M., Dubbert, P., et al. (2007). Psychometric evaluation of a Coping Strategies Inventory—Short Form (CSI-SF) in the Jackson Heart Study Cohort. *International Journal of Environmental Research and Public Health, 4,* 289–295.

Amirkhan, J. H. (1990). A factor analytically derived measure of coping: The Coping Strategy Indicator. *Journal of Personality and Social Psychology, 59,* 1066–1074.

Baider, L., Andritsch, E., Uziely, B., Goldzweig, G., Ever-Hadani, P., Hofman, G., et al. (2003). Effects of age on coping and psychological distress in women diagnosed with breast cancer: Review of literature and analysis of two different geographical settings. *Critical Reviews in Oncology/Hematology, 46,* 5–16.

Baker, J. P., & Berenbaum, H. (2007). Emotional approach and problem-focused coping: A comparison of potentially adaptive strategies. *Cognition and Emotion, 21,* 95–118.

Barnoy, S., Bar-Tal, Y., & Zisser, B. (2006). Correspondence in informational coping styles: How important is it for cancer patients and their spouses? *Personality and Individual Differences, 41,* 105–115.

Bell, P. A., & Byrne, D. (1978). Repression–sensitization. In H. London & J. E. Exner (Eds.), *Dimensions of personality* (pp. 449–485). New York: Wiley.

Bijttebier, P., Vertommen, H., & Vander Steene, G. (2001). Assessment of cognitive coping styles: A closer look at situation-response inventories. *Clinical Psychology Review, 21,* 85–104.

Billings, A. G., & Moos, R. H. (1981). The role of coping resources in attenuating the stress of life events. *Journal of Behavioral Medicine, 4,* 139–157.

Billings, A. G., & Moos, R. H. (1984). Coping, stress and social resources among adults with unipolar depression. *Journal of Personality and Social Psychology, 46,* 877–891.

Brown, G. K., & Nicassio, P. M. (1987). Development of a questionnaire for the assessment of active and passive coping strategies in chronic pain patients. *Pain, 31,* 53–64.

Cano García, F. J., Rodríguez Franco, L., & García Martínez, J. (2007). Spanish version of the Coping Strategies Inventory. *Actas Españolas de Psiquiatría, 35,* 29–39.

Carver, C. S. (1997). You want to measure coping but your protocol's too long: Consider the brief COPE. *International Journal of Behavioral Medicine, 4,* 92–100.

Carver, C. S., Scheier, M. F., & Weintraub, J. K. (1989). Assessing coping strategies: A theoretically based approach. *Journal of Personality and Social Psychology, 56,* 267–283.

Clark, K. K., Bormann, C. A., Cropanzano, R. S., & James, K. (1995). Validation evidence for three coping measures. *Journal of Personality Assessment, 65,* 434–455.

Constant, A., Castera, L., Quintard, B., Bernard, P. H., de Ledinghen, V., Couzigou, P., et al. (2005). Psychosocial factors associated with perceived disease severity in patients coping with hepatitis C: Relationship with information sources and attentional coping style. *Psychosomatics, 46,* 25–33.

Costa-Requena, G., & Gil, F. (2009). The Mental Adjustment to Cancer scale: A psychometric analysis in Spanish cancer patients. *Psycho-Oncology, 18,* 984–991.

Danhauer, S. C., Crawford, S. L., Farmer, D. F., & Avis, N. E. (2009). A longitudinal investigation of coping strategies and quality of life among younger women with breast cancer. *Journal of Behavioral Medicine, 32,* 371–379.

Davis, L. C., Sander, A. M., Struchen, M. A., Sherer, M., Nakase-Richardson, R., & Malec, J. F. (2009). Medical and psychosocial predictors of caregiver distress and perceived burden following traumatic brain injury. *Journal of Head Trauma Rehabilitation, 24,* 145–154.

Dunkel-Schetter, C., Feinstein, L. G., Taylor, S. E., & Falke, R. L. (1992). Patterns of coping with cancer. *Health Psychology, 11,* 79–87.

Eisengart, S. P., Singer, L. T., Kirchner, H. L., Min, M. O., Fulton, S., Short, E. J., et al. (2006). Factor structure of coping: Two studies of mothers with high levels of life stress. *Psychological Assessment, 18,* 278–288.

Elfstrom, M. L., Ryden, A., Kreuter, M., Taft, C., & Sullivan, M. (2005). Relations between coping strategies and health-related quality of life in patients with spinal cord lesion. *Journal of Rehabilitative Medicine, 37,* 9–16.

Endler, N. S., & Parker, J. D. A. (1990a). *Coping Inventory for Stressful Situations (CISS): Manual.* Toronto, Ontario, Canada: Multi-Health Systems.

Endler, N. S., & Parker, J. D. A. (1990b). Multidimensional assessment of coping: A critical evaluation. *Journal of Personality and Social Psychology, 58,* 844–854.

Endler, N. S., & Parker, J. D. A. (1994). Assessment of multidimensional coping: Task, emotion, and avoidance strategies. *Psychological Assessment, 6,* 50–60.

Feifel, H., Strack, S., & Nagy, V. T. (1987). Coping strategies and associated features of medically ill patients. *Psychosomatic Medicine, 49,* 616–625.

Folkman, S., & Lazarus, R. S. (1980). An analysis of coping in a middle-aged community sample. *Journal of Health and Social Behavior, 21,* 219–239.

Folkman, S., & Lazarus, R. S. (1985). If it changes it must be a process: Study of emotion and coping during three stages of a college examination. *Journal of Personality and Social Psychology, 48,* 150–170.

Folkman, S., & Moskowitz, J. T. (2004). Coping: Pitfalls and promise. *Annual Review of Psychology, 55,* 745–774.

Geirdal, A. O., & Dahl, A. A. (2008). The relationship between coping strategies and anxiety in women from families with familial breast-ovarian cancer in the absence of demonstrated mutations. *Psycho-Oncology, 17,* 49–57.

Harland, N. J., & Georgieff, K. (2003). Development of the Coping Strategies Questionnaire 24, a clinically utilitarian version of the Coping Strategies Questionnaire. *Rehabilitation Psychology, 48,* 296–300.

Harrington, S., McGurk, M., & Llewellyn, C. D. (2008). Positive consequences of head and neck cancer: Key correlates of finding benefit. *Journal of Psychosocial Oncology, 26,* 43–62.

Heiden, L. A., Larkin, K. T., & Knowlton, G. E. (1991). Cognitive response to a cold pressor challenge in high and low blood pressure reactive subjects. *Journal of Psychosomatic Research, 35,* 679–685.

Jalowiec, A., Murphy, S. P., & Powers, M. J. (1984). Psychometric assessment of the Jalowiec Coping Scale. *Nursing Research, 33,* 157–161.

Jensen, M. P., Turner, J. A., Romano, J. M., & Strom, S. E. (1995). The Chronic Pain Coping Inventory: Development and preliminary validation. *Pain, 60,* 203–216.

Kershaw, T., Northouse, L., Kritpracha, C., Schafenacker, A., & Mood, D. (2004). Coping strategies and quality of life in women with advanced breast cancer and their family caregivers. *Psychology and Health, 19,* 139–155.

Kershaw, T. S., Wood, D. W., Newth, G., Ronis, D. L., Sanda, M. G., Vaishampayan, U., et al. (2008). Longitudinal analysis of a model to predict quality of life in prostate cancer patients and their spouses. *Annals of Behavioral Medicine, 36,* 117–128.

Klein, D. M., Turvey, C. L., & Pies, C. J. (2007). Relationship of coping styles with quality of life and depressive symptoms in older heart failure patients. *Journal of Aging and Health, 19,* 22–38.

Koehler, M., Koeningsmann, M., & Frommer, J. (2009). Coping with illness and subjective theories of illness in adult patients with haematological malignancies: Systematic review. *Critical Reviews in Oncology/Hematology, 69,* 237–257.

Krohne, H. W., de Bruin, J. T., El-Giamal, M., & Schmukle, S. C. (2000). The assessment of surgery-related coping: The Coping with Surgical Stress Scale (COSS). *Psychology and Health, 15,* 135–149.

Krohne, H. W., Egloff, B., Varner, L. J., Burns, L. R., Weidner, G., & Ellis, H. C. (2000). The assessment of dispositional vigilance and cognitive avoidance: Factorial structure, psychometric properties and validity of the Mainz Coping Inventory. *Cognitive Therapy and Research, 24,* 297–311.

Lazarus, R. S., & Folkman, S. (1984). *Stress, appraisal, and coping.* New York: Springer.

Maes, S., & Bruggemans, E. (1990). Approach–avoidance and illness behavior in coronary heart patients. In L. R. Schmidt, P. Schwenkmezger, J. Weinman, & S. Maes (Eds.), *Theoretical and applied aspects of health psychology* (pp. 297–308). Amsterdam: Harwood Academic.

Maes, S., Leventhal, H., & de Ridder, D. T. (1996). Coping with chronic diseases. In M. Zeidner & N. S. Endler (Eds.), *Handbook of coping* (pp. 221–251). New York: Wiley.

Maes, S., & Schlosser, M. (1987). The role of cognition and coping in health behavior outcomes of asthmatic patients. *Current Psychological Research and Reviews, 6,* 79–90.

Manuel, J. C., Burwell, S. R., Crawford, S. L., Lawrence, R. H., Farmer, D. F., Hege, A., et al. (2007). Younger women's perceptions of coping with breast cancer. *Cancer Nursing, 30,* 85–94.

McCracken, L. M., & Eccleston, C. (2006). A comparison of the relative utility of coping and acceptance-based measures in a sample of chronic pain sufferers. *European Journal of Pain, 10,* 23–29.

McCracken, L. M., Eccleston, C., & Bell, L. (2005). Clinical assessment of behavioral coping responses: Preliminary results from a brief inventory. *European Journal of Pain, 9,* 69–78.

McCracken, L. M., Vowles, K. E., & Eccleston,

C. (2004). Acceptance of chronic pain: Component analysis and a revised assessment method. *Pain, 107,* 159–166.

Miller, S. M. (1987). Monitoring and blunting: Validation of a questionnaire to assess styles of information seeking under threat. *Journal of Personality and Social Psychology, 52,* 345–353.

Miller, S. M., & Mangan, C. E. (1983). Interacting effects of information and coping style in adapting to gynecologic stress: Should the doctor tell all? *Journal of Personality and Social Psychology, 45,* 223–236.

Muris, P., & Schouten, E. (1994). Monitoring and blunting: A factor analysis of the Miller Behavioural Style Scale. *Personality and Individual Differences, 17,* 285–287.

Myers, L. B., & Derakshan, N. (2000). Monitoring and blunting and an assessment of different coping styles. *Personality and Individual Differences, 28,* 111–121.

Nolen-Hoeksema, S., & Larson, J. (1999). *Coping with loss.* Mahwah, NJ: Erlbaum.

O'Connell, K. A., Gerkovich, M. M., Cook, M. R., Shiffman, S., Hickcox, M., & Kakolewski, K. E. (1998). Coping in real time: Using ecological momentary assessment techniques to assess coping with the urge to smoke. *Research in Nursing and Health, 21,* 487–497.

O'Donnell, K., Badrick, E., Kumari, M., & Steptoe, A. (2008). Psychological coping styles and cortisol over the day in healthy older adults. *Psychoneuroendocrinology, 33,* 601–611.

Oxlad, M., Miller-Lewis, L., & Wade, T. D. (2004). The measurement of coping responses: Validity of the Billings and Moos Coping Checklist. *Journal of Psychosomatic Research, 57,* 477–484.

Pargament, K. I., Koenig, H. G., & Perez, L. M. (2000). The many methods of religious coping: Development and initial validation of the RCOPE. *Journal of Clinical Psychology, 56,* 519–543.

Park, D. C. (1994). Self-regulation and control of rheumatic disorders. In S. Maes, H. Leventhal, & M. Johnston (Eds.), *International review of health psychology* (pp. 189–217). Chichester, UK: Wiley.

Parker, J. D. A., & Endler, N. S. (2006). Coping with coping assessment: A critical review. *European Journal of Personality, 6,* 321–344.

Penedo, F. J., Gonzalez, J. S., Davis, C., Dahn, J., Antoni, M. H., Ironson, G., et al. (2003). Coping and psychological distress among symptomatic HIV+ men who have sex with men. *Annals of Behavioral Medicine, 25,* 203–213.

Petersson, L. M., Nordin, K., Glimelius, B., Brekkan, E., Sjödén, P. O., & Berglund, G. (2002). Differential effects of cancer rehabilitation depending on diagnosis and patients' cognitive coping style. *Psychosomatic Medicine, 64,* 971–980.

Ptacek, J. T., Pierce, G. R., & Thompson, E. L. (2006). Finding evidence of dispositional coping. *Journal of Research in Personality, 40,* 1137–1151.

Ramirez-Maestre, C., Esteve, R., & Lopez, A. E. (2008). Cognitive appraisal and coping in chronic pain patients. *European Journal of Pain, 12,* 749–756.

Riley, J. L., III, & Robinson, M. E. (1997). CSQ: Five factors or fiction? *Clinical Journal of Pain, 13,* 156–162.

Rodrigue, J. R., Jackson, S. I., & Perri, M. G. (2000). Medical Coping Modes Questionnaire: Factor structure for adult transplant candidates. *International Journal of Behavioral Medicine, 7,* 89–110.

Rosenstiel, A. K., & Keefe, F. J. (1983). The use of coping strategies in chronic low back pain patients: Relationship to patient characteristics and current adjustment. *Pain, 17,* 33–44.

Roth, S., & Cohen, L. J. (1986). Approach, avoidance, and coping with stress. *American Psychologist, 41,* 813–819.

Sachs, B. C. (1991). Coping with stress. *Stress Medicine, 7,* 61–63.

Schoen, E., Altmaier, E. M., & Tallman, B. (2007). Coping after bone marrow transplantation: The predictive roles of optimism and dispositional coping. *Journal of Clinical Psychology in Medical Settings, 14,* 123–129.

Schwartz, J. E., Neale, J., Marco, C., Shiffman, S. S., & Stone, A. A. (1999). Does trait coping exist?: A momentary assessment approach to the evaluation of traits. *Journal of Personality and Social Psychology, 77,* 360–369.

Schwarzer, R., & Schwarzer, C. (1996). A critical survey of coping instruments. In M. Zeidner & N. S. Endler (Eds.), *Handbook of coping* (pp. 107–132). New York: Wiley.

Shapiro, D. E., Rodrigue, J. R., Boggs, S. R., & Robinson, M. E. (1994). Cluster analysis of the Medical Coping Modes Questionnaire: Evidence for coping with cancer styles? *Journal of Psychosomatic Research, 38,* 151–159.

Sideridis, G. D. (2006). Coping is not an "either" "or": The interaction of coping strategies in regulating affect, arousal, and performance. *Stress and Health, 22,* 315–327.

Sinclair, V. G., & Scroggie, J. (2005). Effects of a cognitive-behavioral program for women with multiple sclerosis. *Journal of Neuroscience Nursing, 37,* 249.

Skinner, E. A., Edge, K., Altman, J., & Sherwood, H. (2003). Searching for the structure of coping: A review and critique of category systems for classifying ways of coping. *Psychological Bulletin, 129,* 216–269.

Smith, R. E., Schutz, R. W., Smoll, F. L., & Ptacek, J. T. (1995). Development and validation of a multidimensional of sport-specific psychological skills: The Athletic Coping Skills Inventory—28. *Journal of Exercise and Sport Psychology, 17,* 379–398.

Sorgen, K. E., & Manne, S. L. (2002). Coping in children with cancer: Examining the goodness-of-fit hypothesis. *Children's Health Care, 31,* 191–207.

Steed, L. G. (1998). A critique of coping scales. *Australian Psychologist, 33,* 193–202.

Steptoe, A. (1989). An abbreviated version of the Miller Behavioral Style Scale. *British Journal of Clinical Psychology, 28,* 183–184.

Suls, J., & Fletcher. B. (1985). The relative efficacy of avoidant and nonavoidant coping strategies: A meta-analysis. *Health Psychology, 4,* 249–288.

Sun, H. M., Zhang, J. J., & Fu, X. D. (2007). Psychological status, coping, and social support of people living with HIV/AIDS in central China. *Public Health Nursing, 24,* 132–140.

Tercyak, K. P., Lerman, C., Peshkin, B. N., Hughes, C., Main, D., Isaacs, C., et al. (2001). Effects of coping style and BRCA1 and BRCA2 test results on anxiety among women participating in genetic counseling and testing for breast and ovarian cancer risk. *Health Psychology, 20,* 217–222.

Terry, D. J. (1994). Determinants of coping: The role of stable and situational factors. *Journal of Personality and Social Psychology, 66,* 895–910.

Tobin, D. L., Holroyd, K. A., Reynolds, R. V., & Wigul, J. K. (1989). The hierarchical factor structure of the Coping Strategies Inventory. *Cognitive Therapy and Research, 13,* 343–361.

Ulvik, B., Johnsen, T. B., Nygard, O., Hanestad, B. R., Wahl, A. K., & Wentzel-Larsen, T. (2008). Factor structure of the revised Jalowiec Coping Scale in patients admitted for elective coronary angiography. *Scandinavian Journal of the Caring Sciences, 22,* 596–607.

Utne, I., San, C., Miaskowski, C., Bjordal, K., Cooper, B. A., Valeberg, B. T., et al. (2009). Confirmatory factor analysis of the Coping Strategies Questionnaire—Revised in samples of oncology outpatients and inpatients with pain. *Clinical Journal of Pain, 25,* 391–400.

van Zuuren, F. J., de Groot, K. I., Mulder, N. L., & Muris, P. (1996). Coping with medical threat: An evaluation of the Threatening Medical Situations Inventory (TMSI). *Personality and Individual Differences, 21,* 21–31.

Voss, U., Kolling, T., & Heidenreich, T. (2006). Role of monitoring and blunting coping styles in primary insomnia. *Psychosomatic Medicine, 68,* 110–115.

Voss, U., Muller, H., & Schermelleh-Engel, K. (2006). Towards the assessment of adaptive vs. rigid coping styles: Validation of the Frankfurt Monitoring Blunting Scale by means of confirmatory factor analysis. *Personality and Individual Differences, 41,* 295–306.

Vowles, K. E., McCracken, L. M., McLeod, C., & Eccleston, C. (2008). The Chronic Pain Acceptance Questionnaire: Confirmatory analysis and identification of patient subgroups. *Pain, 140,* 284–291.

Wakefield, C. E., Homewood, J., Mahmut, M., Taylor, A., & Meiser, B. (2007). Usefulness of the Threatening Medical Situations Inventory in individuals considering genetic testing for cancer risk. *Patient Education and Counseling, 69,* 29–38.

Walker, K., Lindner, H., & Noonan, M. (2009). The role of coping in the relationship between depression and illness severity in chronic fatigue syndrome. *Journal of Allied Health, 38,* 91–99.

Warburton, L. A., Fishman, B., & Perry, S. W. (1997). Coping with the possibility of testing HIV-positive. *Personality and Individual Differences, 22,* 459–464.

Watson, M., Greer, S., Young, J., Inayat, Q., Burgess, C., & Robertson, C. (1988). Development of a questionnaire measure of adjustment to cancer: The MAC scale. *Psychological Medicine, 18,* 203–209.

Watson, M., & Homewood, J. (2008). Mental Adjustment to Cancer Scale: Psychometric properties in a large cancer cohort. *Psycho-Oncology, 17,* 1146–1151.

Willoughby, D. F., Kee, C. C., Demi, A., & Parker, V. (2000). Coping and psychosocial adjustment of women with diabetes. *Diabetes Educator, 26,* 105–112.

Zuckerman, M., & Gagne, M. (2003). The COPE revised: Proposing a 5-factor model of coping strategies. *Journal of Research in Personality, 37,* 169–204.

CHAPTER 10

Physical Activity

Patricia M. Dubbert
Todd A. Smitherman
Jeanne Gabriele

Recent studies of physical activity, exercise, and health have substantially increased the range of variables that are of interest. Regular vigorous sports participation has been linked to many health benefits, but everyday activities such as leisure walking and household and yard work also contribute significantly to health promotion and disease prevention (Dubbert, 2002; Haskell et al., 2007). In this chapter, *physical activity* includes the broad range of "bodily movement produced by skeletal muscle that results in energy expenditure" (Caspersen, Powell, & Christenson, 1985). *Exercise* is the subset of physical activity that is "planned, structured, and performed for the purpose of improving physical fitness" (Caspersen et al., 1985). We present a subset of the array of methods of assessing physical activity, exercise, physical fitness, and related variables that are relevant to the practice of clinical health psychology. Measures are presented in three groups: self-report questionnaires and surveys, objective measures of activity, and measures of physical fitness.

Self-Report Measures of Physical Activity and Related Variables

The most commonly used measures for physical activity, exercise, and related variables are interviewer- or self-administered instruments that assess activity type, intensity, frequency, and duration over a defined period of time. These types of self-report instruments are familiar to clinical psychologists, generally easy to use, and have good face validity with clients or research participants; however, they have the disadvantages of error due to inaccurate recall and variable interpretation of items. Many such instruments have been developed, and the best choice for any specific application depends on the specific behavior and time frame that is of interest. Table 10.1 summarizes information about several standardized self-report instruments that are useful in a variety of situations, ranging from assessment of individuals seen in clinical settings to large samples in epidemiological studies.

TABLE 10.1. Characteristics of Selected Self-Report Measures of Physical Activity and Exercise for Adults and Older Adults

Measure	Content assessed and time frame	Number and types of items	Reliability[a]	Validity[a]
International Physical Activity Questionnaire (IPAQ; Craig et al., 2003)	Time spent in moderate and vigorous PA, walking, and sitting during past 7 days or usual week	Short (9 items) and long (31 items) forms for telephone interviewer or self-administration query number of days and time in work, household, work, and transportation PA and sitting	3- to 7-day test–retest reliability = about .80	Correlations = .33 for long form and .30 for short form with accelerometer data
Behavioral Risk Factor Surveillance Survey (BRFSS; Yore et al., 2007)	Time spent in moderate and vigorous leisure and occupational PA in a usual week	11 interviewer- (telephone-) administered items on moderate and vigorous intensity PA, walking, muscle strengthening, and occupational PA	Test–retest = .35–.53 for moderate, .80–.86 for vigorous PA	Correlations = .31 with accelerometer for moderate, .17 for vigorous PA
Seven-Day Physical Activity Recall (PAR; Sallis, 1997; Dubbert et al., 2004)	Time spent in moderate and higher intensity leisure and occupational PA past 7 days to compute PA energy expenditure	Interviewer administered; 8 items plus estimates of time spent in sleep, moderate, hard, and very hard activity each of past 7 days	2-week test–retest for hard/vigorous PA about .30; for moderate PA from .10 to .50; 2- to 4-week test–retest intraclass correlation for PA energy expenditure = .89 in older men	Correlation with activity log = .36 to .71; correlations with maximal fitness tests = .30 to .61; correlation with 6-minute walk .22 in older men
Community Healthy Activity Model Program for Seniors (CHAMPS; Stewart et al., 2001)	Time spent in light, moderate, and vigorous activities in past 4 weeks; can compute PA energy expenditure	40 items for interview or self-administration, including 13 activities other than PA	6-month intraclass correlation =.67 for moderate and greater caloric expenditure	Correlation = .27 with 6-minute walk
Kaiser Physical Activity Survey (KPAS; Ainsworth, Sternfeld, et al., 2000)	PA in work, sports, and nonsports leisure during past year; KPAS added home/yard section	Items in KPAS produce four index scores; index scores can be summed for total score	1-month test–retest for KPAS = .79–.91	Correlations for KPAS with activity monitor = .30–.44
Paffenbarger Physical Activity Questionnaire (Paffenbarger et al., 1978)	Sport and leisure time PA during past week or past year; can compute PA energy expenditure	8 interview-administered items including pace of walking, stairs, sports, times per week of vigorous and moderate PA, usual exertion level in PA	2-week test–retest correlations = .23–.68 for specific items, .34 for PA energy expenditure	Total index correlations = .52 with maximal fitness tests, .30 with activity monitor
Yale Physical Activity Survey for Older Persons (YPAS; DiPietro et al., 1993)	Time spent in various activities used to compute summary indices for total time, energy expenditure, and activity dimensions scores for vigorous, leisurely, moving, standing, and sitting PA	40 interviewer-administered items covering work/household, yardwork, caretaking, sport and recreation, leisure walking, moving, standing, sitting	2-week test–retest .42 for total time	Correlations for summary index = .20–.58 with maximal fitness tests, .37 with activity monitor

Note. PA., physical activity.
[a] Values are from references shown in column 1 and/or summary tables for the instrument in special issue of *Medicine and Science in Sports and Exercise* (Kriska & Caspersen, 1997).

To evaluate adherence to current public health guidelines for adequate physical activity (Haskell et al., 2007), the International Physical Activity Questionnaire (IPAQ; Craig et al., 2003) or recent physical activity modules of the Centers for Disease Control and Prevention's Behavioral Risk Factor Surveillance Survey (BRFSS; *www.cdc.gov/brfss/about.htm*; Yore et al., 2007) provide easy-to-use assessments that can be administered in person or by telephone interview. The Seven-Day Physical Activity Recall (PAR; Sallis, 1997) requires more time (20–30 minutes) to administer, but it can provide very detailed descriptions of the types, intensity, and duration of physical activity during the preceding week. Simple modifications of the PAR allow estimation of physical activity time and energy expenditure (EE) for light–moderate as well as moderate and hard–vigorous intensities (Dubbert, Vander Weg, Kirchner, & Shaw, 2004). The Community Healthy Activity Model Program for Seniors (CHAMPS) survey (Resnicow et al., 2003; Stewart et al., 2001) can be self- or interview-administered and is very user friendly for older persons or other populations, including relatively inactive people. The Yale Physical Activity Survey (YPAS; DiPietro, Caspersen, Ostfeld, & Nadel, 1993) was also specifically developed for older populations and samples light to moderate and home/yard-oriented activities, as well as sports participation.

Using an instrument that allows direct comparison with data collected in earlier studies is important in longitudinal cohort studies and for determining population trends over time. Modifications of the Baecke Questionnaire of Habitual Physical Activity (Baecke, Burema, & Fritjers, 1982), which provide physical activity index scores for sport, occupational, nonsport leisure, and household/family/garden activities, have been validated and used in several large-scale epidemiological studies. These include the instrument used in the Atherosclerosis Risk in Communities study (ARIC/Baecke; Richardson, Ainsworth, Wu, Jacobs, & Leon, 1995), the Kaiser Physical Activity Survey (KPAS; Ainsworth, Sternfeld, Richardson, & Jackson, 2000) used in a multiethnic study of women, and the Jackson Heart Study Cohort survey (J-PAC; Dubbert et al., 2005; Smitherman et al., 2009)

used in a study of cardiovascular disease in African Americans. The Paffenbarger Physical Activity Questionnaire (Paffenbarger, Wing, & Hyde, 1978) includes several items that have been individually related to health outcomes, including pace of walking, city blocks walked, and intensity of usual physical activity participation (scale of 0–10).

Useful compilations of physical activity survey measures have been published, including a special issue of *Medicine and Science in Sports and Exercise* (Pereira et al., 1997) that provided a collection of important measures that were available in the late 1990s and frequently used in epidemiologic and clinical studies. Subsequently, special issues of *Research Quarterly for Exercise and Sport* (Wood, 2000) and *Medicine and Science in Sports and Exercise* (Montoye, 2000) included reviews of conceptual issues and current self-report and objective physical activity assessment methodologies. Another useful resource is the most recent update of the *Compendium of Physical Activity* (Ainsworth, Haskell, et al., 2000), which provides a comprehensive list of physical activities and their estimated energy expenditure values. Because space is limited in this chapter, readers are encouraged to consult these and more recent reviews for additional detailed information. Researchers are continually developing new instruments and evaluating psychometric data on older instruments for previously understudied populations, such as ethnic and racial minorities and persons with physical and mental disabilities. A recent study found that both the CHAMPS and BRFSS physical activity module had adequate reliability and correlated with accelerometer physical activity data in a group of men with stable serious mental illness (Dubbert, White, Grothe, O'Jile, & Kirchner, 2006). A Physical Activity Scale for Individuals with Physical Disability is available (Washburn, Zhu, McAuley, Frogley, & Figoni, 2002) and has acceptable psychometric qualities (van der Ploeg et al., 2007).

In addition to the standardized measures such as those just described, for many clinical purposes, simple activity logs or diaries can be devised to assess the variables important to the situation. Typical logs that we use provide for recording of the date, time, type of activity, and its duration. Additional information, such as estimated EE, intensity, pain, enjoyment, mood, self-efficacy, and/or presence of exercise companions may also be recorded depending on the purpose of the self-monitoring assignment and the client's or participant's goals for engaging in the physical activity.

Assessment of Correlates of Physical Activity and Exercise

Research on physical activity and exercise has traditionally reflected a biopsychosocial approach, with studies assessing not only physical activity but also cognitive and social correlates. Theory-based instruments are available for a variety of hypothesized correlates and mediators of physical activity change and sports/exercise motivation, including exercise self-efficacy, decisional balance, processes of physical activity/exercise change, perceived barriers, exercise enjoyment, exercise feeling states, sports team cohesiveness, body image, and social support for exercise (Duda, 1998; Marcus & Owen, 1992; Marcus, Selby, Niaura, & Rossi, 1992; Sallis, Grossman, Pinski, Patterson, & Nader, 1987). These instruments can be used to assess motivational readiness and to enhance tailoring of interventions for individuals and groups.

The context in which physical activity occurs has become a focus of interest only in very recent years. These measures are beyond the scope of many clinical health psychology practices, but, used in conjunction with physical activity self-report, objective activity, and fitness measures, the incorporation of environmental measures allows a more complete biopsychosocial assessment. Environmental measures include community audit measures and park audit measures, the former assessing features of communities and neighborhoods and the latter assessing features of public recreation locations. Assessment typically focuses on domains such as safety, accessibility, attributes and quality of the environment, and aesthetics. Community audit measures include the Neighborhood Environment Walkability Scale (NEWS; Saelens, Sallis, Black, & Chen, 2003), the Irvine–Minnesota Inventory (Day, Boarnet, Alfonzo, & Forsyth, 2006), and Systematic Pedestrian and

Cycling Environment Scan (SPACES; Pikora et al., 2002). The Path Environment Audit Tool (PEAT; Troped et al., 2006) is an example of a park audit tool. Satisfactory reliability has been reported for many of these measures, but much work remains in validating these measures and determining their ease of use. More information about these and other audit tools can be found in a 2006 supplement of the *Journal of Physical Activity and Health*, as well as on the Active Living website (*www.activelivingresearch.org*).

Objective Methods of Assessing Physical Activity

Recent decades have witnessed a growth of interest in methods for assessing physical activity that are objective, quantifiable, and less prone to error and bias than self-report measures. Electronic motion sensors (activity monitors) such as pedometers and accelerometers are the most commonly used tools for directly assessing daily physical activity. Their use provides quantitative data on real-time physical activity over a user-specified period of time. These monitors are generally unobtrusive and thus can be worn in both laboratory and field settings, throughout the day, and during virtually all activities except those in which the wearer might come into contact with water (e.g., showering, swimming). Because they do not assess psychological constructs or environmental factors related to activity, these objective measures are best used in conjunction with self-report measures about other activity-related variables. Table 10.2 summarizes information about pedometer and accelerometer assessment of physical activity.

Pedometers have been used for decades to count steps taken during the course of routine physical activity (Sallis & Owen, 1999). They are inexpensive, unobtrusive, and readily available commercially, making them of particular use in large-scale epidemiological studies and clinical practice. Typically, a pedometer is affixed by a clip to the waist (tethers with an additional clip are highly recommended to prevent loss). An internal sensor detects vertical acceleration caused by ambulatory movement (e.g., walking, jogging) and registers each significant acceleration (above a certain threshold) as a step.

TABLE 10.2. Objective Methods of Measuring Physical Activity

Assessment type	Purpose	Reliability/validity	Comments
Pedometer	Count steps taken and/or distance walked	*Reliability*: Intraclass correlation (ICC) = .72 for 12-week test–retest (Felton et al., 2006); ICC = .51–.92 across different activities (Jago et al., 2006) *Validity*: median r = .86 with accelerometer data, .82 with observed activity, .68 with energy expenditure, and .33 with self-report measures (summary data from Tudor–Locke et al., 2002, review of 25 studies)	Inexpensive, easy to interpret, and reusable; unable to assess intensity, duration, or patterns of activity
Accelerometer	Assess free-living movement in one-, two-, or three-dimensional space (uniaxial vs. biaxial vs. triaxial)	*Reliability*: high interinstrument reliability when worn simultaneously (r = .89–.94; Montoye et al., 1996) and high test–retest reliability (ICC = .85–.96; Welk et al., 2000) *Validity*: moderate correlations with heart rate recording (r = .55), doubly labeled water (r = .69), and direct observation of adults (r = .69) and children (r = .40; from Montoye et al., 1996); strong correlations between raw counts and metabolic variables (r = .62–.91; cited in Welk, 2000)	Assesses frequency, intensity, duration, and patterns of activity; lack of consensus on cut point algorithms; battery life limited on some models; moderate correlations with energy expenditure; instruments are relatively expensive and software licenses required to download and analyze data from some research-quality instruments

Steps are cumulatively tallied and displayed throughout the course of wearing the device and may require a manual reset at the end of each day. Most modern electronic pedometers also calculate the distance walked by allowing stride length to be estimated and input into the device prior to wearing. If the pedometer is not programmed with a memory function, wearers are usually instructed to record their cumulative daily counts (or distance walked) in a provided pedometer log.

Good pedometers exhibit adequate test–retest reliability over a 3-month interval (Felton, Tudor-Locke, & Burkett, 2006). Several studies have evaluated the utility of pedometer-derived data, many of which were summarized in an important review of 25 articles assessing the convergent validity of pedometers with accelerometers, direct observation, self-report measures, and energy expenditure (Tudor-Locke, Williams, Reis, & Pluto, 2002). Although there was considerable variability in the studies, overall pedometer data displayed adequate validity with the other measures (see Table 10.2). Pedometer counts correlated strongly with accelerometer data (median r = .86) and observed activity (median r = .82), moderately with measures of EE (median r = .68), and modestly with the various self-report instruments (median r = .33). Subsequent studies have confirmed the strong validity of pedometer data compared with other objective activity measures. However, users should be aware that pedometers underestimate steps taken at very slow walking speeds (Cyarto, Meyers, & Tudor-Locke, 2004). Normative pedometer data (mean steps/day) exist for virtually all age groups and for individuals with disabilities (Cyarto et al., 2004). A minimum of 3 days' worth of pedometer data is recommended to provide a sufficient estimate of weekly physical activity (Tudor-Locke et al., 2005). Studies indicate that pedometer results are not negatively affected by participant reactivity (Matevery, Rogers, Dawson, & Tudor-Locke, 2006) nor prone to a high frequency of data errors (Schmidt, Blizzard, Venn, Cochrane, & Dwyer, 2007). Other practical concerns include whether and how to adjust for wear time and missing days of data, ways of handling extreme values, and the brand of pedometer to use (Schmidt et al., 2007). Inexpensive pedometers are often unreliable. We recommend having participants test their pedometers by counting 100 steps at different walking speeds to assess the reliability and validity of their instrument.

Accelerometers are the most widely used activity monitors (Sallis & Owen, 1999). Similar to pedometers, accelerometers quantify real-time movement and are usually worn at waist level. Unlike pedometers, however, movement detected by accelerometers is represented as a value of electrical current proportional to the force of acceleration (Welk, 2002). Accelerometers thus quantify not only activity frequency but also its intensity and duration as a continuous variable. Moreover, accelerometers possess a memory capability that allows continuous recording for several days at regular intervals. Current recommendations are that 3–5 days of monitoring are needed to estimate habitual activity among adults, although children may need to be monitored for 7 or more days (Trost, McIver, & Pate, 2005; Ward, Evenson, Vaughn, Rodger, & Troiano, 2005). Although some accelerometers detect vertical movement only (uniaxial), accelerometers now exist that detect movement in multidimensional space (vertical, horizontal, and lateral). However, triaxial accelerometers are typically somewhat larger in size, and whether they provide more accurate data than uniaxial accelerometers is still a matter of some contention (Welk, 2002).

Raw accelerometer counts are usually interpreted after conversion into minutes of light, moderate, and vigorous physical activity and/or estimated physical activity EE. Light activity is that requiring a rate of energy expenditure less than 3 times the resting rate, or the metabolic equivalent (MET) of sitting quietly (1–3 METs). Moderate activity is that requiring a rate of 3–6 METs, and vigorous physical activity is that requiring > 6 METs (Haskell et al., 2007). Numerous accelerometer cut point values and conversion equations have been proposed to convert raw counts into these categories of EE for adults (Freedson, Melanson, & Sirard, 1998; Hendelman, Miller, Baggett, DeBold, & Freedson, 2000; Swartz et al., 2000). No standard practice yet exists, and the vari-

ous cut points result in widely varied estimates of EE, with under- and overestimations largely dependent upon type of activity being performed. Further information about the appropriate use of accelerometers and suggested practices can be found in a recent review by Ward et al. (2005).

The utility of motion sensors, such as pedometers and accelerometers, may be compromised by their difficulty in detecting upper body movements or changes in load, incline, and terrain, as well as by their reduced accuracy in field settings. Accelerometers have the benefit of being able to quantify activity intensity and duration, whereas pedometers provide a cheaper, easily interpretable, and more global estimate of physical activity. Both are appropriate for use in large-scale studies, as well as clinical practice, although the choice of measure will depend on factors such as cost, methodological considerations, and the activity of interest.

Assessment of Physical Fitness

Physical fitness is "a set of attributes that people have or achieve that relates to the ability to perform physical activity" (Caspersen et al., 1985). Components of physical fitness include body composition, cardiorespiratory endurance, muscular strength, muscular endurance, and flexibility. Measures of cardiorespiratory endurance assess oxygen uptake during maximal exercise, or VO_2 max, and are often considered the gold standard in fitness testing. VO_2 max is the maximum rate at which oxygen can be taken up, distributed, and used by the body during physical activity. Maximal oxygen uptake may be measured directly (e.g., volume of air inhaled; change of oxygen concentration from inspired to expired air) or estimated through maximal or submaximal graded exercise tests. Table 10.3 displays several examples of tests used for cardiorespiratory endurance, including classic treadmill tests. In selecting a test, the research or diagnostic question being assessed, the age and risk stratification of the individual being tested, the equipment available, the availability of qualified personnel to conduct testing, the number of individuals being tested, time, and accuracy are all important consider-

TABLE 10.3. Example Physical Fitness Tests for Adults and Older Adults

Test	Type of test	Protocol
Modified Bruce Protocol (Bruce, 1971; Bruce et al., 1973)	Maximal treadmill	• Stage 1 (minutes 1–3): 1.7 mph and 0% grade • Stage 2 (minutes 4–6): 1.5 mph and 5% grade • Additional stages (3 minutes each): speed increased by 0.8–0.9 mph and grade increased by 2% • Use prediction equation or nomogram to estimate VO_2 max.
One-Mile Walking Test (Kline et al., 1987)	Community track	• Walk 1 mile as quickly as possible on a track or level surface. • Heart rate is measured in the final minute during last ¼ mile.
6-minute walk test (Sadaria & Bohannon, 2001)	Clinic or community track	• Walk as far as possible in 6 minutes; rest stops may be permitted; instructions and motivational statements according to protocol selected.

ations. More information on fitness tests and measuring VO_2 max can be found in the American College of Sports Medicine's *Guidelines for Exercise Testing and Prescription* (American College of Sports Medicine, 2013). Although psychologists usually rely on colleagues with appropriate technical expertise and professional certification to oversee physical fitness measures, knowledge of the advantages and limitations of these methods is very helpful in interpreting data for individual patients or clinical trials.

Graded exercise testing, which involves walking or running on a treadmill or cycling at increasing levels of intensity or workload, is the most common method of assessing cardiorespiratory endurance. Treadmill tests such as the Balke (Balke & Ware, 1959) and the Bruce or modified Bruce (Bruce, 1971; Bruce, Kusumi, & Hosmer, 1973) protocols have been used for several decades in clinical settings. These tests may be performed to help determine whether coronary heart disease is present in asymptomatic individuals, to evaluate the progress of an individual with cardiovascular disease, to assess the safety of beginning an exercise program, or to use as a motivational tool. Graded exercise tests can be maximal or submaximal. Maximal tests are performed until an individual reaches fatigue, whereas submaximal tests are performed until an individual reaches a predetermined end point such as 85% of age-predicted maximal heart rate.

Field tests provide a means of testing fitness in community settings and/or for large groups of people. Running or walking and step tests are the most common types of field tests. Advantages of field tests are the low cost and ability to be used for group testing. Disadvantages of field tests are that they are less accurate and are more influenced by motivation than graded exercise tests. When assessing physical fitness in intervention studies, the mode of exercise testing should match the mode of activity targeted in the intervention (i.e., treadmill or other walking test for walking interventions; arm ergometer for interventions in individuals with physical disabilities or who engage in upper body exercises). Selection of a test should also be based on the population being assessed. For example, treadmill protocols that have a constant speed and small, consistent increments in grade may be a better alternative for individuals with low fitness levels (Skinner, 1993). Additionally, if individuals are not accustomed to cycling, muscle fatigue can result in an underestimate of cardiorespiratory endurance. Walking tests such as the one-mile walk (Kline et al., 1987) or the 6-minute walk are often preferred to step tests for obese adults because they exert less stress on the knee joints. The 6-minute walk test, which can be conducted in community settings and does not require medical supervision, has good reliability and validity and can be a good alternative for older individuals (Rikli & Jones, 1999).

Safety Considerations for Physical Activity and Fitness Testing

The American College of Sports Medicine (2013) lists contraindications for exercise testing and indications for stopping testing that should be reviewed before commencing testing. Individuals with recent health changes suggesting new or worsening heart and blood vessel disease, neuromuscular, musculoskeletal, or rheumatoid disorders exacerbated by exercise, or uncontrolled chronic or infectious disease should not be subjected to maximal tests. In low-risk individuals, tests should be terminated for chest pain, drop in blood pressure or failure of blood pressure to rise, excessive rise in blood pressure, signs of poor circulation, failure of heart rate to increase with increased intensity, noticeable change in heart rhythm, a request by the person to stop, physical or verbal manifestations of extreme fatigue, or failure of testing equipment. Psychologists without appropriate training and supervision should not perform fitness testing, and individuals being tested must be properly screened to determine whether they meet the criteria for the test being used.

Fitness testing is usually not necessary prior to increasing light to moderate physical activity, but testing is generally recommended before large increases in activity or vigorous exercise for persons with certain heart disease risk factors, signs, or symptoms and other chronic disease (Haskell et al., 2007). The Physical Activity Readiness Questionnaire (Canadian Society for Exercise Physiology, 1994) is a self-report instrument that has been widely used for screening to determine whether adults should seek medical advice prior to increasing their physical activity.

Summary

There are now a number of reliable and valid self-report and objective measures that can be used for physical activity assessment. Clinical health psychologists can combine these with measures of physical fitness and psychosocial correlates to achieve sophisticated biopsychosocial assessments of physical activity and related variables. Because there are so many good options, careful consideration should be given to the purposes for the measures, time available for data collection and processing, overall participant burden, costs for copyrighted instruments and equipment, and comparability to other data in the literature when making decisions about what measures to use. Consultation with exercise experts can be very helpful and may be a necessity when the assessment methodology includes fitness testing and/or accelerometer data.

REFERENCES

Ainsworth, B. E., Haskell, W. L., Whitt, M. C., Irwin, M. L., Swartz, A. M., Strath, S. J., et al. (2000). Compendium of physical activities: An update of activity codes and MET intensities. *Medicine and Science in Sports and Exercise, 32,* S498–S516.

Ainsworth, B. E., Sternfeld, B., Richardson, M. T., & Jackson, K. (2000). Evaluation of the Kaiser Physical Activity Survey in women. *Medicine and Science in Sports and Exercise, 32*(7), 1327–1338.

American College of Sports Medicine. (2013). *ACSM's guidelines for exercise testing and prescription* (9th ed.). Philadelphia: Lippincott, Williams, and Wilkins.

Baecke, J. A. H., Burema, J., & Fritjers, J. E. R. (1982). A short questionnaire for the measurement of habitual activity in epidemiological studies. *American Journal of Clinical Nutrition, 36,* 936–942.

Balke, B., & Ware, R. W. (1959). An experimental study of physical fitness of Air Force personnel. *U.S. Armed Forces Medical Journal, 10,* 675–682.

Bruce, R. A. (1971). Exercise testing of patients with coronary artery disease. *Annals of Clinical Research, 3,* 323–330.

Bruce, R. A., Kusumi, F., & Hosmer, D. (1973). Maximal oxygen intake and nomographic assessment of functional aerotic impairment in cardiovascular disease. *American Heart Journal, 85,* 545–562.

Canadian Society for Exercise Physiology. (1994). *PAR-Q and You.* Ottawa, Ontario, Canada: Author. Available at *www.csep.ca/cmfiles/publications/parq/par-q.pdf.*

Caspersen, C. J., Powell, K. E., & Christenson, G. M. (1985). Physical activity, exercise, and physical fitness: Definitions and distinctions for health-related research. *Public Health Reports, 100*(2), 126–131.

Craig, C. L., Marshal, A. L., Sjostrom, M., Bauman, A. E., Booth, M. L., Ainsworth, B. E., et al. (2003). International physical activity questionnaire: 12-country reliability and validity.

Medicine and Science in Sports and Exercise, 35(8), 1381–1395.

Cyarto, E. V., Meyers, A. M., & Tudor-Locke, C. (2004). Pedometer accuracy in nursing home and community-dwelling older adults. *Medicine and Science in Sports and Exercise, 36*, 144–150.

Day, K., Boarnet, M., Alfonzo, M., & Forsyth, A. (2006). The Irvine–Minnesota Inventory to measure built environments: Development. *American Journal of Preventive Medicine, 30*, 144–152.

DiPietro, L., Caspersen, C. J., Ostfeld, A. M., & Nadel, E. R. (1993). A survey for assessing physical activity among older adults. *Medicine and Science in Sports and Exercise, 25*(5), 628–642.

Dubbert, P. M. (2002). Physical activity and exercise: Recent advances and current challenges. *Journal of Consulting and Clinical Psychology, 70*(3), 526–536.

Dubbert, P. M., Carithers, T., Ainsworth, B. E., Taylor, H. A., Wilson, G., & Wyatt, S. B. (2005). Physical activity assessment methods in the Jackson Heart Study. *Ethnicity and Disease, 15*, S6-56–S6-61.

Dubbert, P. M., Vander Weg, M., Kirchner, K., & Shaw, B. (2004). Evaluation of the 7-day physical activity recall in urban and rural men. *Medicine and Science in Sports and Exercise, 36*(9), 1646–1654.

Dubbert, P. M., White, J. D., Grothe, K. B., O'Jile, J., & Kirchner, K. A. (2006). Physical activity in patients who are severely mentally ill: Feasibility of assessment for clinical and research applications. *Archives of Psychiatric Nursing, 20*(5), 205–209.

Duda, J. L. (1998). *Advances in Sport and Exercise Psychology Measurement*. Morgantown, WV: Fitness Information Technology.

Felton, G. M., Tudor-Locke, C., & Burkett, L. (2006). Reliability of pedometer-determined free-living physical activity data in college women. *Research Quarterly for Exercise and Sport, 77*, 304–308.

Freedson, P. S., Melanson, E., & Sirard, J. (1998). Calibration of the Computer Science and Applications, Inc., accelerometer. *Medicine and Science in Sports and Exercise, 30*(5), 777–781.

Haskell, W. L., Lee, I., Pate, R. R., Powell, K. E., Blair, S. N., Franklin, B. A., et al. (2007). Physical activity and public health: Updated recommendations for adults from the American College of Sports Medicine and the American Heart Association. *39*(8), 1423–1434.

Hendelman, D., Miller, K., Baggett, C., DeBold, E., & Freedson, P. (2000). Validity of accelerometry for the assessment of moderate intensity physical activity in the field. *Medicine and Science in Sports and Exercise, 32*(9, Suppl.), S442–S449.

Jago, R., Watson, K., Baranowski, T., Zakeri, I., Yoo, S., Baranowski, J., et al. (2006). Pedometer reliability, validity and daily activity targets among 10- to 15-year-old boys. *Journal of Sports Sciences, 24*, 241–251.

Kline, G. M., Porcari, J. P., Hintermeister, R., Freedson, P. S., Ward, A., McCarron, R. F., et al. (1987). Estimation of VO_2max from a one-mile track walk: Gender, age, and body weight. *Medicine and Science in Sports and Exercise, 19*(3), 253–259.

Kriska, A. M., & Caspersen, C. J. (1997). Introduction to a collection of physical activity questionnaires. *Medicine and Science in Sports and Exercise, 29*(6, Suppl.), S5–S9.

Marcus, B. H., & Owen, N. (1992). Motivational readiness, self-efficacy and decision-making for exercise. *Journal of Applied Social Psychology, 22*, 3–16.

Marcus, B. H., Selby, V. C., Niaura, R. S., & Rossi, J. S. (1992). Self-efficacy and the stages of exercise behavior change. *Research Quarterly for Exercise and Sport, 63*, 60–64.

Matevery, C., Rogers, L. Q., Dawson, E., & Tudor-Locke, C. (2006). Lack of reactivity during pedometer self-monitoring in adults. *Measurement in Physical Education and Exercise Science, 10*, 1–11.

Montoye, H. J. (2000). Introduction: Evaluation of some measurements of physical activity and energy expenditure. *Medicine and Science in Sports and Exercise, 32*(9, Suppl.), S439–S441.

Montoye, H. J., Kemper, H. C., Saris, W. H. M., & Washburn, R. A. (1996). *Measuring physical activity and energy expenditure*. Champaign, IL: Human Kinetics.

Paffenbarger, R. S., Wing, A. L., & Hyde, R. T. (1978). Physical activity as an index of heart attack risk in college alumni. *American Journal of Epidemiology, 108*, 161–175.

Pereira, M. A., Fitzgerald, S. J., Gregg, E. W., Joswiak, M. L., Ryan, W. J., Suminski, R. R., et al. (1997). A collection of physical activity questionnaires for health-related research. *Medicine and Science in Sports and Exercise, 29*, S1–S205.

Pikora, T. J., Bull, F. C., Jamrozik, K., Knuiman, M., Giles-Corti, B., & Conovan, R. J. (2002). Developing a reliable audit instrument to measure the physical environment for physical activity. *American Journal of Preventive Medicine, 23*, 187–194.

Resnicow, K., McCarty, F., Blissett, D., Wang, T., Heitzler, C., & Lee, R. F. (2003). Validity of a modified CHAMPS physical activity questionnaire among African Americans. *Medicine and Science in Sports and Exercise, 35*, 1537–1545.

Richardson, M. T., Ainsworth, B. E., Wu, H., Jacobs, D. R., Jr., & Leon, A. S. (1995). Ability of the Atherosclerosis Risk in Communities (ARIC)/Baecke Questionnaire to assess leisure-time physical activity. *International Journal of Epidemiology, 24*(4), 685–693.

Rikli, R. E., & Jones, C. J. (1999). Development and validation of a functional fitness test for community-residing older adults. *Journal of Aging and Physical Activity, 7*, 129–161.

Sadaria, K. S., & Bohannon, R. W. (2001). The 6-minute walk test: A brief review of literature. *Clinical Exercise Physiology, 3*, 127–132.

Saelens, B. E., Sallis, J. F., Black, J. B., & Chen, D. (2003). Preliminary evaluation of the Neighborhood Environment Walkability Scale and neighborhood-based differences in physical activity. *American Journal of Public Health, 93*(9), 1552–1558.

Sallis, J. F. (1997). Seven-Day Physical Activity Recall. *Medicine and Science in Sport and Exercise, 29*(6), S89–S103.

Sallis, J. F., Grossman, R. M., Pinski, R. B., Patterson, T. L., & Nader, P. R. (1987). The development of scales to measure social support for diet and exercise behaviors. *Preventive Medicine, 16*, 825–836.

Sallis, J. F., & Owen, N. (1999). *Physical activity and behavioral medicine.* Thousand Oaks, CA: Sage.

Schmidt, M. D., Blizzard, C. L., Venn, A. J., Cochrane, J. A., & Dwyer, T. (2007). Practical considerations when using pedometers to assess physical activity in population studies: Lessons from the Burni Take Heart Study. *Research Quarterly for Exercise and Sport, 78*, 162–170.

Skinner, J. S. (1993). *Exercise testing and exercise prescription for special cases.* Philadelphia: Lea & Febiger.

Smitherman, T. A., Dubbert, P. M., Grothe P. M., Sung, J. H., Kendzor, D. E., Reis, J. P., et al. (2009) Validity of the Jackson Heart Study physical activity survey in African Americans. *Journal of Physical Activity and Health, 6*(Suppl.), S124–S132.

Stewart, A. L., Mills, K. M., King, A. C., Haskell, W. L., Gillis, D., & Ritter, P. L. (2001). CHAMPS physical activity questionnaire for older adults: Outcomes for interventions. *Medicine and Science in Sports and Exercise, 33*, 1126–1141.

Swartz, A. M., Strath, S. J., Bassett, D. R., Jr., O'Brien, W. L., King, G. A., & Ainsworth, B. E. (2000). Estimation of energy expenditure using CSA accelerometers at hip and waist sites. *Medicine and Science in Sports and Exercise, 32*(9, Suppl.), S450–S456.

Troped, P. J., Croey, E. K., Fragala, M. S., Melly, S. J., Hasbrouck, H. H., Gortmaker, S. L., et al. (2006). Development and reliability testing of an audit tool for trail/path characteristics: The Path Environment Audit Tool (PEAT). *Journal of Physical Activity and Health, 3*(Suppl. 1), S158–S175.

Trost, S. G., McIver, K. L., & Pate, R. R. (2005). Conducting accelerometer-based activity assessments in field-based research. *Medicine and Science in Sports and Exercise, 37*(11, Suppl.), S531–S543.

Tudor-Locke, C., Burkett, L., Reis, J. P., Ainsworth, B. E., Macera, C. A., & Wilson, D. K. (2005). How many days of pedometer monitoring predict weekly physical activity in adults? *Preventive Medicine, 40*, 293–298.

Tudor-Locke, C., Williams, J. E., Reis, J. P., & Pluto, D. (2002). Utility of pedometers for assessing physical activity: Convergent validity. *Sports Medicine, 32*(12), 795–808.

van der Ploeg, H. P., Streppel, K. R., van der Beek, A. J., van der Woude, L. H., Vollenbroek-Hutten, M., & van Mechelen, W. (2007). The Physical Activity Scale for Individuals with Physical Disabilities: Test–retest reliability and comparison with an accelerometer. *Journal of Physical Activity and Health, 4*, 96–100.

Ward, D. S., Evenson, K. R., Vaughn, A., Rodger, A. G., & Troiano, R. P. (2005). Accelerometer use in physical activity: Best practices and research recommendations. *Medicine and Science in Sports and Exercise, 37*(11, Suppl.), S582–S588.

Washburn, R. A., Zhu, W., McAuley, E., Frogley, M., & Figoni, S. F. (2002). The Physical Activity Scale for Individuals with Physical Disabilities: Development and evaluation. *Archives of Physical Medicine and Rehabilitation, 83,* 193–200.

Welk, G. J. (2002). Use of accelerometry-based activity monitors to assess physical activity. In G. J. Welk (Ed.), *Physical activity assessments for health-related research* (pp. 125–141). Champaign, IL: Human Kinetics.

Welk, G. J., Blair, S. N., Wood, K., Jones, S., & Thompson, R. W. (2000). A comparative evaluation of three accelerometry-based physical activity monitors. *Medicine and Science in Sports and Exercise, 32* (9, Suppl.), S489–S497.

Wood, T. M. (2000). Issues and future directions in assessing physical activity: An introduction to the conference proceedings. *Research Quarterly for Exercise and Sport, 71*(2, Suppl.), ii.

Yore, M. M., Ham, S. A., Ainsworth, B. E., Kruger, J., Reis, J. P., Kohl, H. W., III, et al. (2007). Reliability and validity of the instrument used in BRFSS to assess physical activity. *Medicine and Science in Sports and Exercise, 39*(8), 1267–1274.

CHAPTER 11

Quality of Life

Jan Passchier
Jan Busschbach

The past five decades saw an exponential increase in the number of articles involving quality of life in medical sciences. Until the beginning of the 1960s, the impact of a disease and its treatment was mainly expressed in measures of morbidity and mortality. The need to know the consequences of intrusive interventions such as kidney dialysis, transplantation, and aggressive cancer treatments (Elkinton, 1966) led to the expanding development of quality-of-life-related measures. Nowadays, almost each disease and treatment evaluation includes a quality-of-life instrument. Parallel with this development, it became clear that the quality of life of a patient should be judged by the patient and not, like his or her physical condition, by the physician. This was put into words powerfully by one of the pioneers of quality-of-life research, Neil Aaronson: "Given its inherently subjective nature, consensus was quickly reached that quality of life ratings should, whenever possible, be elicited directly from patients themselves" (Aaronson, Cull, Kaasa, & Sprangers, 1996, p. 180). This brings quality of life directly within the domain of the discipline of psychology, as the self-report of the patient is a behavior and is thus influenced by emotions, cognitions, abilities, and personality.

So far, most quality-of-life measurement has been carried out in research. In clinical practice, formal quality-of-life measures are rarely implemented, although one could argue that the self-reported health states as used in mental health care could be seen as an operational clinical quality-of-life assessment. In somatic clinical practice, formal quality-of-life assessment has not yet found a clear position, but there are signs that this will change. The use of quality-of-life assessment and, more generally, that of patient-reported outcomes (PROs) in routine outcome monitoring has now been established in order to test the performance of medical departments and complete hospitals (Revicki et al., 2009). Several studies and reviews have already been published about the effect of presenting quality-of-life data to the treating physicians and/or patients on patient care, satisfaction, and treatment outcome (Gutteling et al., 2008; Haverman et al., 2013; Engelen et al., 2012).

Definitions

Like the concept of intelligence, "quality of life" (QoL) can be defined in many ways, and, also like the concept of intelligence, it is "operationally defined": It is the specific operationalization of this concept that defines its meaning. For instance, it is often said that "intelligence is what an intelligence test measures." In that line of reasoning, QoL is what "a quality-of-life questionnaire or interview measures." One could argue that this is a rather loose, nonscientific way of defining a concept in the absence of a clear definition. On the other hand, although readers of this chapter may not use a common definition of the concept "time," they nevertheless will not question the status of the clock as a scientific instrument. Through consensus about the instrument, we are able to reproduce experimental results. If we are able to reproduce results, the subject of the research becomes independent of the researcher and thus becomes "objective." By introducing formalized QoL measures, the "subjective evaluation of the quality of life by the patient" becomes independent of the observation skills and of the researcher and brings QoL into the scientific domain. Because the concept of QoL leans so heavily on its operationalization, we spend a considerable part of this chapter focusing on the applications of the QoL measurement. As this measurement is performed in different fields of the health sciences, clinical, epidemiology, and health economics, we also introduce the different "perspectives" of QoL measurements.

One difference in perspectives is between that on life in general and that on "just health." The first perspective is often referred to as "happiness research" (Veenhoven, n.d.). For instance, the World Health Organization Quality of Life (WHOQoL) research group defined QoL as a concept that encompasses and summarizes the satisfaction of individuals with all aspects of life (World Health Organization, 1993). The latter perspective focuses more on health and is referred to as "health-related QoL" or "health status" (Davis et al., 2006). Because this volume is concerned with clinical health psychology, we describe QoL from the "health" perspective.

QoL can be conceived as a multidimensional or as a unidimensional concept. Another differentiation can be made between "generic" and "disease-specific." As a multidimensional concept, QoL is often conceived as consisting of three dimensions (physical, psychological, and social), reflected in one or more scores for each.[1] The unidimensional conception of QoL tries to capture the concept in just one value. A generic perspective of QoL assessment tries to capture all aspects relevant in (health-related) QoL, whereas, when viewed as a disease-specific concept, QoL focuses on the specific life problems that are associated with a specific disease. Generic instruments make it possible to compare the outcomes over different diseases, whereas disease-specific measures hold the promise of being sensitive to the specific illness. A third difference in perspective concerns the distinction between the societal perspective, the group (of patients) perspective, and the perspective of the individual patient. In the next section we elaborate on the relevance of the societal, group, and individual perspectives on the measurement of health-related QoL.

Social, Group, and Individual Perspectives

The *societal* perspective of QoL concerns the measurement and comparison of differences in QoL between groups of patients in the populations. Its purpose is usually to set priorities between these groups of patients, for instance, in health policy. An example of such a question is, "Should we, as a government, invest in the prevention of lung cancer, home care for the elderly, or cholesterol medication?"

Typically, in the answer to that question, QoL is made dependent upon the number of patients involved and the duration of the losses in QoL. For instance, a relevant research question here is, "Which patient category has the highest needs: migraine—with its high prevalence—or Huntington's disease, with its high burden but relatively lower prevalence?" This idea of measurement is adopted by the World Health Organization in their Burden of Disease studies,

---

[1] World Health Organization, Preamble to the Constitution of the World Health Organization as adopted by the International Health Conference, New York, 19–22 June, 1946; signed on 22 July 1946 by the representatives of 61 States (Official Records of the World Health Organization, no. 2, p. 100) and entered into force on 7 April 1948.

which integrate mortality and morbidity in disability-adjusted life years (DALYs; U.S. Burden of Disease Collaborators, 2013). When the costs of cure are related to the increase in QoL, QoL becomes an outcome in cost-effectiveness, usually in the form of quality-adjusted life years (QALYs; discussed further later in the chapter), often referred to as cost-utility analysis. As the name suggests, DALYs and QALYs are related, as they are each other's complement (see Figure 11.1).

The perspective of the *patient group* concerns the interest of a patient group with a specific disease or illness, irrespective of other patient groups. Its focus is on the impact of this disease on the life of the patients in the relevant category only. Another application is the evaluation of the effect of the different treatment options on QoL within the same group of patients, to see which treatment improves the QoL of these patients most. The research question here can be, "Is treatment *A* more effective than treatment *B* in bringing the patients with a myocardial infarction back to a normal quality of life, also as related to different expressions of myocardial infarction?" Understandably, in most effectiveness studies, measures of mortality and morbidity in terms of physical dysfunctions are taken as the primary outcome (here, for instance, the number of patients who die or who will have a reinfarction) and the effect on QoL are weighted as secondary outcome. However, when no cure can be expected, such as in the case of palliative treatment of patients in the final phase of their disease, the purpose can be to maintain the QoL of the patient at the

highest level. Here QoL becomes a primary outcome variable, as it is the primary objective of treatment.

The *individual patient perspective* concerns the QoL of the individual patient. Its measurement has a function in, for instance, the decision on the best treatment for this particular patient. The answer to the question, "Will the life of Mrs. Jones be more improved by chemotherapy than by radiotherapy?" is not just dependent on the life expectancy associated with each of these treatments, given her age and physical condition. It is also important to consider how she estimates her QoL for the period during and after each of these treatments, knowing the consequences of each and the problems she will have to face. *Decision analysis* is an important tool to translate a person's estimations into the optimal policy for a patient like Mrs. Jones, and individual weighted QoL assessment tools provide helpful reflections.

So, each perspective has its own associated set of questions, and each question requires its own specific outcome measure. These outcomes are elucidated in the next section.

Perspective and QoL Measures

As we discuss, most but not all QoL instruments are self-report questionnaires that have to be completed by the patient. These instruments can take different forms, because the instruments may approach QoL from different perspectives. Next we describe these differences, following the same classi-

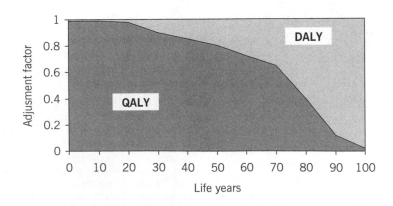

FIGURE 11.1. QALYs and DALYs across life years.

fication of division of perspectives as above: societal, group, and individual. This division translates into *generic, disease-specific,* and *individual weighted* measures.

Generic Measures

Suppose that a cardiologist is interested in the effect of open-heart surgery on the lives of her patients with myocardial infarction. She wants to know which aspects of the patients' lives show most improvement and which the least. In addition, she wants to know how good or bad the QoL of her patients is in comparison with that of the healthy population.

To answer questions on these different aspects, she needs a QoL instrument that consists of different subscales, each covering an important dimension of the life of the patient. Such an instrument measures QoL in a *multidimensional* way, generally by a questionnaire. Most of these questionnaires include at least the following three dimensions: physical, psychological, and social functioning/well-being. As she also wants to know what the lives of her patients with myocardial infarction are like in comparison with those of a group of healthy people, this questionnaire should be *generic.* For both research questions, the cardiologist is in need of a generic instrument, measuring a broad spectrum of QoL dimensions relevant for both patients with myocardial infarction and the general public. Examples of such generic items might be "Due to my health, I feel depressed" or "My health impedes my functioning at work." Well-known generic multidimensional QoL instruments and their dimensions include the Short Form–36 (SF-36; *www.sf-36.org*; Ware & Gandek, 1998) and the Nottingham Health Profile (NHP; McKenna, Hunt, &Tennant, 1993).

Our cardiologist might be interested, however, in just one of these dimensions. She may want to know in particular the effect of open-heart surgery on the emotional well-being of the patients. Or she might be interested in a specific domain within the emotional dimension, such as negative emotions. Emotional well-being as measured by one of the generic questionnaires is relatively global, and the number of items devoted to each dimension is, due to space restrictions, limited to a few. It is better, therefore, for her to use a domain-specific questionnaire. This is a generic questionnaire, but it focuses only on the relevant dimension of interest and provides more detail and is more reliable due to the larger number of items. In her case, she might use a questionnaire that measures the negative emotions she is interested in, such as the Hospital Anxiety and Depression Scale (HADS; Zigmond & Snaith, 1983).[2]

Disease-Specific Measures

Suppose our cardiologist is not so much interested in comparing the QoL of her patients with that of other groups. Rather, she wants to know how the treatment influences the specific problems that her patients experience because of their cardiac disease. Has the patient less fear of a heart attack? Has the patient resumed sports? The cardiologist needs a questionnaire that zooms in on such specific problems. This questionnaire belongs to the family of *disease-specific* questionnaires, which act like a magnifying glass and have a good resolution for detecting the differences between the problems of patients with the same disease and the changes in such disease-related problems. Note the subtle difference with domain-specific questionnaires: These questionnaires also zoom in on a specific aspect, but that aspect is not necessarily related to a specific disease, such as anxiety. Disease-specific questionnaires are therefore more sensitive for detecting changes (have a higher response sensitivity) than generic questionnaires. Like generic questionnaires, disease-specific questionnaires are usually multidimensional. Whereas the number of generic questionnaires is relatively small, the number of disease-specific questionnaires is very high; for almost every common disease a disease-specific questionnaire has been constructed. A well-known disease-specific questionnaire is the QoL measure for cancer patients developed by the European Organization for Research and Treatment of Cancer (EORTC). The EORTC QLQ-30, which has been translated into more than 80 languages, can be supplemented by modules specifically for patients with breast cancer,

---

[2]These types of measures are commonly used in clinical health psychology.

lung cancer, esophageal cancer, and many others (Cull et al., 2001).

Individual Weighted Measures

The inherent value of QoL varies considerably between patients: QoL is called "subjective" for good reason. There are specific instruments that measure this variance at an individual level. The patient is not only asked to indicate any problems in specific domains of QoL but is also asked to indicate how important that domain of QoL is from his or her perspective. An important example of such an instrument is the Schedule for the Evaluation of Individual Quality of Life (SEIQoL). When using the SEIQoL—mostly in an interview format—the individual starts by naming the five most important areas of his or her life. Next, the person rates the importance of each one and finally rates his or her own current position with respect to each of these areas. These ratings thus correspond with how good or poor the person's life is in these personal aspects[3] (O'Boyle, 1994). The applicability of patient-generated outcome measures in a clinical trial setting is not obvious, as there is not yet a clear consensus about summation of the different weightings of the individual patients. Nevertheless, patient-generated outcome measures are promising in guiding individual patient treatment decisions (Patel, Veenstra, & Patrick, 2003).

The Application of QoL in Decision Making

Suppose that an oncologist has the choice between two interventions for patients with prostate cancer, the first being surgery and the second being chemotherapy. The first treatment is associated with a remaining life expectancy of 15 years, the second with a life expectancy of 10 years. On the basis of that information only, a surgery treatment should be preferred. However, this surgery can have side effects, such as impotence. When making a decision about the best option, not only

the duration of the patient's remaining life but also its quality is important. It is, therefore, important to know the QoL of the patients who have received these interventions and the perception of the patient who is confronted with the decision about the QoL of each group. For this, there are several *valuation* procedures or methods for quantifying the QoL associated with the remaining estimated life duration. A simple method is to give the patient information about the conditions that can be expected for his or her life during and after each treatment option. Next, he or she is asked to rate this expectation on a visual analogue scale (VAS). The VAS is usually a line of about 10 centimeters with the extremes (often) defined as "perfect health" (100) or "dead" (0). Suppose that the patient gives a rating of 60 to the remaining life associated with the intervention surgery and 70 to that associated with the intervention chemotherapy. This results in a QoL corrected survival of $0.6 \times 15 = 9$ QALYs for surgery and $0.7 \times 10 = 7$ QALYs for chemotherapy. It will be clear that on basis of this calculation, surgery treatment is still to be preferred to chemotherapy.[4]

There are a number of other valuation methods apart from the VAS, for which we refer to the specialized literature (Green, Brazier, & Deverill, 2000). Some multidimensional generic instruments come with specific scoring algorithms that provide unidimensional values on the basis of former validation research. Most notable are the EuroQoL EQ-5D (*www.euroqol.org*), the Health Utility Index (HUI; *http://fhs.mcmaster.ca/hug*) and the SF-6D (Brazier, Roberts, Tsuchiya, & Busschbach, 2004). The latter reference also provides a comparison between the sensitivity of the EQ-5D and the SF-6D: The EQ-5D seems more sensitive than the SF-6D when used with patients who are severely ill, whereas the SF-6D seems to perform better in patients who have mild complaints.

Health Economics and the Societal Perspective

A specific feature of QoL research in health economics is that the general public deter-

---

[3]Although the areas often differ between individuals and render a comparison difficult, the overall SEIQoL Index across areas can be grouped, thus enabling the calculation of group averages as well.

[4]Because the real figures change across time, we have presented imaginary figures here.

mines the value of a health state, not the patient. As health economics almost always relates to health insurance, the measurement is accomplished from an insurance perspective. When using the insurance perspective, one has to judge at the outset what is valuable and what is not. For instance, when someone's house is on fire, it has no meaning to ask the person to express how he values fire insurance. From this insurance perspective, the general public is seen as the potential patients, who are anticipating that they themselves might one day be those patients. Noneconomists, such as psychologists and physicians, are often reluctant to accept this societal perspective. Moreover, the psychometrics of the questionnaire are different from standard psychometrics as applied to standard questionnaires, such as IQ and attitude tests in psychology. For instance, a key feature of a validated IQ test is a known distribution of scores in the general population. This key feature in "normal" validity is hardly relevant in health economics: A validated test is a test that can determine health state in patients, and for which the societal values of these health states are known, irrespective of the distribution of these health states. Much of the debate about the validity of health economic tests and the related QALY concept arises from a misunderstanding of the societal perspective of health economics. It is of the utmost importance for noneconomists to first familiarize themselves with this societal perspective before judgments about validity are made, as normal psychometrics can be misleading (Green et al., 2000; de Wit, Busschbach, & Charro, 2000).

In a *cost-effectiveness* study, the number of QALYs that accrue from a specific treatment is compared with the costs of treatment and possible savings that are lost and/or gained. For instance, when the surgery and its related costs for prostate cancer is $9,000 and the number of QALYs is three more than the option of doing nothing, its costs are $3,000 per QALY. When chemotherapy costs $1,500 and its number of QALYs is one more than doing nothing, then this implies a cost per QALY of $1,500, which indicates a more cost-effective treatment than surgery. On the basis of cost-effectiveness arguments alone, we would prefer the chemotherapy intervention, which

gives us QALYs for half the price. Obviously, criteria other than economics need consideration in the decision-making process, chiefly those based on humane and political values. Nevertheless, the QALY concept has made a valuable contribution to health care decision making, as it has moved the discussions of cost-effectiveness away from "subjective value judgments" to formal and validated evaluation methods. This is also an example in which the QoL research has lifted the "subjective" aspects of QoL to a level on which observations can be made in a scientifically verifiable, objective manner.

Specific Topics and Recent Developments

Construction of QoL Questionnaires

The development of a standardized psychological instrument follows a number of well-described steps: collection of items, item reduction, and testing of reliability, validity, and (sometimes) of responsiveness to change. Broadly speaking, the construction of an instrument of QoL does not differ from that of other psychological measures. Some aspects are, however, different or deserve more emphasis. First, health-related QoL reflects the evaluation of the patient (or healthy person) on his or her health. That means that the first step in gathering items involves interviewing patients about their experience concerning the different life aspects in relation to the illness. Further, because the instrument often needs also to be answered by patients in a severe phase of a disease that is often accompanied by pain and fatigue, it has to be short. *Feasibility* is, therefore, an important requirement of QoL measures. Consequently, QoL measures often have only a limited number of items per domain, as reliability is a trade-off for feasibility. Moreover, before undergoing psychometric testing, the concept version of a QoL instrument first receives an extensive tryout among the patient group in order to see whether the items are understandable, applicable, and written in common wording (McKenna et al., 1993). When a lot of normative data are available and the instrument can be completed using a computer, the use of methods derived from item response theory enables the researcher/clinician to obtain a reliable and valid score of the patient by using just a few items.[5] For a specific demographic subgroup within the general population, such as older people, existing questionnaires can be tested first to see whether their psychometric properties also hold for these groups (Haywood, Garrat, & Fitzpatrick, 2005). For a group of children or their parents, specific QoL questionnaires are developed, such as the Child Health Questionnaire (CHQ; Raat, Bonsel, Essink-Bot, Landgraf, & Gemke, 2002) or the Pediatric Quality of Life Inventory (PedsQL; Varni, Seid, & Kurtin, 2001).

Measurement Formats

Patients with severe and debilitating afflictions who are bedridden, as in the final stages of cardiac disease or cancer, can be too fatigued to answer a paper-and-pencil questionnaire. It is not uncommon to present these questionnaires in the form of a structured interview, though most of the available evidence about reliability and validity does not apply to this way of administration. Feasibility in this case again has priority over psychometric background and comparability with previous findings based on the (original) questionnaire format.

QoL questionnaires differ in their instructions regarding the recall time. The recall time is dependent on the research question (Is it about the past day or the past year?), the specific disease of the patients (Is it a fluctuating or a stable disease?), and the attention span of the patients (Is it for children or adults?). The recall times range from "at the moment" (as in the NHP) to the preceding 4 weeks (several items from the SF-36). As another example, the Migraine Disability Assessment Scale (MIDAS; Stewart et al., 2000) looks back across a 3-month period, whereas the Migraine-Specific Quality of Life Questionnaire (MSQoLQ; Hartmaier, Santanello, Epstein, & Silberstein, 1995) covers the 24-hour period around a migraine attack, to be used in trials of acute medication to alleviate the symptoms of separate attacks.

The necessary number of assessments depends on the stability of the condition of the patient. For cancer patients at the end of life, in whom dramatic changes can be expected in a short time, more frequent assessments are recommended, for instance every week (Tang & McCorkle, 2002). In most patients, the frequency of assessments is much lower, as QoL is a more obvious outcome in chronic diseases with a stable course than in diseases with an acute manifestation. A modern development is the use of "experience sampling" methods, by which patients answer the questions on their physical and mental states with the help of an electronic diary on a mobile phone at different times during the day. Scores on these measures are averaged into an overall score.

From Outcome to Screener and Target

So far, QoL measures are often found as an outcome measure of a disease or an intervention. A new development is the use of QoL measures as the target of an intervention or as a screening tool (Espallargues, Valderas, & Alonso, 2000). An example of this application is the medical procedure in which patients with liver disease complete a computerized version of the SF-36 as part of the intake procedure. The scores are presented to their physicians as background information in order to enable the physicians to adapt their policies on the basis of these outcomes in order to improve the patients' QoL (Gutteling et al., 2008).

The discussion about the use of QoL measures in clinical practice is related to that about patient-reported outcome measures (PROs or PROMS). PROs are defined as "reports coming directly from patients about how they feel or function in relation to a health condition and its therapy without interpretation by healthcare professionals or anyone else" (Patrick, Guyatt, & Acquadro, 2011). QoL measures form an important category within PROs.

The application of QoL measures to guide the clinician in the treatment of patients has been studied and reviewed quite a lot, in particular in patients with cancer. So far, its effect on the process of care is promising, but the effect on patient outcome is limited (Valderas et al., 2008; Luckett, Butow,

---

[5]The description of item response theory and its application is outside the scope of this chapter. We refer the reader to Ware, Bjorner, and Kosinski (2000).

& King, 2009). A recent review in oncology on PROs in general indicated "strong evidence that the well-implemented PRO's improved patient–provider communication and patient satisfaction" (Chen, Ou, & Hollis, 2013). Methodological issues, for instance the limited use of the information by the doctors and the variation in contexts and interventions, prevent us from drawing too-firm conclusions. But the introduction of electronic methods for the measurement of PROs ("e-PROs"), such as computers and smart phones, has enhanced its feasibility in clinical practice enormously, and an abundance of data will be ready for giving definite answers to questions about its clinical effects.

There is also an increasing tendency for public health service agencies and health insurance companies to demand the routine collection of PROs from the institutions with which they have a cooperative agreement. For instance, the British National Health Service recommends and supports the routine collection of PROs for hip or knee replacement, groin hernia, and varicose vein surgery (U.K. Department of Health, 2009–2010). Apart from condition-specific measures, a generic measure (the EQ-5D) is used here as well. It can be applied to evaluate the clinical quality of an institute (for benchmarks and audits).

Another example, using a domain-specific QoL instrument as both a screening device and a treatment target, lies in the treatment of patients with migraine. A common strategy in the treatment of patients with migraine is to start with common analgesics first and, if this is not successful, to continue with migraine-specific medication ("stepped care"). However, Lipton, Stewart, Stone, Lainez, and Sawyer (2000) followed another strategy. They asked the patients at intake to complete the MIDAS so they could determine the severity of their migraine-related disability. The type of medication chosen was then based on the grade of the disability (following a "stratified care" approach). Patients with more severe migraine received migraine-specific medication immediately. The authors found that this "stratified care" procedure resulted in improved migraine relief and lesser disability than the alternative stepped-care treatment.

Response Shift

A salient phenomenon that struck researchers at the beginning of QoL research was the normalization of QoL scores of patients with life-threatening diseases, such as cancer, or with other severe disabilities. It was noted that these patients often reported a level of QoL similar to that of healthy people (Breetvelt & Van Dam, 1991). Apart from feeling better due to the beneficial effects of treatment, this phenomenon can be explained by a change in the patient's perception of what "health" now means for them. In most occasions this change consists of a lowering of their standards for a good QoL, and, consequently, patients start to consider a lower QoL as normal. In health-related QoL research this phenomenon is referred to as "response shift," and it is associated with an underestimation of treatment effects. Response shift relates to cognitive dissonance reduction in cognitive psychology, to preference drift in economics, and to coping in medical or health psychology. The idea that preference drift reduces the treatment effect on QoL suggests that the patient may not be the best assessor of the "true" QoL. On the other hand, one could argue that response shift is a part of the real evaluation of QoL in patients and should therefore be viewed as a true representation of the patient's preferences. A meta-analysis of studies on response shift indicated that its magnitude varied a lot but that it was small on average (Schwartz et al., 2006). In health economics and epidemiology research, the problem of response shift is less pronounced. In epidemiology, the value of a health state is often determined by physicians, and in health economics the general public values health states, as health economics adopts the societal perspective and not the patient perspective. As both the general public and physicians have a fixed perspective in time, preference drift is eliminated (de Wit et al., 2000).

Minimal Clinical Difference

An important question is what size of change in QoL is needed to be considered meaningful. It is a question that is relevant for other outcome measures as well. Several methods are available to compute a minimally important change for QoL instruments. In most circumstances half a standard deviation is considered to be a relevant threshold for changes in QoL for chronic diseases (Norman, Sloan, & Wyewich, 2003).

Andrasik (2001) summarized in a review on QoL a number of approaches to determine clinically meaningful and significant treatment effects that were derived from Jacobson and Truax (1991). A preferred approach is one in which the patient achieves a level of functioning that, after treatment, falls within the normative range. Clinical change would be demonstrated when post-intervention QoL results in the patient's (1) falling outside the range of the dysfunctional group, defined as being 2 standard deviations away from the mean; (2) falling within the range of the functional group, defined as being less than 2 standard deviations away from the mean; or (3) being closer to the mean of the functional group than to that of the dysfunctional group. For this approach, the collection of adequate normative data is of paramount importance.

Cross-Cultural Application

QoL measures are sometimes used for comparing the QoL between different nations and to estimate the global burden of a specific disease worldwide. Also, a clinical trial may be designed multinationally and involve the outcomes from patients in several countries. Going from the different national scores to a summarizing figure across the countries can only be accomplished when each local instrument measures the same concept in the same degree. One method of obtaining this required uniformity is to use formal translation protocols to translate existing reliable and valid instruments from their original versions into other languages. These protocols are not simple procedures that can be performed with just the use of a dictionary. The process often consists of a sequence of procedures, such as forward and backward translation, use of several independent translators, or development of translated versions that are the outcome of panel meetings. Next, the translated questionnaires have to be tested in a pilot study by administering them to an appropriate number of participants (about 15–20) from the target population who are asked to comment on the content and comprehensibility of the translated instrument.

When this has led to the necessary adaptations, the translated version has to be evaluated psychometrically, and its internal consistency, test–retest reliability, validity, and, if applicable, responsiveness to change need to be evaluated (Peters & Passchier, 2006).

An even more elaborate procedure to design a questionnaire that is comparable between nations or cultures was used by the World Health Organization (1993). They started the development of a QoL questionnaire from scratch by having focus groups, composed of representatives from each of the countries in question, define the life domains that were relevant for their country. After the definitions of the relevant common domains were obtained, items within each domain were determined and formulated in these focus groups. This procedure resulted in a final questionnaire of 100 items (the WHOQOL) that might be extended with modules that are relevant for a specific country (or culture) only.[6] It is available in many language versions.

Conclusion

QoL is a concept that has "won" its position during the past 50 years in health care. Its methods of measurement vary and are dependent on the purpose of the researcher or clinician. The goals of measuring QoL are mainly to measure the impact of a disease on the patient's life, to measure the effect of a treatment, to choose between treatments, and to screen and determine an intervention strategy. Traditional psychometric indices are applicable on most QoL measures, but feasibility merits specific attention. Validation of QoL instruments in health economics requires a nonclassical design, as norms are not determined by the distribution of scores but by the general public that values the health states. QoL measures are nowadays well accepted in research, and their application in clinical practice is slowly but steadily increasing. Recent developments include the use of computerized versions that allow a reliable and valid measurement of the QoL with a reduced number of items.

---

[6] A shorter version, the WHOQoL-BREF, consisting of 26 items, is now available as well (World Health Organization, 1998).

REFERENCES

Aaronson, N. K., Cull, A. M., Kaasa, S., & Sprangers, M. A. G. (1996). The European Organization for Research and Treatment of Cancer (EORTC) modular approach to quality of life assessment in oncology: An update. In B. Spilker (Ed.), *Quality of life and pharmacoeconomics in clinical trials* (2nd ed., pp. 179–189). Philadelphia: Lippincott-Raven.

Andrasik, F. (2001). Migraine and quality of life: Psychological considerations. *Journal of Headache and Pain, 2,* S1–S9.

Brazier, J., Roberts, J., Tsuchiya, A., & Busschbach, J. (2004). A comparison of the EQ-5D and SF-6D across seven patient groups. *Health Economics, 13,* 873–884.

Breetvelt, I., & Van Dam, F. (1991). Underreporting by cancer patients: The case of response-shift. *Social Science and Medicine, 32,* 981–987.

Chen, J., Ou, L., & Hollis, S. J. (2013). A systematic review of the impact of routine collection of patient reported outcome measures on patients, providers and health organisations in an oncologic setting. *BMC Health Services Research, 13,* 211. Available at *www.biomedcentral.com/1472-6963/13/211.*

Cull, A., Howat, S., Greimel, E., Waldenstrom, A. C., Arraras, J., Kudelka, A., et al. (2001). Development of a European Organization for Research and Treatment of Cancer questionnaire module to assess the quality of life of ovarian cancer patients in clinical trials: A progress report. *European Journal of Cancer, 37,* 47–53.

Davis, E., Waters, E., Mackinnon, A., Reddihough, M., Kerr Graham, H., Mehmet-Radji, O., et al. (2006). Paediatric quality of life instruments: A review of the impact of the conceptual framework on outcomes. *Development Medicine and Child Neurology, 48,* 311–318.

de Wit, G., Busschbach, J. J., & Charro, F. de (2000). Sensitivity and perspective in the valuation of health status: Whose values count? *Health Economics, 9,* 109–126.

Elkinton, J. R. (1966). Medicine and the quality of life. *Annals of Internal Medicine, 64,* 711–714.

Engelen, V., Detmar, S., Koopman, H., Maurice-Stam, H., Caron, H., Hoogerbrugge, P., et al. (2012). Reporting health-related quality of life scores to physicians during routine follow-up visits of pediatric oncology patients: Is it effective? *Pediatric Blood Cancer, 58*(5), 766–774.

Espallargues, M., Valderas, J., & Alonso, J. (2000). Provision of feedback on perceived health status to health care professionals: A systematic review of its impact. *Medical Care, 38,* 175–186.

Green, C., Brazier, J., & Deverill, M. (2000). Valuing health-related quality of life: A review of health state valuation techniques. *Pharmacoeconomics, 17,* 151–165.

Gutteling, J. J., Darlington, A. S., Janssen, H. L., Duivenvoorden, H. J., Busschbach, J. J., & de Man, R. A. (2008). Effectiveness of health-related quality-of-life measurement in clinical practice: A prospective, randomized controlled trial in patients with chronic liver disease and their physicians. *Quality of Life Research, 17*(2), 195–205.

Hartmaier, S. L., Santanello, C., Epstein, R. S., & Silberstein, S. D. (1995). Development of a brief 24-hours migraine-specific quality of life questionnaire. *Headache, 35,* 320–329.

Haverman, L., van Rossum, M. A. J., van Veenendaal, M., van den Berg, J. M., Dolman, K. M., Swart, J., et al. (2013) Effectiveness of a web-based application to monitor health-related quality of life. *Pediatrics, 131,* e533.

Haywood, K., Garrat, A., & Fitzpatrick, R. (2005). Quality of life in older people: A structured review of generic self-assessed health instruments. *Quality of Life Research, 14,* 1651–1668.

Jacobson, N. S., & Truax, P. (1991). Clinical significance: A statistical approach to defining meaningful change in psychotherapy research. *Journal of Consulting and Clinical Psychology, 59,* 12–19.

Lipton, R. B., Stewart, W. F., Stone, A. M., Lainez, M. J. A., & Sawyer, J. P. C. (2000). Stratified care vs step care strategies for migraine: The Disability in Strategies of Care (DISC) Study: A randomized trial. *Journal of the American Medical Association, 284,* 2599–2605.

Luckett, T., Butow, P. N., & King, M. T. (2009). Improving patient outcomes through the routine use of patient-reported data in cancer clinics: Future directions. *Psycho-Oncology, 18,* 1129–1138.

McKenna, S. P., Hunt, S. M., & Tennant, A. (1993). The development of a patient-completed index of distress from the Nottingham Health Profile: A new measure for use in cost-utility studies. *British Journal of Medical Economics, 6,* 13–24.

Norman, G., Sloan, J., & Wyewich, K. (2003). Point/counterpoint: Interpretation of changes in health-related quality of life: The remarkable universality of half a standard deviation. *Medical Care, 41,* 582–592.

O'Boyle, C. A. (1994). The Schedule for the Evaluation of Individual Quality of Life (SEIQoL). *International Journal of Mental Health, 23,* 3–23.

Patel, K., Veenstra, D., & Patrick, D. (2003). A review of selected patient-generated outcome measures and their application in clinical trials. *Value Health, 6,* 595–603.

Patrick, D., Guyatt, G. H., & Acquadro, C. (2011). Patient-reported outcomes. In J. P. T. Higgins & S. Green (Eds.), *Cochrane handbook for systematic reviews of interventions* (Version 5.1.0, Chapter 17). Available at *www.cochrane-handbook.org.*

Peters, M., & Passchier, J. (2006). Translating instruments for cross-cultural studies in headache research. *Headache, 46,* 82–91.

Raat, H., Bonsel, G. J., Essink-Bot, M.-L., Landgraf, J. M., & Gemke, R. J. (2002). Reliability and validity of comprehensive health status measures in children: The Child Health Questionnaire in relation to the Health Utilities Index. *Journal of Clinical Epidemiology, 55,* 67–76.

Revicki, D. A., Kawata, A. K., Harnam, N., Chen, W. H., Hays, R. D., & Cella, D. (2009). Predicting EuroQol (EQ-5D) scores from the patient-reported outcomes measurement information system (PROMIS) global items and domain item banks in a United States sample. *Quality of Life Research, 18*(6), 783–791.

Schwartz, C., Bode, R., Repucci, N., Becker, J., Sprangers, M., & Fayers, P. (2006). The clinical significance of adaptation to changing health: A meta-analysis of response shift. *Quality of Life Research, 15,* 1533–1550.

Stewart, W. F., Lipton, R. B., Kolodner, K. B., Sawyer, J., Lee, C., & Liberman, J. N. (2000). Validity of the Migraine Disability Assessment (MIDAS) score in comparison to a diary-based measure in a population sample of migraine sufferers. *Pain, 88,* 41–52.

Tang, S., & McCorkle, R. (2002). Appropriate time frames for data collection in quality of life research among cancer patients at the end of life. *Quality of Life Research, 11,* 145–155.

U.K. Department of Health. (2009–2010). *Guidance on the routine collection of patient reported outcome measures.* Available at *http://webarchive.nationalarchives.gov.uk/+/www.dh.gov.uk/en/Publicationsandstatistics/Publications/PublicationsPolicyAndGuidance/DH_092647.*

U.S. Burden of Disease Collaborators. (2013). The state of U.S. Health, 1990–2010: Burden of diseases, injuries, and risk factors. *Journal of the American Medical Association, 310*(6), 591–606. Available at *http://jama.jamanetwork.com/article.aspx?articleid=1710486.*

Valderas, J. M., Kotzeva, A., Espallargues, M., Guyatt, G., Ferrans, C. E., Halyard, M. Y., et al. (2008). The impact of measuring patient-reported outcomes in clinical practice: A systematic review of the literature. *Quality of Life Research, 17,* 179–193.

Varni, J. W., Seid, M., & Kurtin, P. (2001). PedsQL 4.0: Reliability and validity of the Pediatric Quality of Life Inventory Version 4.0 Generic Core Scales in healthy and patient populations. *Medical Care, 39,* 800–812.

Veenhoven, R. (n.d.) *World database of happiness.* Rotterdam, The Netherlands: Erasmus University, Institute of Health Policy and Management, Happiness Economics Research Organization. Retrieved June 16, 2014, from *http://worlddatabaseofhappiness.eur.nl.*

Ware, J. J., Bjorner, J., & Kosinski, M. (2000). Response to Hays et al. and McHorney and Cohen: Practical implications of item response theory and computerized adaptive testing: A brief summary of ongoing studies of widely used headache impact scales. *Medical Care, 38*(Suppl. II), II-73–II-82.

Ware, J. J., & Gandek, B. (1998). Overview of the SF-36 Health Survey and the International Quality of Life Assessment (IQoLA) Project. *Journal of Clinical Epidemiology, 51,* 903–912.

World Health Organization. (1993). Study protocol for the World Health Organization project to develop a quality of life assessment instrument (WHOQoL). *Quality of Life Research, 2,* 153–159.

World Health Organization. (1998). Development of the World Health Organization WHOQoL-BREF quality of life assessment. *Psychological Medicine, 28,* 551–558.

Zigmond, A., & Snaith, R. (1983). The Hospital Anxiety and Depression Scale. *Acta Psychiatrica Scandinavica, 67,* 361–370.

PART III

Assessment
of Clinical
Problems

CHAPTER 12

Cancer

Tammy A. Schuler
Thomas M. Atkinson
Errol J. Philip

Psychosocial assessment is integral to oncology clinical care and research. Assessment may provide diagnostic data; inform treatment; describe patient outcomes; aid in the development, implementation, and dissemination of research protocols; and/or bolster the conceptualization and refinement of theoretical models. Ultimately, the foundation of psychosocial assessment rests on the use of psychometrically sound instruments (Cook Gotay & Stern, 1995; Derogatis & Spencer, 1984). This chapter describes a biobehavioral model of cancer stress and disease course for a comprehensive illustration of areas for assessment, delineate cancer-specific considerations for assessment of the oncology patient, and provide an updated review of relevant assessment tools with acceptable psychometric properties (defined herein).

Areas to Assess According to the Biobehavioral Model

The Biobehavioral Model

The biobehavioral model of cancer stress and disease course (Figure 12.1; Andersen, Kiecolt-Glaser, & Glaser, 1994) is a conceptual framework in which psychological, biological, and behavioral aspects of cancer diagnosis interact and may ultimately influence disease course. Other factors, such as life stressors, social support, and personality, are also hypothesized to influence these relationships (Andersen, 2002). According to the biobehavioral model, acute stress is present at cancer diagnosis and during treatment. As patients adjust to diagnosis, stress often diminishes over time. However, stress may remain present during other critical periods, such as a prolonged recovery, or even with the transition to survivorship. Stress is also acute with declining health and disease progression (Andersen, Shapiro, Farrar, Crespin, & Wells-DiGregorio, 2005). Stress can, in turn, contribute to lowered quality of life (QoL; Golden-Kreutz et al., 2005), emotional distress (Golden-Kreutz & Andersen, 2004), and reduced meaning in life (Jim, Richardson, Golden-Kreutz, & Andersen, 2006).

Regarding considerations for assessment, cancer-specific stress questionnaires (e.g., the Impact of Event Scale [IES]; Horowitz, Wilner, & Alvarez, 1979) may provide precise insight into the cancer experience compared with general or psychiatric measures. Cancer-specific stress questionnaires are used not only for screening studies but also in routine clinical care—particularly when the objective is to identify patients

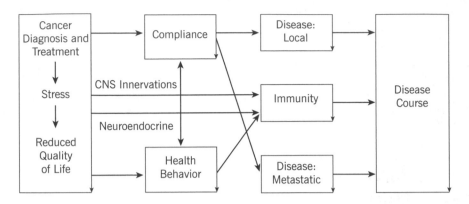

FIGURE 12.1. The biobehavioral model of cancer stress and disease course is depicted, showing inter-relations between psychological, biological, and behavioral sequelae of cancer diagnosis. These may ultimately influence disease course. CNS, central nervous system. From Andersen, Kiecolt-Glaser, and Glaser (1994). Copyright 1994 by the American Psychological Association. Reprinted by permission. The use of APA information does not suggest endorsement by APA.

who may benefit from additional support (Herschbach et al., 2004). Assessing health-related QoL has become a critical point in the development of tailored treatment modalities in clinical and supportive cancer care (Cella, Chang, Lai, & Webster, 2002). An individual's self-reported QoL reflects the impact of disease and its treatment and can provide important information beyond individual symptom scales. It is most frequently assessed across a number of domains, including physical, social, emotional, and functional well-being (e.g., the European Organization for Research and Treatment of Cancer QLQ-C30 [EORTC QLQ-C30] cancer-specific scales; Aaronson et al., 1993).

In addition to lowered QoL, emotional distress, and reduced meaning, stress also covaries with neuroendocrine changes (e.g., hypothalamic–pituitary–adrenal axis dys-regulation [Raison & Miller, 2001]; sym-pathomedullary pathway dysregulation [Miller, Chen, & Zhou, 2007]; decreased secretion of human growth hormone). These neuroendocrine changes may be related to lowered immunity (Bergmann & Sautner, 2002; Röntgen, Sablotzki, Simm, Silber, & Czeslick, 2004). Down-regulation of the immune system is, itself, related to cancer-specific stress (Andersen et al., 1998), emotional distress (e.g., depressive symptoms [Thornton, Andersen, Schuler, & Carson, 2009] and anxiety [Stein, Keller, & Schleifer,

1988]), as well as "sickness behaviors" related to emotional distress, such as fatigue and anorexia (Anisman & Merali, 2003). Moreover, emotional distress can also contribute to hypothalamic–pituitary–adrenal axis dysregulation (Miller et al., 2007), an increased inflammatory response (Elenkov, Iezzoni, Daly, Harris, & Chrousos, 2005), and lowered immunity (Zorrilla et al., 2001).

Stress may increase negative health behaviors (e.g., smoking, alcohol use [Goeders, 2004; Ng & Jeffery, 2003]) and decrease positive health behaviors (e.g., regular exercise; Stetson, Rahn, Dubbert, Wilner, & Mercury, 1997). Negative health behaviors, such as alcohol use, are linked to lowered immunity (Frank, Witte, Schrödl, & Schütt, 2004). Further, combined emotional distress and negative health behaviors may syner-gistically affect immunity more than either alone, as in the case of depressive symptoms and smoking (Jung & Irwin, 1999). However, reducing negative health behaviors, such as smoking, and increasing positive health behaviors, such as exercise, has been shown to improve mood and bolster immunity (Fairey et al., 2005; Trivedi, Greer, Grannemann, Chambliss, & Jordan, 2006). Smoking abstinence, even for 1 day, has been found to reduce cortisol levels (Steptoe & Ussher, 2006). Stress is linked with sleep disturbances (Steptoe, O'Donnell, Marmot, & Wardle, 2008), which may affect sym-pathetic arousal and decrease immunity

(Savard, Laroche, Simard, Ivers, & Morin, 2003). Moreover, stress may increase the likelihood of negative dietary changes, such as eating less often or eating meals of poorer nutritional value (Grunberg & Straub, 1992), whereas dietary improvements may enhance immune responses and reduce rates of infection (Galbán et al., 2000). Finally, cancer treatment adherence may be lowered in the context of increased stress and heightened emotional distress (McDonough, Boyd, Varvares, & Maves, 1996). In fact, poor cancer treatment adherence has been cited as a potential mechanism influencing the relationship between emotional distress and disease course (Kissane, 2009).

Other Factors That May Influence Biobehavioral Outcomes

Other factors may influence biobehavioral outcomes. These are variables such as other life stressors, having few social ties and/or low social support, psychiatric history, spirituality, and physical symptom burden. Patients reporting greater life stressors combined with fewer social ties have shown higher mood disturbance (Koopman, Hermanson, Diamond, Angell, & Spiegel, 1998), and those with more precancer traumatic stressors and lower levels of social support exhibit more posttraumatic stress symptoms (Andrykowski & Cordova, 1998). "Aversive" support (e.g., criticism, disrespect) from friends, family, and health care professionals predicts heightened emotional distress (Hampton & Frombach, 2000). Ongoing marital distress, in particular, has been shown to covary longitudinally with greater emotional distress, poorer health behaviors, worse functional status, and more physical symptoms (Yang & Schuler, 2009). Ongoing marital distress combined with depressive symptoms may be linked to decreased immunity (Schuler, Yang, Thornton, Andersen, & Carson, 2014). Couples who report precancer marital distress are those most likely to endorse postdiagnostic marital distress (Hagedoorn, Sanderman, Bolks, Tuinstra, & Coyne, 2008).

Side effects from cancer treatments may affect intimate relationships (Kornblith & Ligibel, 2003; Manne, 2011). For example, as the survival rate for many common cancer types has increased, greater focus has been afforded to QoL concerns such as sexual functioning and body image disturbances. Sexual dysfunction in particular has been reported in a number of cancer cohorts (Morreale, 2011; Reese, 2011), including rectal cancer (Hendren et al., 2005), breast cancer (Alder & Bitzer, 2010), prostate cancer (Ruiz-Aragon, Marquez-Pelaez, & Luque Romero, 2010) and gynecological cancer (Onujiogu et al., 2011; Tsai et al., 2011), and has been associated with impaired QoL (Di Fabio, Koller, Nascimbeni, Talarico, & Salerni, 2008). In addition, sexual dysfunction is often underreported and undertreated and can be a difficult topic for patients to bring up in clinical visits.

Dysfunctional family interaction patterns, such as greater conflict and lower cohesion, confer risk for psychosocial morbidity. This has been shown to be particularly evident during palliative care and bereavement (Kissane et al., 1996). Young families in which the wife/mother has cancer and in which young children are present are at heightened risk for relationship difficulties (Vess, Moreland, & Schwebel, 1985). Family strain itself is affected by disease variables (e.g., stage, prognosis), family-specific variables (e.g., socioeconomic status, other life stressors), and relational variables (e.g., marital distress; Sales, Schulz, & Biegel, 1992).

The context in which diagnostic and treatment information is disclosed is important (Carpenter & Andersen, 2008). Physicians who communicate hope have patients who are, in turn, more hopeful and experience better psychological adjustment. Alternatively, communicating "false hope" is unwelcome (Sardell & Trierweiler, 1993). In a study of gynecological cancer patients, Roberts, Brown, Elkins, and Larson (1997) indicated that, although patients expect compassion, 89% prefer "straight talk" about their prognosis. Thus patients' previous experiences with their providers may provide information regarding their psychological adjustment trajectory, as well as potential future communication issues with their treatment team. Empirical studies providing communications training to physicians have resulted in patients reporting fewer depressive symptoms and higher levels of trust in their physicians, satisfaction with the interaction, and feelings of personal control after consultation (Beck & Beck, 1972;

Bylund et al., 2010; Rutter, Iconomou, & Quine, 1996; Tulsky et al., 2011).

Regarding other factors that may influence biobehavioral outcomes, history of psychiatric disorder—particularly depression—places an individual at increased risk of depression beyond the general population base rate (Plumb & Holland, 1981). Personality is another factor that may influence interactions between biobehavioral components, such as that between cancer treatment adherence and such positive health behaviors as dietary practices (Andersen, 2002; Friedman et al., 1995). Moreover, optimism, a sense of control, and greater use of active coping strategies may confer decreased risk of emotional distress (Carver et al., 1993; Taylor, Lichtman, & Wood, 1984).

Spiritual and religious beliefs and practices can play an important role in coping with life stressors. In the United States, religious and spiritual beliefs are held by the majority of the population (Hodge, 1996) and are a frequently employed coping mechanism by individuals diagnosed with life-threatening diseases such as cancer (Vachon, 2008). Religious coping has been associated with positive outcomes (Weaver & Flannelly, 2004), including improved adjustment, hope and meaning, access to social networks, and greater acceptance of illness.

The physical symptom burden associated with cancer diagnosis and treatment has been widely documented (Henry et al., 2008). In addition, there is growing recognition of the potential for survivors to experience persistent symptomatology long after treatment ends (Harrington, Hansen, Moskowitz, Todd, & Feuerstein, 2010). Frequently reported symptoms can include, for example, persistent pain, fatigue, sexual dysfunction, poorer body image, and cognitive difficulties. These symptoms have the ability to impact QoL, an individual's ability to return to personal and professional roles, and his or her ability to engage in follow-up care and healthy lifestyle practices, and they are therefore critical to routinely assess in the care of cancer patients and survivors. A consistent relationship has been shown between fatigue and the availability of social resources (Smets et al., 1998), severity of psychiatric symptoms such as depression and anxiety (Hann et al., 1999), and muscle weakness, numbness, sleep disturbances,

and concentration difficulties (Jacobsen et al., 1999).

Demographic factors may also put oncology patients at higher risk for emotional distress or psychiatric symptoms. These include younger age (i.e., < 60 years, possibly due to factors such as the diagnosis being less expected Bloom & Kessler, 1994) and lower socioeconomic status (SES; Ramirez et al., 1993). Patients with lower SES are also at greater risk for decreased adherence with cancer treatments, as are patients with hectic work schedules, with children, or with transportation difficulties (Formenti et al., 1995). Lower education has been shown to predict poorer QoL outcomes for women of Asian heritage (Chan et al., 2001).

Summary

Taken together, the biobehavioral sequelae of cancer diagnosis and treatment, as well as other influencing factors, may exercise individual or symbiotic effects on disease course (Andersen et al., 1994; Lutgendorf & Sood, 2011). The areas targeted for assessment will, of course, be influenced by the assessment's aim (e.g., to provide diagnostic data in a clinical setting; for randomized clinical trial outcome analyses). Nevertheless, a working knowledge of the biobehavioral framework and its influencing factors can direct well-informed, comprehensive assessment.

Symptom Clusters

Symptom clusters are those that tend to aggregate, or occur concurrently (Dodd et al., 2001). A working understanding of symptom clusters is another knowledge base that may bolster comprehensive assessment. If a patient exhibits one symptom from a cluster, he or she may have an increased likelihood of exhibiting other symptoms from the cluster. Symptom clusters may or may not share a common etiology (Dodd, Miaskowski, & Lee, 2004), and may also reflect disease or treatment characteristics, such as diagnostic site, time since diagnosis, or specific hormone therapy regimen.

Pain, depression, and fatigue are among the most distressing symptoms in advanced breast cancer, and these have a high rate of co-occurrence (Miller, Ancoli-Israel, Bower, Capuron, & Irwin, 2008). The pain, depression, and fatigue symptom cluster has been shown to relate to cortisol and epinephrine levels (Thornton, Andersen, & Blakely, 2010), as well as inflammatory reactions (Dantzer, O'Connor, Freund, Johnson, & Kelley, 2008). Moreover, sleep disturbances and cognitive dysfunction have also been proposed as related symptoms, forming a cytokine-induced "sickness-behavior" symptom cluster, due to a potentially common inflammatory etiology (Miller et al., 2008). Symptom cluster data are fewer for diagnostic sites other than the breast; however, longitudinal data also suggest a fatigue, dyspnea, and cough cluster among 5-year lung cancer survivors (Cheville et al., 2011). Consistent with clinical reports, a gastrointestinal cluster (composed of nausea and vomiting) has been identified among recipients of chemotherapy (Dodd et al., 2004).

Cancer-Specific Considerations for Biobehavioral Assessment

Special considerations are warranted for disease and treatment characteristics that may influence biobehavioral assessment. This chapter provides an overview of such considerations. However, due to the heterogeneous nature of cancer diagnoses and corresponding treatments, recommendations cannot be offered for all possible assessment scenarios. Nevertheless, it is vital that assessments be informed by data relevant to specific cancer diagnoses and treatments.

Disease and Treatment Characteristics

Diagnostic Site

Different diagnostic sites are linked with variable biobehavioral histories and post-diagnostic trajectories. Individuals diagnosed with lung cancer often report higher levels of distress than those with other cancers and represent a unique population on a number of levels (Cooley, Lynch, Fox, & Sarna, 2010). First, there currently exists no reliable method by which to detect lung cancer, and therefore the majority of patients are diagnosed with advanced disease. This fact, along with the subsequent poor prog-

nosis and significant symptom burden, accounts in part for the increased rates of psychosocial and existential concerns (Zabora, BrintzenhofeSzoc, Curbow, Hooker, & Piantadosi, 2001). Further, the well-known and publicized association between cigarette smoking and lung cancer has resulted in significant stigma and blame surrounding this particular disease. This is notable both for individuals with a history of smoking who may therefore experience guilt and receive blame and for those without a history of smoking who may be required to frequently address assumptions concerning the etiology of their disease.

Patients diagnosed with cancers of the gastrointestinal tract must often manage short- and long-term changes to their eating habits, nutritional status, bowel function, and sexual health. For some individuals, this will also involve adjustment to a temporary or permanent ostomy pouch as part of their course of treatment and follow-up care. This pouch allows for feces to be removed from the body from an opening in the digestive tract and requires special care. It has also been associated with distress and impaired QoL for some individuals (Jansen, Koch, Brenner, & Arndt, 2010). The management of an ostomy device can require careful cleaning and emptying procedures, can restrict involvement in certain activities, and can prompt concerns about body image and sexual functioning (American Cancer Society, 2011b; Charua-Guindic et al., 2011). It is therefore important to keep these issues in mind when assessing and treating an individual who is managing changes in digestive or bowel functioning or an ostomy device as a result of their cancer (Krouse, 2010).

Breast cancer is one of the most common female cancer diagnoses in the United States, with over 230,000 cases estimated in 2011 (American Cancer Society, 2011a). Treatment can often involve a combination of therapies, including surgery, radiation, and chemotherapy. Surgical interventions can include a lumpectomy (targeted tissue removal) or mastectomy (entire breast removal) and, despite the often positive prognosis, can be associated with significant distress (Rowland & Massie, 2010). Treatment can also prompt or exacerbate concerns surrounding self-esteem, body image, and sexual function and can interfere in intimate relationships (e.g., Kornblith & Ligibel, 2003). These issues can therefore be important to consider in the assessment and treatment of breast cancer patients and survivors.

Patients with gynecological cancers are at particular risk for lowered psychological adjustment and marital distress. Patients with gynecological cancer often experience major, or even permanent, changes in sexual functioning related to associated emotional disturbances, magnitude of disease, and cancer treatment (Carpenter & Andersen, 2008). Patients with particularly aggressive treatment regimens, such as for ovarian cancer, may be at risk for poorer QoL outcomes (Miller, Pittman, Case, & McQuellon, 2002).

Extent of Cancer

Patients with persistent or disseminated cancer also show postdiagnostic biobehavioral trajectories that differ from those of newly diagnosed patients or those with early-stage disease. Cancer recurrence is devastating, characterized by emotional distress similar to that present at initial diagnosis (Andersen et al., 2005). Similar to the stress experienced at first diagnosis, the levels of cancer-specific stress and global stress is equivalent to that of patients seeking psychiatric treatment for anxiety disorders (Yang, Thornton, Shapiro, & Andersen, 2008). However, the emotional distress tends to abate sooner than that of initial diagnosis. Compared with initial diagnosis, cancer recurrence is generally associated with greater functional impairment and more physical symptoms from disease and treatment (Andersen et al., 2005; Yang et al., 2008). Typical physical sequelae include pain (Sarenmalm, Odén, & Gaston-Johansson, 2008), and appetitive difficulties (e.g., cachexia; Body, Lossignol, & Ronson, 1997). Some cancer types are more likely to recur than others. Ovarian cancer is one example, partially due to its low rate of early detection (Goff, Mandel, Melancon, & Muntz, 2004).

Cancer stage appears to predict psychological distress in that higher stage tends to confer greater physical symptomatology or extent of treatment (Edgar, Rosberger, & Nowlis, 1992; Ramirez et al., 1993). Patients with more advanced cancers generally show higher rates of depression (Kornblith et al., 1995), as do those who perceive their illness as severe (Marks, Richardson, Graham, & Levine, 1986). Compared with early-stage cancer patients and their partners, advanced cancer patients and their partners report more physical symptoms from cancer and its treatment and greater restriction of activities and also that these problems persist across a lengthier span of time (Cook Gotay, 1984).

Cancer Treatments

Differing cancer treatment types (e.g., surgery, radiation, chemotherapies, hormone therapies) and subtypes (e.g., various chemotherapy regimens) are associated with a range of symptom profiles. Further, symptom profiles may vary as an interaction of type and extent of the cancer and corresponding treatment. For example, the surgical site may portend lower levels of sexual activity and responsiveness, as in women with gynecological cancers and men with prostate cancer (Andersen, 2002; Andersen, Woods, & Copeland, 1997; Manne, 2011; Shrader-Bogen, Kjellberg, McPherson, & Murray, 1997).

Symptom profiles may also change as a function of treatment phase. Initially, patients may experience a great deal of stress over choosing a treatment (Carpenter & Andersen, 2008). Broadly, once treatment is initiated, common side effects of surgery, radiation, chemotherapies, and hormone treatment include nausea and vomiting, pain, and fatigue. Cancer surgery patients may be distinguished by higher overall levels of emotional distress and slower rates of emotional recovery compared with patients who undergo benign surgery (Carpenter & Andersen, 2008). Gottesman and Lewis (1982) reported greater and more enduring experiences of crisis and feelings of helplessness among cancer patients compared with benign surgery patients. Medical factors associated with poorer psychological adjustment include more postoperative symptoms or side effects of adjuvant treatment (Razavi et al., 1993), more physical impairment (Vinokur, Threatt, Vinokur-Kaplan, & Satariano, 1990), and other comorbid chronic illnesses (Stewart et al., 1989).

Importantly, psychological symptoms may cause more distress than physical symptoms (Formenti et al., 1995) and have been shown to predict treatment response (Wallace, Priestman, Dunn, & Priestman, 1993). Compared with patients undergoing or recovering from cancer treatment, lower rates of depression have been shown in patients who are, instead, ambulatory with better functional status (Kornblith et al., 1995; Levine, Jones, & Sack, 1993; Massie & Holland, 1990). Inpatient status, compared with ambulatory patients in treatment at outpatient clinics or patients not in treatment, may confer characteristics such as severe physical symptoms, greater functional impairment, comorbid medical or psychiatric conditions, cognitive impairment, or lower available social support (e.g., having no possibilities for care at home). Some treatment sequelae may affect social support and intimate relationships (Kornblith & Ligibel, 2003) or disrupt employment and contribute to financial strain (Arndt, Merx, Stegmaier, Ziegler, & Brenner, 2004; Bradley, Neumark, Bednarek, & Schenk, 2005), thereby heightening emotional distress and reducing QoL.

Emotional distress from the trauma of diagnosis and treatment may linger for a small subset of cancer patients (5–7%; Carpenter & Andersen, 2008; Smith, Redd, Peyser, & Vogl, 1999), and this distress has been likened to that of posttraumatic stress disorder. This tends to occur in patients who have undergone the most difficult treatment regimens (e.g., hematopoietic stem cell transplantation), lengthy chemotherapies with debilitating side effects, and disfiguring treatments (e.g., pelvic exenteration; Carpenter & Andersen, 2008). Longitudinal correlates of treatment have been shown for certain chemotherapies. Thornton et al. (2009) reported greater nurse-reported physical symptom burden in breast cancer patients during treatment with Taxol (paclitaxel) compared with those not treated with Taxol. Though the two groups showed convergence on physical symptom burden following treatment, patients treated with Taxol showed significantly higher rates of probable clinical depression at 1-year follow-up. Patients treated with Taxol also showed delayed emotional recovery, with emotional distress persisting for 1 year past that of patients not treated with Taxol. Early and late effects of other, more novel thera-

pies may be unknown. It is thus vital for assessors to remain informed as these data become available.

Measurement Instruments by Domain[1]

Table 12.1 includes measurement instruments selected based on a review of their key psychometric properties (e.g., reliability, validity), as well as their prevalence of use in the clinical setting. For clinician-administered measures, preference was given to those with established interrater and test–retest reliability. With regard to patient-reported outcome (PRO) measures, instruments were selected based on the psychometric guidelines described in the U.S. Food and Drug Administration (2009) guidance for industry on the use of PRO measures in medical product development to support labeling claims. Most notably, the instruments selected exhibit reasonable internal consistency, have appropriately high test–retest reliability, have a clearly defined statement of the relationships between concepts, domains, and items, and contain clear and appropriate response options. In instances in which there were multiple suitable measures, we selected the most parsimonious instruments, so as to ultimately minimize patient burden.

Implications for Further Assessment and Intervention

The wide range of domains to be considered for psychosocial assessment of the oncology patient precludes us, of course, from describing an exhaustive list of possible measurement tools. We chose not to include other acceptable measures for the sake of brevity. As described previously, specific instruments were chosen for inclusion in the chapter based on their psychometric rigor, prevalence of use in the clinical setting, and parsimony. These inclusion criteria may serve as a guide by which assessment tools not listed in Table 12.1 may be chosen.

Additionally, we present measurement tools that cover a number of domains per-

---

[1]Prior to selection of a given instrument, confirm that you are using the most current version and be certain to adhere to all potential copyright restrictions.

TABLE 12.1. Psychometric Properties of Biopsychosocial Cancer Assessment Tools

Name	Domain	Brief description/constructs measured	No. of items, subscales, and scoring information	Psychometric properties
Hamilton Anxiety Rating Scale (HAM-A; Hamilton, 1959)	Anxiety	Brief clinician-administered measure of psychic anxiety and somatic anxiety.	14 items measured on a 5-point (i.e., 0 = *not present*, 4 = *severe*) scale. Score range 0–56. Mild severity < 17; mild to moderate severity 18–24; moderate to severe 25–30; severe > 30.	Interrater reliability range .70–.74 (Maier, Buller, Philipp, & Heuser, 1988).
Generalized Anxiety Disorder–7 (GAD-7; Spitzer, Kroenke, Williams, & Lowe, 2006)	Anxiety (screening)	Brief patient-reported screening measure of generalized anxiety disorder.	7 items scored on 0–3 Likert-type scale (i.e., 0 = *not at all*, 3 = *nearly every day*). Score range 0–21. Mild ≥ 5; moderate ≥ 10; severe ≥ 15.	Overall Cronbach's alpha value = 0.92. Test–retest reliability = .83.
Mini-Mental Status Exam (MMSE; Folstein, Folstein, & McHugh, 1975)	Cognitive function (screening)	Brief clinician-administered screening measure of cognitive function (i.e., orientation to time, orientation to place, registration of three words, attention and calculation, recall of three words, language, visual construction).	Score range 0–30. Severe cognitive impairment, 0–17; 18–23, mild cognitive impairment; 24–30, no cognitive impairment.	Cronbach's alpha values range 0.68–0.96. Test–retest reliability (2 months) range .80–.95 (Tombaugh & McIntyre, 1992).
Brief COPE (Carver, 1997)	Coping strategies	Brief measure of coping strategies aimed at capturing self-distraction, active coping, denial, substance use, use of emotional support, use of instrumental support, behavioral disengagement, venting, positive reframing, planning, humor, acceptance, religion, and self-blame.	28 items (2 per dimension) scored on 1–4 Likert-type scale (i.e., 1 = *I haven't been doing this at all*, 4 = *I have been doing this a lot*).	Cronbach's alpha values range 0.50–0.90.
Religious/Spiritual Coping Short Form (Brief RCOPE; Pargament, Koenig, & Perez, 2000)	Coping strategies (religious)	Patient-reported measure of a patient's positive and negative religious coping methods.	14 items rated using a 1–4 Likert-type scale (i.e., 1 = *not at all*, 4 = *a great deal*).	Cronbach's alpha values range 0.61–0.96.

Measure	Construct	Description	Psychometrics
Hamilton Depression Rating Scale (HAM-D; Hamilton, 1960)	Depression	Brief clinician-administered measure of depressed mood, suicide, work and loss of interest, retardation, agitation, general somatic symptoms, hypochondriasis, insight, and loss of weight.	17 items measured on 3-point (i.e., 0 = absent, 2 = clearly present) and 5-point (i.e., 0 = absent, 4 = severe) Likert-type scales. Mild depression, 8–13; moderate depression, 14–18; severe depression, 19–22; very severe depression, ≥ 23.	Cronbach's alpha values range 0.46–0.92. Interrater reliability range 0.65–0.98. Test–retest reliability ranges .81–.98 (Bagby, Ryder, Schuller, & Marshall, 2004).
Patient Health Questionnaire–9 (PHQ-9; Kroenke, Spitzer, & Williams, 2001)	Depression (screening)	Brief patient-reported screening measure of depression severity.	9 items scored on 0–3 Likert-type scale (i.e., 0 = not at all, 3 = nearly every day). Score range 0–27. Mild depression ≥ 5; moderate ≥ 10; moderately severe ≥ 15; severe ≥ 20.	Cronbach's alpha values range 0.86–0.89. Test–retest reliability at 48 hours = .84.
Multidimensional Fatigue Symptom Inventory—Short Form (MFSI-SF; Stein, Jacobsen, Blanchard, & Thors, 2004)	Fatigue	Patient-reported measure of global, somatic, affective, cognitive, and behavioral symptoms of fatigue.	30 items rated using a 0–4 Likert-type scale (i.e., 0 = not at all, 4 = extremely).	Cronbach's alpha values range 0.87–0.96.
Insomnia Severity Index (ISI; Morin, 1993)	Insomnia	Brief screening measure of insomnia.	7 items scored on 0–4 Likert-type scale (i.e., 0 = not at all, 4 = extremely). Score range 0–28. Subthreshold insomnia ? 8; moderate clinical insomnia ≥ 15; severe clinical insomnia ≥ 21.	Overall Cronbach's alpha value = 0.90. Test–retest reliability = 0.83 (1 month), 0.77 (2 months), and 0.73 (3 months; Savard, Savard, Simard, & Ivers, 2005).
Brief Pain Inventory (BPI; Daut, Cleeland, & Flanery, 1983)	Pain	Brief patient-reported measure of pain intensity and pain interference.	11 items (4 pain intensity, 7 pain interference). All items scored on 0–10 NRS (e.g., no pain, pain as bad as you can imagine).	Cronbach's alpha values range 0.78–0.96. Test–retest reliability estimates range .62–.97 (Atkinson et al., 2010).
Perceived Stress Scale (PSS; Cohen, Kamarck, & Mermelstein, 1983)	Perceived stress	Brief patient-reported measure of the degree to which situations from the past month are appraised by patient as stressful.	10 items scored 0–4. Score range 0–40. Higher scores indicate greater distress.	All Cronbach's alpha values ≥ 0.70.

(continued)

TABLE 12.1. *(continued)*

Name	Domain	Brief description/constructs measured	No. of items, subscales, and scoring information	Psychometric properties
Karnofsky Performance Status (KPS; Karnofsky & Burchenal, 1949)	Performance status	Physician rating scale of patient's ability to perform normal activity and do active work and of need for assistance.	0–100 NRS. Unable to care for self ≥ 40; unable to work, varying degree of assistance needed > 40 ≥ 70; Normal > 70.	Interrater reliability = .89 (Schag, Heinrich, & Ganz, 1984).
NEO Five-Factor Inventory (NEO-FFI; Costa & McCrae, 1992)	Personality	Brief measure of neuroticism, extraversion, openness to experience, agreeableness, and conscientiousness.	60 items (12 per domain).	Cronbach's alpha values range from 0.30 (Openness to Experience) to 0.83 (Conscientiousness; Hull, Beaujean, Worrell, & Verdisco, 2010).
Brief Symptom Inventory (BSI; Derogatis & Melisaratos, 1983)	Psychiatric symptomatology	Patient-reported measure of somatization, obsessive–compulsive, interpersonal sensitivity, depression, anxiety, hostility, phobic anxiety, paranoid ideation, and psychoticism domains.	53 items rated on a 0–4 Likert-type scale (i.e., 0 = *not at all*, 4 = *extremely*). Items form General Severity Index, Positive Symptom Total, and Positive Symptom Distress Index.	Cronbach's alpha values ranges 0.71–0.85. Test–retest reliability ranges .68–.91.
Psychosocial Adjustment to Illness Scale (PAIS; Derogatis, 1986)	Psychological and social adjustment	Semistructured clinical interview to assess the psychological/social adjustment of medical patients or their immediate families to the patient's illness.	7 domains (i.e., health care orientation, vocational environment, domestic environment, sexual relationships, extended family relationships, social environment, and psychological distress) across 45 items.	Cronbach's alpha values range 0.12–0.93. Interrater reliability range .33–.86.

Measure	Construct	Description	Items and scoring	Reliability
European Organization for Research and Treatment of Cancer QLQ-C30 (EORTC QLQ-C30; Aaronson et al., 1993)	Quality of life	Patient-reported measure of physical, role, cognitive, emotional and social functioning and global quality of life.	30 total items. 28 rated on 1–4 Likert-type scale (i.e., 1 = *not at all*, 4 = *very much*). 2 items rated 1–7 NRS (i.e., 1 = very poor; 7 = excellent).	All Cronbach's alpha values ≥ 0.70.
Female Sexual Function Index (FSFI; Rosen et al., 2000)	Sexual functioning (female)	Brief patient-reported measure of female sexual desire, arousal, lubrication, orgasm, satisfaction, and pain/discomfort.	19 items (desire and subjective arousal, lubrication, orgasm, satisfaction, pain/discomfort). All items scored on 1–5 or 0–5 Likert-type scale. Score range 0–36. Sexual dysfunction ≥ 26.55.	Cronbach's alpha values range 0.82–0.95. Test–retest reliability estimates range .62–.91.
International Index of Erectile Function (IIEF; Rosen et al., 1997)	Sexual functioning (male)	Brief patient-reported measure of male sexual desire, erectile function, orgasmic function, intercourse satisfaction, and overall satisfaction.	15 items scored on 1–5 or 0–5 Likert-type scale.	All Cronbach's alpha values ≥ 0.70. Test–retest reliability estimates range .64–.84.
Pittsburgh Sleep Quality Index (PSQI; Buysse, Reynolds, Monk, Berman, & Kupfer, 1989)	Sleep quality	Measure of subjective sleep quality, sleep latency, sleep duration, habitual sleep efficiency, sleep disturbances, use of sleeping medication, and daytime dysfunction.	19 items measuring 7 domains. Each domain scored 0–3. Score range 0–21. Administered across 1-month interval. Poor sleepers > 5.	Overall Cronbach's alpha value = 0.83. Test–retest reliability ranges .65–.84.
Interpersonal Support Evaluations List (ISEL; Cohen & Hoberman, 1983)	Social support	Brief measure of tangible, belonging, self-esteem, appraisal domains.	40 items (10 per domain) rated using NRS (i.e., −3 = extremely negative, +3 = extremely positive).	Cronbach's alpha values range 0.60–0.77.
Impact of Events Scale—Revised (IES-R; Weiss & Marmar, 1997)	Traumatic stress	Brief measure of subjective distress attributed to traumatic events.	22 items rated on a 0–4 Likert-type scale (i.e., 0 = *not at all*, 4 = *extremely*). Intrusion, Avoidance and Hyperarousal subscales included. Score range 0–88.	Cronbach's alpha values range 0.81–0.93.

Note. NRS, Numeric Rating Scale.

tinent to the assessment of individuals diagnosed with cancer. Whereas the goal was to present the most psychometrically rigorous measures available, it was beyond the scope of the chapter to provide detailed information regarding the populations for which measures were validated and the potential availability of measures in alternate languages. The potential impact of race, ethnicity, language, and culture on assessment has been well established in the literature (Groth-Marnat, 2009), and it is therefore important that the potential limitations of selected measures be considered. Further, many tools described in this chapter have been translated and validated in languages other than English—for example, the Brief Pain Inventory is currently available in 50 languages (23 languages psychometrically validated) as of last review (Cleeland, 2012)—and are frequently being updated.

Whether in the context of research or clinical care, the overarching aim of psychosocial assessment is to inform patient care. The biobehavioral model underscores the importance of assessment at the time of initial diagnosis and treatment, as well as during other critical periods, such as during declining health and disease progression. For occasions on which distress may warrant further assessment (e.g., Holland et al., 2010) and psychosocial intervention, recommendations (e.g., Andersen, Golden-Kreutz, Emery, & Thiel, 2009; Jacobsen & Jim, 2008) have been published. In brief, a primary goal of psychosocial intervention is to improve patients' QoL. Similar to our recommendations for assessment tools, we recommend psychosocial interventions supported by empirical research data. Examples include biobehavioral (e.g., Andersen et al., 2009) and cognitive-behavioral (e.g., Antoni et al., 2001) stress management, relaxation training (e.g., Redd, Montgomery, & DuHamel, 2001), and supportive-expressive group interventions (e.g., Kissane et al., 2004; Redd et al., 2001). In the scope of clinical care, psychosocial assessment results and cancer-specific considerations may assist in determining the best intervention match. To illustrate, patients with heightened depressive symptoms may show improvement in a cognitive-behavioral intervention (Antoni et al., 2001), and patients experiencing anticipatory nausea and vomiting from chemotherapies may particularly benefit from relaxation training (Redd et al., 2001).

Future Directions

Two future directions for the field of biobehavioral assessment in cancer patients are noted here. First, with the recent publication of the fifth edition of the *Diagnostic and Statistical Manual of Mental Disorders* (DSM-5; American Psychiatric Association, 2013), shifts in diagnostic criteria for mental disorders have occurred. Given this circumstance, clinical assessment and research tools that assist with diagnostic decision making, such as the Hamilton Depression Rating Scale (HAM-D; Hamilton, 1960), may require further qualitative and psychometric studies. Second, recent paradigm shifts have occurred, with the offering of large banks of items designed to assess patient-reported health status effectively and efficiently. These have undergone rigorous evaluation and refinement with epidemiological samples. An example is the Patient-Reported Outcomes Measurement Information System network (PROMIS; Cella et al., 2010). Tools from the PROMIS network have been described as for use in clinical, observational, comparative effectiveness, health services, and health policy research studies, as well as to assist with diagnosis in clinical settings. Research to expand these item banks continues.

ACKNOWLEDGMENTS

We thank Katherine N. DuHamel and Barbara L. Andersen for reviews of this chapter.

REFERENCES

Aaronson, N. K., Ahmedzai, S., Bergman, B., Bullinger, M., Cull, A., Duez, N. J., et al. (1993). The European Organization for Research and Treatment of Cancer QLQ-C30: A quality-of-life instrument for use in international clinical trials in oncology. *Journal of the National Cancer Institute, 85*(5), 365–376.

Alder, J., & Bitzer, J. (2010). Sexualität nach Brustkrebs [Sexuality after breast cancer]. *Therapeutische Umschau, 67*(3), 129–133.

American Cancer Society. (2011a). *Cancer facts and figures 2011*. Atlanta, GA: Author.

American Cancer Society. (2011b). *Colostomy: A guide*. Atlanta, GA: Author.

American Psychiatric Association. (2013). *Diagnostic and statistical manual of mental disorders* (5th ed.). Arlington, VA: Author.

Andersen, B. L. (2002). *Cancer*. Oxford, UK: Blackwell.

Andersen, B. L., Farrar, W. B., Golden-Kreutz, D., Kutz, L. A., MacCallum, R., Courtney, M. E., et al. (1998). Stress and immune responses after surgical treatment for regional breast cancer. *Journal of the National Cancer Institute, 90*(1), 30–36.

Andersen, B. L., Golden-Kreutz, D. M., Emery, C. F., & Thiel, D. L. (2009). Biobehavioral intervention for cancer stress: Conceptualization, components, and intervention strategies. *Cognitive and Behavioral Practice, 16*(3), 253–265.

Andersen, B. L., Kiecolt-Glaser, J. K., & Glaser, R. (1994). A biobehavioral model of cancer stress and disease course. *American Psychologist, 49*(5), 389–404.

Andersen, B. L., Shapiro, C. L., Farrar, W. B., Crespin, T., & Wells-DiGregorio, S. (2005). Psychological responses to cancer recurrence. *Cancer, 104*(7), 1540–1547.

Andersen, B. L., Woods, X. A., & Copeland, L. J. (1997). Sexual self-schema and sexual morbidity among gynecologic cancer survivors. *Journal of Consulting and Clinical Psychology, 65*(2), 221–229.

Andrykowski, M. A., & Cordova, M. J. (1998). Factors associated with PTSD symptoms following treatment for breast cancer: Test of the Andersen model. *Journal of Traumatic Stress, 11*(2), 189–203.

Anisman, H., & Merali, Z. (2003). Cytokines, stress and depressive illness: Brain-immune interactions. *Annals of Medicine (Helsinki), 35*(1), 2–11.

Antoni, M. H., Lehman, J. M., Klibourn, K. M., Boyers, A. E., Culver, J. L., Alferi, S. M., et al. (2001). Cognitive-behavioral stress management intervention decreases the prevalence of depression and enhances benefit finding among women under treatment for early-stage breast cancer. *Health Psychology, 20*(1), 20–32.

Arndt, V., Merx, H., Stegmaier, C., Ziegler, H., & Brenner, H. (2004). Quality of life in patients with colorectal cancer 1 year after diagnosis compared with the general population: A population-based study. *Journal of Clinical Oncology, 22*(23), 4829–4836.

Atkinson, T. M., Mendoza, T. R., Sit, L., Passik, S., Scher, H. I., Cleeland, C., et al. (2010). The Brief Pain Inventory and its "pain at its worst in the last 24 hours" item: Clinical trial endpoint considerations. *Pain Medicine, 11*, 337–346.

Bagby, R. M., Ryder, A. G., Schuller, D. R., & Marshall, M. B. (2004). The Hamilton Depression Rating Scale: Has the gold standard become a lead weight? *American Journal of Psychiatry, 161*, 2163–2177.

Beck, A. T., & Beck, R. W. (1972). Screening depressed patients in family practice: A rapid technic. *Postgraduate Medicine, 52*(6), 81–85.

Bergmann, M., & Sautner, T. (2002). Immunomodulatory effects of vasoactive catecholamines. *Wiener Klinische Wochenschrift, 114*(17–18), 752–761.

Bloom, J. R., & Kessler, L. (1994). Risk and timing of counseling and support interventions for younger women with breast cancer. *Journal of the National Cancer Institute*, Monographs (No. 16), 199.

Body, J.-J., Lossignol, D., & Ronson, A. (1997). The concept of rehabilitation of cancer patients. *Current Opinion in Oncology, 9*(4), 332.

Bradley, C. J., Neumark, D., Bednarek, H. L., & Schenk, M. (2005). Short-term effects of breast cancer on labor market attachment: Results from a longitudinal study. *Journal of Health Economics, 24*(1), 137.

Buysse, D. J., Reynolds, C. F., Monk, T. H., Berman, S. R., & Kupfer, D. J. (1989). The Pittsburgh Sleep Quality Index: A new instrument for psychiatric practice and research. *Psychiatry Research, 28*, 193–213.

Bylund, C. L., Brown, R., Gueguen, J. A., Diamond, C., Bianculli, J., & Kissane, D. W. (2010). The implementation and assessment of a comprehensive communication skills training curriculum for oncologists. *Psycho-Oncology, 19*(6), 583–593.

Carpenter, K. M., & Andersen, B. L. (2008). *Psychological and sexual aspects of gynecologic cancer*. Global Library of Women's Medicine. Retrieved from *www.glowm.com/section_view/heading/Psychological%20and%20Sexual%20Aspects%20of%20Gynecologic%20Cancer/item/276*.

Carver, C. S. (1997). You want to measure coping but your protocol's too long: Consider the brief COPE. *International Journal of Behavioral Medicine, 4*(1), 92–100.

Carver, C. S., Pozo, C., Harris, S., Noriega, V., Scheier, M., Robinson, D., et al. (1993). How coping mediates the effect of optimism on distress: A study of women with early stage breast cancer. *Journal of Personality and Social Psychology, 65*(2), 375–390.

Cella, D. F., Chang, C. H., Lai, J. S., & Webster, K. (2002). Advances in quality of life measurements in oncology patients. *Seminars in Oncology, 29*(3, Suppl. 8), 60–68.

Cella, D. F., Riley, W., Stone, A., Rothrock, N., Reeve, B., Yount, S., et al. (2010). The Patient-Reported Outcomes Measurement Information System (PROMIS) developed and tested its first wave of adult self-reported health outcome item banks: 2005–2008. *Journal of Clinical Epidemiology, 63*(11), 1179–1194.

Chan, Y. M., Ngan, H. Y., Yip, P. S., Li, B. Y., Lau, O. W., & Tang, G. W. (2001). Psychosocial adjustment in gynecologic cancer survivors: A longitudinal study on risk factors for maladjustment. *Gynecologic Oncology, 80*(3), 387–394.

Charua-Guindic, L., Benavides-Leon, C. J., Villanueva-Herrero, J. A., Jimenez-Bobadilla, B., Abdo-Francis, J. M., & Hernandez-Labra, E. (2011). Quality of life in ostomized patients. *Cirugia y Cirujanos, 79*(2), 149–155.

Cheville, A. L., Novotny, P. J., Sloan, J. A., Basford, J. R., Wampfler, J. A., Garces, Y. I., et al. (2011). Fatigue, dyspnea, and cough comprise a persistent symptom cluster up to five years after diagnosis with lung cancer. *Journal of Pain and Symptom Management, 42*(2), 202–212.

Cleeland, C. S. (2012). *The Brief Pain Inventory (BPI)*. Houston: University of Texas, M. D. Anderson Cancer Center. Retrieved March 5, 2012, from *www.mdanderson.org/education-and-research/departments-programs-and-labs/departments-and-divisions/symptom-research/symptom-assessment-tools/brief-pain-inventory.html*.

Cohen, S., & Hoberman, S. (1983). Positive events and social supports as buffers of life change stress. *Journal of Applied Social Psychology, 13*(2), 99–125.

Cohen, S., Kamarck, T., & Mermelstein, R. (1983). A global measure of perceived stress. *Journal of Health and Social Behavior, 24*, 386–396.

Cook Gotay, C. C. (1984). The experience of cancer during early and advanced stages: The views of patients and their mates. *Social Science and Medicine, 18*(7), 605–613.

Cook Gotay, C. C., & Stern, J. D. (1995). Assessment of psychological functioning in cancer patients. *Journal of Psychosocial Oncology, 13*, 123–160.

Cooley, M. E., Lynch, J., Fox, K., & Sarna, L. (2010). Lung cancer. In J. Holland, W. Breitbart, P. Jacobsen, M. Lederberg, M. Loscalzo, & R. McCorkle (Eds.), *Psycho-oncology*. New York: Oxford University Press.

Costa, P. T., Jr., & McCrae, R. R. (1992). *Revised NEO Personality Inventory (NEO-PI-R) and NEO Five Factor Inventory (NEO-FFI) professional manual*. Odessa, FL: Psychological Assessment Resources.

Dantzer, R., O'Connor, J. C., Freund, G. G., Johnson, R. W., & Kelley, K. W. (2008). From inflammation to sickness and depression: When the immune system subjugates the brain. *Nature Reviews Neuroscience, 9*(1), 46–56.

Daut, R. L., Cleeland, C. S., & Flanery, R. C. (1983). Development of the Wisconsin Brief Pain Questionnaire to assess pain in cancer and other diseases. *Pain, 17*, 197–210.

Derogatis, L. R. (1986). The Psychological Adjustment to Illness Scale (PAIS). *Journal of Psychosomatic Research, 30*(1), 77–91.

Derogatis, L. R., & Melisaratos, N. (1983). The Brief Symptom Inventory: An introductory report. *Psychological Medicine, 13*, 596–605.

Derogatis, L. R., & Spencer, P. M. (1984). Psychometric issues in the psychological assessment of the cancer patient. *Cancer, 53*, 2228–2234.

Di Fabio, F., Koller, M., Nascimbeni, R., Talarico, C., & Salerni, B. (2008). Long-term outcome after colorectal cancer resection: Patients' self-reported quality of life, sexual dysfunction and surgeons' awareness of patients' needs. *Tumori, 94*(1), 30–35.

Dodd, M. J., Janson, S., Facione, N., Faucett, J., Froelicher, E. S., Humphreys, J., et al. (2001). Advancing the science of symptom management. *Journal of Advanced Nursing, 33*(5), 668–676.

Dodd, M. J., Miaskowski, C., & Lee, K. A. (2004). Occurrence of symptom clusters. *Journal of the National Cancer Institute*. Monographs (No. 32), 76–78.

Edgar, L., Rosberger, Z., & Nowlis, D. (1992). Coping with cancer during the first year after diagnosis: Assessment and intervention. *Cancer, 69*(3), 817–828.

Elenkov, I. J., Iezzoni, D. G., Daly, A., Harris, A. G., & Chrousos, G. P. (2005). Cytokine dysregulation, inflammation and well-being. *Neuroimmunomodulation, 12*(5), 255–269.

Fairey, A. S., Courneya, K. S., Field, C. J., Bell, G. J., Joncs, L. W., & Mackey, J. R. (2005). Randomized controlled trial of exercise and blood immune function in postmenopausal breast cancer survivors. *Journal of Applied Physiology, 98*(4), 1534–1540.

Folstein, M. F., Folstein, S. E., & McHugh, P. R. (1975). "Mini-mental State": A practical method for grading the cognitive state of patients for the clinician. *Journal of Psychiatry Research, 12,* 189–198.

Formenti, S. C., Meyerowitz, B. E., Ell, K., Muderspach, L., Groshen, S., Leedham, B., et al. (1995). Inadequate adherence to radiotherapy in latina immigrants with carcinoma of the cervix: Potential impact on disease-free survival. *Cancer, 75*(5), 1135–1140.

Frank, J., Witte, K., Schrödl, W., & Schütt, C. (2004). Chronic alcoholism causes deleterious conditioning of innate immunity. *Alcohol and Alcoholism, 39*(5), 386–392.

Friedman, H. S., Tucker, J. S., Schwartz, J. E., Tomlinson-Keasey, C., Martin, L. R., Wingard, D. L., et al. (1995). Psychosocial and behavioral predictors of longevity: The aging and death of the "Termites." *American Psychologist, 50*(2), 69–78.

Galbán, C., Montejo, J. C., Mesejo, A., Marco, P., Celaya, S., Sánchez-Segura, J. M., et al. (2000). An immune-enhancing enteral diet reduces mortality rate and episodes of bacteremia in septic intensive care unit patients. *Critical Care Medicine, 28*(3), 643–648.

Goeders, N. E. (2004). Stress, motivation, and drug addiction. *Current Directions in Psychological Science, 13*(1), 33–35.

Goff, B. A., Mandel, L. S., Melancon, C. H., & Muntz, H. G. (2004). Frequency of symptoms of ovarian cancer in women presenting to primary care clinics. *Journal of the American Medical Association, 291*(22), 2705–2712.

Golden-Kreutz, D. M., & Andersen, B. L. (2004). Depressive symptoms after breast cancer surgery: Relationships with global, cancer-related, and life event stress. *Psycho-Oncology, 13*(3), 211–220.

Golden-Kreutz, D. M., Thornton, L. M., Wells-Di Gregorio, S., Frierson, G. M., Jim, H. S., Carpenter, K. M., et al. (2005). Traumatic stress, perceived global stress, and life events: Prospectively predicting quality of life in breast cancer patients. *Health Psychology, 24*(3), 288–296.

Gottesman, D., & Lewis, M. S. (1982). Differences in crisis reactions among cancer and surgery patients. *Journal of Consulting and Clinical Psychology, 50*(3), 381–388.

Groth-Marnat, G. (2009). *Handbook of psychological assessment* (5th ed.). Hoboken, NJ: Wiley.

Grunberg, N. E., & Straub, R. O. (1992). The role of gender and taste class in the effects of stress on eating. *Health Psychology, 11*(2), 97–100.

Hagedoorn, M., Sanderman, R., Bolks, H. N., Tuinstra, J., & Coyne, J. C. (2008). Distress in couples coping with cancer: A meta-analysis and critical review of role and gender effects. *Psychological Bulletin, 134*(1), 1–30.

Hamilton, M. (1959). The assessment of anxiety states by rating. *British Journal of Medical Psychology, 32,* 50–55.

Hamilton, M. (1960). A rating scale for depression. *Journal of Neurology, Neurosurgery and Psychiatry, 23,* 56–62.

Hampton, M. R., & Frombach, I. (2000). Women's experience of traumatic stress in cancer treatment. *Health Care for Women International, 21*(1), 67–76.

Hann, D. M., Garovoy, N., Finkelstein, B., Jacobsen, P. B., Azzarello, L. M., & Fields, K. K. (1999). Fatigue and quality of life in breast cancer patients undergoing autologous stem cell transplantation: A longitudinal comparative study. *Journal of Pain and Symptom Management, 17*(5), 311–319.

Harrington, C. B., Hansen, J. A., Moskowitz, M., Todd, B. L., & Feuerstein, M. (2010). It's not over when it's over: Long-term symptoms in cancer survivors—a systematic review. *International Journal of Psychiatry Medicine, 40*(2), 163–181.

Hendren, S. K., O'Connor, B. I., Liu, M., Asano, T., Cohen, Z., Swallow, C. J., et al. (2005). Prevalence of male and female sexual dysfunction is high following surgery for rectal cancer. *Annals of Surgery, 242*(2), 212–223.

Henry, D. H., Viswanathan, H. N., Elkin, E. P., Traina, S., Wade, S., & Cella, D. (2008). Symptoms and treatment burden associated with cancer treatment: Results from a cross-sectional national survey in the U.S. *Support Care Cancer, 16*(7), 791–801.

Herschbach, P., Keller, M., Knight, L., Brandl, T., Huber, B., Henrich, G., et al. (2004). Psychological problems of cancer patients: A cancer distress screening with a cancer-specific questionnaire. *British Journal of Cancer, 91*(3), 504–511.

Hodge, D. R. (1996). Religion in America: The demographics of belief and affiliation. In E. P. Shafranske (Ed.), *Religion and the clinical practice of psychology* (pp. 21–41). Washington, DC: American Psychological Association.

Holland, J. C., Andersen, B., Breitbart, W. S., Compas, B., Dudley, M. M., Fleishman, S., et al. (2010). Distress management. *Journal of the National Comprehensive Cancer Network, 8*(4), 448–485.

Horowitz, M., Wilner, N., & Alvarez, W. (1979). Impact of Event Scale: A measure of subjective stress. *Psychosomatic Medicine, 41*(3), 209–218.

Hull, D. M., Beaujean, A. A., Worrell, F. C., & Verdisco, A. E. (2010). An item-level examination of the factorial validity of NEO Five-Factor Inventory Scores. *Educational and Psychological Measurement, 70*, 1021–1041.

Jacobsen, P. B., Hann, D. M., Azzarello, L. M., Horton, J., Balducci, L., & Lyman, G. H. (1999). Fatigue in women receiving adjuvant chemotherapy for breast cancer: Characteristics, course, and correlates. *Journal of Pain and Symptom Management, 18*(4), 233–242.

Jacobsen, P. B., & Jim, H. S. (2008). Psychosocial interventions for anxiety and depression in adult cancer patients: Achievements and challenges. *CA: A Cancer Journal for Clinicians, 58*(4), 214–230.

Jansen, L., Koch, L., Brenner, H., & Arndt, V. (2010). Quality of life among long-term (≥ 5 years) colorectal cancer survivors—systematic review. *European Journal of Cancer, 46*(16), 2879–2888.

Jim, H. S., Richardson, S. A., Golden-Kreutz, D. M., & Andersen, B. L. (2006). Strategies used in coping with a cancer diagnosis predict meaning in life for survivors. *Health Psychology, 25*(6), 753–761.

Jung, W., & Irwin, M. (1999). Reduction of natural killer cytotoxic activity in major depression: Interaction between depression and cigarette smoking. *Psychosomatic Medicine, 61*(3), 263–270.

Karnofsky, D. A., & Burchenal, J. H. (1949). The clinical evaluation of chemotherapeutic agents in cancer. In C. M. Macleod (Ed.), *Evaluation of chemotherapeutic agents* (pp. 199–205). New York: Columbia University Press.

Kissane, D. W. (2009). Beyond the psychotherapy and survival debate: The challenge of social disparity, depression and treatment adherence in psychosocial cancer care. *Psycho-Oncology, 18*(1), 1–5.

Kissane, D. W., Bloch, S., Onghena, P., McKenzie, D. P., Snyder, R. D., & Dowe, D. L. (1996). The Melbourne Family Grief Study: II. Psychosocial morbidity and grief in bereaved families. *American Journal of Psychiatry, 153*(5), 659–666.

Kissane, D. W., Grabsch, B., Clarke, D. M., Christie, G., Clifton, D., Gold, S., et al. (2004). Supportive-expressive group therapy: The transformation of existential ambivalence into creative living while enhancing adherence to anti-cancer therapies. *Psycho-Oncology, 13*(11), 755–768.

Koopman, C., Hermanson, K., Diamond, S., Angell, K., & Spiegel, D. (1998). Social support, life stress, pain and emotional adjustment to advanced breast cancer. *Psycho-Oncology, 7*(2), 101–111.

Kornblith, A. B., & Ligibel, J. (2003). Psychosocial and sexual functioning of survivors of breast cancer. *Seminars in Oncology, 30*(6), 799–813.

Kornblith, A. B., Thaler, H. T., Wong, G., Vlamis, V., McCarthy Lepore, J., Loseth, D. B., et al. (1995). Quality of life of women with ovarian cancer. *Gynecologic Oncology, 59*(2), 231–242.

Kroenke, K., Spitzer, R. L., & Williams, J. B. W. (2001). The PHQ-9: Validity of a brief depression severity measure. *Journal of General Internal Medicine, 16*, 606–613.

Krouse, R. (2010). Gastrointestinal cancer. In J. Holland, W. Breitbart, P. Jacobsen, M. Lederberg, M. Loscalzo, & R. McCorkle (Eds.), *Psycho-oncology*. New York: Oxford University Press.

Levine, S. H., Jones, L. D., & Sack, D. A. (1993). Evaluation and treatment of depression, anxiety, and insomnia in cancer patients. *Oncology, 7*, 119–125.

Lutgendorf, S. K., & Sood, A. K. (2011). Biobehavioral factors and cancer progression: Physiological pathways and mechanisms. *Psychosomatic Medicine, 73*(9), 724–730.

Maier, W., Buller, R., Philipp, M., & Heuser, I. (1988). The Hamilton Anxiety Scale: Reliability, validity and sensitivity to change in anxiety and depressive disorders. *Journal of Affective Disorders, 14*, 61–68.

Manne, S. (2011). Restoring intimacy in relationships affected by cancer. In J. P. Mulhall, L. Incrocci, I. Goldstein & R. Rosen (Eds.), *Cancer and sexual health* (pp. 739–750). New York: Humana Press.

Marks, G., Richardson, J. L., Graham, J. W.,

& Levine, A. (1986). Role of health locus of control beliefs and expectations of treatment efficacy in adjustment to cancer. *Journal of Personality and Social Psychology, 51*(2), 443–450.

Massie, M. J., & Holland, J. C. (1990). Depression and the cancer patient. *Journal of Clinical Psychiatry, 51*(Suppl.), 12–19.

McDonough, E. M., Boyd, J. H., Varvares, M. A., & Maves, M. D. (1996). Relationship between psychological status and compliance in a sample of patients treated for cancer of the head and neck. *Head and Neck, 18*(3), 269–276.

Miller, A. H., Ancoli-Israel, S., Bower, J. E., Capuron, L., & Irwin, M. R. (2008). Neuroendocrine-immune mechanisms of behavioral comorbidities in cancer patients. *Journal of Clinical Oncology, 26*(6), 971–982.

Miller, B. E., Pittman, B., Case, D., & McQuellon, R. P. (2002). Quality of life after treatment for gynecologic malignancies: A pilot study in an outpatient clinic. *Gynecologic Oncology, 87*(2), 178–184.

Miller, G. E., Chen, E., & Zhou, E. S. (2007). If it goes up, must it come down?: Chronic stress and the hypothalamic–pituitary–adrenocortical axis in humans. *Psychological Bulletin, 133*(1), 25–45.

Morin, C. M. (1993). *Insomnia: Psychological assessment and management.* New York: Guilford Press.

Morreale, M. K. (2011). The impact of cancer on sexual function. *Advances in Psychosomatic Medicine, 31*, 72–82.

Ng, D. M., & Jeffery, R. W. (2003). Relationships between perceived stress and health behaviors in a sample of working adults. *Health Psychology, 22*(6), 638–642.

Onujiogu, N., Johnson, T., Seo, S., Mijal, K., Rash, J., Seaborne, L., et al. (2011). Survivors of endometrial cancer: Who is at risk for sexual dysfunction? *Gynecologic Oncology, 123*(2), 356–359.

Pargament, K. I., Koenig, H. G., & Perez, L. M. (2000). The many methods of religious coping: Development and initial validation of the RCOPE. *Journal of Clinical Psychology, 56*(4), 519–543.

Plumb, M., & Holland, J. (1981). Comparative studies of psychological function in patients with advanced cancer: II. Interviewer-rated current and past psychological symptoms. *Psychosomatic Medicine, 43*(3), 243–254.

Raison, C. L., & Miller, A. H. (2001). The neuroimmunology of stress and depression. *Seminars in Clinical Neuropsychiatry, 6*(4), 277–295.

Ramirez, A. J., Pinder, K. L., Black, M. E., Richardson, M. A., Gregory, W. M., & Rubens, I. D. (1993). Psychiatric disorder with patients with advanced breast cancer: Prevalence and associated factors. *European Journal of Cancer, 29*, 524–527.

Razavi, D., Delvaux, N., Farvacques, C., De Brier, F., Van Heer, C., Kaufman, L., et al. (1993). Prevention of adjustment disorders and anticipatory nausea secondary to adjuvant chemotherapy: A double-blind, placebo-controlled study assessing the usefulness of alprazolam. *Journal of Clinical Oncology, 11*(7), 1384–1390.

Redd, W. H., Montgomery, G. H., & DuHamel, K. N. (2001). Behavioral intervention for cancer treatment side effects. *Journal of the National Cancer Institute, 93*(11), 810–823.

Reese, J. B. (2011). Coping with sexual concerns after cancer. *Current Opinion in Oncology, 23*(4), 313–321.

Roberts, J. A., Brown, D., Elkins, T., & Larson, D. B. (1997). Factors influencing views of patients with gynecologic cancer about end-of-life decisions. *American Journal of Obstetrics and Gynecology, 176*(1, Part 1), 166–172.

Röntgen, P., Sablotzki, A., Simm, A., Silber, R.-E., & Czeslick, E. (2004). Effect of catecholamines on intracellular cytokine synthesis in human monocytes. *European Cytokine Network (Montrouge), 15*(1), 14.

Rosen, R., Brown, C., Heiman, J., Leiblum, C., Meston, C., Shabsigh, R., et al. (2000). The Female Sexual Function Index (FSFI): A multidimensional self-report instrument for the assessment of female sexual function. *Journal of Sex and Marital Therapy, 26*(2), 191–208.

Rosen, R., Riley, A., Wagner, G., Osterloh, I. H., Kirkpatrick, J., & Mishra, A. (1997). The International Index of Erectile Function (IIEF): A multidimensional scale for assessment of erectile dysfunction. *Urology, 49*, 822–830.

Rowland, J. H., & Massie, M. J. (2010). Breast cancer. In J. Holland, W. Breitbart, P. Jacobsen, M. Lederberg, M. Loscalzo, & R. McCorkle (Eds.), *Psycho-oncology* (pp. 177–186). New York: Oxford University Press.

Ruiz-Aragon, J., Marquez-Pelaez, S., & Luque Romero, L. G. (2010). Erectile dysfunction in patients with prostate cancer who have undergone surgery: Systematic review of literature [in Spanish]. *Actas Urologicas Españolas, 34*(8), 677–685.

Rutter, D. R., Iconomou, G., & Quine, L. (1996). Doctor–patient communication and outcome in cancer patients: An intervention. *Psychology and Health, 12*(1), 57–71.

Sales, E., Schulz, R., & Biegel, D. (1992). Predictors of strain in families of cancer patients: A review of the literature. *Journal of Psychosocial Oncology, 10*(2), 1–26.

Sardell, A. N., & Trierweiler, S. J. (1993). Disclosing the cancer diagnosis: Procedures that influence patient hopefulness. *Cancer, 72*(11), 3355–3365.

Sarenmalm, K., Odén, A., & Gaston-Johansson, F. (2008). Experience and predictors of symptoms, distress, and health-related quality of life over time in postmenopausal women with recurrent breast cancer. *Psycho-Oncology, 17*, 497–505.

Savard, J., Laroche, L., Simard, S., Ivers, H., & Morin, C. M. (2003). Chronic insomnia and immune functioning. *Psychosomatic Medicine, 65*(2), 211–221.

Savard, M. H., Savard, J., Simard, S., & Ivers, H. (2005). Empirical validation of the Insomnia Severity Index in cancer patients. *Psycho-Oncology, 14*, 429–441.

Schag, C. C., Heinrich, R. L., & Ganz, P. A. (1984). Karnofsky Performance Status revisited: Reliability, validity, and guidelines. *Journal of Clinical Oncology, 2*(3), 187–193.

Schuler, T. A., Yang, H.-C., Thornton, L. M., Andersen, B. L., & Carson, W. E., III. (2014). *Depressive symptoms moderate the relationship between marital distress and immunity trajectories in five-year breast cancer survivors.* Columbus: Ohio State University.

Shrader-Bogen, C. L., Kjellberg, J. L., McPherson, C. P., & Murray, C. L. (1997). Quality of life and treatment outcomes. *Cancer, 79*(10), 1977–1986.

Smets, E. M. A., Visser, M. R. M., Garssen, B., Frijda, N. H., Oosterveld, P., & de Haes, J. C. J. M. (1998). Understanding the level of fatigue in cancer patients undergoing radiotherapy. *Journal of Psychosomatic Research, 45*(3), 277–293.

Smith, M. Y., Redd, W. H., Peyser, C., & Vogl, D. (1999). Post-traumatic stress disorder in cancer: A review. *Psycho-Oncology, 8*(6), 521–537.

Spitzer, R. L., Kroenke, K., Williams, J. B. W., & Lowe, B. (2006). A brief measure for assessing generalized anxiety disorder: The GAD-7.

Archives of Internal Medicine, 166, 1092–1097.

Stein, K. D., Jacobsen, P. B., Blanchard, C. M., & Thors, C. (2004). Further validation of the Multidimensional Fatigue Symptom Inventory—Short Form. *Journal of Pain and Symptom Management, 27,* 14–23.

Stein, M., Keller, S. E., & Schleifer, S. J. (1988). Immune system: Relationship to anxiety disorders. *Psychiatric Clinics of North America, 11*(2), 349–360.

Steptoe, A., O'Donnell, K., Marmot, M., & Wardle, J. (2008). Positive affect, psychological well-being, and good sleep. *Journal of Psychosomatic Research, 64*(4), 409–415.

Steptoe, A., & Ussher, M. (2006). Smoking, cortisol and nicotine. *International Journal of Psychophysiology, 59*(3), 228–235.

Stetson, B. A., Rahn, J. M., Dubbert, P. M., Wilner, B. I., & Mercury, M. G. (1997). Prospective evaluation of the effects of stress on exercise adherence in community-residing women. *Health Psychology, 16*(6), 515–520.

Stewart, A. L., Greenfield, S., Hays, R. D., Wells, K., Rogers, W. H., Berry, S. D., et al. (1989). Functional status and well-being of patients with chronic conditions. *Journal of the American Medical Association, 262*(7), 907–913.

Taylor, S. E., Lichtman, R. R., & Wood, J. V. (1984). Attributions, beliefs about control, and adjustment to breast cancer. *Journal of Personality and Social Psychology, 46*(3), 489–502.

Thornton, L. M., Andersen, B. L., & Blakely, W. P. (2010). The pain, depression, and fatigue symptom cluster in advanced breast cancer: Covariation with the hypothalamic–pituitary–adrenal axis and the sympathetic nervous system. *Health Psychology, 29*(3), 333–337.

Thornton, L. M., Andersen, B. L., Schuler, T. A., & Carson, W. E. (2009). A psychological intervention reduces inflammatory markers by alleviating depressive symptoms: Secondary analysis of a randomized controlled trial. *Psychosomatic Medicine, 71*(7), 715–724.

Tombaugh, T. N., & McIntyre, N. J. (1992). The Mini-Mental State Examination: A comprehensive review. *Journal of the American Geriatrics Society, 40*(9), 922–935.

Trivedi, M. H., Greer, T. L., Grannemann, B. D., Chambliss, H. O., & Jordan, A. N. (2006). Exercise as an augmentation strategy for treatment of major depression. *Journal of Psychiatric Practice, 12*(4), 205–213.

Tsai, T. Y., Chen, S. Y., Tsai, M. H., Su, Y. L., Ho, C. M., & Su, H. F. (2011). Prevalence and associated factors of sexual dysfunction in cervical cancer patients. *Journal of Sexual Medicine, 8*(6), 1789–1796.

Tulsky, J. A., Arnold, R. M., Alexander, S. C., Olsen, M. K., Jeffreys, A. S., Rodriguez, K. L., et al. (2011). Enhancing communication between oncologists and patients with a computer-based training program. *Annals of Internal Medicine, 155*(9), 593–601.

U.S. Department of Health and Human Services Food and Drug Administration. (2009). Guidance for industry patient-reported outcome measures: Use in medical product development to support labeling claims. Retrieved from *www.fda.gov/downloads/Drugs/Guidances/UCM193282.pdf*.

Vachon, M. L. (2008). Meaning, spirituality, and wellness in cancer survivors. *Seminars in Oncology Nursing, 24*(3), 218–225.

Vess, J. D., Moreland, J. R., & Schwebel, A. I. (1985). A follow-up study of role functioning and the psychological environment of families of cancer patients. *Journal of Psychosocial Oncology, 3*(2), 1–14.

Vinokur, A. D., Threatt, B. A., Vinokur-Kaplan, D., & Satariano, W. A. (1990). The process of recovery from breast cancer for younger and older patients: Changes during the first year. *Cancer, 65*(5), 1242–1254.

Wallace, L. M., Priestman, S. G., Dunn, J. A., & Priestman, T. J. (1993). The quality of life of early breast cancer patients treated by two different radiotherapy regimens. *Clinical Oncology, 5*(4), 228–233.

Weaver, A. J., & Flannelly, K. J. (2004). The role of religion/spirituality for cancer patients and their caregivers. *Southern Medical Journal, 97*(12), 1210–1214.

Weiss, D. S., & Marmar, C. R. (1997). The Impact of Event Scale—Revised. In J. P. Wilson & T. M. Keane (Eds.), *Assessing psychological trauma and PTSD* (pp. 98–135). New York: Guilford Press.

Yang, H.-C., & Schuler, T. A. (2009). Marital quality and survivorship. *Cancer, 115*(1), 217–228.

Yang, H.-C., Thornton, L. M., Shapiro, C. L., & Andersen, B. L. (2008). Surviving recurrence: Psychological and quality-of-life recovery. *Cancer, 112*(5), 1178–1187.

Zabora, J., BrintzenhofeSzoc, K., Curbow, B., Hooker, C., & Piantadosi, S. (2001). The prevalence of psychological distress by cancer site. *Psycho-Oncology, 10*(1), 19–28.

Zorrilla, E. P., Luborsky, L., McKay, J. R., Rosenthal, R., Houldin, A., Tax, A., et al. (2001). The relationship of depression and stressors to immunological assays: A meta-analytic review. *Brain, Behavior, and Immunity, 15*(3), 199–226.

CHAPTER 13

Cardiovascular Disease

Benson M. Hoffman
Amy Goetzinger
James A. Blumenthal

Cardiovascular disease (CVD) refers to a broad range of diseases that affect the heart and blood vessels and is the number one health problem in the United States today. Approximately one in three adults suffers from CVD (Rosamond et al., 2007). In 2004, CVD accounted for 36% of all deaths in the United States and was the primary diagnosis in more than 72 million physician office visits, 6 million hospitalizations, and 4 million emergency room visits, with direct costs estimated to exceed $283 billion in 2007 (Rosamond et al., 2007).

In addition to the traditional risk factors of smoking, hypertension, hyperlipidemia, and diabetes, psychosocial risk factors have been recognized as contributing to the initiation and progression of CVD (Rozanski, Blumenthal, Davidson, Saab, & Kubzansky, 2005; Rozanski, Blumenthal, & Kaplan, 1999). In turn, a CVD diagnosis and subsequent treatment can elicit significant psychosocial changes and have a profound impact on quality of life (QoL; Rothenhausler et al., 2005; Sumanen, Suominen, Koskenvuo, Sillanmaki, & Mattila, 2004). A comprehensive psychosocial evaluation can provide valuable information critical for optimal disease management, treatment planning, and outcome evaluation.

This chapter presents a framework for clinical health psychologists to use in the psy-chosocial evaluation of patients with CVD. First, a brief overview of CVDs and psychosocial risk factors is presented, followed by suggested instruments for assessing key psychosocial risk factors. The chapter concludes with a discussion of the evaluation of specialized CVD patient populations, including patients with end-stage heart disease who are preparing for heart transplantation, and their respective caregivers.

Epidemiology and Pathophysiology of CVD

Hypertension is the most prevalent of all cardiovascular diseases; 90% of all people with CVD have hypertension (Rosamond et al., 2007). Hypertension and CVD risk factors such as smoking, obesity, physical inactivity, diabetes, and hyperlipidemia promote atherosclerosis, which causes the coronary arteries to develop a build up of fatty deposits or plaque. Coronary atherosclerosis is the underlying cause of coronary heart disease (CHD), which results in angina pectoris (chest pain), myocardial infarction (MI; heart attack), and sudden cardiac death. CVD progression also results in greater risk for stroke, renal insufficiency, and peripheral vascular disease (Dzau et al., 2006). Eventually, the heart can lose the ability to effectively pump blood, resulting in end-stage organ disease, or heart failure (HF; Dzau et al., 2006). HF can be classified as ischemic or nonischemic; 6% of patients with CVD suffer from HF (Rosamond et al., 2007) and approximately 1 in 5 patients with newly diagnosed HF die within 1 year (Rosamond et al., 2007).

The most common treatment options for CVD include medication, surgery, and behavioral or lifestyle interventions such as diet and exercise. Hypertension, CHD, and HF can be treated pharmacologically (e.g., ACE inhibitors, beta blockers, and diuretics for hypertension; warfarin and aspirin to reduce clotting; statins to reduce elevated lipids; and nitroglycerine to vasodilate constricted arteries). In more advanced cases, CVD can be treated surgically (e.g., coronary bypass surgery, coronary angioplasty, pacemaker implantation, and, in the most serious cases, heart transplantation).

Behavioral and psychosocial interventions are used to treat the entire spectrum of CVD, from "prehypertension" (i.e., blood pressures from 120–139/80–89 mm Hg) through HF. For example, so-called lifestyle interventions (e.g., diet—including a diet low in sodium and high in fruits, vegetables, and low-fat dairy products known as the DASH diet—weight loss, smoking cessation, physical activity, and moderate intake of alcohol) are widely advocated for primary prevention (P. K. Whelton et al., 2002) and initial treatment of hypertension and have been shown to be particularly effective when combined (Appel et al., 2003). A number of clinical trials have demonstrated that cardiac rehabilitation for CHD patients reduces mortality and improves QoL (Jolliffe et al., 2000), and psychosocial interventions may provide added benefit when included in standard cardiac rehabilitation (Linden, 2000). For CHD patients, stand-alone psychosocial interventions (i.e., without cardiac rehabilitation) also have been shown to reduce cardiac mortality and morbidity (Friedman et al., 1986; Frasure-Smith & Prince, 1985). For patients with HF, exercise-based rehabilitation has been associated with improved survival and QoL (Rees, Taylor, Singh, Coats, & Ebrahim, 2004). Because psychosocial factors affect prognosis and because most CVD patients can potentially benefit from psychosocial interventions, clinical health psychol-

ogy psychosocial assessments can be useful for CVD patients and their families.

Psychosocial Assessment of CVD

The primary objectives of a psychosocial assessment for patients with CVD are to characterize patients' psychosocial adjustment and to evaluate behavioral and psychological risk factors for future CVD events. The traditional risk factors include older age, male gender, family history of heart disease, hypertension, cigarette smoking, diabetes mellitus, hypercholesterolemia, physical inactivity, and obesity (Grundy et al., 1998; Chobanian et al., 2003). With the exception of older age, family history, and male gender, all of these other risk factors have a behavioral component and can be modified through lifestyle interventions (Chobanian et al., 2003). In addition to these behavioral factors, CVD disease progression has been linked to psychosocial factors such as depression, anxiety, hostility, and stress, as well as low social support (Rozanski et al., 2005). These psychosocial risk factors appear to add significantly to the risk for CVD events. For example, a multisite international case-controlled study of nearly 30,000 patients with acute MI and controls revealed that high levels of psychosocial distress were associated with an increased risk of MI that was similar in size to that of smoking and diabetes and even greater than hypertension and obesity (Yusuf et al., 2004).

A thorough psychosocial assessment of behavioral, emotional, social, and cognitive risk factors can be accomplished through clinical interview, medical record review, and psychometric testing. The interview permits the clinical health psychologist to place the patient in the context of a narrative, to understand patients' perceptions of their situations, to observe patient's style of relating, and to gather ideographic data. Psychological testing increases the reliability and validity of the clinical interview and can quantitate patients' self-reported attitudes, feelings, and behaviors. Also, by using validated measures, the clinical health psychologist can rapidly evaluate an individual patient's functioning relative to normative data. A summary of measures recommended for the psychosocial evaluation of patients with CVD can be found in Table 13.1.

TABLE 13.1. Summary of the Measures Recommended for the Psychosocial Evaluation of Patients with CVD

Measure	Content area	Description	Validity/reliability
Physical Activity Recall (PAR; Sallis et al., 1985)	Exercise	15-minute semistructured interview of moderate or high-intensity physical activity over a 7-day period.	Interrater reliability, $r = .78–.86$; correlation with activity monitors, $r = .26–.57$; correlation with aerobic fitness, $r = .22–.61$
Diet History Questionnaire (DHQ; Subar et al., 2001)	Diet	124-item list of food categories; respondents indicate frequency and amount eaten in the past month; can be scored to provide estimated nutritional and caloric intake.	Correlation with 24-hour dietary recalls, $r = .60–.70$ for 26 dietary variables
Alcohol Use Disorders Identification Test (AUDIT; Saunders et al., 1993)	Alcohol consumption	10 multiple-choice and yes–no questions on quantity and frequency of alcohol consumption, symptoms of dependency, and hazardous drinking.	Internal reliability, alpha > 0.80; test–retest reliability, $r > .85$; detection of problematic drinking, sensitivity $> .90$, specificity $> .80$
Brief Medical Questionnaire (BMQ; Svarstad et al., 1999)	Medication regimen adherence	Semistructured interview of medication names, dosages, indications, missed doses, and barriers to adherence over the past 7 days. Subscales: Adherence, Uncertainty/Side Effects, Recall.	Sensitivity and specificity coefficients $\geq .80$ with electronic pill monitoring system; correlation with MEMS Cap measured adherence, $r = .67–.71$
Structured Hamilton Depression Rating Scale (HAM-D; Williams, 1988)	Depression	Semistructured interview of depressive symptoms frequency and severity.	Interrater reliability intraclass correlation coefficients $= .82–.99$
Beck Depression Inventory–II (BDI; Beck et al., 1996)	Depression	Self-report 21-item questionnaire measuring the severity of cognitive, affective, and somatic symptoms of depression.	Test–retest reliability $r > .90$
Abbreviated Cook–Medley Hostility Scale (Ho; Barefoot et al., 1989)	Hostility	Self-report measure consisting of 39 true–false questions that measure cynicism, hostile attributions, hostile affect, and aggressive responding.	Internal reliability, alpha > 0.85; test–retest reliability, $r > .84$
State–Trait Anxiety Inventory (STAI; Spielberger, 1983)	Anxiety	Self-report 40-item questionnaire measuring the frequency and severity of anxiety symptoms; scored to produce measures of state and trait anxiety.	Internal reliability, alpha > 0.90; test–retest reliability, $r > .71$

Measure	Construct	Description	Psychometric properties
Perceived Stress Scale (PSS; Cohen, Kanarck, & Mermelstein, 1983)	Perceived stress	Self-report 14-item measure of unpredictability, lack of control, burden overload, and stressful life circumstances.	Internal reliability, alpha ≥ 0.84; test–retest reliability, $r \geq .55$
Job Content Questionnaire (JCQ; Karasek et al., 1998)	Occupational stress	Self-report 49-item measure of job decision latitude, psychological job demands, job-related social support, job physical demands, and job insecurity.	Internal reliability, alpha = 0.73–0.74; subscale Internal reliability, alpha = 0.68
Abbreviated COPE scale (Carver, 1997)	Coping	A 28-item multidimensional measure of coping; respondents indicate the frequency with which they employ coping strategies.	Inconsistent internal structure
Perceived Social Support Scale (PSSS; Blumenthal et al., 1987)	Perceived social support	Self-report 12-item measure of the degree to which respondents agree with statements about perceived social support.	Internal reliability, alpha = 0.88; test–retest reliability, $r = .85$
Mini-Mental State Examination (MMSE; Folstein et al., 1975)	Mental status	An 11-item semistructured interview assessing orientation, registration, attention and calculation, recall, and language.	Test–retest reliability, $r = .83$–$.89$; sensitivity of 87% and specificity of 82% for detecting delirium or dementia
Kansas City Cardiomyopathy Questionnaire (KCCQ; Green et al., 2000)	Quality of life—HF	Self-report, measures physical functioning, HF disease-specific symptoms, QoL, social limitations, self-efficacy, and disease knowledge; 23 items.	Subscale internal reliability, alpha = .62–.95; sensitivity greater than the Minnesota Living with Heart Failure Questionnaire or the SF-36
Psychosocial Assessment of Candidates for Transplantation (PACT; Olbrisch et al., 1989)	Psychosocial suitability for transplant	Rated by trained clinician, measures psychosocial risk factors for transplant: social support, personality and psychopathology, lifestyle and behavioral factors, including substance abuse and compliance and understanding of transplant surgery and follow-up procedures; 8 items.	Interrater reliability, $k = .85$; correlates with Transplant Evaluation Rating Scale
Caregiver Subjective and Objective Burden Scale (CSOB; Montgomery et al., 1985)	Caregiver burden	Self-report, measures objective (potentially negative experiences) and subjective (distress in response to these experiences) caregiver burden; 22 items.	Internal reliability: objective burden, alpha = 0.85; subjective burden, alpha = 0.86

Assessment of Behavioral Risk Factors

Physical Activity

The relationship between higher levels of aerobic fitness and reduced CVD risk has been firmly established in large-scale studies (Blair et al., 1995, 1996). Among healthy adults, low levels of fitness have been associated with greater risk for CVD mortality (Blair et al., 1996), and even small improvements in fitness have been associated with reduced risk for CVD mortality (Blair et al., 1995; Mora, Cook, Buring, Ridker, & Lee, 2007), independent of other CVD risk factors. Aerobic exercise has been associated with improvements in traditional CVD risk factors, including blood pressure (S. P. Whelton, Chin, Xin, & He, 2002; Pescatello et al., 2004), lipids (Leon & Sanchez, 2001), and weight (Shaw, Gennat, O'Rourke, & Del, 2006), as well as emotional CVD risk factors, such as depression (Barbour & Blumenthal, 2005) and anxiety (Petruzzello, Landers, Hatfield, Kubitz, & Salazar, 1991).

Physical activity can be measured by using the Seven-Day Physical Activity Recall (PAR) semistructured interview (Sallis et al., 1985). Using the PAR, the interviewer asks patients to describe their activity level over a 7-day period. Each day is divided into three segments (morning, afternoon, and evening). Physical activities of at least moderate intensity and at least 15 minutes in length are noted. Patients are instructed to consider an activity to be of moderate intensity if that activity feels similar to walking at a normal pace, of very hard intensity if it feels like running, and of hard intensity if it falls in between. These data are sufficient for a clinical health psychologist to understand whether a patient's level of exercise activity achieves recommended levels (i.e., at least 30 minutes per day of moderate-intensity exercise, at least 5 days per week; Haskell et al., 2007), and to then work with a patient and his or her cardiologist or primary care provider to progress toward safe exercise goals. The PAR has been validated in a number of studies. Interrater reliability coefficients have been reported between .78 and .86 (Sallis, Patterson, Buono, & Nader, 1988; Gross, Sallis, Buono, Roby, & Nelson, 1990). Also, the Seven-Day PAR total activity level and very hard activity levels have been observed to significantly correlate with activity monitors (r's between .26 and .57; Rauh, Hovell, Hofstetter, Sallis, & Gleghorn, 1992; Jacobs, Ainsworth, Hartman, & Leon, 1993) and aerobic fitness (r's between .22 and .61; Blair et al., 1985; Dishman & Steinhardt, 1988).

There are a number of other instruments for the measurement of physical activity as well, ranging from single-item questionnaires to detailed exercise diaries (Lagerros & Lagiou, 2007). For example, the short form of the International Physical Activity Questionnaire (IPAQ) is a 7-item self-report instrument that asks patients to recall the number of days and hours per day that they engaged in vigorous, moderate, light, and sedentary activity (Booth, 2000). The IPAQ has been observed to be a reliable and valid measure of physical activity and has been validated internationally (Craig et al., 2003).

Diet

Dietary advice for the reduction of CVD risk generally includes reduced salt and fat intake and increased intake of fruit, vegetables, and fiber (Brunner, Thorogood, Rees, & Hewitt, 2005). Such dietary advice has been shown to reduce CVD risk factors including blood pressure, total cholesterol, and low-density lipoprotein (LDL) cholesterol (Brunner et al., 2005). Such advice has been consolidated into the Dietary Approaches to Stop Hypertension (DASH) eating plan (Sacks et al., 2001), which recommends a diet high in fruits, vegetables, potassium, and low-fat dairy products and low in sodium. The DASH diet (Sacks et al., 2001), as well as nutritional advice based upon similar principles (Brunner et al., 2005), has been associated with improvements in CVD risk factors, especially reduced blood pressure. Although detailed nutritional advice is usually provided by other health professionals (e.g., dieticians and nutritionists), health psychologists can obtain a general impression of patient dietary habits with such instruments as food frequency questionnaires (FFQs) and food diaries.

FFQs are self-report measures that provide a list of foods and ask respondents to indicate the frequency with which they typically consume each food. The responses can then be used to produce an estimate of nutritional and caloric intake (Willett, 1998). FFQs provide less detailed data than food diaries, and they have been criticized for this reason (Posner et al., 1992). However, FFQs are easy to complete, provide data that correlate with food diary results (Thompson & Byers, 1994), and are generally considered useful for the purposes of categorical classification (Posner et al., 1992; Kant, Graubard, & Schatzkin, 2004). The most widely used and well-validated FFQs are the 106-item Block FFQ (Block et al., 1986) and the 126-item Willett FFQ (Willett, 1998). However, researchers at the National Cancer Institute recently developed the Diet History Questionnaire (DHQ), a 124-item FFQ designed to measure diet with greater accuracy by providing clearer questions (Subar et al., 2001). Correlation coefficients between 24-hour dietary recalls and each of these three measures generally varied between .60 and .70 for 26 dietary variables (Subar et al., 2001). The DHQ and an easy-to-use scoring program are available online at *http://riskfactor.cancer.gov/DHQ*.

Food diaries provide respondents with a structured form on which they record their daily food intake for a specified number of days. Food diaries are viewed as accurate and correlate well with biochemical measures of nutritional intake (Bentley, 2006). However, they are burdensome for respondents (Bentley, 2006), and interpretation of the data requires a level of expertise in diet and nutrition that may be beyond the competence of many health psychologists.

Smoking

Nicotine use is a firmly established CVD risk factor (Grundy et al., 1998; Chobanian et al., 2003). Among patients with CHD, cigarette smoking has been shown to independently predict both cardiac and noncardiac death (Dankner, Goldbourt, Boyko, & Reicher-Reiss, 2003). Furthermore, patients with cardiac disease who quit smoking reduce their risk of death by at least one-third (Critchley & Capewell, 2004). In general, research has shown that self-reported smoking behavior, when validated against biochemical assessment, is accurate (Rebagliato, 2002; Vartiainen, Seppala, Lillsunde, & Puska, 2002). For example, in a recent study of more than 4,500 American adults,

only 1.3% of self-reported nonsmokers had positive cotinine (a nicotine metabolite) tests (West, Zatonski, Przewozniak, & Jarvis, 2007). However, self-report may be less reliable in medical populations, where there is pressure not to admit smoking (Twardella, Rothenbacher, Hahmann, Wusten, & Brenner, 2006). Objective measures of nicotine use, such as urine or salivary cotinine tests (SRNT Subcommittee on Biochemical Verification, 2002), are not routinely used but should be considered in high-risk situations (e.g., a heart transplant patient who recently quit smoking).

Alcohol Consumption

The effect of excessive alcohol consumption on hypertension is well documented (Beilin & Puddey, 1993). Furthermore, a recent research review determined that heavy drinkers (averaging 3–6 drinks per day) can significantly reduce their blood pressure by reducing their intake of alcohol (Xin et al., 2001). Based on this literature, it has been recommended that alcohol use be restricted to a maximum of 1 ounce per day (Chobanian et al., 2003). The Alcohol Use Disorders Identification Test (AUDIT) is a quick and effective self-report measure for detection of elevated alcohol use (Saunders, Aasland, Babor, & de la Fuente, 1993). The AUDIT consists of 10 multiple-choice and yes–no questions: three on the quantity and frequency of alcohol consumption, three on symptoms of dependency, and four on hazardous drinking. Each question is scored on a scale of 0–4, and the scores are summed to produce a total score between 0 and 40. The AUDIT is the alcohol screening instrument used by the World Health Organization. The AUDIT has demonstrated high levels of internal reliability (Cronbach's alpha (α) > 0.80; Fleming, Barry, & MacDonald, 1991; Bergman & Kallmen, 2002) and test–retest reliability (r's > .85; Bergman & Kallmen, 2002; Sinclair, McRee, & Babor, 1992). In the validation studies, a cutoff of 8 was associated with sensitivities in the .90s and specificities in the .80s as compared with various indices of problematic drinking (Saunders et al., 1993).

The CAGE questionnaire is a simple, brief, commonly used alternative to the AUDIT (Ewing, 1984). The CAGE consists of four yes–no questions, and one or more "yes" responses is considered to be a positive screen. The CAGE is sensitive to lifetime prevalence of alcoholism (Magruder-Habib, Stevens, & Alling, 1993). The word "CAGE" is a useful mnemonic for the four CAGE questions: (1) Have you ever felt you should *c*ut down on your drinking? (2) Have people *a*nnoyed you by criticizing your drinking? (3) Have you ever felt bad or *g*uilty about your drinking? (4) Have you ever had a drink for thing in the morning to steady your nerves or to get rid of a hangover (*e*ye-opener)?

Treatment Adherence

Adherence can be defined as the extent to which patients follow the instructions they are given for prescribed treatments. Medications can work only if patients take them. On average, approximately 50% of patients fail to adhere to their medication protocols (Clark & Becker, 1998; Rand & Weeks, 1998; Haynes et al., 2005). For patients with CVD, medication nonadherence is a significant and independent risk factor for cardiovascular events (Gehi, Ali, Na, & Whooley, 2007) and death (Rasmussen, Chong, & Alter, 2007; Horwitz et al., 1990). Patient adherence to medication can most easily be adequately measured by self-report (Stephenson, Rowe, Haynes, Macharia, & Leon, 1993). Self-reported adherence has a high degree of specificity for nonadherence, but social desirability and vaguely worded questions can result in an overestimation of adherence (Vitolins, Rand, Rapp, Ribisl, & Sevick, 2000; Farmer, 1999). The Brief Medical Questionnaire (BMQ) is a semistructured interview designed to improve on previous self-report measures by using nonjudgmental language and clear, concretely worded questions (Svarstad, Chewning, Sleath, & Claesson, 1999). The BMQ asks patients to reconstruct their medication regimens over the preceding 7 days, including the names of their medications, dosages, indications, and self-report of missed doses and also asks several questions about barriers to adherence, such as memory difficulty or side effects. The BMQ is then scored on three scales: a five-item Regimen Screen (self-reported adherence), a two-item Belief screen (uncertainty about regimen, side effects), and a two-item Recall screen (regimen complexity, barriers to adherence). When the BMQ was validated against an electronic pill monitoring system (i.e., MEMS Cap), the Regimen and Belief screens were each found to have sensitivity and specificity coefficients at or above .80 for the detection of greater than 20% deviation from prescription, and the Recall screen was found to be at or above .80 sensitivity and specificity for the prediction of nonadherence of less than 20%. Also, the Regimen and Belief screens each correlated with MEMS-measured adherence over the previous week (r's = .67 and .71, respectively; Svarstad et al., 1999).

An important factor in the successful rehabilitation of patients with cardiac disease is not simply taking medications as prescribed but also adhering to recommended lifestyle changes, including stopping smoking, losing weight, or changing dietary habits and increasing levels of physical exercise. In the last decade, researchers and clinicians have increasingly focused on the processes by which patients adopt and maintain healthy lifestyle changes (Marcus et al., 2006). Among the various theories of health behavior change, the transtheoretical model of change (TTM) has received particular attention (Prochaska & DiClemente, 1983, 1984). TTM postulates that behavior change occurs through five stages: precontemplation (there is no intention to change), contemplation (there is intention to change sometime in the future), preparation (there is intention to change in the immediate future), action (behavior is changing), and maintenance (change is established). The TTM also postulates intermediate constructs (e.g., decisional balance, self-efficacy; Velicer, Rossi, DiClemente, & Prochaska, 1996) and cognitive and behavioral processes (Prochaska, Velicer, DiClemente, & Fava, 1988) through which behavior changes occur. Improved rates of patient adherence to lifestyle change recommendations have been observed when those recommendations are tailored to the patient's stage of change with respect to smoking cessation (DiClemente et al., 1991; Pallonen et al., 1994), exercise (Cardinal & Sachs, 1996; Peterson & Aldana, 1999), dietary changes (Brug, Glanz, Van, Kok, & van Breukelen, 1998), and multiple behavioral changes (Prochaska et al., 2005), although positive results from brief, education-only interventions have not been consistently observed across studies (Riemsma et al., 2002). TTM often has been used in conjunction with motivational interviewing (Miller, 1983; Miller & Rollnick, 1991), the client-centered counseling approach originally used in the addiction field (Rollnick, Heather, Gold, & Hall, 1992; Berg-Smith et al., 1999), and more recently used by public health and medical practitioners to address various health-related behaviors (Colby et al., 1998; Dunn, Deroo, & Rivara, 2001). Motivational interviewing interventions have been associated with increased patient adherence to health-related behavior recommendations in the areas of cigarette smoking, alcohol use, diet, and exercise (Burke, Arkowitz, & Menchola, 2003; Hyman, Pavlik, Taylor, Goodrick, & Moye, 2007; Ahluwalia et al., 2007).

A patient's readiness to make a behavioral change can quickly be ascertained by using brief stage of change (SOC) questionnaires. Brief SOC questionnaires describe a specific health-related behavior and present a series of statements that reflect the various stages of change (e.g., "I currently do not exercise, and I do not intend to start in the next 6 months" for precontemplative, "I currently do not exercise, but I am thinking about starting exercising in the next 6 months" for contemplative). Respondents then select the statement with which they most agree or indicate the degree to which they agree with each statement. Brief SOC questionnaires have been generated for health-related behaviors such as exercise (Marcus, Selby, Niaura, & Rossi, 1992), smoking cessation (DiClemente et al., 1991), and weight loss (O'Connell & Velicer, 1988). Donovan and colleagues created a flexible SOC scale on which respondents describe a specific, positive, health-related behavioral change and then select which stage-related statement most applies to them ("I am not thinking of making this change," "I am trying to make this change at the moment," etc.; Donovan, Jones, Holman, & Corti, 1998). A scale such as this might be particularly useful in clinical practice, as it permits providers and patients to determine individually tailored health-related behavioral goals.

There also are a number of self-report instruments that clinicians can use to measure the intermediate processes hypothesized by TTM to be associated with forward stage movement. For example, a patient's perception of the costs and benefits of exercise can be measured with the Exercise Decisional Balance Scale (Nigg, Rossi, Norman, & Benisovich, 1998). A patient's confidence in his or her ability to engage in regular exercise can be measured with the Exercise Self-Efficacy Scale (Marcus et al., 1992). The frequency with which a patient reports using the cognitive and behavioral processes associated with forward stage movement can be measured with the Processes of Behavioral Change scale (Nigg, Norman, Rossi, & Benisovich, 1999). Each of these instruments has been shown to be reliable and valid, although support for the relationship between these intermediate processes and forward stage movement has not been consistently observed between studies (Spencer, Adams, Malone, Roy, & Yost, 2006).

Assessment of Emotional Risk Factors

The primary emotional factors that have been shown to promote CHD and are associated with increased morbidity and mortality in CHD patients include depression, anxiety, and anger/hostility (Rozanski et al., 2005; Kubzansky, 2007). The mechanisms underlying the relationship between negative emotions and cardiac events remain unclear. Commonly studied physiological mechanisms include chronic stimulation of the sympathetic nervous system and hypothalamic–pituitary–adrenal (HPA) axis (Carney, Freedland, & Veith, 2005). There may be psychosocial mechanisms as well. For example, patients with depression are less likely to take their medication (Carney et al., 2004; DiMatteo, Lepper, & Croghan, 2000) and more likely to be physically inactive (Barbour & Blumenthal, 2005). Patients with CHD and depression are more likely to smoke (Lehto et al., 2000) and less likely to quit smoking (Glassman et al., 1990).

Depression

Depression is the most widely studied emotional risk factor for cardiac events. Rates of depression are disproportionately high among patients with heart disease, as compared with the general population (Rozanski et al., 1999; Lett et al., 2004). Major depressive disorder (MDD) has been linked with cardiac events, both for healthy individuals and for individuals with preexisting heart disease (Lett et al., 2004). Furthermore, recent observational data suggest that depressive symptom severity is a powerful and independent predictor of future cardiac death, even when depressive symptoms are subclinical (Davidson et al., 2006; Lesperance, Frasure-Smith, Talajic, & Bourassa, 2002).

Despite the evidence linking depression to increased mortality, there is currently no evidence to indicate that depression treatment reduces the risk for future cardiac events. Observational studies have observed that a decline in depressive symptom severity may be associated with lowered cardiovascular risk (Lesperance et al., 2002). The ENRICHD study compared the effects of individual cognitive-behavioral therapy (CBT) with usual care for MI patients with depression or low social support. CBT was associated with modest improvements in depression and social support, but the intervention did not reduce mortality or recurrent cardiac events (Berkman et al., 2003). However, post hoc analyses revealed that patients in the CBT condition who showed reduced depressive symptoms (Carney et al., 2004) and patients who received treatment with antidepressants (Taylor et al., 2005) were observed to be at decreased risk for death and reinfarction. The randomized trial known as SADHART compared the effects of sertraline to placebo for patients with MDD and unstable angina or recent MI (Glassman et al., 2002). Sertraline was associated with greater improvements in depressive symptoms in patients with more severe depression, and there was a tendency for patients receiving sertraline to have fewer serious adverse cardiac events than those receiving placebo.

In general, depression is diagnosed by clinical interview, but symptom severity can be assessed by self-report questionnaire. Clinical interview is the most common approach to depression diagnosis, and the structured clinical interview is considered to be the gold standard. Interview permits direct observation of behavior and questions to clarify the impact of mood symptoms on functioning, both of which are essential components of a diagnosis (American Psychiatric Association, 2000). When attempting to establish the severity of depression, we recommend the structured Hamilton Depression Rating Scale (HAM-D; Hamilton, 1960). We suggest the 17-item structured HAM-D that is scored by a trained clinical interviewer (Williams, 1988). The severity of each symptom is rated on either a 3-point or a 5-point scale, permitting both classification (i.e., depressed vs. nondepressed) and rating of depression severity. The HAM-D generally requires 15–20 minutes to administer. The HAM-D originally was published without interview guidelines, and it has been criticized over the years for variable interrater reliability. Subsequent publication of a semistructured interview version of the HAM-D yielded increased interrater reliability, with intraclass correlation coefficients ranging between .82 (Williams, 1988) and .99 (Moberg et al., 2001).

Clinicians have long been advised to use a multimethod approach to assessments (Campbell & Fiske, 1959). Given the critical importance of depression to CVD, we recommend supplementing the interview with a self-report depression measure to quantitate the severity of depressive symptoms. The Beck Depression Inventory-II (BDI) is a self-report scale consisting of 21 items, each corresponding to a specific category of symptoms and attitudes (Beck, Steer, & Brown, 1996). The severity of each symptom is rated on a 4-point scale. The BDI-II can be separated into two subscales: an 8-item "cognitive" subscale (e.g., pessimism, past failures, self-dislike, suicidal thoughts) and a 13-item "affective/somatic" subscale (e.g., sadness, loss of interest, loss of appetite, loss of energy; Steer, Ball, Ranieri, & Beck, 1999). Items on the somatic subscale can overlap with symptoms of physical illness (e.g., fatigue, loss of appetite), resulting in "false positives" (Steer, Cavalieri, Leonard, & Beck, 1999). The BDI has been studied extensively since it was first developed in 1961 (Beck & Steer, 1961) and has been widely used in the study of heart disease (McGee, Hevey, & Horgan, 1999). With the advent of the BDI-II, the instrument has become increasingly reliable, with Cronbach's alpha and test–retest reliability coefficients above .90 (Beck et al., 1996).

Two widely used alternatives to the BDI are the Zung Self-Rating Depression Scale

(SDS; Zung, 1965) and the Center for Epidemiologic Studies Depression Scale (CES-D; Radloff, 1977). The SDS is a 20-item scale measuring four characteristics of depression: pervasive effect, physiological equivalents, other disturbances, and psychomotor activities. Each item is scored on a scale of 1–4 (*a little of the time* to *most of the time*), and scores are summed to produce an overall score of 20–80. The CES-D is a 20-item scale that draws its items from several other scales, including the SDS and BDI. Participants rate each item on a scale from 0 to 3 answering the question "How often have you felt this way during the past week?" using the anchors of 0 = *rarely or none of the time (less than 1 day)* and 4 = *most or all of the time (5–7 days)*. The CES-D produces scores from 0 to 60. In a recent study, both the SDS and the CES-D were observed to be internally consistent (alpha > 0.90) and reliable (test–retest r > .70; Fountoulakis et al., 2007). The CES-D has been shown to be associated with increased mortality in patients who have undergone cardiac surgery, with scores > 27 before surgery or scores > 16 that persist for 6 months following surgery being associated with more than a doubling of risk (Blumenthal et al., 2003).

A recent scientific advisory panel commissioned by the American Heart Association (Lichtman et al., 2009) recommended that medical professionals screen cardiac patients for possible depression using the Patient Health Questionnaire (PHQ). Specifically, the panel recommended the two-item PHQ-2 as a screen, followed by the full PHQ-9 for patients who screen positive on the PHQ-2. The PHQ-9 is a self-report questionnaire that presents patients with each of the nine symptoms used to diagnose MDD. Patients indicate whether they have experienced each symptom on a 4-point scale anchored by *not at all* and *nearly every day*. Consequently, health psychologists who work with cardiac patients are likely to encounter the PHQ-9 and are advised to be familiar with the instrument.

Trait Anger and Hostility

The relationship between trait anger and/or chronic hostility and CVD has received considerable attention (Smith, Glazer, Ruiz, & Gallo, 2004). Early findings of a relation-

ship between the Type A behavior pattern (i.e., ambitious, competitive, time-urgent, and quick-tempered) and subsequent development of CHD (Rosenman et al., 1975) were not confirmed by subsequent studies (Shekelle, Gale, & Norusis, 1985). However, components of Type A behavior, including hostility and anger, have proven to be predictive of cardiac-related events. For example, a meta-analytic review found that chronic anger/hostility is an independent risk factor for the development of CHD and premature mortality, although the effect size was noted to be small (Miller, Smith, Turner, Guijarro, & Hallet, 1996). A recent study of 1,328 patients with CHD found that a very large (i.e., 2 standard deviations) difference in hostility scores was associated with a modest increase in the odds of death from CHD or all-cause mortality over a 14-year period, independent of disease severity (Boyle et al., 2004). Although the relationship between hostility and hard cardiac endpoints has been small, the consistency of this finding across studies, as well as the observed relationships between hostility and other CHD risk factors, such as body mass index (BMI), lipids, triglycerides, glucose, alcohol consumption, and smoking (Bunde & Suls, 2006), serves as an argument for its measurement and treatment.

Hostility is generally considered to be a multidimensional construct that taps attitudes as well as emotions and behavioral tendencies. At this time, there is no consensus about the structure of this construct. For example, researchers examining the Cook–Medley Hostility Scale of the Minnesota Multiphasic Personality Inventory (MMPI) determined that hostility consists of cynicism, hostile attributions, hostile affect, and aggressive responding (Barefoot, Dodge, Peterson, Dahlstrom, & Williams, 1989). In contrast, a recent factor analytic study determined that hostility consists of anger-out, negative affect, coping, and anger-in (Donker, Breteler, & van der Staak, 2000). Other studies have identified as many as eight factors (Miller, Jenkins, Kaplan, & Salonen, 1995). Across studies, factors tend to overlap on a conceptual level and have been observed to strongly correlate with one another (Donker et al., 2000).

The Cook–Medley Hostility Scale (Ho) from the MMPI (Cook & Medley, 1954) is the most widely used self-report measure of hostility (Smith et al., 2004). The original scale consists of 50 true–false questions, 9 of which were updated for the MMPI-2 due to outdated language, male-oriented language, or awkward wording (Han, Weed, Calhoun, & Butcher, 1995). These 50 items were selected on an empirical rather than on a theoretical basis. As a result, the content covered by this scale is diverse (Han et al., 1995), covering constructs such as cynicism, hostile attributions, hostile affect, and aggressive responding (Barefoot et al., 1989). Nevertheless, it has been observed to be an internally consistent instrument (alpha = 0.85; Martin, Watson, & Wan, 2000). A large prospective study observed a 4-year test–retest correlation coefficient of .84 (Shekelle, Gale, Ostfeld, & Paul, 1983). An abbreviated 39-item version was created by removing 11 items that were thought to be unrelated to hostility (Barefoot et al., 1989) and may be more desirable for clinical use than the longer version.

The Ho scale has been associated with CVD risk factors such as BMI, insulin resistance, lipids, triglycerides, glucose, alcohol consumption, and smoking (Bunde & Suls, 2006), as well as CVD mortality independent of such risk factors (Miller et al., 1996; Boyle et al., 2005). Compared with the 50-item version, the 39-item abbreviated Ho scale has been found to be a more powerful predictor of survival among healthy adults (Barefoot et al., 1989) and coronary patients (Boyle et al., 2004, 2005). Although associations between cardiovascular outcomes and hostility generally are stronger when hostility is measured by structured interview (Miller et al., 1996), the requisite time and expertise to administer structured interviews make them impractical for clinical practice.

Large studies using the updated Cook–Medley Ho items have observed mean scores between 18 and 20, with standard deviations of approximately 8 (Boyle et al., 2005; Han et al., 1995), and abbreviated Ho mean score of 16.25, with a standard deviation of 7 (Boyle et al., 2005). It is important to note that significant results have generally been obtained by looking at large differences (Colligan & Offord, 1988), and health psychologists are encouraged to interpret the significance of Ho scores within 1 standard deviation of normal with caution.

Anxiety

Relative to the data available for depression and hostility, less is known about the relationship between anxiety and CVD. The relationship between high levels of anxiety and worry and increased risk for cardiovascular mortality has been supported by large epidemiological studies of healthy adults (Kawachi, Sparrow, Vokonas, & Weiss, 1994; Kubzansky et al., 1997; Thurston, Kubzansky, Kawachi, & Berkman, 2006), and smaller studies of individuals with heart disease (Shibeshi, Young-Xu, & Blatt, 2007; Denollet & Brutsaert, 1998).

The instrument used most often to measure anxiety is the State–Trait Anxiety Inventory (STAI; Borkovec, Castonguay, & Newman, 1997). The STAI is a self-report instrument with two 20-item subscales designed to capture anxiety both as a state (i.e., in the moment) and as a trait (i.e., a stable, general tendency; Spielberger, 1983). The two subscales differ in item wording, in response format (the state form asks for symptom intensity, whereas the trait form asks for symptom frequency), and in instructions for how to respond ("right now" vs. "generally"). The STAI was revised in order to better differentiate between anxiety and depression, although the original and revised STAI are highly correlated measures (r's < .96; Spielberger, 1983). The STAI has been found to be reliable, with 30-day test–retest reliability coefficients for trait anxiety above .71 (Spielberger, 1983), and internally stable, with Cronbach's alpha coefficients for each subscale above 0.90 among healthy participants (Spielberger, 1983), as well as participants with cardiac disease (Frasure-Smith & Lesperance, 2003; An et al., 2004).

In addition to more general levels of anxiety, phobic anxiety specifically has been associated with ventricular arrhythmias and sudden cardiac death (Haines, Imeson, & Meade, 1987; Albert, Chae, Rexrode, Manson, & Kawachi, 2005; Kawachi et al., 1994). One instrument that has been widely used to assess phobic anxiety is the Phobic Anxiety subscale of the Crown–Crisp Experiential Index (Crown & Crisp, 1966) and is recommended for use.

Assessment of Stress

Acute psychological stress induces hemo-dynamic and neuroendocrine responses, including release of catecholamines and cor-ticosteroids, increases in heart rate, cardiac output, and blood pressure, and changes in biological processes related to clotting of blood (Krantz & McCeney, 2002). Over time, these pathophysiological change pro-cesses may lead to the development or pro-gression of CVD. A recent international case-controlled study of nearly 30,000 patients with acute MI and controls deter-mined that a composite measure of work stress, financial stress, stressful life events, perceived inability to control life circum-stances, and mood was associated with a risk of MI that was similar in size to those of smoking and diabetes and larger than those of hypertension and obesity (Yusuf et al., 2004). Similarly, occupational stress (Karasek et al., 1988; Schnall et al., 1990), job loss (Gallo et al., 2006), social isola-tion (Bland, Krogh, Winkelstein, & Trev-isan, 1991; Case, Moss, Case, McDermott, & Eberly, 1992), and lower socioeconomic status (McDonough, Duncan, Williams, & House, 1997; Marmot, Shipley, & Rose, 1984) have been associated with increased risk of coronary disease and mortality.

Perceived Stress

Perceived stress refers to one's subjective experience that life situations are "unpre-dictable, uncontrollable, and overloading" (Cohen, Kamarck, & Mermelstein, 1983). Perceived stress has been associated with the development of CHD (Strodl, Kenardy, & Aroney, 2003), and cardiovascular mortality (Iso et al., 2002). Perceived stress is most fre-quently measured with the Perceived Stress Scale (PSS; Cohen et al., 1983). This scale consists of 14 items that assess the stress domains of unpredictability, lack of control, burden overload, and stressful life circum-stances. Respondents indicate the frequency with which they experienced symptoms of stress over the past month on a 1- to 5-point scale, anchored by *never* and *very often*. Items are summed to produce a total score between 0 and 56. In the validation stud-ies, Cronbach's alphas were observed to be between 0.84 and 0.86, and test–retest cor-relation coefficients were observed to be .85 after 2 days and .55 after 6 weeks (Cohen et al., 1983). Validity was established by the observation of correlation coefficients between PSS scores and physical symptom burden of between .52 and .70; note that these correlation coefficients were supe-rior to the correlation coefficients between stressful life event scales and physical symp-tom burden (Cohen et al., 1983).

Occupational Stress

Occupational stress has been associated with increased risk of CVD, all-cause mor-tality, and CVD risk factors such as hyper-tension (Schnall, Landsbergis, & Baker, 1994). Among individuals with CVD or CVD risk factors, recent studies have found occupational stress to be associated with an increased risk of recurrent CHD (Aboa-Eboule et al., 2007) and CVD mortality (Matthews & Gump, 2002). Recent studies also have linked occupational stress to future coronary events among individuals who were healthy at baseline (Kuper & Marmot, 2003). However, the association between job strain and CHD risk has not always been observed among cohorts that were healthy at baseline (Eaker, Sullivan, Kelly-Hayes, D'Agostino, & Benjamin, 2004; De Bacquer et al., 2005).

Occupational stress is thought to arise primarily from "job strain," in which job demands far exceed job latitude (Karasek, Baker, Marxer, Ahlbom, & Theorell, 1981), and from "job imbalance," in which job effort far exceeds job rewards (Siegrist, 1996). Job strain and job imbalance inde-pendently predict cardiovascular outcomes (Bosma, Peter, Siegrist, & Marmot, 1998), and their predictive ability appears to be similar (Peter et al., 2002).

Occupational stress is most commonly measured with the Job Content Question-naire (JCQ; Karasek et al., 1998). This self-report questionnaire was constructed for the Framingham Offspring Study, and therefore designed to be rapid and easy to complete. The most widely used version contains 49 items covering the domains of job decision latitude (i.e., skill variety, decision-making authority), psychological job demands, job-related social support, job physical demands, and job insecurity. Respondents are presented with statements about their jobs (e.g., "My job requires that I learn new things") and asked to respond on a 1–4 Likert scale, anchored by 1 = *strongly disagree* and 4 = *strongly agree*. National normative data are available. Job strain is indicated by scores above the median on psychological demands and below the median on decision latitude (Karasek et al., 1998). Large-scale studies have observed the JCQ to be an internally consistent scale (alpha = 0.73–0.74; Karasek et al., 1998), with internally consistent subscales (alpha > 0.68; Pelfrene et al., 2003).

Laboratory Stress

Although he use of mental stress testing in patients with cardiac disease has not been widely adopted in medical practice, there is considerable evidence that mental stressors such as public speaking and mental arithmetic can produce robust increases in cardiovascular responses, including blood pressure and heart rate, and that such mental stress can elicit myocardial ischemia in susceptible individuals (Blumenthal et al., 1995). Moreover, prospective studies have demonstrated that patients with cardiac disease who exhibit mental stress ischemia are more likely to suffer adverse cardiac events, including death and nonfatal infarction (Jiang et al., 1996; Sheps et al., 2002).

Coping

The impact of stress can be affected by patients' coping styles (Lazarus & Folkman, 1984). Among patients with CHD, active, problem-focused coping has been associated with superior adjustment to health-related problems (Suls & Fletcher, 1985) and increased QoL (Shen, Myers, & McCreary, 2006), whereas avoidant coping has been associated with increased psychological distress (Maes & Bruggemans, 1990). However, individual differences in coping styles in patients with CVD have rarely been studied, and to our knowledge coping styles have not been shown to be predictive of CVD outcomes.

Coping is most frequently measured with either the 50-item Ways of Coping Questionnaire (WCQ; Folkman & Lazarus, 1980) or the 28-item abbreviated version of the COPE scale (Carver, 1997). Both scales include a number of subscales (8 for the WCQ, 14 for the COPE), and both ask respondents to use a 0–3 scale to indicate the frequency with which they employ sample coping strategies. Both scales define coping as a complex, multidimensional construct. Given the complexity of the underlying construct, neither scale produces a total score (Folkman & Lazarus, 1980; Carver, 1997). Both scales have produced inconsistent results in factor analyses (Parker & Endler, 1992; Zeidner & Hammer, 1992). Because the COPE is shorter and has been used in the cardiovascular disease literature cited previously (Shen et al., 2006), we recommend its use.

Assessment of Social Support

Social support is a multidimensional construct that includes *structural* aspects of social support, such as marital status and number of friends and family members (Case et al., 1992), and *functional* aspects of social support, such as perceived emotional support, instrumental support, and tangible support (Berkman et al., 2003) . The literature shows that low levels of social support are associated with increased risk of cardiac death in healthy adults and in patients with CHD (Lett et al., 2005). For example, in a study of approximately 730 women, both perceived social support and social network size predicted MI or CHD death among initially healthy individuals (Orth-Gomér, Rosengren, & Wilhelmsen, 1993). Similarly, among patients with CHD, both structural support (Ruberman, Weinblatt, Goldberg, & Chaudhary, 1984) and perceived support (Woloshin et al., 1997) have been shown to be predictive of mortality, although functional social support is generally considered more important in predicting clinical outcomes in patients with cardiac disease. Several studies have shown that higher levels of perceived social support may "buffer" the negative impact of stress and depression on CHD (Orth-Gomér et al., 1993). For example, in data from the ENRICHD trial, high perceived social support was associated with reduced mortality and nonfatal MI among patients with low depression but not high depression (Lett et al., 2007). Therefore, it is important to measure social support as a potential psychosocial risk factor for CVD events.

The Perceived Social Support Scale (PSSS; Blumenthal et al., 1987) is a brief self-report questionnaire that can be specifically recommended for use in populations with CVD. The PSSS includes 12 items on which respondents use a 5-point Likert-type format to indicate the degree to which they agree with statements about perceived support from family, friends, and significant others. The PSSS has been observed to be internally consistent (alpha = 0.88) and reliable (2–3 month test–retest reliability coefficient = .85). Also, the PSSS is noteworthy for its frequent use in recent cardiovascular studies (Lett et al., 2007; Aquarius, De, Henegouwen, & Hamming, 2006; Hintsanen et al., 2005; Barefoot et al., 2003).

There are several other well-validated instruments available for measuring social support that should be mentioned. The most frequently cited instruments include the Social Support Questionnaire (SSQ; Sarason, Levine, Basham, & Sarason, 1983), a 27-item measure that asks respondents to list people available to support them in hypothetical scenarios; the Perceived Social Support (PSS) scales (Procidano & Heller, 1983), two 20-item measures on which respondents indicate whether or not they agree with declarative statements about received support from family (PSS-Fa) or friends (PSS-Fr); and the Interpersonal Support Evaluation List (ISEL; Cohen & Hoberman, 1983), a 40-item scale on which respondents indicate the degree to which first-person statements about tangible support, belonging support, self-esteem support, and appraisal support are true. All three scales have been observed to be internally reliable (alpha > 0.75), and all have been widely used and validated (Sarason et al., 1983; Procidano & Heller, 1983; Cohen & Hoberman, 1983).

An additional scale, the ENRICHD Social Support Inventory (ESSI; Mitchell et al., 2003), was specifically designed to quickly measure aspects of social support that are most predictive of poor outcomes in patients with MI and CHD. The ESSI consists of 7 questions about the frequency with which social support is available, with response options anchored by 1 = none of the time and 5 = all of the time. The ESSI has been observed to be an internally reliable scale (alpha = 0.87), to correlate with the PSSS (r = .63; ENRICHD Investigators, 2000).

Assessment of Neurocognitive Impairment

CVD is a risk factor for neurocognitive impairment (Waldstein & Elias, 2001). Coronary events, such as MI, bypass surgery, and stroke, can cause neurological damage (Vingerhoets, 2001; Newman et al., 2001). Over time, CVD can result in vascular dementia (Lezak, Howieson, Loring, Hannay, & Fischer, 2004). A complete neuropsychological battery is beyond the scope of a typical health psychologist's evaluation. However, a clinical health psychologist can screen for impairment and refer impaired patients for a more complete neurocognitive evaluation.

The most widely used instrument for the measurement of general cognitive functional deficits is the Mini-Mental State Examination (Folstein, Folstein, & McHugh, 1975). The MMSE is a formalized mental status examination that simply and quickly samples various domains of cognitive functioning to produce a general cognitive functioning score (Lezak et al., 2004). The MMSE consists of 11 items that test orientation, registration, attention and calculation, recall, and language. One point is awarded for each correct answer to produce a total score between 0 and 30. In the original validation study, the MMSE was able to distinguish the various clinical groups from one another and from the control group. Test–retest reliability was r = .89 over 24 hours, and interrater reliability was r = .83 over 24 hours with different testers (Folstein et al., 1975). In a large validation study of more than 15,000 adults, a cutoff score of 24 captured 95% of the general population. On general medical units, a cutoff score of 24 produced sensitivity of 87% and specificity of 82% when looking for delirium or dementia (Folstein, Fetting, Lobo, Niaz, & Capozzoli, 1984). The MMSE has been criticized as being insensitive to subtle, mild cognitive impairment.

The Blessed Dementia Scale (BDS) is a useful alternative to the MMSE. The BDS consists of two scales: a caregiver scale, which inquires about activities of daily living and personality changes, and a patient scale, which consists of brief tests of information/orientation, memory, and concentration (Blessed, Tomlinson, & Roth, 1968). Like the MMSE, the BDS is quick to administer, and it has been shown to be sensitive to dementia (Erkinjuntti, Hokkanen, Sulkava, & Palo, 1988).

Psychosocial Assessment in Special Cardiac Populations

Health psychologists may also work with unique cardiac populations requiring specialized assessment. Several notable populations include patients with heart failure (HF), patients who are preparing for heart transplantation, and caregivers of patients with CVD.

Heart Failure

HF is a condition in which the heart is unable to pump sufficient blood throughout the body, resulting in inadequate blood supply to major organs that is a significant cause of morbidity and mortality (Davis, Hobbs, & Lip, 2000). Due to a lack of sufficient oxygen and nutrients, organ damage and loss of functioning result. Although HF can sometimes develop suddenly, for example, in response to a viral infection, it is more commonly a result of ischemic heart disease (Hunt et al., 2005). HF is associated with numerous physical symptoms, which are often chronic and progressively worsen throughout the course of the illness. Of particular importance, many of the HF physical symptoms represent clinically relevant symptoms of depression and anxiety, highlighting the need for careful diagnostic assessment and differential diagnosis. Thus health psychologists need to assess psychiatric symptoms in the context of the course of the patient's heart disease and progression of symptoms.

The most commonly reported physical symptoms associated with HF include edema, shortness of breath, and fatigue. Other symptoms include persistent coughing or wheezing, loss of appetite and nausea, increased heart rate, and confusion or impaired cognition. In the course of HF, as blood flow out of the heart slows, blood returning to the heart backs up, causing congestion in the tissues. This congestion often results in swelling, or edema, which most often builds up in the legs and ankles (peripheral edema); however, fluid can also collect in other areas of the body, including the abdomen and lungs (pulmonary edema). Pulmonary edema interferes with breathing, causing shortness of breath (dyspnea), and sometimes results in persistent coughing or wheezing. In addition, HF can affect the kidneys' ability to dispose of sodium and water, resulting in worsening edema. Fatigue results when blood flow is diverted away from less vital organs, particularly muscles in the limbs, in order to direct blood flow to vital organs, including the heart and brain. Moreover, when blood flow is diverted from the digestive system, loss of appetite, nausea, and other gastrointestinal problems can occur. The heart attempts to pump faster to make up for the loss of pumping capacity, leading it to beat faster.

QoL in HF patients can be measured by two disease-specific instruments. The Kansas City Cardiomyopathy Questionnaire (KCCQ) is a 23-item HF-specific questionnaire used to measure physical functioning, HF disease-specific symptoms, QoL, social limitations, self-efficacy, and disease knowledge (Green, Porter, Bresnahan, & Spertus, 2000). The Minnesota Living with Heart Failure Questionnaire (MLHFQ) is a 21-item questionnaire using a 5-point Likert scale to measure ways in which the HF affects patient's lives (Rector, Kubo, & Cohn, 1987). The MLHFQ measures both physical and emotional aspects of QoL, and it has proven reliability and validity (Rector et al., 1995; Rector & Cohn, 1992). The KCCQ, however, also has been shown to be an internally reliable instrument (subscales alpha = 0.62–0.95), and it has shown substantially greater sensitivity than the MLHFQ and the SF-36 (Green et al., 2000).

Cardiac Transplantation

Heart transplant represents a major advancement in extending the life of patients with end-stage cardiomyopathies. According to the United Network for Organ Sharing (UNOS), the organization that coordinates the U.S. organ transplant system, 2,063 patients with some form of CVD underwent heart transplantation in 2005, and another 3,861 patients were listed on the waiting list for heart transplant (Organ Procurement and Transplantation Network [OPTN], 2006). Depending on disease severity and numerous other factors, the length of time a heart transplant candidate spends on the waiting list may vary. Of the current patients listed and waiting for transplant, 67% have been waiting for 1 year or more (*www. unos.org*), and this waiting period can add another dimension of stress for patients and their families.

The shortage of donor organs creates significant pressure for just and efficient allocation of organs. The ultimate goals of transplant from a medical perspective are survival of the organ (graft), as well as survival of the patient. Decisions regarding the appropriate selection of patients for organ transplant typically involve a multidisciplinary team approach including surgeons, nurses, social workers, psychologists, and financial specialists.

As part of a multidisciplinary team, psychologists are often called on to perform psychosocial assessments to evaluate a patient's suitability for transplant. These assessments typically include a semistructured diagnostic interview and battery of psychometric questionnaires. The purpose of the psychosocial evaluation is to identify relevant psychosocial issues that may affect a candidate's readiness for transplantation and/or affect his or her postoperative course. In addition to summarizing relevant medical and mental health history and current functioning, the psychosocial evaluation aims to provide an integrated assessment, or summary of relevant issues to be addressed, as well as recommendations for improved functioning and transplant readiness. Although programs may differ in terms of interview format and selection of psychometric measures, evaluations typically assess the following domains: behavioral risk factors, psychological and personality functioning, availability of a primary caregiver and social support, medical adherence, cognitive functioning, knowledge of transplant, and motivation to pursue transplant.

Two scaled formats are available for summarizing the results of psychosocial evaluations of transplant candidates: the Psychosocial Assessment of Candidates for Transplantation (PACT; Olbrisch, Levenson, & Hamer, 1989) and the Transplant Evaluation Rating Scale (TERS; Twillman, Manetto, Wellisch, & Wolcott, 1993). The PACT was developed to assess whether a patient is an acceptable candidate for transplant, and, if so, how good a candidate. The PACT is an eight-item rating scale that examines the predictive validity of psychosocial assessments relative to transplant outcomes and assesses patients with regard to social support, personality and psychopathology, lifestyle, and behavioral factors, including substance abuse and compliance, and their understanding of transplant surgery and follow-up procedures. The TERS is a 10-item measure, based on DSM-III taxonomy, producing subscale scores for Axis I and Axis II history, substance use/abuse, compliance, health behaviors, social support quality, coping history, coping with disease and treatment, quality of affect, and mental status. Psychometrics for the PACT and TERS with heart transplant patients are not well established. Interrater reliability of the PACT ($k = .85$) and TERS ($k = .77$) have been shown in other transplant populations, and both measures correlate with one another (Hoodin & Kalbfleisch, 2001; Olbrisch et al., 1989).

Caregivers

Patients with chronic CVD often require assistance in taking care of themselves, especially following surgery. Although patients undergoing bypass surgery usually only spend 4–7 days in the hospital and may resume most activities within 4–6 weeks, patients undergoing heart transplantation often require more intensive assistance. Because the perioperative period requires considerable care, transplant candidates are asked to identify a primary caregiver, as well as backup caregivers, who would be able to provide emotional and tangible support during this period. Caregivers tend to be family members and sometimes close friends.

During the perioperative period, the primary caregiver is responsible for providing instrumental support, which may include transportation to medical appointments, assistance with medication management, assistance with activities of daily living such as bathing, dressing, and meal preparation, and assistance with instrumental activities of daily living such as filling prescriptions, grocery shopping, and cleaning. In addition, caregivers commonly provide emotional and social support to the patient during this stressful period.

Caring for patients having chronic health conditions, including patients awaiting transplantation, is widely recognized as demanding and stressful. Medical psychologists and/or social workers typically meet with the primary caregivers and possibly backup caregivers to assess the adequacy of the patient's care plan. Caregivers often take part in a short, semistructured clinical interview and also complete a similar battery of psychometric questionnaires. The purpose of this evaluation is to assess the caregiver's commitment level and ability to provide adequate care. The caregiver's level of stress, current coping, and psychological functioning are important factors to assess, as caregivers are more likely to feel stressed and burdened and to exhibit higher levels of psychiatric symptoms and psychopathology.

Caregiver stress can be measured in terms of objective burdens (i.e., actual demands of caregiving) and subjective burdens (i.e., subjective appraisal of stress and burden). Given the demands of the situation, caregivers may not prioritize their own needs and may not devote adequate time to their own self-care. In addition, caregivers who report higher levels of objective and subjective burden and distress may not be able to provide adequate care for the patient. As such, it is important that patients identify backup caregivers who would be able to provide needed respite for the primary caregiver. In addition to measures from the transplant candidate battery of self-report instruments, caregivers commonly complete measures of objective and subjective burden.

The Caregiver Subjective and Objective Burden Scale (CSOB) is a 22-item self-report instrument with response options on a 5-point Likert scale (Montgomery, Gonyea, & Hooyman, 1985). The scale was the first to provide subscale scores for both objective (number of potentially negative experiences) and subjective (caregivers' reported distress in response to these experiences) caregiver burden, and both subscales have been observed to be internally reliable (alpha = 0.85–0.86). Caregiver stress also can be measured with the Caregiver Strain Index (CSI), a 13-item self-report instrument measuring five domains of objective caregiver burden, including employment, financial, physical, social, and time-related

strain (Robinson, 1983). This measure has produced adequate internal reliability (alpha = 0.85), as well as construct validity, and it was originally developed with a sample that included patients having arteriosclerotic heart disease.

Summary and Conclusions

Research has documented the importance of psychosocial risk factors in patients with CVD. Lifestyle factors such as diet and exercise, adherence to prescribed medical therapies, the presence of social support, and depression, hostility, and other emotional factors also have been associated with clinical outcomes in patients with CVD and have been shown to affect the course of recovery in patients participating in cardiac rehabilitation. Because psychosocial factors affect patients' prognosis and QoL, it is important that health psychologists routinely provide a comprehensive psychological, behavioral, and social evaluation of cardiac patients in a wide range of clinical settings.

ACKNOWLEDGMENTS

The writing of this chapter was supported, in part, by Grant Nos. HL 080664 and MH 49679 from the National Institutes of Health.

REFERENCES

Aboa-Eboule, C., Brisson, C., Maunsell, E., Masse, B., Bourbonnais, R., Vezina, M., et al. (2007). Job strain and risk of acute recurrent coronary heart disease events. *Journal of the American Medical Association, 298,* 1652–1660.

Ahluwalia, J. S., Nollen, N., Kaur, H., James, A. S., Mayo, M. S., & Resnicow, K. (2007). Pathway to health: Cluster-randomized trial to increase fruit and vegetable consumption among smokers in public housing. *Health Psychology, 26,* 214–221.

Albert, C. M., Chae, C. U., Rexrode, K. M., Manson, J. E., & Kawachi, I. (2005). Phobic anxiety and risk of coronary heart disease and sudden cardiac death among women. *Circulation, 111,* 480–487.

American Psychiatric Association. (2000). *Diagnostic and statistical manual of mental disorders.* (4th ed., text rev.) Washington, DC: Author.

An, K., De Jong, M. J., Riegel, B. J., McKinley, S., Garvin, B. J., Doering, L. V., et al. (2004). A cross-sectional examination of changes in anxiety early after acute myocardial infarction. *Heart and Lung, 33,* 75–82.

Appel, L. J., Champagne, C. M., Harsha, D. W., Cooper, L. S., Obarzanek, E., Elmer, P. J., et al. (2003). Effects of comprehensive lifestyle modification on blood pressure control: Main results of the PREMIER clinical trial. *Journal of the American Medical Association, 289,* 2083–2093.

Aquarius, A. E., De, V. J., Henegouwen, D. P., & Hamming, J. F. (2006). Clinical indicators and psychosocial aspects in peripheral arterial disease. *Archives of Surgery, 141,* 161–166.

Barbour, K. A., & Blumenthal, J. A. (2005). Exercise training and depression in older adults. *Neurobiology of Aging, 26,* S119–S123.

Barefoot, J. C., Burg, M. M., Carney, R. M., Cornell, C. E., Czajkowski, S. M., Freedland, K. E., et al. (2003). Aspects of social support associated with depression at hospitalization and follow-up assessment among cardiac patients. *Journal of Cardiopulmonary Rehabilitation, 23,* 404–412.

Barefoot, J. C., Dodge, K. A., Peterson, B. L., Dahlstrom, W. G., & Williams, R. B., Jr. (1989). The Cook–Medley hostility scale: Item content and ability to predict survival. *Psychosomatic Medicine, 51,* 46–57.

Beck, A. T., & Steer, R. A. (1961). An inventory of measuring depression. *Archives of General Psychiatry, 4,* 53–63.

Beck, A. T., Steer, R. A., & Brown, G. K. (1996). *Manual for the Beck Depression Inventory—II.* San Antonio, TX: Psychological Corporation.

Beilin, L. J., & Puddey, I. B. (1993). Alcohol, hypertension and cardiovascular disease: Implications for management. *Clinical and Experimental Hypertension, 15,* 1157–1170.

Bentley, B. (2006). A review of methods to measure dietary sodium intake. *Journal of Cardiovascular Nursing, 21,* 63–67.

Berg-Smith, S. M., Stevens, V. J., Brown, K. M., Van Horn, L., Gernhofer, N., Peters, E., et al. (1999). A brief motivational intervention to improve dietary adherence in adolescents. *Health Education Research, 14,* 399–410.

Bergman, H., & Kallmen, H. (2002). Alcohol use among Swedes and a psychometric evaluation of the Alcohol Use Disorders Identification Test. *Alcohol and Alcoholism, 37,* 245–251.

Berkman, L. F., Blumenthal, J., Burg, M., Carney, R. M., Catellier, D., Cowan, M. J., et al. (2003). Effects of treating depression and low perceived social support on clinical events after myocardial infarction: The Enhancing Recovery in Coronary Heart Disease Patients (ENRICHD) randomized trial. *Journal of the American Medical Association, 289,* 3106–3116.

Blair, S. N., Haskell, W. L., Ho, P., Paffenbarger, R. S., Jr., Vranizan, K. M., Farquhar, J. W., et al. (1985). Assessment of habitual physical activity by a seven-day recall in a community survey and controlled experiments. *American Journal of Epidemiology, 122,* 794–804.

Blair, S. N., Kampert, J. B., Kohl, H. W., III, Barlow, C. E., Macera, C. A., Paffenbarger, R. S., Jr., et al. (1996). Influences of cardiorespiratory fitness and other precursors on cardiovascular disease and all-cause mortality in men and women. *Journal of the American Medical Association, 276,* 205–210.

Blair, S. N., Kohl, H. W., III, Barlow, C. E., Paffenbarger, R. S., Jr., Gibbons, L. W., & Macera, C. A. (1995). Changes in physical fitness and all-cause mortality: A prospective study of healthy and unhealthy men. *Journal of the American Medical Association, 273,* 1093–1098.

Bland, S. H., Krogh, V., Winkelstein, W., & Trevisan, M. (1991). Social network and blood pressure: A population study. *Psychosomatic Medicine, 53,* 598–607.

Blessed, G., Tomlinson, B. E., & Roth, M. (1968). The association between quantitative measures of dementia and of senile change in the cerebral grey matter of elderly subjects. *British Journal of Psychiatry, 114,* 797–811.

Block, G., Hartman, A. M., Dresser, C. M., Carroll, M. D., Gannon, J., & Gardner, L. (1986). A data-based approach to diet questionnaire design and testing. *American Journal of Epidemiology, 124,* 453–469.

Blumenthal, J. A., Burg, M. M., Barefoot, J., Williams, R. B., Haney, T., & Zimet, G. (1987). Social support, Type A behavior, and coronary artery disease. *Psychosomatic Medicine, 49,* 331–340.

Blumenthal, J. A., Jiang, W., Waugh, R. A., Frid, D. J., Morris, J. J., Coleman, R. E., et al. (1995). Mental stress-induced ischemia in the laboratory and ambulatory ischemia during daily life: Association and hemodynamic features. *Circulation, 92,* 2102–2108.

Blumenthal, J. A., Lett, H. S., Babyak, M. A., White, W., Smith, P. K., Mark, D. B., et al. (2003). Depression as a risk factor for mortality after coronary artery bypass surgery. *Lancet, 362,* 604–609.

Booth, M. (2000). Assessment of physical activity: An international perspective. *Research Quarterly for Exercise and Sport, 71,* S114–S120.

Borkovec, T. D., Castonguay, L. G., & Newman, M. G. (1997). Measuring treatment outcome for posttraumatic stress disorder and social phobia: A review of current instruments and recommendations for future research. In H. H. Strupp, L. M. Horowitz, & M. J. Lambert (Eds.), *Measuring patient changes in mood, anxiety, and personality disorders: Toward a core battery* (pp. 117–154). Washington DC: American Psychological Association.

Bosma, H., Peter, R., Siegrist, J., & Marmot, M. (1998). Two alternative job stress models and the risk of coronary heart disease. *American Journal of Public Health, 88,* 68–74.

Boyle, S. H., Williams, R. B., Mark, D. B., Brummett, B. H., Siegler, I. C., & Barefoot, J. C. (2005). Hostility, age, and mortality in a sample of cardiac patients. *American Journal of Cardiology, 96,* 64–66.

Boyle, S. H., Williams, R. B., Mark, D. B., Brummett, B. H., Siegler, I. C., Helms, M. J., et al. (2004). Hostility as a predictor of survival in patients with coronary artery disease. *Psychosomatic Medicine, 66,* 629–632.

Brug, J., Glanz, K., Van, A. P., Kok, G., & van Breukelen, G. J. (1998). The impact of computer-tailored feedback and iterative feedback on fat, fruit, and vegetable intake. *Health Education and Behavior, 24,* 517–531.

Brunner, E. J., Thorogood, M., Rees, K., & Hewitt, G. (2005). Dietary advice for reducing cardiovascular risk. *Cochrane Database of Systematic Reviews,* Issue 4, Article No. CD002128.

Bunde, J., & Suls, J. (2006). A quantitative analysis of the relationship between the Cook–Medley Hostility Scale and traditional coronary artery disease risk factors. *Health Psychology, 25,* 493–500.

Burke, B. L., Arkowitz, H., & Menchola, M. (2003). The efficacy of motivational interviewing: A meta-analysis of controlled clinical trials. *Journal of Consulting and Clinical Psychology, 71,* 843–861.

Campbell, D. T., & Fiske, D. W. (1959). Convergent and discriminant validation by the multitrait–multimethod matrix. *Psychological Bulletin, 56,* 81–105.

Cardinal, B. J., & Sachs, M. L. (1996). Effects of mail-mediated, stage-matched exercise behavior change strategies on female adults' leisure-time exercise behavior. *Journal of Sports Medicine and Physical Fitness, 36,* 100–107.

Carney, R. M., Blumenthal, J. A., Freedland, K. E., Youngblood, M., Veith, R. C., Burg, M. M., et al. (2004). Depression and late mortality after myocardial infarction in the Enhancing Recovery in Coronary Heart Disease (ENRICHD) study. *Psychosomatic Medicine, 66,* 466–474.

Carney, R. M., Freedland, K. E., & Veith, R. C. (2005). Depression, the autonomic nervous system, and coronary heart disease. *Psychosomatic Medicine, 67*(Suppl. 1), S29–S33.

Carver, C. S. (1997). You want to measure coping but your protocol's too long: Consider the brief COPE. *International Journal of Behavioral Medicine, 4,* 92–100.

Case, R. B., Moss, A. J., Case, N., McDermott, M., & Eberly, S. (1992). Living alone after myocardial infarction. Impact on prognosis. *Journal of the American Medical Association,, 267,* 515–519.

Chobanian, A. V., Bakris, G. L., Black, H. R., Cushman, W. C., Green, L. A., Izzo, J. L., Jr., et al. (2003). Seventh Report of the Joint National Committee on Prevention, Detection, Evaluation, and Treatment of High Blood Pressure. *Hypertension, 42,* 1206–1252.

Clark, N. M., & Becker, M. H. (1998). Theoretical models and strategies for improving adherence and disease management. In S. A. Shumaker, E. B. Schron, J. K. Ockene, & W. L. McBee (Eds.), *The handbook of health behavior change* (2nd ed., pp. 5–32). New York: Springer.

Cohen, S., & Hoberman, H. M. (1983). Positive events and social supports as buffers of life change stress. *Journal of Applied Social Psychology, 13,* 99–125.

Cohen, S., Kamarck, T., & Mermelstein, R. (1983). A global measure of perceived stress. *Journal of Health and Social Behavior, 24,* 385–396.

Colby, S. M., Monti, P. M., Barnett, N. P., Rohsenow, D. J., Weissman, K., Spirito, A., et al. (1998). Brief motivational interviewing in a hospital setting for adolescent smoking: A preliminary study. *Journal of Consulting and Clinical Psychology, 66,* 574–578.

Colligan, R. C. & Offord, K. P. (1988). The risky use of the MMPI Hostility scale in assessing risk for coronary heart disease. *Psychosomatics, 29,* 188–196.

Cook, W. W., & Medley, D. M. (1954). Proposed Hostility and Pharisaic-Virtue scales for the MMPI. *Journal of Applied Psychology, 38,* 414–418.

Craig, C. L., Marshall, A. L., Sjostrom, M., Bauman, A. E., Booth, M. L., Ainsworth, B. E., et al. (2003). International Physical Activity Questionnaire: 12-country reliability and validity. *Medicine and Science in Sports and Exercise, 35,* 1381–1395.

Critchley, J., & Capewell, S. (2004). Smoking cessation for the secondary prevention of coronary heart disease. *Cochrane Database of Systematic Reviews,* Issue 1, Article No. CD003041.

Crown, S., & Crisp, A. H. (1966). A short clinical diagnostic self-rating scale for psychoneurotic patients: The Middlesex Hospital Questionnaire (MHQ). *British Journal of Psychiatry, 112,* 917–923.

Dankner, R., Goldbourt, U., Boyko, V., & Reicher-Reiss, H. (2003). Predictors of cardiac and noncardiac mortality among 14,697 patients with coronary heart disease. *American Journal of Cardiology, 91,* 121–127.

Davidson, K. W., Kupfer, D. J., Bigger, J. T., Califf, R. M., Carney, R. M., Coyne, J. C., et al. (2006). Assessment and treatment of depression in patients with cardiovascular disease: National Heart, Lung, and Blood Institute working group report. *Annals of Behavioral Medicine, 32,* 121–126.

Davis, R. C., Hobbs, F. D., & Lip, G. Y. (2000). ABC of heart failure: History and epidemiology. *BMJ, 320,* 39–42.

De Bacquer, D., Pelfrene, E., Clays, E., Mak, R., Moreau, M., De Smet P., et al. (2005). Perceived job stress and incidence of coronary events: 3-year follow-up of the Belgian Job Stress Project cohort. *American Journal of Epidemiology, 161,* 434–441.

Denollet, J., & Brutsaert, D. L. (1998). Personality, disease severity, and the risk of long-term cardiac events in patients with a decreased ejection fraction after myocardial infarction. *Circulation, 97,* 167–173.

DiClemente, C. C., Prochaska, J. O., Fairhurst, S. K., Velicer, W. F., Velasquez, M. M., &

Rossi, J. S. (1991). The process of smoking cessation: An analysis of precontemplation, contemplation, and preparation stages of change. *Journal of Consulting and Clinical Psychology, 59,* 295–304.

DiMatteo, M. R., Lepper, H. S., & Croghan, T. W. (2000). Depression is a risk factor for noncompliance with medical treatment: Meta-analysis of the effects of anxiety and depression on patient adherence. *Archives of Internal Medicine, 160,* 2101–2107.

Dishman, R. K., & Steinhardt, M. (1988). Reliability and concurrent validity for a 7-d recall of physical activity in college students. *Medicine and Science in Sports and Exercise, 1,* 14–25.

Donker, F. J., Breteler, M. H., & van der Staak, C. P. (2000). Assessment of hostility in patients with coronary heart disease. *Journal of Personality Assessment, 75,* 158–177.

Donovan, R. J., Jones, S., Holman, C. D., & Corti, B. (1998). Assessing the reliability of a stage of change scale. *Health Education Research, 13,* 285–291.

Dunn, C., Deroo, L., & Rivara, F. P. (2001). The use of brief interventions adapted from motivational interviewing across behavioral domains: A systematic review. *Addiction, 96,* 1725–1742.

Dzau, V. J., Antman, E. M., Black, H. R., Hayes, D. L., Manson, J. E., Plutzky, J., et al. (2006). The cardiovascular disease continuum validated: Clinical evidence of improved patient outcomes. Part I: Pathophysiology and clinical trial evidence (risk factors through stable coronary artery disease). *Circulation, 114,* 2850–2870.

Eaker, E. D., Sullivan, L. M., Kelly-Hayes, M., D'Agostino, R. B., Sr., & Benjamin, E. J. (2004). Does job strain increase the risk for coronary heart disease or death in men and women?: The Framingham Offspring Study. *American Journal of Epidemiology, 159,* 950–958.

ENRICHD Investigators. (2000). Enhancing recovery in coronary heart disease patients (ENRICHD): Study design and methods. *American Heart Journal, 139,* 1–9.

Erkinjuntti, T., Hokkanen, L., Sulkava, R., & Palo, J. (1988). The Blessed Dementia Scale as a screening test for dementia. *International Journal of Geriatric Psychiatry, 3,* 267–273.

Ewing, J. A. (1984). Detecting alcoholism: The CAGE questionnaire. *Journal of the American Medical Association, 252,* 1905–1907.

Farmer, K. C. (1999). Methods for measuring and monitoring medication regimen adherence in clinical trials and clinical practice. *Clinical Therapeutics, 21,* 1074–1090.

Fleming, M. F., Barry, K. L., & MacDonald, R. (1991). The Alcohol Use Disorders Identification Test (AUDIT) in a college sample. *International Journal of the Addictions, 26,* 1173–1185.

Folkman, S., & Lazarus, R. S. (1980). An analysis of coping in a middle-aged community sample. *Journal of Health and Social Behavior, 21,* 219–239.

Folstein, M. F., Fetting, J. H., Lobo, A., Niaz, U., & Capozzoli, K. D. (1984). Cognitive assessment of cancer patients. *Cancer, 53,* S2250–S2257.

Folstein, M. F., Folstein, S. E., & McHugh, P. R. (1975). Mini-mental state: A practical method for grading the cognitive state of patients for the clinician. *Journal of Psychiatric Research, 12,* 189–198.

Fountoulakis, K. N., Bech, P., Panagiotidis, P., Siamouli, M., Kantartzis, S., Papadopoulou, A., et al. (2007). Comparison of depressive indices: Reliability, validity, relationship to anxiety and personality and the role of age and life events. *Journal of Affective Disorders, 97,* 187–195.

Frasure-Smith, N., & Lesperance, F. (2003). Depression and other psychological risks following myocardial infarction. *Archives of General Psychiatry, 60,* 627–636.

Frasure-Smith, N., & Prince, R. (1985). The ischemic heart disease life stress monitoring program: Impact on mortality. *Psychosomatic Medicine, 47,* 431–445.

Friedman, M., Thoresen, C. E., Gill, J. J., Ulmer, D., Powell, L. H., Price, V. A., et al. (1986). Alteration of type A behavior and its effect on cardiac recurrences in post myocardial infarction patients: Summary results of the recurrent coronary prevention project. *American Heart Journal, 112,* 653–665.

Gallo, W. T., Teng, H. M., Falba, T. A., Kasl, S. V., Krumholz, H. M., & Bradley, E. H. (2006). The impact of late career job loss on myocardial infarction and stroke: A 10-year follow-up using the Health and Retirement Survey. *Occupational and Environmental Medicine, 63,* 683–687.

Gehi, A. K., Ali, S., Na, B., & Whooley, M. A. (2007). Self-reported medication adherence and cardiovascular events in patients with stable coronary heart disease: The heart and soul study. *Archives of Internal Medicine, 167,* 1798–1803.

Glassman, A. H., Helzer, J. E., Covey, L. S., Cottler, L. B., Stetner, F., Tipp, J. E., et al. (1990). Smoking, smoking cessation, and major depression. *Journal of the American Medical Association, 264,* 1546–1549.

Glassman, A. H., O'Connor, C. M., Califf, R. M., Swedberg, K., Schwartz, P., Bigger, J. T., Jr., et al. (2002). Sertraline treatment of major depression in patients with acute MI or unstable angina. *Journal of the American Medical Association, 288,* 701–709.

Green, C. P., Porter, C. B., Bresnahan, D. R., & Spertus, J. A. (2000). Development and evaluation of the Kansas City Cardiomyopathy Questionnaire: A new health status measure for heart failure. *Journal of the American College of Cardiology, 35,* 1245–1255.

Gross, L. D., Sallis, J. F., Buono, M. J., Roby, J. J., & Nelson, J. A. (1990). Reliability of interviewers using the Seven-Day Physical Activity Recall. *Research Quarterly for Exercise and Sport, 61,* 321–325.

Grundy, S. M., Balady, G. J., Criqui, M. H., Fletcher, G., Greenland, P., Hiratzka, L. F., et al. (1998). Primary prevention of coronary heart disease: Guidance from Framingham: A statement for healthcare professionals from the AHA Task Force on Risk Reduction. *Circulation, 97,* 1876–1887.

Haines, A. P., Imeson, J. D., & Meade, T. W. (1987). Phobic anxiety and ischaemic heart disease. *BMJ, 295,* 297–299.

Hamilton, M. (1960). A rating scale for depression. *Journal of Neurology, Neurosurgery and Psychiatry, 23,* 56–62.

Han, K., Weed, N. C., Calhoun, R. F., & Butcher, J. N. (1995). Psychometric characteristics of the MMPI-2 Cook-Medley Hostility Scale. *Journal of Personality Assessment, 65,* 567–585.

Haskell, W. L., Lee, I. M., Pate, R. R., Powell, K. E., Blair, S. N., Franklin, B. A. et al. (2007). Physical activity and public health: Updated recommendation for adults from the American College of Sports Medicine and the American Heart Association. *Circulation, 116,* 1081–1093.

Haynes, R. B., Yao, X., Degani, A., Kripalani, S., Garg, A., & McDonald, H. P. (2005). Interventions to enhance medication adherence. *Cochrane Database of Systematic Reviews,* Issue 4, Article No. CD00011.

Hintsanen, M., Kivimaki, M., Elovainio, M.,

Pulkki-Raback, L., Keskivaara, P., Juonala, M., et al. (2005). Job strain and early atherosclerosis: The Cardiovascular Risk in Young Finns study. *Psychosomatic Medicine, 67,* 740–747.

Hoodin, F., & Kalbfleisch, K. R. (2001). How psychometrically sound is the Transplant Evaluation Rating Scale for bone marrow transplant recipients? *Psychosomatics, 42,* 490–496.

Horwitz, R. I., Viscoli, C. M., Berkman, L., Donaldson, R. M., Horwitz, S. M., Murray, C. J., et al. (1990). Treatment adherence and risk of death after a myocardial infarction. *Lancet, 336,* 542–545.

Hunt, S. A., Abraham, W. T., Chin, M. H., Feldman, A. M., Francis, G. S., Ganiats, T. G., et al. (2005). ACC/AHA 2005 guideline update for the diagnosis and management of chronic heart failure in the adult: A report of the American College of Cardiology/American Heart Association Task Force on Practice Guidelines. *Circulation, 112,* 154–235.

Hyman, D. J., Pavlik, V. N., Taylor, W. C., Goodrick, G. K., & Moye, L. (2007). Simultaneous vs. sequential counseling for multiple behavior change. *Archives of Internal Medicine, 167,* 1152–1158.

Iso, H., Date, C., Yamamoto, A., Toyoshima, H., Tanabe, N., Kikuchi, S., et al. (2002). Perceived mental stress and mortality from cardiovascular disease among Japanese men and women. *Circulation, 106,* 1229–1236.

Jacobs, D. R., Ainsworth, B. E., Hartman, T. J., & Leon, A. S. (1993). A simultaneous evaluation of 10 commonly used physical activity questionnaires. *Medicine and Science in Sports and Exercise, 25,* 81–91.

Jiang, W., Babyak, M., Krantz, D. S., Waugh, R. A., Coleman, R. E., Hanson, M. M., et al. (1996). Mental stress-induced myocardial ischemia and cardiac events. *Journal of the American Medical Association, 275,* 1651–1656.

Jolliffe, J. A., Rees, K., Taylor, R. S., Thompson, D., Oldridge, N., & Ebrahim, S. (2000). Exercise-based rehabilitation for coronary heart disease. *Cochrane Database of Systematic Reviews,* Issue 4, Article No. CD001800.

Kant, A. K., Graubard, B. I., & Schatzkin, A. (2004). Dietary patterns predict mortality in a national cohort: The National Health Interview Surveys, 1987 and 1992. *Journal of Nutrition, 134,* 1793–1799.

Karasek, R., Baker, D., Marxer, F., Ahlbom, A., & Theorell, T. (1981). Job decision latitude, job demands, and cardiovascular disease: A prospective study of Swedish men. *American Journal of Public Health, 71,* 694–705.

Karasek, R., Brisson, C., Kawakami, N., Houtman, I., Bongers, P., & Amick, B. (1998). The Job Content Questionnaire (JCQ): An instrument for internationally comparative assessments of psychosocial job characteristics. *Journal of Occupational Health Psychology, 3,* 322–355.

Karasek, R. A., Theorell, T., Schwartz, J. E., Schnall, P. L., Pieper, C. F., & Michela, J. L. (1988). Job characteristics in relation to the prevalence of myocardial infarction in the U.S. Health Examination Survey (HES) and the Health and Nutrition Examination Survey (HANES). *American Journal of Public Health, 78,* 910–918.

Kawachi, I., Colditz, G. A., Ascherio, A., Rimm, E. B., Giovannucci, E., Stampfer, M. J., et al. (1994). Prospective study of phobic anxiety and risk of coronary heart disease in men. *Circulation, 89,* 1992–1997.

Kawachi, I., Sparrow, D., Vokonas, P. S., & Weiss, S. T. (1994). Symptoms of anxiety and risk of coronary heart disease: The Normative Aging Study. *Circulation, 90,* 2225–2229.

Krantz, D. S., & McCeney, M. K. (2002). Effects of psychological and social factors on organic disease: A critical assessment of research on coronary heart disease. *Annual Review of Psychology, 53,* 369.

Kubzansky, L. D. (2007). Sick at heart: The pathophysiology of negative emotions. *Cleveland Clinic Journal of Medicine, 74,* S67–S72.

Kubzansky, L. D., Kawachi, I., Spiro, A., III, Weiss, S. T., Vokonas, P. S., & Sparrow, D. (1997). Is worrying bad for your heart?: A prospective study of worry and coronary heart disease in the Normative Aging Study. *Circulation, 95,* 818–824.

Kuper, H., & Marmot, M. (2003). Job strain, job demands, decision latitude, and risk of coronary heart disease within the Whitehall II study. *Journal of Epidemiology and Community Health, 57,* 147–153.

Lagerros, Y. T., & Lagiou, P. (2007). Assessment of physical activity and energy expenditure in epidemiological research of chronic diseases. *European Journal of Epidemiology, 22,* 353–362.

Lazarus, R. S., & Folkman, S. (1984). *Stress, appraisal, and coping.* New York: Springer.

Lehto, S., Koukkunen, H., Hintikka, J., Viinamaki, H., Laakso, M., & Pyorala, K. (2000). Depression after coronary heart disease events. *Scandinavian Cardiovascular Journal, 34,* 580–583.

Leon, A. S., & Sanchez, O. A. (2001). Response of blood lipids to exercise training alone or combined with dietary intervention. *Medicine and Science in Sports and Exercise, 33,* S502–S515.

Lesperance, F., Frasure-Smith, N., Talajic, M., & Bourassa, M. G. (2002). Five-year risk of cardiac mortality in relation to initial severity and one-year changes in depression symptoms after myocardial infarction. *Circulation, 105,* 1049–1053.

Lett, H. S., Blumenthal, J. A., Babyak, M. A., Catellier, D. J., Carney, R. M., Berkman, L. F., et al. (2007). Social support and prognosis in patients at increased psychosocial risk recovering from myocardial infarction. *Health Psychology, 26,* 418–427.

Lett, H. S., Blumenthal, J. A., Babyak, M. A., Sherwood, A., Strauman, T., Robins, C., et al. (2004). Depression as a risk factor for coronary artery disease: Evidence, mechanisms, and treatment. *Psychosomatic Medicine, 66,* 305–315.

Lett, H. S., Blumenthal, J. A., Babyak, M. A., Strauman, T. J., Robins, C., & Sherwood, A. (2005). Social support and coronary heart disease: Epidemiologic evidence and implications for treatment. *Psychosomatic Medicine, 67,* 869–878.

Lezak, M. D., Howieson, D. B., Loring, D. W., Hannay, H. J., & Fischer, J. S. (2004). *Neuropsychological assessment* (4th ed.). New York: Oxford University Press.

Lichtman, J. H., Bigger, J. T., Jr., Blumenthal, J. A., Frasure-Smith, N., Kaufmann, P. G., Lesperance, F., et al. (2009). AHA science advisory. Depression and coronary heart disease. *Progress in Cardiovascular Nursing, 24,* 19–26.

Linden, W. (2000). Psychological treatments in cardiac rehabilitation: Review of rationales and outcomes. *Journal of Psychosomatic Research, 48,* 443–454.

Maes, S., & Bruggemans, E. (1990). Approach–avoidance and illness behavior in coronary heart patients. In L. R. Schmidt, P. Schwenkmezger, J. Weinman, & S. Maes (Eds.), *Theoretical and applied aspects of health psychology* (pp. 297–308). Amsterdam, The Netherlands: Harwood Academic.

Magruder-Habib, K., Stevens, H. A., & Alling, W. C. (1993). Relative performance of the MAST, VAST, and CAGE versus DSM-III-R criteria for alcohol dependence. *Journal of Clinical Epidemiology, 46,* 435–441.

Marcus, B. H., Selby, V. C., Niaura, R. S., & Rossi, J. S. (1992). Self-efficacy and the stages of exercise behavior change. *Research Quarterly for Exercise and Sport, 63,* 60–66.

Marcus, B. H., Williams, D. M., Dubbert, P. M., Sallis, J. F., King, A. C., Yancey, A. K., et al. (2006). Physical activity intervention studies: What we know and what we need to know. *Circulation, 114,* 2739–2752.

Marmot, M. G., Shipley, M. J., & Rose, G. (1984). Inequalities in death: Specific explanations of a general pattern? *Lancet, 1,* 1003–1006.

Martin, R., Watson, D., & Wan, C. K. (2000). A three-factor model of trait anger: Dimensions of affect, behavior, and cognition. *Journal of Personality, 68,* 869–897.

Matthews, K. A., & Gump, B. B. (2002). Chronic work stress and marital dissolution increase risk of posttrial mortality in men from the Multiple Risk Factor Intervention Trial. *Archives of Internal Medicine, 162,* 309–315.

McDonough, P., Duncan, G. J., Williams, D., & House, J. (1997). Income dynamics and adult mortality in the United States, 1972 through 1989. *American Journal of Public Health, 87,* 1476–1483.

McGee, H. M., Hevey, D., & Horgan, J. H. (1999). Psychosocial outcome assessments for use in cardiac rehabilitation service evaluation: A 10-year systematic review. *Social Science and Medicine, 48,* 1373–1393.

Miller, T. Q., Jenkins, C. D., Kaplan, G. A., & Salonen, J. T. (1995). Are all hostility scales alike?: Factor structure and covariation among measures of hostility. *Journal of Applied Social Psychology, 25,* 1142–1168.

Miller, T. Q., Smith, T. W., Turner, C. W., Guijarro, M. L., & Hallet, A. J. (1996). A meta-analytic review of research on hostility and physical health. *Psychological Bulletin, 119,* 322–348.

Miller, W. R. (1983). Motivational interviewing with problem drinkers. *Behavioural Psychotherapy, 11,* 147–172.

Miller, W. R., & Rollnick, S. (1991). *Motivational interviewing: Preparing people to change addictive behavior.* New York: Guilford Press.

Mitchell, P. H., Powell, L., Blumenthal, J., Norten, J., Ironson, G., Pitula, C. R., et al.

(2003). A short social support measure for patients recovering from myocardial infarction: The ENRICHD Social Support Inventory. *Journal of Cardiopulmonary Rehabilitation, 23,* 398–403.

Moberg, P. J., Lazarus, L. W., Mesholam, R. I., Bilker, W., Chuy, I. L., Neyman, I., et al. (2001). Comparison of the standard and structured interview guide for the Hamilton Depression Rating Scale in depressed geriatric inpatients. *American Journal of Geriatric Psychiatry, 9,* 35–40.

Montgomery, R. J., Gonyea, J. G., & Hooyman, N. R. (1985). Caregiving and the experience of subjective and objective burden. *Family Relations, 34,* 19–26.

Mora, S., Cook, N., Buring, J. E., Ridker, P. M., & Lee, I. M. (2007). Physical activity and reduced risk of cardiovascular events: Potential mediating mechanisms. *Circulation, 116,* 2110–2118.

Newman, M. F., Kirchner, J. L., Phillips-Bute, B., Gaver, V., Grocott, H., Jones, R. H., et al. (2001). Longitudinal assessment of neurocognitive function after coronary-artery bypass surgery. *New England Journal of Medicine, 344,* 395–402.

Nigg, C. R., Norman, G. J., Rossi, J. S., & Benisovich, S. V. (1999, March). *Processes of exercise behavior change: Redeveloping the scale.* Poster presented at the meeting of the Society of Behavioral Medicine, San Diego, CA.

Nigg, C. R., Rossi, J. S., Norman, G. J., & Benisovich, S. V. (1998). Structure of decisional balance for exercise adoption. *Annals of Behavioral Medicine, 20,* S211.

O'Connell, D., & Velicer, W. F. (1988). A decisional balance measure for weight loss. *International Journal of Addictions, 23,* 729–750.

Olbrisch, M. E., Levenson, J. L., & Hamer, R. (1989). The PACT: A rating scale for the study of clinical decision-making in psychosocial screening of organ transplant candidates. *Clinical Transplantation, 3,* 164–169.

Organ Procurement and Transplantation Network. (2006). *Annual report of the U.S. Organ Procurement and Transplantation Network and the Scientific Registry of Transplant Recipients: Transplant data 1996–2005.* Rockville, MD: Department of Health and Human Services, Health Resources and Services Administration, Healthcare Systems Bureau, Division of Transplantation; Richmond, VA: United Network for Organ Sharing; Ann Arbor, MI: University Heart Research and Education Association.

Orth-Gomér, K., Rosengren, A., & Wilhelmsen, L. (1993). Lack of social support and incidence of coronary heart disease in middle-aged Swedish men. *Psychosomatic Medicine, 55,* 37–43.

Pallonen, U. E., Leskinen, L., Prochaska, J. O., Willey, C. J., Kaariainen, R., & Salonen, J. T. (1994). A 2-year self-help smoking cessation manual intervention among middle-aged Finnish men: An application of the transtheoretical model. *Preventive Medicine, 23,* 507–514.

Parker, J. D., & Endler, N. S. (1992). Coping with coping assessment: A critical review. *European Journal of Personality, 6,* 321–344.

Pelfrene, E., Clays, E., Moreau, M., Mak, R., Vokonas, P., Kornitzer, M., et al. (2003). The Job Content Questionnaire: Methodological considerations and challenges for future research. *Archives of Public Health, 61,* 53–74.

Pescatello, L. S., Franklin, B. A., Fagard, R., Farquhar, W. B., Kelley, G. A., Ray, C. A., et al. (2004). American College of Sports Medicine position stand: Exercise and hypertension. *Medicine and Science in Sports and Exercise, 36,* 533–553.

Peter, R., Siegrist, J., Hallqvist, J., Reuterwall, C., Theorell, T., & SHEEP Study Group. (2002). Psychosocial work environment and myocardial infarction: Improving risk estimation by combining two complementary job stress models in the SHEEP Study. *Journal of Epidemiology and Community Health, 56,* 294–300.

Peterson, T. R., & Aldana, S. G. (1999). Improving exercise behavior: An application of the stages of change model in a worksite setting. *American Journal of Health Promotion, 13,* 229–232.

Petruzzello, S. J., Landers, D. M., Hatfield, B. D., Kubitz, K. A., & Salazar, W. (1991). A meta-analysis on the anxiety-reducing effects of acute and chronic exercise: Outcomes and mechanisms. *Sports Medicine, 11,* 143–182.

Posner, B. M., Martin-Munley, S. S., Smigelski, C., Cupples, L. A., Cobb, J. L., Schaefer, E., et al. (1992). Comparison of techniques for estimating nutrient intake: The Framingham Study. *Epidemiology, 3,* 171–177.

Prochaska, J. O., & DiClemente, C. C. (1983). Stages and processes of self-change of smoking: Toward an integrative model of change. *Journal of Consulting and Clinical Psychology, 51,* 390–395.

Prochaska, J. O., & DiClemente, C. C. (1984). Self-change processes, self-efficacy and decisional balance across five stages of smoking cessation. *Progress in Clinical and Biological Research, 156,* 131–140.

Prochaska, J. O., Velicer, W. F., DiClemente, C. C., & Fava, J. (1988). Measuring processes of change: Applications to the cessation of smoking. *Journal of Consulting and Clinical Psychology, 56,* 520–528.

Prochaska, J. O., Velicer, W. F., Redding, C., Rossi, J. S., Goldstein, M., DePue, J., et al. (2005). Stage-based expert systems to guide a population of primary care patients to quit smoking, eat healthier, prevent skin cancer, and receive regular mammograms. *Preventive Medicine, 14,* 406–416.

Procidano, M. E., & Heller, K. (1983). Measures of perceived social support from friends and from family: Three validation studies. *American Journal of Community Psychology, 11,* 1–24.

Radloff, L. S. (1977). The CES-D Scale: A self-report depression scale for research in the general population. *Applied Psychological Measurement, 1,* 385–401.

Rand, C. S., & Weeks, K. (1998). Measuring adherence with medication regimens in clinical care and research. In S. A. Shumaker, E. B. Schron, J. K. Ockene, & W. L. McBee (Eds.), *Handbook of health behavior change* (2nd ed., pp. 114–132). New York: Springer.

Rasmussen, J. N., Chong, A., & Alter, D. A. (2007). Relationship between adherence to evidence-based pharmacotherapy and long-term mortality after acute myocardial infarction. *Journal of the American Medical Association, 297,* 177–186.

Rauh, M. J., Hovell, M. F., Hofstetter, C. R., Sallis, J. F., & Gleghorn, A. (1992). Reliability and validity of self-reported physical activity in Latinos. *International Journal of Epidemiology, 21,* 966–971.

Rebagliato, M. (2002). Validation of self-reported smoking. *Journal of Epidemiology and Community Health, 56,* 163–164.

Rector, T. S., & Cohn, J. N. (1992). Assessment of patient outcome with the Minnesota Living with Heart Failure Questionnaire: Reliability and validity during a randomized, double-blind, placebo-controlled trial of pimobendan. *American Heart Journal, 124,* 1017–1025.

Rector, T. S., Kubo, S. H., & Cohn, J. N. (1987, October/November). Patients' self-assessment of their congestive heart failure. *Heart Failure,* pp. 198–209.

Rector, T. S., Tschumperlin, L. K., Kubo, S. H., Bank, A. J., Francis, G. S., McDonald, K. M., et al. (1995). Use of the Living with Heart Failure questionnaire to ascertain patients' perspectives on improvement in quality of life versus risk of drug-induced death. *Journal of Cardiac Failure, 1,* 201–206.

Rees, K., Taylor, R. S., Singh, S., Coats, A. J., & Ebrahim, S. (2004). Exercise-based rehabilitation for heart failure. *Cochrane Database of Systematic Reviews,* Issue 3, Article No. CD003331.

Riemsma, R. P., Pattenden, J., Bridle, C., Sowden, A. J., Mather, L., Watt, I. S., et al. (2002). A systematic review of the effectiveness of interventions based on a stages-of-change approach to promote individual behaviour change. *Health Technology Assessment, 6,* 1–231.

Robinson, B. C. (1983). Validation of a Caregiver Strain Index. *Journal of Gerontology, 38,* 344–348.

Rollnick, S., Heather, N., Gold, R., & Hall, W. (1992). Development of a short "readiness to change" questionnaire for use in brief, opportunistic interventions among excessive drinkers. *British Journal of Addiction, 87,* 743–754.

Rosamond, W., Flegal, K., Friday, G., Furie, K., Go, A., Greenlund, K., et al. (2007). Heart Disease and Stroke Statistics—2007 update: A report from the American Heart Association Statistics Committee and Stroke Statistics Subcommittee. *Circulation, 115,* 169–171.

Rosenman, R. H., Brand, R. J., Jenkins, D., Friedman, M., Straus, R., & Wurm, M. (1975). Coronary heart disease in Western Collaborative Group Study: Final follow-up experience of 8½ years. *Journal of the American Medical Association, 233,* 872–877.

Rothenhausler, H. B., Grieser, B., Nollert, G., Reichart, B., Schelling, G., & Kapfhammer, H. P. (2005). Psychiatric and psychosocial outcome of cardiac surgery with cardiopulmonary bypass: A prospective 12-month follow-up study. *General Hospital Psychiatry, 27,* 18–28.

Rozanski, A., Blumenthal, J. A., Davidson, K. W., Saab, P. G., & Kubzansky, L. (2005). The epidemiology, pathophysiology, and management of psychosocial risk factors in cardiac practice: The emerging field of behavioral cardiology. *Journal of the American College of Cardiology, 45,* 637–651.

Rozanski, A., Blumenthal, J. A., & Kaplan, J. (1999). Impact of psychological factors on the pathogenesis of cardiovascular disease and implications for therapy. *Circulation, 99,* 2197–2217.

Ruberman, W., Weinblatt, E., Goldberg, J. D., & Chaudhary, B. S. (1984). Psychosocial influences on mortality after myocardial infarction. *New England Journal of Medicine, 311,* 552–559.

Sacks, F. M., Svetkey, L. P., Vollmer, W. M., Appel, L. J., Bray, G. A., Harsha, D., et al. (2001). Effects on blood pressure of reduced dietary sodium and the Dietary Approaches to Stop Hypertension (DASH) diet. *New England Journal of Medicine, 344,* 3–10.

Sallis, J. F., Haskell, W. L., Wood, P. D., Fortmann, S. P., Rogers, T., Blair, S. N., et al. (1985). Physical activity assessment methodology in the Five-City Project. *American Journal of Epidemiology, 121,* 91–106.

Sallis, J. F., Patterson, T. L., Buono, M. J., & Nader, P. R. (1988). Relation of cardiovascular fitness and physical activity to cardiovascular disease risk factors in children and adults. *American Journal of Epidemiology, 127,* 933–941.

Sarason, I. G., Levine, H. M., Basham, R. B., & Sarason, B. R. (1983). Assessing social support: The Social Support Questionnaire. *Journal of Personality and Social Psychology, 44,* 127–139.

Saunders, J. B., Aasland, O. G., Babor, T. F., & de la Fuente, G. M., Jr. (1993). Development of the Alcohol Use Disorders Identification Test (AUDIT): WHO Collaborative Project on Early Detection of Persons with Harmful Alcohol Consumption: II. *Addiction, 88,* 791–804.

Schnall, P. L., Landsbergis, P. A., & Baker, D. (1994). Job strain and cardiovascular disease. *Annual Review of Public Health, 15,* 381–411.

Schnall, P. L., Pieper, C., Schwartz, J. E., Karasek, R. A., Schlussel, Y., Devereux, R. B., et al. (1990). The relationship between "job strain," workplace diastolic blood pressure, and left ventricular mass index: Results of a case-control study. *Journal of the American Medical Association, 263,* 1929–1935.

Shaw, K., Gennat, H., O'Rourke, P., & Del, M. C. (2006). Exercise for overweight or obesity. *Cochrane Database of Systematic Reviews,* Issue 4, Article No. CD003817.

Shekelle, R. B., Gale, M., & Norusis, M. (1985).

Type A score (Jenkins Activity Survey) and risk of recurrent coronary heart disease in the aspirin myocardial infarction study. *American Journal of Cardiology, 56,* 221–225.

Shekelle, R. B., Gale, M., Ostfeld, A. M., & Paul, O. (1983). Hostility, risk of coronary heart disease, and mortality. *Psychosomatic Medicine, 45,* 109–114.

Shen, B. J., Myers, H. F., & McCreary, C. P. (2006). Psychosocial predictors of cardiac rehabilitation quality-of-life outcomes. *Journal of Psychosomatic Research, 60,* 3–11.

Sheps, D. S., McMahon, R. P., Becker, L., Carney, R. M., Freedland, K. E., Cohen, J. D., et al. (2002). Mental stress-induced ischemia and all-cause mortality in patients with coronary artery disease: Results from the Psychophysiological Investigations of Myocardial Ischemia study. *Circulation, 105,* 1780–1784.

Shibeshi, W. A., Young-Xu, Y., & Blatt, C. M. (2007). Anxiety worsens prognosis in patients with coronary artery disease. *Journal of the American College of Cardiology, 49,* 2021–2027.

Siegrist, J. (1996). Adverse health effects of high-effort/low-reward conditions. *Journal of Occupational Health Psychology, 1,* 27–41.

Sinclair, M., McRee, B., & Babor, T. F. (1992). *Evaluation of the reliability of AUDIT.* Unpublished manuscript, University of Connecticut School of Medicine, Alcohol Research Center.

Smith, T. W., Glazer, K., Ruiz, J. M., & Gallo, L. C. (2004). Hostility, anger, aggressiveness, and coronary heart disease: An interpersonal perspective on personality, emotion, and health. *Journal of Personality, 72,* 1217–1270.

Spencer, L., Adams, T. B., Malone, S., Roy, L., & Yost, E. (2006). Applying the transtheoretical model to exercise: A systematic and comprehensive review of the literature. *Health Promotion Practice, 7,* 428–443.

Spielberger, C. D. (1983). *Manual for the State–Trait Anxiety Inventory (STAI Form Y).* Palo Alto, CA: Mind Garden.

SRNT Subcommittee on Biochemical Verification. (2002). Biochemical verification of tobacco use and cessation. *Nicotine and Tobacco Research, 4,* 149–159.

Steer, R. A., Ball, R., Ranieri, W. F., & Beck, A. T. (1999). Dimensions of the Beck Depression Inventory—II in clinically depressed outpatients. *Journal of Clinical Psychology, 55,* 117–128.

Steer, R. A., Cavalieri, T. A., Leonard, D. M., & Beck, A. T. (1999). Use of the Beck Depression Inventory for Primary Care to screen for major depression disorders. *General Hospital Psychiatry, 21*, 106–111.

Stephenson, B. J., Rowe, B. H., Haynes, R. B., Macharia, W. M., & Leon, G. (1993). The rational clinical examination: Is this patient taking the treatment as prescribed? *Journal of the American Medical Association, 269*, 2779–2781.

Strodl, E., Kenardy, J., & Aroney, C. (2003). Perceived stress as a predictor of the self-reported new diagnosis of symptomatic CHD in older women. *International Journal of Behavioral Medicine, 10*, 205–220.

Subar, A. F., Thompson, F. E., Kipnis, V., Midthune, D., Hurwitz, P., McNutt, S., et al. (2001). Comparative validation of the Block, Willett, and National Cancer Institute food frequency questionnaires: The Eating at America's Table Study. *American Journal of Epidemiology, 154*, 1089–1099.

Suls, J., & Fletcher, B. (1985). The relative efficacy of avoidant and nonavoidant coping strategies: A meta-analysis. *Health Psychology, 4*, 249–288.

Sumanen, M. P., Suominen, S. B., Koskenvuo, M. J., Sillanmaki, L. H., & Mattila, K. J. (2004). Occurrence of symptoms and depressive mood among working-aged coronary heart disease patients. *Health and Quality of Life Outcomes*. Available at *www.hqlo.com/content/2/1/60*.

Svarstad, B. L., Chewning, B. A., Sleath, B. L., & Claesson, C. (1999). The Brief Medication Questionnaire: A tool for screening patient adherence and barriers to adherence. *Patient Education and Counseling, 37*, 113–124.

Taylor, C. B., Youngblood, M. E., Catellier, D., Veith, R. C., Carney, R. M., Burg, M. M., et al. (2005). Effects of antidepressant medication on morbidity and mortality in depressed patients after myocardial infarction. *Archives of General Psychiatry, 62*, 792–798.

Thompson, F. E., & Byers, T. (1994). Dietary assessment resource manual. *Journal of Nutrition, 124*, S2245–S2317.

Thurston, R. C., Kubzansky, L. D., Kawachi, I., & Berkman, L. F. (2006). Do depression and anxiety mediate the link between educational attainment and CHD? *Psychosomatic Medicine, 68*, 25–32.

Twardella, D., Rothenbacher, D., Hahmann, H., Wusten, B., & Brenner, H. (2006). The underestimated impact of smoking and smoking cessation on the risk of secondary cardiovascular disease events in patients with stable coronary heart disease: Prospective cohort study. *Journal of the American College of Cardiology, 47*, 887–889.

Twillman, R. K., Manetto, C., Wellisch, D. K., & Wolcott, D. L. (1993). The Transplant Evaluation Rating Scale: A revision of the Psychosocial Levels System for evaluating organ transplant candidates. *Journal of Consultation Liason Psychiatry, 34*, 144–153.

Vartiainen, E., Seppala, T., Lillsunde, P., & Puska, P. (2002). Validation of self-reported smoking by serum cotinine measurement in a community-based study. *Journal of Epidemiology and Community Health, 56*, 167–170.

Velicer, W. F., Rossi, J. S., DiClemente, C. C., & Prochaska, J. O. (1996). A criterion measurement model for health behavior change. *Addictive Behaviors, 21*, 555–584.

Vingerhoets, G. (2001). Cognitive consequences of myocardial infarction, cardiac arrhythmias, and cardiac arrest. In S. R. Walstein & M. F. Elias (Eds.), *Neuropsychology of cardiovascular disease* (pp. 143–163). Mahwah, NJ: Erlbaum.

Vitolins, M. Z., Rand, C. S., Rapp, S. R., Ribisl, P. M., & Sevick, M. A. (2000). Measuring adherence to behavioral and medical interventions. *Controlled Clinical Trials, 21*, S118–S194.

Waldstein, S. R., & Elias, M. F. (2001). *Neuropsychology of cardiovascular disease.* Mahwah, NJ: Erlbaum.

West, R., Zatonski, W., Przewozniak, K., & Jarvis, M. J. (2007). Can we trust national smoking prevalence figures?: Discrepancies between biochemically assessed and self-reported smoking rates in three countries. *Cancer Epidemiology, Biomarkers and Prevention, 16*, 820–822.

Whelton, P. K., He, J., Appel, L. J., Cutler, J. A., Havas, S., Kotchen, T. A., et al. (2002). Primary prevention of hypertension: Clinical and public health advisory from the National High Blood Pressure Education Program. *Journal of the American Medical Association, 288*, 1882–1888.

Whelton, S. P., Chin, A., Xin, X., & He, J. (2002). Effect of aerobic exercise on blood pressure: A meta-analysis of randomized, controlled trials. *Annals of Internal Medicine, 136*, 493–503.

Willett, W. (1998). *Nutritional epidemiology: Monographs in epidemiology and biostatistics* (2nd ed.). Oxford, UK: Oxford University Press.

Williams, J. B. (1988). A structured interview guide for the Hamilton Depression Rating Scale. *Archives of General Psychiatry, 45,* 742–747.

Woloshin, S., Schwartz, L. M., Tosteson, A. N., Chang, C. H., Wright, B., Plohman, J., et al. (1997). Perceived adequacy of tangible social support and health outcomes in patients with coronary artery disease. *Journal of General Internal Medicine, 12,* 613–618.

Xin, X., He, J., Frontini, M. G., Ogden, L. G., Motsamai, O. I., & Whelton, P. K. (2001). Effects of alcohol reduction on blood pressure: A meta-analysis of randomized controlled trials. *Hypertension, 38,* 1112–1117.

Yusuf, S., Hawken, S., Ounpuu, S., Dans, T., Avezum, A., Lanas, F., et al. (2004). Effect of potentially modifiable risk factors associated with myocardial infarction in 52 countries (the INTERHEART study): Case-control study. *Lancet, 364,* 937–952.

Zeidner, M., & Hammer, A. L. (1992). Coping with missile attack: Resources, strategies, and outcomes. *Journal of Personality, 60,* 709–746.

Zung, W. W. (1965). A self-rating depression scale. *Archives of General Psychiatry, 12,* 63–70.

CHAPTER 14

Chronic Pain

Donald D. McGeary
Robert J. Gatchel
Cindy A. McGeary
Monica Escamilla

The evaluation of chronic musculoskeletal pain (CMP) conditions is a primary concern for all treatment practitioners, and CMP assessment can pose unique challenges requiring careful thought and planning. The goal of this chapter is to identify some of the more important domains in chronic pain assessment, highlight the reasons why assessment of each domain is important, point the reader to some of the available assessment resources touching on each domain, and (when applicable) examine how assessment information and tools can be used to meaningfully track outcomes.

There are a number of reasons why CMP assessment can be a significant challenge, one of the foremost of which is inconsistency in how musculoskeletal pain is defined. Definitions of CMP vary along several dimensions, including the longevity (or chronicity) of the pain, the contribution of physical and psychosocial factors to the pain experience, and the presence or absence of a clear pathophysiological etiology of pain. For example, Wright and Gatchel (2002) offer one comprehensive definition citing the U.S. Department of Labor, which defines a musculoskeletal disorder as "an injury or disorder of the muscles, tendons, ligaments, joints, cartilage, and spinal discs" (p. 349). Although definitions may vary, it is reasonable to assume that CMP is an enduring pain associated with initial damage to the musculoskeletal system with pain duration of sufficient length to result in chronic psychosocial distress and behavioral change.

Statistics on the prevalence and cost of musculoskeletal disorders vary between sources due to differences in the definition of musculoskeletal disorder, but all sources agree that the prevalence of musculoskeletal disorders is disturbingly high. The U.S. Department of Labor (2000) noted that 593,000 musculoskeletal disorders were reported in the United States in 1998, with an average of 5 work days lost per injury claim (Wright & Gatchel, 2002). Andersson, Pope, Frymoyer, and Snook (1991) found a lifetime incidence of spinal disorders ranging from 51.4 to 70%, and a report by the National Research Council (NRC; 2001) revealed that 15% of the American population had suffered from at least one musculoskeletal disorder in 1990, resulting in a treatment cost of $215 billion. The NRC also warned that pain-related costs are expected to rise as the incidence of musculoskeletal pain continues to increase in the future. In terms of spinal pain alone, annual expenditures rose 65% during the period from 1997 to 2005, without any measurable improvement in outcomes (Martin et al., 2008). The Bureau of Labor Statistics (2009) found that 195,150 back injuries and 379,340 work-related injuries involving sprains, strains, or tears were diagnosed in 2009. Furthermore, a recent report from the National Institute of Arthritis and Musculoskeletal and Skin Diseases (NIAMS; 2010) noted that one-fourth of the adult U.S. population will experience at least 1 day of low back pain in a 3-month period.

CMP has been linked to several etiological factors, including physical stress, psychosocial variables, job strain, social variables, and even smoking, all of which should be considered in assessment (Bergman et al., 2001). As a result, assessment for CMP can be complex and multifaceted. Price, McGrath, Rafii, and Buckingham (1983) noted that a "good" pain assessment battery should measure specific aspects of the complex pain concept in a valid and reliable way. This revelation represented a significant change in the way in which pain assessment was conceptualized. The earliest measure of pain was based on the patient's subjective report upon presentation for medical treatment, often consisting of a simple and unidimensional assessment (Kast & Collins, 1966). This assessment was later supplemented by experimental attempts to develop a more objective measurement of pain through the use of an animal pain model, which was evaluated based on reflexive behavioral responses to painful stimuli. Animal models were primarily studied in the hopes of identifying specific pain-related behavioral and physiological responses that could be used to better quantify the human pain experience (cf. Chapman et al., 1985). These reflexive animal pain behaviors were considered an indirect measure of pain resulting from both sensory and motor processes and contributed little to our understanding of human pain. Chapman et al. (1985) found that animal models of pain only provided basic information about specific physiological responses to pain, neglecting more high-level cognitive pain responses more likely to be implicated in human pain processing. Later animal research began to focus more on voluntary behaviors in response to painful or aversive stimuli, including writhing,

vocalizing, escape, avoidance, and stimulus discrimination (Chapman et al., 1985). Although these data were more applicable to a human model of pain, they focused purely on motivational aspects of pain, neglecting the important affective component of the pain response.

Attempts to evaluate pain based on a human model began with a psychophysical model of pain in which a stimulus "threshold" was conceptualized. It was surmised that an aversive stimulus with adequate intensity to overcome one's pain threshold would be considered "painful" (Chapman et al., 1985). Research investigating the pain threshold concept was easy for health care professionals to understand, but the pain threshold theory was found to be fairly insensitive to analgesic effects (Beecher, 1957), and it produced inconsistent experimental outcomes (Chapman et al., 1985). Correlates of these simple pain report measures, including pain-related behaviors and autonomic physiological responses, were eventually added to more comprehensive models of pain to better capture the complexity of pain assessment (Ohnhaus & Adler, 1975). Through these efforts, pain measurement has evolved from its infancy of estimating and scientifically testing a person's pain threshold and tolerance to a more complex assessment using various psychosocial and physiological methods (Price et al., 1983). Even today there is still a great need to isolate the best measures for monitoring therapeutic gains and outcomes for specific treatment modalities and patient groups (Wittink & Carr, 2008).

This chapter explores a number of different concerns relevant to the assessment of CMP. For each area discussed, specific targets for assessment are reviewed, reliable methods of assessment are suggested, and interpretive guidance is provided. Though there is a great breadth of assessment options for all pain domains, only a few assessment options are discussed for each (for brevity's sake). For the reader's convenience, Table 14.1 summarizes many of the measures discussed. Furthermore, the recently published fifth edition of the *Diagnostic and Statistical Manual of Mental Disorders* (DSM-5; American Psychiatric Association, 2013) has resulted in some changes to assessment and diagnosis for pain-related conditions. Where

TABLE 14.1. Common Chronic Pain Measures

Domain	Measure	Interpretation/outcome
Demographics	Demo sheet	• Higher pain prevalence among elderly • Younger pain sufferers more likely to use cognitive coping strategies • Female sufferers more likely to have endured childhood abuse • Consider race- and SES-based differences in health care access
Socioeconomic outcomes	Follow-up interview	• Disability venue and case settlement • Financial situation • Planned health care utilization • Employment history posttreatment
Depression	Beck Depression Inventory	• Use two-factor approach (Poole et al., 2009) • Increased depression is associated with worsening pain • Concern about high number of somatic items
	Hamilton Depression Rating Scale	• Score ≥ 25 suggests significant depression
	Center for Epidemiologic Studies Depression Scale	• Total score ≥ 19 suggests notable depression
Anxiety	Hospital Anxiety and Depression Scale	• Anxiety scale score ≥ 8, suspicious for anxiety • Anxiety scale score ≥ 11, anxiety definitely present
	Beck Anxiety Inventory	• Total score ≥ 11 suggestive of some anxiety • Concerns about high number of somatic items
	Pain Anxiety Symptoms Scale	• Four-factor structure • Improvements on scale related to increased physical functioning and decreased self-reported disability
Personality	Minnesota Multiphasic Personality Inventory (MMPI-2)	• Disability profile (four or more significantly elevated clinical scales) associated with significantly greater psychopathology (Gatchel et al., 2006)
	Personality Assessment Inventory (PAI)	• Four pain-specific factors identified (Karlin et al., 2005)
Pain quality/ intensity assessment	Visual analogue scale Numeric Rating Scale	• Should have at least 11 points • Should have behavioral anchors at extremes and center • Need at least one-third decrease in pain intensity for clinical significant difference
	McGill Pain Questionnaire	• Higher scores associated with higher pain
Health-related quality of life	Short Form–36	• MCS ≤ 35 indicative of significant risk for depression
Pain coping	Multidimensional Pain Inventory	• Coping profiles are useful to assess environmental/social factors contributing to pain
Fear avoidance	Fear Avoidance Beliefs Questionnaire	• Physical Activity (PA) and Work (W) subscales • PA score > 15, significant physical fear avoidance • W score ≥ 34 suggests poor outcomes of treatment
	Tampa Scale of Kinesiophobia	• Higher scores predict greater functional disability • Two- and four-factor interpretations available
Pain acceptance	Chronic Pain Acceptance Questionnaire	• Higher scores indicate higher levels of pain acceptance and more likely treatment engagement

(continued)

TABLE 14.1. *(continued)*

Domain	Measure	Interpretation/outcome
Pain catastrophizing	Pain Catastrophizing Scale	• Total score ≥ 30 indicates clinically significant catastrophizing, suggesting need for cognitive therapy
Pain behaviors	Observation	• Pain behaviors rarely indicate malingering
	Waddell signs	• Pain behaviors usually suggest a pain sufferer's serious concerns about pain
Pain-related disability	Oswestry	• Designed for back pain but adapted for other musculoskeletal pain conditions • Score indicates percent of disability at site
	Million Visual Analogue Scale	• Scores > 85 suggest "severe" disability • Decreased scores after treatment suggest improvement

relevant, we include a description of changes to assessment and interpretation based on DSM-5.

Self-Reported Pain Measures

At the outset, it should be noted that Worzer, Theodore, Rogerson, and Gatchel (2008) have provided a comprehensive review of commonly used self-report measures of pain and disability, as well as a comparison of their respective effect sizes in different pain populations. Some information on these measures is presented later, but additional information can be found in Worzer et al. (2008). Additionally, the reader will find an excellent, detailed overview of chronic pain assessment in the most recent edition of the *Handbook of Pain Assessment* (Turk & Melzack, 2011).

Pain Intensity Rating Scales

Because of the frequency with which they are used, pain ratings deserve specific attention. It seems that the vast majority of pain treatment providers often rely on a brief pain intensity rating as both a diagnostic and outcome measure for pain treatment (Zanoli, Stromqvist, & Jonsson, 2001). Despite the widespread use of these ratings, few practitioners seem to have a clear idea about the best mechanism for assessing pain intensity and how the resultant data should be interpreted, a situation that is particularly troublesome due the significant increase in the use of pain ratings among medical providers

after the Joint Commission identified pain as "the fifth vital sign" (Lorenz et al., 2009). This section describes existing options for assessing pain intensity, examines available information on how to develop a "good" pain intensity rating system, and provides guidance on how these ratings should be interpreted.

Scott and Huskisson (1976) observed that "the measurement of pain must always be subjective since pain is a subjective phenomenon—only the patient can therefore measure its severity" (p. 184). Although early rating schemes for pain involved an ordinal measure in which pain was assessed as "mild," "moderate," or "severe," these ratings have been replaced by visual analogue scales (VASs) and numerical rating scales (NRSs). These measures offer a statistical improvement over categorical ratings because they can generate interval or ratio data, allowing for a more sensitive measure. It must be noted, however, that categorical ratings of pain do still offer some value, especially at their extremes. For example, McGeary, Mayer, and Gatchel (2006) found that "extreme" pain ratings (reflected as a pain rating of either 9 or 10 out of 10 on an NRS) are significantly predictive of future surgical interventions, even after successful completion of a pain management program.

The VAS of pain assessment, described as "a straight line, the ends of which are defined as the extreme limits of the sensation or response being measured" (Scott & Huskisson, 1976, p. 175), represents a truly continuous scale of pain intensity. VASs can be modified with descriptive terms placed at equal intervals along the line to give patients anchors for rating their pain on the line; this adaptation has been classified as a graphic rating scale (GRS; Scott & Huskisson, 1976). The GRS improves on the VAS by helping patients choose where to make a mark on the VAS line, resulting in more reliable responding among groups of patients. A good VAS or GRS should specifically define the sensation being evaluated, with definite cutoff points at the median response thought to occur in the exact center of the line (Scott & Huskisson, 1976). Captions at either end of the VAS line should not be extremely worded (e.g., "terribly severe"), and descriptors should be short and easily understood.

In an effort to strike a balance between the benefits of the GRS and VAS, Jensen, Turner, and Romano (1994) explored the use of NRSs of pain. An NRS is the most common metric used for subjective pain assessment and typically involves asking a patient to rate the intensity of his or her pain on an ascending scale ranging from 0 or 1 up to 5 or 10. To address disagreement about the most valid and reliable format of an NRS, Jensen and colleagues (1994) evaluated NRSs of various increments with a sample of patients with chronic pain. Jensen et al. (1994) concluded that NRSs with 11 and 21 points are comparable to the VAS psychometrically and should be used preferentially because they are easier for patients to complete. The authors replicated these results in a sample of patients with low back pain.

Further studies have sought to examine the clinical significance of changes in pain rating scores. Stahmer, Shofer, Marino, Shepherd, and Abbuhl (1998) evaluated an NRS measure of pain intensity, along with a measure of patient treatment satisfaction and pain relief. They concluded that an NRS reduction of 57% represented a clinically significant change in pain intensity based on a comparison with patient reports of pain relief and satisfaction. However, further investigation revealed that the amount of pain reduction necessary for significant clinical changes in pain is dependent on the patient's pretreatment pain levels. Patients with initial NRS ratings of less than 5 out of 10 needed an 84% decrease in pain in order to consider the relief significant. Conversely, patients with pretreatment pain of 5 or more out of 10 needed only a 29% reduction in

pain by the NRS measurement to achieve clinically significant relief. The authors hypothesized that there may be a threshold above which even small decreases in pain can bring relief, but below which greater decreases in pain are needed to be clinically significant. It should be noted, though, that a 2005 consensus report concluded that only a minimum of a one-third decrease in self-reported pain should be considered clinically significant (Dworkin et al., 2005).

Quantified Pain Drawing

Early evaluations of pain involved the use of "pain charts," which allowed physicians to make quick evaluations of pain severity and location, as well as to determine the origin of pain (Ohlund, Eek, Palmblad, Areskoug, & Nachemson, 1996). These charts have since been improved as more scientific quantified pain drawings with multiple scoring techniques yielding a wide range of information about pain. The Quantified Pain Drawing (QPD; Mooney, 1984) is a nonverbal measure of pain location and pain severity. The resultant output of the QPD is a three-part score indicating overall pain intensity, as well as pain intensity scores specific to the trunk and extremities. A second component of the QPD includes a brief visual analogue measure of pain intensity. This second portion comprises a 10-centimeter horizontal line on which the patient is asked to make a mark to rate his or her pain intensity. The established cutoff scores for this portion of the instrument are as follows: ratings between 0 and 4 indicate no or mild pain, ratings from 4 to 6 indicate moderate pain, and ratings from 7 to 10 indicate severe pain (McGeary et al., 2006).

McGill Pain Questionnaire

The McGill Pain Questionnaire (MPQ; McGill pain index) is a self-administered questionnaire that was developed by Melzack and Torgerson in 1971. Although it was originally used in evaluating pain therapies, its application has extended to monitoring pain over time and to measuring the effectiveness of any intervention. To date it has been translated into most European languages, including Spanish, as well as Arabic and Canadian French. Results of the questionnaire provide a subjective description of pain based on sensory qualities (skin color, temperature changes), affective qualities (tension, fear), and evaluative concerns that can help gauge intensity of pain. The questionnaire takes 15–20 minutes to administer.

The questionnaire is divided into three sections that quantify experience of pain, change of pain over time, and intensity of pain. It includes a list of 102 words describing pain, organized into 20 categories, with each word assigned a value. Patients are asked to circle only the words that best describe their present pain. Four scoring and interpretation methods are proposed that include sum of scale value for words in a category or across all categories, rank placement of each word within its category, number of selected words, and present pain intensity score (PPI). Tests of validity indicate that PPI scores do not agree closely with other scores. Tests of reliability (test–retest method) have yielded an average consistency of 70.3%. Degree of correlation between sensory and affective scores was found to be independent of type of pain evaluated. The MPQ was shortened and revised into the second edition short-form MPQ (SF-MPQ-2; Dworkin et al., 2009). The SF-MPQ-2 includes only 22 items while maintaining the excellent validity and reliability of the original measure. The revision of the MPQ also enhanced its validity and reliability in the assessment of neuropathic pain (Dworkin et al., 2009).

Social and Cognitive Factors

There are a number of social and cognitive variables to consider when assessing chronic pain. In the social domain, primary consideration is often given to the measurement of quality of life and approaches to coping with CMP. Although a number of cognitive variables contribute to chronic pain experience, the concepts of fear avoidance, pain catastrophizing, and pain acceptance are starting to receive a great deal of attention.

Health-Related Quality of Life

Health-related quality of life is a significant concern for any individual struggling with a chronic health condition. The Medical

Outcomes Survey, Short Form (SF-36), is a comprehensive health survey of 36 items, originally created for clinical and research use in the assessment of health-related quality of life. The SF-36 includes two multi-item scales that assess eight health-related concepts, including physical functioning, role limitations due to physical health, social limitations, role limitations due to emotional health, bodily pain, general mental health, vitality, and general physical health perceptions (Ware & Sherbourne, 1992). Krishnan et al. (1985) note that the SF-36 serves as a specifically good measure of health status among pain sufferers and can be additionally used as a reliable indicator of significant depression among patients with pain (Mental Component Summary; MCS ≤ 35 indicates significant depression). A second version of the SF-36 (SF-36 Version 2) was published in 2000 to address international concerns about the sensitivity of the measure to patient populations outside of the United States (Hawthorne, Osborne, Taylor, & Sansoni, 2007).

Measures of Pain Coping

The Multidimensional Pain Inventory (MPI) was developed by Kerns, Turk, and Rudy in 1985 as a self-report measure of the impact of pain on various aspects of one's life based on 12 subscales measuring participation in activities of daily living, response of others to a patient with pain, and a patient's communication of his or her pain. Turk and Rudy have also developed a system of classifying MPI score profiles into categories of coping, primarily interpersonally distressed copers, adaptive copers, and dysfunctional copers (Turk & Rudy, 1988). The MPI has been widely used in studies of chronic pain and chronic pain treatment and has been shown to have good psychometric properties. Scoring programs are available for the MPI through the University of Pittsburgh Pain Medicine Program (see *www.pain.pitt. edu/mpi*), the most recent of which relies on Rasch scoring methods to improve the psychometrics of MPI scale scores. There have been some concerns about the stability of the MPI coping profiles (McKillop & Nielson, 2011), which have prompted more recent research exploring the clinical utility of the MPI. Although MPI coping profiles have been questioned as pain intervention outcomes, a recent study found that these profiles can reliably and validly classify patients with pain who may not respond well to "typical" pain intervention (Choi, Mayer, Williams, & Gatchel, 2013).

Fear Avoidance

The concept of fear avoidance has started to move to the fore of significance in pain-related treatment, assessment, and research. Briefly, the term "fear avoidance" refers to a purposeful decrease in functional activity due to concerns about harm that may result from the activity, even when these concerns are not substantiated. Fear avoidance accompanies a confusion regarding activity-related increases in pain intensity. Pain sufferers who experience an increase in pain during physical activity may confuse this pain increase with harm, when, in fact, the pain increase represents natural muscle soreness due to physical deconditioning or other non-harmful activity-related pain. Activity may be unnecessarily decreased due to these concerns, further contributing to deconditioning and removing the pain sufferer from access to external coping resources that may help her or him better manage pain. Measures of fear avoidance have started to proliferate, but the two most common measures in use today are described next.

Fear Avoidance Beliefs Questionnaire

The Fear Avoidance Beliefs Questionnaire (FABQ) was developed by Waddell, Mewton, Henderson, Somerville, and Main (1993), and it has two components: one that assesses a general fear of physical activity (FABQ-PA), and the other assessing fear of work-related activities (FABQ-W). All items are rated on a 0–6 scale on which a 0 rating represents complete disagreement with a statement and 6 represents complete agreement. The FABQ-PA subscale consists of four items with a scale score ranging from 0 to 24; the FABQ-W subscale consists of seven items with scale scores ranging from 0 to 42. The Work component of the FABQ seems to show a strong association with pain-related lost work time, suggesting that the FABQ-W scale may have a great value in assessing psychosocial factors that could interfere with return to work in patients

with chronic pain. Some attempts to establish cutoff scores for the FABQ have already been undertaken, though more work may be necessary to identify the most meaningful cutoffs. Crombez, Vlaeyen, Heuts, and Lysens (1999) identified a FABQ-PA score greater than 15 points as a "high" level of activity-related fear avoidance; Burton, Waddell, Tillotson, and Summerton (1999) echoed this. Fritz and George (2002) identified the FABQ-W as the best measure of predicting work return and pain chronicity for those with acute low back pain. They determined that a FABQ-W score of 29 or below was predictive of recovery and work return, whereas a score of 34 or more on the FABQ-W subscale was indicative of worse outcomes (see also George, Bialosky, & Fritz, 2004).

Research is already accumulating in support of the FABQ as a measure of fear avoidance in pain. Grotle, Vollestad, and Brox (2006) found that fear avoidance, as measured by the FABQ, can be an effective predictor of long-term problems with chronic pain and disability, even after adjusting for possible confounding sociodemographic and pain variables. They also noted that fear avoidance seemed to play a role in the development of pain chronicity and the onset of pain-related disability. Coudeyre and colleagues (2007) further state that fear avoidance may begin to develop early in the process of pain chronicity (at least for low back pain). The authors indicate that those patients with pain who endorse higher scores on the Physical Activity subscale of the FABQ are more likely to endorse more self-imposed limitations on active recreational activity (i.e., sports), whereas those with occupational back injuries are likely to exhibit higher FABQ–Work subscale scores. In a novel contribution to fear avoidance research, Poiraudeau et al. (2006) and Coudeyre et al. (2007) found that physicians who endorse high levels of fear avoidance related to physical activity (FABQ-PA) are more likely to have patients with pain who endorse high levels of both physical and work-related fear avoidance beliefs.

Tampa Scale for Kinesiophobia

The Tampa Scale for Kinesiophobia (TSK) is another widely used measure of activity-related fears among those with chronic pain.

The TSK specifically measures fears of reinjury associated with movement among those with existing pain using a 17-item format in which each item is rated on a 4-point Likert scale with values ranging from "strongly agree" to "strongly disagree" (Kori, Miller, & Todd, 1990). High TSK scores are typically associated with greater levels of fear of movement due to concerns about reinjury. Further, high TSK scores have been found to significantly predict functional disability among pain sufferers (Vlaeyen, Kole-Snijders, Boeren, & van Eek, 1995). Several attempts have been made to identify a meaningful factor structure for the TSK. Vlaeyen and colleagues identified four factors in the Dutch version of the TSK, including concerns about Harm, Fear of Reinjury, Avoidance of Activity, and the Importance of Exercise. Clark, Kori, and Brockel (1996) identified two TSK factors: Avoidance of Activity and Pathological Focus on Somatic Symptoms. Goubert, Vlaeyen, Crombez, and Craig (2011) relied on confirmatory factor analysis to better substantiate the factor structure of the TSK. The authors found that Clark et al.'s (1996) two-factor model of the TSK was the best fit and defined the two factors as Harm and Fear Avoidance.

Pain Acceptance

Acceptance of CMP can play a significant role in how an individual responds to pain and engages in pain treatment. Often, those with chronic pain conditions will experience initial difficulty accepting that the condition is chronic and focus on treatment with a short-term view, often with the hope of finding a "cure" or "fix" to the pain condition. This may result in a hesitancy to engage in chronic pain treatment modalities that are designed for long-term management. Developing a sense of pain acceptance likely contributes to motivation to engage in pain management treatment and may have an impact on catastrophic thinking about pain. Studies are currently under way to explore the relationship between catastrophic thoughts about CMP and acceptance of chronic pain.

Chronic Pain Acceptance Questionnaire

The Chronic Pain Acceptance Questionnaire (CPAQ; McCracken, Vowles, & Eccleston, 2004) is designed to assess the acceptance of chronic pain. Acceptance of chronic pain is described as living a meaningful life despite feeling sensations of pain (Vowles, McCracken, & Eccleston, 2008). The CPAQ is a 20-item self-report measure. It has two subscales: Activities Engagement and Pain Willingness. With these two subscales, it assesses both the degree to which pain influences behavior ("It's a relief to realize that I don't have to change my pain to get on with my life") and the degree of effort an individual puts forth in an attempt to control pain ("I have to struggle to do things when I have pain"). Patients are asked to rate how true each statement is related to their own experience of pain. Items are scored on a 7-point Likert scale (ranging from 0, *never true*, to 6, *always true*). A total score is obtained by summing the two subscale scores together, with scores ranging from 0 to 120. When interpreting the CPAQ, higher scores indicate greater levels of pain acceptance. The CPAQ shows very good to excellent internal consistency and shows moderate to high correlations with measures of avoidance, distress, and daily functioning (McCracken et al., 2004).

Pain Catastrophizing

Pain catastrophizing is best defined as "an exaggerated negative mental set brought to bear during actual or anticipated painful experience" (Sullivan et al., 2001, p. 53). Sullivan, Thorn, Rodgers, and Ward (2004) suggest that there is a link between catastrophic thinking and the development of chronic pain. They stated that catastrophic thinking contributes to higher levels of pain and emotional distress, increasing the likelihood that a pain condition will persist over an extended period of time. Further, Picavet, Vlaeyen, and Schouten (2002) found that catastrophic thoughts about pain are significantly related to pain fear avoidance even when one controls for the possible impacts of pain severity and duration. The authors also documented that high levels of premorbid pain catastrophizing are predictive of chronic low back pain development later in life.

Pain Catastrophizing Scale

The Pain Catastrophizing Scale (PCS) was developed in 1995 by Michael Sullivan and his colleagues at the University Centre for Research on Pain and Disability (Sullivan, Bishop, & Pivik, 1995). It is one of the most widely administered scales for examining the impact of catastrophic thinking on pain symptoms. The PCS measures three elements of catastrophizing, including rumination ("I can't stop thinking about how much it hurts"), magnification ("I worry that something serious may happen"), and helplessness ("It's awful and I feel that it overwhelms me"). Participants are asked to reflect on 13 statements describing different thoughts and feelings that may be associated with pain. Participants are asked to respond to which degree they have experienced each statement on a 5-point Likert scale. The Likert scale includes the following responses: 0, *not at all*; 1, *to a slight degree*; 2, *to a moderate degree*; 3, *to a great degree*; and 4, *all the time*. PCS scoring results in both a total score and three subscale scores (Rumination, Magnification, and Helplessness). The total score is computed by summing the responses to all items. PCS total scores can range from 0 to 52. PCS scores are normally distributed (suggesting that people experience different levels of catastrophizing); however, a total PCS score of 30 is indicative of a clinically relevant level of catastrophizing. The PCS has been shown to have adequate to excellent internal consistency (Sullivan et al., 1995). Clinicians can easily use this measure to evaluate catastrophic thinking, keeping in mind that people who score highly on this measure may have an increased risk of developing chronic pain. PCS total score can be broken into three subscales measuring rumination about pain, magnification of pain, and helpless thoughts about pain. This scale, which takes less than 5 minutes to complete and score, is publicly available and free to duplicate and use.

Behavioral Factors

The assessment of behavioral symptoms associated with CMP can add a great deal to one's understanding of how a chronic pain condition is developed and maintained. Evidence of muscular bracing through static postures or purposeful limitation of movement may suggest increased muscle tension that can add to pain intensity. Changes in gait or posture in response to pain may be interpreted in light of subjective disability and functional measures to help describe the impact of pain on functioning. Audible utterances in response to pain exacerbation may be a sign of distress or a way of eliciting help when it is needed. All of these behaviors are relevant to musculoskeletal pain assessment and should be documented. Some behaviors may even help a treating practitioner identify how much of a role behavioral manifestations of distress play in functional impairment; examples of these behaviors include Waddell signs (see the next subsection).

Pain Behaviors

"Waddell signs" refers to a short list of behaviors and signs first developed by Waddell, Gordon, Kummel, and Venner (1980) as a brief measure of a pain sufferer's communicated pain intensity. Though commonly interpreted as an assessment of malingering among pain patients, Waddell signs were originally intended to help pain treatment providers establish an objective metric for distress associated with the experience of chronic pain and to identify predictors of secondary gain through exaggerated pain report. Specifically, Main and Waddell (1998) describe five behavioral signs indicating that a patient with pain is trying to purposefully communicate seriousness about his or her pain experience to others. These five signs include superficial tenderness, pain response elicited from activity that should not induce pain (e.g., exerting downward pressure on the top of the head), difference in pain report when distracted during manipulation, regional weakness or sensory variation that are manifested in an unexpected manner, and exaggerated response to physical examination.

Data supporting the usefulness of Waddell signs are mixed, and these mixed results are likely attributable to differences in how individuals interpret Waddell signs. For example, there are some who suggest that Waddell signs offer some information about "psychological overlay" to chronic pain, but they do not completely rule out the impact of physical factors (Waddell et al., 1980; Main & Waddell, 1998). Though some support the use of Waddell sign assessment to detect malingering in pain sufferers, others have suggested that there is no association between Waddell sign assessments and malingering in pain (Fishbain, Cutler, Rosomoff, & Rosomoff, 2004). This casts some doubt on conclusions drawn from Waddell and similar behavioral assessments. Based on the current state of the evidence, behavioral assessment of chronic pain should be limited to observation of pain behaviors and a cautious interpretation of pain behaviors as indicators of distress and possibly poor pain coping rather than egregious attempts to malinger.

Disability and Physical Function

The assessment of disability and physical function among pain sufferers is a complex endeavor and can help to improve a behavioral health practitioner's understanding of the impact of pain on a patient's daily living. However, it can be quite difficult to accomplish. Before discussing disability assessment, it is helpful to consider the meaning of disability for those suffering with pain. Stanos, McLean, and Rader (2007) point out that the term "disability" can actually be better understood when considered in juxtaposition to similar concepts such as "impairment" and "handicap." According to the authors, "disability" is a concept that is actually rooted in a patient's "impairment," which refers to a deleterious change in either psychological or physical capacity associated with a pain condition. "Disability," then, represents changes in the pain sufferer's ability to complete activities of daily living and tasks necessary to contribute to home, work, and recreation life based on his or her level of "impairment." "Handicap" is, according to Stanos et al. (2007), a broader concept describing the disruption of the pain sufferer's ability to fulfill his or her societal role due to "disability"-related restrictions in functional activity.

Based on these definitions, it is clear that disability and handicap can be quantified functionally (through an assessment of physical impairment) and behaviorally (through an assessment of psychological impairment), but a strong subjective component is also worth considering. As a result, an assessment of disability and handicap should include a subjective assessment of limitations and contributions by the patient. Fortunately, there are good self-report measures available that can contribute to this assessment; two of the most commonly used are reviewed next.

Measures of Self-Reported Disability

Oswestry Disability Inventory

The Oswestry Disability Inventory (OSW or ODI), originally developed by Fairbank, Couper, Davies, and O'Brien (1980), evaluates the degree of functional impairment a patient with chronic pain is experiencing. It consists of 10 questions assessing multiple domains of daily physical function, with responses for each scored from 0 to 5 (higher scores indicating greater impairment). The total ODI score can be doubled to produce a percent disability rating related to pain. Due to its ease of use and interpretation, the ODI has been used in more than 100 studies of back pain to date and cited more than 200 times in the pain research literature as of 2000. A PubMed search on the instrument in 2008 yielded more than 1,000 references citing the measure. Recent reviews of ODI scoring have supported its use as a disability screener for chronic pain and offered scoring alternatives (Mehra, Baker, Disney, & Pynsent, 2008). The assessor then sums the values of all 10 items and doubles the resulting sum, which is often interpreted as the respondent's percentage of disability (Fairbank et al., 1980). ODI scores have been found to be significantly related to subjective pain report and quantified physical functioning (see Ohnmeiss, 2000, for an example of one such finding). Though originally developed specifically for back pain, the ODI has been successfully adapted to a number specific pain conditions, including neck and knee pain.

Million Visual Analogue Scale

The Million Visual Analogue Scale (MVAS), originally developed by Million, Hall, Nilsen, and Baker in 1982, is now composed of 15 VAS questions evaluating the intensity of the patient's pain, the etiological factors of the pain, activities that exacerbate patient pain, and 10 measures of spinal movement (Helliwell, Moll, & Wright, 1992). The MVAS is a British-designed instrument that has been revised with idioms more appropriate to U.S. patients (Gatchel, Polatin, & Mayer, 1995). Because of its reliance on

VAS data for responses to each question, the patients are able to convey their pain and disability in a nonverbal way (Gatchel et al., 1995). Helliwell et al. (1992) note that an observer usually administers the MVAS, and the intra- and interrater reliability of the instrument has been found to be adequate, with good sensitivity to change in physical measures over an 8-week interval. The two end points of the scale are *No Problems,* representing a score of 0, and *Totally Cannot Work,* representing a score of 10. Scores for the 15 items are summed to generate a total score, which can range from 0 to 150 points. MVAS total score cutoffs have been established as follows: < 39, "mildly disabling"; 40–84, "moderately disabling"; and > 85, "severely disabling" (Gatchel et al., 1995).

Demographics

Pain-related demographic factors can be a vital component of pain assessment. CMP symptoms have shown systematic variance along demographic dimensions such as age, gender, race, and socioeconomic class (Kelsey, Mundt, & Golden, 1992). All of these potential demographic contributors can be easily assessed through a comprehensive clinical interview or the completion of a brief demographics sheet. Relevant demographic variables are briefly discussed next.

Age

The incidence of chronic pain increases as we age, with older adults more likely to report musculoskeletal pain (Elliot, Smith, Penny, Smith, & Chambers, 1999). The first back pain episode typically does not appear until middle age, although the frequency of back pain episodes has been shown to be fairly equal for all age groups during the working years (Bigos et al., 1986; Kelsey et al., 1992). Although older adults are more likely to report experiencing chronic pain, younger adults also report CMP. Arola, Nicholls, Mallen, and Thomas (2010) reported an estimated prevalence of chronic pain among the elderly ranging from 40 to 65%. In their survey of more than 4,000 pain sufferers over the age of 50, the investigators found that chronic pain symptoms (particularly interference of pain in functioning) were

significantly related to depression and anxiety symptom development. The prevalence of chronic pain among children is also on the rise, with recent estimates of childhood chronic pain ranging from 19.5 to 30.4% (Perquin et al., 2000). Lewandowski, Palermo, De la Motte, S., and Fu (2010) identified unique factors contributing to chronic pain in children, including family functioning and dyadic parent–child variables, which should be considered when assessing for pain in children. For those interested in assessing chronic pain in child and adolescent populations, there are specific measures available that can tap the constructs unique to these groups (e.g., the Adolescent Pain Behavior Questionnaire; Lynch-Jordan, Kashikar-Zuck, & Goldschneider, 2010).

Age affects not only the incidence of pain but also how sufferers cope with and respond to their pain. For example, Sorkin, Rudy, Hanlon, Turk, and Stieg (1990), found that older patients with pain utilize fewer cognitive strategies for coping with pain in comparison with younger patients with pain. Also, older adults may have difficulty accurately reporting the presence and severity of pain due, in part, to increased prevalence of cognitive impairment with older age (Fox, Raina, & Jadad, 1999). For patients with cognitive impairment, providers may need to pay particular attention to pain-related behaviors to accurately assess these cases.

Gender

Studies of gender have shown variable results in the frequency of CMP disorders. Males have shown a higher rate of low back pain involving workers' compensation benefits, likely due to a higher concentration of males in jobs requiring greater physical exertion (Kelsey et al., 1992; Snook, 1987). However, in a population-based survey of the Dutch population, Wijnhoven, de Vet, and Picavet (2006) found a 45% prevalence of musculoskeletal pain complaints among women compared with only 39% among men. The higher prevalence of CMP among women remained even after controlling for pain duration.

There is also evidence that the relationship between gender and pain may have roots in childhood abuse. Some have hypothesized that emotional distress associated with childhood trauma (physical and sexual abuse) may make one less resilient to trauma later, leaving the person increasingly vulnerable to the development of the chronic pain syndrome. McMahon, Gatchel, Polatin, and Mayer (1997), for example, found that female patients with chronic pain reported a rate of abuse five times higher than that of a healthy comparison group, including higher rates of sexual abuse involving the use of threat/injury/weapons and higher rates of father–daughter incest. Male patients with chronic pain did not evidence a similar relationship between chronic pain incidence and childhood abuse history. These data indicate that chronic pain assessment should include not only the assessment of gender but also consideration of childhood physical or sexual abuse.

Race and Socioeconomic Status

Race/ethnicity and socioeconomic status (SES) play a significant role in the assessment and treatment of a number of health conditions, including chronic pain. Fuentes, Hart-Johnson, and Green (2007) aptly point out that the impact of these factors on physical health spans individual, health system, and societal domains. They cite past research indicating a possible overlap between race and SES, though their own analysis of a pain population revealed that these two constructs are far too complicated to be used interchangeably. Instead, the researchers recommend the assessment of both race/ethnicity and SES separately when trying to describe and understand a pain population. They additionally suggest that the assessment of poverty, education, and employment strengthen the reliability and validity of SES as it relates to chronic pain course and treatment.

Some have identified a relationship between low SES, race, and an increased frequency of chronic pain symptoms (including disability), though the exact nature of this relationship seems to be complex and difficult to clearly discern (Fuentes et al., 2007; Gerstle, All, & Wallace, 2001). Fuentes and colleagues found that black race was related to lower levels of SES in their sample, but race was not always an SES mediator. They did point out that race seemed to contribute to higher levels of pain-related affective disorders (possibly mediated by SES) and that age and gender may also play contributing roles in the complex pain–SES relationship.

Race may also contribute to pain coping through racially based differences in health care utilization and attitudes toward health care. Green, Baker, and Ndao-Brumblay (2004) found that racial differences in health care coverage and the overall ability to pay for health care services for pain contribute to race-based differences in health care utilization for pain management. In their sample, the researchers found that African American sufferers had greater difficulty paying for pain care and were more likely to report their pain and related treatment as a significant source of financial stress. Similarly, Green et al. (2004) found that racial differences in pain care attitudes and utilization may also contribute to disparities in the quality of care. African American participants in their sample were less likely to have care coordinated through a primary care manager than European American participants and were less likely to identify pain medication as potentially helpful for their pain. The relationship between SES and work serves as another relevant mediator of the impact of SES on pain. A higher frequency of low back pain among those with lower SES has been found, which is likely attributable to a higher rate of physical, labor-intensive jobs in this demographic group (Kelsey et al., 1992).

Socioeconomic Outcomes Assessment

Often, a follow-up interview is a vital and necessary way to identify socioeconomic variables that can serve as an index for treatment effectiveness and the long-term financial and social impacts of chronic pain. Tucker and Mayer (2000) have provided a comprehensive review of how such structured interviews can be conducted. Information gathered during this evaluation can include the following:

- A patients' case settlement venue and status (e.g., lawsuit disposition/consideration, workers' compensation claim consideration, filing for disability).
- The patient's financial situation (e.g. income, disability compensation, litigation outcomes).

- Any additional data relevant to treatment considerations and resource planning (e.g., planned medical treatments, medication use, emergency room visits for pain management).
- Employment history (including the number of jobs the patient has had and the length of time in employ at the patient's current job at the time of injury).

Emotional Factors

Research on the chronic pain syndrome has begun to account for more complex variables playing a role in its onset and maintenance; one such variable is emotional distress. McMahon et al. (1997) stress that emotional psychopathology plays a major role in the development of chronic pain and, as efforts to explore the chronic pain–emotion link have increased, it has become evident that chronic pain assessment must include the assessment of comorbid or contributing psychopathology (Dersh, Gatchel, Polatin, & Mayer, 2002; Rush, Polatin, & Gatchel, 2000). Gatchel (1996) explains that emotional disturbance may not be the product of the onset of pain per se, suggesting that emotional distress may play an active role in vulnerability to chronic pain onset. Emotional factors are substantively implicated in chronic pain (to some extent), and reports show that the incidence of emotional disturbance in the chronic pain literature ranges from 10 to 100% (Polatin, 1991). Acute pain does not appear to be significantly related to an increased prevalence of psychopathology, suggesting that psychosocial problems develop as pain becomes more chronic.

The mere assessment of general emotional distress may not be enough to fully describe the complex relation between emotions and pain; it may be necessary to specify the nature of the emotional disturbance. Individuals with depression and anxiety diagnoses differ according to the amount and nature of intrusion the psychopathology has on pain. Polatin (1991) states, "patients with an anxiety neurosis tend to have a lower pain threshold, whereas depressed patients' thresholds may vary" (p. 152). It has further been suggested that some forms of psychopathology, notably anxiety, may deteriorate one's ability to cope with pain, thereby "greasing the wheels" for the development of chronic pain. Thus emotional assessment of patients with CMP should include measures of both depression and anxiety.

Recent evidence strongly supports the role of depression and anxiety in chronic pain development and maintenance. Depressive disorders are common among chronic pain sufferers, with an estimated prevalence of up to 65% (Poleshuck, Talbot, et al., 2010). High chronic pain severity has been independently associated with increased levels of depressive symptoms (Hooten, Shi, Gazelka, & Warner, 2011), and the presence of chronic pain has been identified as a risk factor for higher symptom severity, suicide risk, and general psychosocial functioning among individuals with depression (Poleshuck, Gamble, et al., 2010). Poleshuck, Talbot, and colleagues (2010) suggest that pain and depression influence one another reciprocally and note that comorbid pain and depression ultimately result in poor treatment outcomes for either condition, making treatment difficult for this population. Asmundson and Katz (2009) offer a comprehensive review of the role of anxiety in chronic pain. The authors cite multiple epidemiological studies of anxiety disorder comorbidity in chronic pain, with a prevalence of around 30%, though some estimates for specific anxiety disorder diagnoses are much higher (e.g., posttraumatic stress disorder [PTSD]). They note that there is little evidence to support the theory that anxiety disorders cause chronic pain to occur, and they describe a mutual maintenance model in which symptoms or characteristics of chronic pain and anxiety maintain and exacerbate each other.

Some of the more commonly used measures of emotional disturbance in chronic pain are included in the following subsection. Because these measures are well described elsewhere, these discussions focus more on the specific implications of these measures on CMP assessment than on basic descriptions of the measures themselves.

Depression Measures

The recent publication of DSM-5 (American Psychiatric Association, 2013) has resulted in slight changes in how mood disorders will be diagnosed. As a result, it will be interesting to monitor how pain assessment and intervention are altered under these new diagnostic categories and specifiers. For example, DSM-5 now includes specifiers for mixed mood symptoms in bipolar and depressive disorders, allowing for representation of manic symptoms occurring in the presence of a depressive episode. Manic symptoms, especially those akin to agitation, may alter pain response in the context of comorbid pain and depression. It will be interesting to see how assessment of mood follows these changes. At the time this chapter was written, there have been no significant strides in reinterpreting mood assessment for pain patients. It is quite likely, however, that future research efforts will result in these changes.

Gatchel and Dersh (2002) note that, among all psychological concomitants of chronic pain, depression has received the most attention. A number of chronic pain symptoms and outcomes likely contribute to the development and maintenance of depression among chronic pain sufferers, including functional disability, perceived lack of control over pain symptoms, lack of understanding about chronic pain on the part of one's family, friends, and coworkers, and so forth (Banks & Kerns, 1996). As a result, it is vital to fully assess depression among chronic pain sufferers.

Beck Depression Inventory

Today, the Beck Depression Inventory (BDI) is one of the most widely used rating scales for depression in the world, and it is becoming one of the most commonly utilized measures of depression in chronic pain. Some have expressed reservations about using the BDI in a chronic pain assessment due to a strong somatic component to the BDI factor structure that results in artificially inflated BDI "depression" scores for the medically injured (Wesley, Gatchel, Garofalo, & Polatin, 1999).

In order to improve the utility of BDI scores for pain sufferers, many have sought to identify a factor structure to the measure that will help differentiate truly depressive symptoms from confounding somatic/pain symptoms. Wesley et al. (1999) evaluated 200 patients with chronic low back pain with the BDI. After factor analyzing their data, the authors noted a unique factor structure for

patients with pain (as compared with that found for psychiatric patients). The two factors that made up the structure for patients with chronic low back pain included a measure of depression severity and a measure of somatic difficulties and disability. This finding serves as evidence that there may have been certain components of depression (as measured by the BDI) that overlapped with pain-specific symptoms, notably, somatic symptoms and perceived disability. Assessing for depression in a musculoskeletal pain population with the BDI was, therefore, likely to result in a confounded measure of depression.

In 1996, the BDI was revised into a second version in response to criticism that the original relied too heavily on somatic symptoms of depression and to allow a measure of depression that was commensurate with the diagnostic criteria of depression present in DSM-IV. Early attempts to develop a pain-related factor structure for the BDI-II once again revealed a two-factor structure similar to that previously identified for the original BDI (Poole, Bramwell, & Murphy, 2009). Poole and colleagues identified factors in BDI-II assessment that tapped two specific domains of depressive symptoms, namely "negative thoughts" and "behaviors." Both of these factors were found to correlate to indices of pain symptoms in opposite directions, suggesting that attempts to pool these factors in interpretation through the use of a total score could result in a misrepresentation of pain-related depression. A two-factor approach, however, might allow for a clearer picture of the role of depression in CMP.

Hamilton Depression Rating Scale

The Hamilton Depression Rating Scale (HAM-D; adapted from Hedlund & Vieweg, 1979) is another oft-used measure of depression among chronic pain populations, based on a 17-question structured interview evaluating various aspects of depression rated on Likert scales ranging from 0 to 2 and 0 to 4. The points generated for each question in the interview are summed, resulting in a total score. Krishnan and colleagues (1985) note that the HAM-D is useful in discriminating between various subtypes of depression, as well as in differentiating patients with and without depression. Dunlop and

Ninan (2003) suggest some caution in using the HAM-D for chronic pain assessment given the inclusion of somatic items in the measure that may artificially raise scores for patients with pain. Typically, a score of 25 or greater is considered clinically significant depression, though no scoring mechanisms seem to have been developed with chronic pain sufferers in mind.

Center for Epidemiologic Studies Depression Scale

The Center for Epidemiologic Studies Depression Scale (CES-D) has long been a preferred measure of depression for those with chronic pain conditions (Radloff, 1977). The reason is the scale's structure, which relies on the assessment of nonsomatic symptoms of depression, possibly leading to a depression index that is less confounded by comorbid pain symptomatology. The CES-D is composed of 20 items with an established cutoff score of 16 for significant depression in most populations. A CES-D score of 19 or greater has been identified as an indicator of notable depressive symptoms for those with chronic spinal pain (see Walsh et al., 2006).

Anxiety Measures

As was the case with depression, the publication of DSM-5 resulted in a few changes in how anxiety disorders are conceptualized and diagnosed that could directly influence pain assessment and intervention. All DSM-5 disorders may now include a panic attack specifier. This change is quite likely to have an impact on pain sufferers because of the widely recognized and long-held recognition of panic as a complicating factor for pain (likely through somatic preoccupation commonly associated with panic symptoms; Kuch, Cox, Woszczyna, Swinson, & Shulman, 1991).

Measuring anxiety in a population with chronic pain can be particularly difficult due to the significant representation of somatic symptoms present in both pain and anxiety sufferers. Teasing pain and anxiety apart requires the selection of a responsible instrument, as well as a thorough biopsychosocial understanding of the patient with pain. Though there are enough anxiety measures used in pain assessment to fill this entire chapter (e.g., the State–Trait Anxiety Inventory), only a few notable examples are discussed here.

The Hospital Anxiety and Depression Scale

The Hospital Anxiety and Depression Scale (HADS; Zigmond & Snaith, 1983) is a 14-item self-report measure assessing both depression and anxiety symptoms. The instrument is specifically tailored for a medical population, with a notable lack of emotional/somatic symptoms among the assessment items. This makes it an attractive option for the assessment of depression and anxiety in chronic pain populations. Greenough and Fraser (1991) examined the validity and reliability of the HADS for a chronic pain sample and found the measure to be appropriate for this population. There are no specific interpretative guidelines available for the HADS, so standard interpretation ($\geq$ 8 for suspicious cases and $\geq$ 11 for safe cases on each subscale; Zigmond & Snaith, 1983) is recommended unless responsible specific guidelines for musculoskeletal pain are noted.

Beck Anxiety Inventory

The Beck Anxiety Inventory (BAI; Beck, Epstein, Brown, & Steer, 1988) is one of the most widely used measures of anxiety and was developed to sensitively discriminate between anxiety and depression symptoms. Multiple studies have confirmed the solid psychometrics of the BAI, and it has been used in a number of studies focused on pain populations. The BAI is a 21-item measure of anxiety symptom severity with some support for its reliability in chronic pain populations (Davidson, Tripp, Fabrigar, & Davidson, 2008). Specific cutoff scores for CMP are not widely available, though scores greater than or equal to 11 indicate some anxiety is present.

Pain Anxiety Symptoms Scale

The Pain Anxiety Symptoms Scale (PASS) is a 40-item measure specifically designed for the assessment of pain-related anxiety across four different dimensions (McCracken, Zayfert, & Gross, 1992). A shortened, 20-item version of this measure is also available.

Studies have supported the four-factor structure of the PASS, which appears to tap into cognitive anxiety, escape–avoidance behaviors, fear of pain, and physiological symptoms of anxiety. The PASS has been widely demonstrated to be a valid and reliable assessment tool for pain-related anxiety symptoms.

Comprehensive Psychopathology Assessment and Somatic Symptom Disorders

The DSM-5 includes some changes to personality disorder diagnoses that may affect patients with chronic pain. However, there are substantive changes to "somatic symptom and related disorder" that are likely to significantly alter how pain is diagnosed and addressed in behavioral health. "Pain disorder" (307.89 in DSM-IV-TR) has been merged with other somatic diagnoses (somatoform disorder, hypochondriasis) into a broad category called "somatic symptom disorder" (McCarron, 2013). The American Psychiatric Association published a 2013 information sheet titled "Highlights of Changes from DSM-IV-TR to DSM-5" (*www.dsm5.org/Documents/changes%20 from%20dsm-iv-tr%20to%20dsm-5.pdf*) that explains that pain disorder has been difficult to diagnose and interpret due to attribution of pain to both physical and psychological factors that are often difficult to clearly disentangle. As a result, DSM-5 now offers three reasonable alternatives to pain disorder, including somatic symptom disorder (with predominant pain), psychological factors affecting other medical conditions, and adjustment disorder. As with other changes to DSM, assessment instruments have not yet been examined for sensitivity to these classifications. It will be interesting to see how future research on pain assessment addresses DSM-5 pain classification.

Many have sought to identify a general or overarching psychological profile of chronic pain sufferers, suggesting that there may be aspects of psychological development (i.e., personality) that contribute to a vulnerability to chronic pain development. Although research in this area has not successfully identified a solid "pain personality" profile, the use of some comprehensive inventories can shed valuable light on how a person's mental life may contribute to his or her chronic pain experience (Karlin et al., 2005).

Minnesota Multiphasic Personality Inventory— 2nd Edition

The two editions of the Minnesota Multiphasic Personality Inventory (MMPI and MMPI-2) have been widely used in the study of chronic pain, resulting in a wealth of research investigating the applications of the MMPI to chronic pain populations (Vendrig, 2000; Karlin et al., 2005). Vendrig notes that the usefulness of the MMPI in differentiating and diagnosing patients with chronic pain has evolved with our understanding of chronic pain, though some doubt was expressed as to the suitability of the instrument for pain screening. Many specific applications of the MMPI to pain assessment have been identified, including the assessment of psychological defense mechanisms that may contribute to the development and intrusion of chronic pain (Monsen & Havik, 2001).

The MMPI was originally used to discriminate between patients with pain of an organic versus a psychogenic origin (Hanvik, 1951). Hanvik found elevations on scales 1 and 3 for patients with psychogenic pain, and his findings have since been replicated many times (see Vendrig, 2000). This line of research led to the introduction of supplemental Low Back (LB) and Dorsal (DOR) scales into the MMPI (Hanvik, 1951; Vendrig, 2000), which were found to differentiate between psychogenic and organic pain, though these findings were not statistically significant.

These early efforts to evaluate chronic pain based on the "disease model" have become outdated with the introduction of Melzack and Wall's (1965) *gate-control theory of pain*. Using the gate-control theory as a guide in interpreting the MMPI, Keller and Butcher (1991) were among the first to note the "Conversion V" pattern of elevation in scales 1, 2, and 3. Vendrig (2000) also noted that MMPI and MMPI-2 data have been found to significantly predict the development of chronic pain per the model set forth by Gatchel et al. (1995). Specifically, Scale 3 was found to be a good primary and secondary chronic pain predictor, and Scale 1 was identified as a good tertiary predictor. More recently, Gatchel, Mayer, and Eddington (2006) have isolated the "disability profile" on the MMPI as predictive of psychopathology in patients with chronic spine pain. In light of these applications, Vendrig (2000) warns that MMPI-2 data cannot be used in a vacuum to evaluate chronic pain. MMPI-2 data need to be used in conjunction with other sources of patient data to be truly valuable in giving information about psychopathology and personality.

Personality Assessment Inventory

The Personality Assessment Inventory (PAI) is an oft-used alternative to the MMPI-2. It is a 344-item measure primarily intended as a comprehensive assessment of psychopathology and personality factors. Though the literature examining the application of the PAI to a chronic pain population is somewhat limited at this time (only one comprehensive paper has been published as of 2013), the measure has been widely applied to a number of health concerns, and a good case has been made regarding the clinical utility of PAI assessment for patients with chronic pain. PAI scoring results in 22 discrete scales, including 11 clinical scales, 4 validity scales, 5 treatment consideration scales, and 2 interpersonal scales. Karlin and colleagues (2005) have published one of the few comprehensive studies of the PAI to date.

Karlin and colleagues (2005) note that the PAI offers a number of advantages over the MMPI-2 for chronic pain assessment, including the measure's relative brevity (344 items compared to 567 items for the MMPI-2) and the fact that only a sixth-grade reading level is needed to complete it (though it must be noted the MMPI-2 has been found to require only a fifth-grade reading level; Paolo, Ryan, & Smith, 1991). The authors factor-analyzed 432 valid PAI profiles from a regional interdisciplinary pain center and identified four pain-related PAI factors. These factors were Nonspecific Psychological Distress, Disconnectedness, Recklessness/Hostility, and Substance Use. Interestingly, Karlin et al. (2005) stress that the recklessness factor did not contain a substance abuse component, suggesting that substance use may have a different meaning among chronic pain sufferers compared with the general population. Interested read-

ers are referred to Karlin et al. (2005) for further details.

Summary and Conclusions

CMP assessment is a vital part of treatment planning and outcome tracking. Due to the complexity of CMP, multiple domains of assessment are needed. Previous attempts to quantify pain through animal models and a biomedical perspective have failed to fully describe the experience of CMP, resulting in a need for more comprehensive assessment approaches. With the recent focus on a biopsychosocial conceptualization of chronic health conditions, CMP assessment has evolved to include not only behavioral and physical variables associated with pain but also psychosocial and environmental concerns that appear to play major roles in the chronic pain experience. This chapter was written to serve as an overview of a comprehensive, biopsychosocial approach to CMP assessment. Though it would be difficult to fully explicate all potential foci of assessment, significant domains of concern were addressed and examples of relevant measures in all domains were introduced.

REFERENCES

American Psychiatric Association. (2013). *Diagnostic and statistical manual of mental disorders* (5th ed.). Arlington, VA: Author.

Andersson, G. B. J., Pope, M. H., Frymoyer, J. W., & Snook, S. (1991). Epidemiology and cost. In J. W. Frymoyer (Ed.), *The adult spine: principles and practice* (pp. 107–146). St. Louis, MO: Mosby.

Arola, H., Nicholls, E., Mallen, C., & Thomas, E. (2010). Self-reported pain interference and symptoms of anxiety and depression in community-dwelling older adults: Can a temporal relationship be determined? *European Journal of Pain, 14,* 966–971.

Asmundson, G. J. G., & Katz, J. (2009). Understanding the co-occurrence of anxiety disorders and chronic pain: State-of-the-art. *Depression and Anxiety, 26,* 888–901.

Banks, S. M., & Kerns, R. D. (1996). Explaining high rates of depression in chronic pain: A diathesis–stress framework. *Psychological Bulletin, 119,* 95–110.

Beck, A. T., Epstein, N., Brown, G., & Steer, R. A. (1988). An inventory for measuring clinical anxiety: Psychometric properties. *Journal of Consulting and Clinical Psychology, 56,* 893–897.

Beecher, H. K. (1957). The measurement of pain. *Pharmacological Review, 9,* 59–209.

Bergman, S., Herrstrom, P., Hogstrom, K., Petersson, I. F., Svensson, B., & Jacobsson, L. T. (2001). Chronic musculoskeletal pain, prevalence rates, and sociodemographic associations in a Swedish population study. *Journal of Rheumatology, 28,* 1369–1377.

Bigos, S. J., Spengler, D. M., Martin, N. A., Zeh, J., Fisher, L. D., Nachemson, A. L., & Wang, M. H. (1986). Back injuries in industry: A retrospective study: II. Injury factors. *Spine, 11,* 246–251.

Bureau of Labor Statistics. (2009). *Occupational injury and illness classification system.* Retrieved from *www.bls.gov/iif/oshoiics.htm.*

Burton, A. K., Waddell, G., Tillotson, K. M., & Summerton, N. (1999). Information and advice to patients with back pain can have a positive effect: A randomized controlled trial of a novel educational booklet in primary care. *Spine, 24,* 2484–2491.

Chapman, C. R., Casey, K. L., Dubner, R., Foley, K. M., Gracely, R. H., & Reading, A. E. (1985). Pain measurement: An overview. *Pain, 22,* 1–31.

Choi, Y., Mayer, T. G., Williams, M., & Gatchel, R. J. (2013). The clinical utility of the Multidimensional Pain Inventory (MPI) in characterizing chronic disabling occupational musculoskeletal disorders. *Journal of Occupational Rehabilitation, 23,* 239–247.

Clark, M. E., Kori, S. H., & Brockel, J. (1996). Kinesiophobia and chronic pain: Psychometrics, characteristics, and factor analysis of the Tampa Scale. *American Pain Society Abstracts, 15,* 77.

Coudeyre, E., Tubach, F., Rannou, F., Baron, G., Coriat, F., Brin, S., et al. (2007). Fear-avoidance beliefs about back pain in patients with acute low back pain. *Annales de Readaption et de Medecine Physique, 50,* 327–336.

Crombez, G., Vlaeyen, J. W., Heuts, P. H., & Lysens, R. (1999). Pain-related fear is more disabling than pain itself: Evidence on the role of pain-related fear in chronic back pain disability. *Pain, 80,* 329–339.

Davidson, M. A., Tripp, D. A., Fabrigar, L. R., & Davidson, P. R. (2008). Chronic pain assessment: A seven-factor model. *Pain Research and Management, 13,* 299–308.

Dersh, J., Gatchel, R. J., Polatin, P. B., & Mayer, T. (2002). Prevalence of psychiatric disorders in patients with chronic work-related musculoskeletal pain disability. *Journal of Occupational and Environmental Medicine, 44,* 459–468.

Dunlop, B. W., & Ninan, P. T. (2003). Pharmacologic considerations in the treatment of severe depression. *Medscape Psychiatry and Mental Health, 8*(2). Retrieved from *www.medscape.com/viewarticle/462603.*

Dworkin, R. H., Turk, D. C., Farrar, J. T., Haythornthwaite, J. A., Jensen, M. P., Katz, N. P., et al. (2005). Core outcome measures for chronic pain clinical trials: IMMPACT recommendations. *Pain, 113,* 9–19.

Dworkin, R. H., Turk, D. C., Revicki, D. A., Harding, G., Coyne, K. S., Peirce-Sandner, S., et al. (2009). Development and initial validation of an expanded and revised version of the Short Form McGill Pain Questionnaire (SF-MPQ-2). *Pain, 144,* 35–42.

Elliott, A. M., Smith, B. H., Penny, K. I., Smith, W. C., & Chambers, W. A. (1999). The epidemiology of chronic pain in the community. *Lancet, 354,* 1248–1252.

Fairbank, J. C. T., Couper, J., Davies, J. B., & O'Brien, J. P. (1980). The Oswestry low back pain disability questionnaire. *Physiotherapy, 66,* 271–273.

Fishbain, D. A., Cutler, R. B., Rosomoff, H. L., & Rosomoff, R. S. (2004). Is there a relationship between non-organic physical findings (Waddell signs) and secondary gain/malingering? *Clinical Journal of Pain, 20,* 399–408.

Fox, P. A., Raina, P., & Jadad, A. R. (1999). Prevalence and treatment of pain in older adults in nursing homes and other long-term care institutions: A systematic review. *Canadian Medical Association Journal, 160,* 329–333.

Fritz, J. M., & George, S. Z. (2002). Identifying psychosocial variables in patients with acute work-related low back pain: The importance of fear-avoidance beliefs. *Physical Therapy, 82,* 973–983.

Fuentes, M., Hart-Johnson, T., & Green, C. R. (2007). The association among neighborhood socioeconomic status, race and chronic pain in black and white older adults. *Journal of the National Medical Association, 99,* 1160–1169.

Gatchel, R. J. (1996). Psychological disorders and chronic pain: Cause-and-effect relationships. In R. J. Gatchel & D. C. Turk (Eds.), *Psychological approaches to pain management: A practitioner's handbook* (pp. 33–52). New York: Guilford Press.

Gatchel, R. J., & Dersh, J. (2002). Psychological disorders and chronic pain: Are there cause-and-effect relationships? In R. J. Gatchel & D. C. Turk (Eds.), *Psychological approaches to pain management: A practitioner's handbook* (pp. 33–52). New York: Guilford Press.

Gatchel, R. J., Mayer, T. G., & Eddington, A. (2006). MMPI disability profile: The least known, most useful screen for psychopathology in chronic occupational spinal disorders. *Spine, 31,* 2973–2978.

Gatchel, R. J., Polatin, P. B., & Mayer, T. G. (1995). The dominant role of psychosocial risk factors in the development of chronic low back pain disability. *Spine, 20,* 2702–2709.

George, S. Z., Bialosky, J. E., & Fritz, J. M. (2004). Physical therapy management of a patient with acute low back pain and elevated fear avoidance beliefs: A case report. *Physical Therapy, 34,* 430–439.

Gerstle, D. S., All, A. S., & Wallace, D. C. (2001). Quality of life and chronic nonmalignant pain. *Pain Management Nursing, 2,* 98–109.

Goubert, L., Vlaeyen, J. W. S., Crombez, G., & Craig, K. D. (2011). Learning about pain from others: An observational learning account. *Journal of Pain, 12,* 167–174.

Green, C. R., Baker, T. A., & Ndao-Brumblay, S. K. (2004). Patient attitudes regarding healthcare utilization and referral: A descriptive comparison in African and Caucasian Americans with chronic pain. *Journal of the National Medical Association, 96,* 31–42.

Greenough, C. G., & Fraser, R. D. (1991). Comparison of eight psychometric instruments in unselected patients with back pain. *Spine, 16,* 1068–1074.

Grotle, M., Vollestad, N. K., & Brox, J. I. (2006). Clinical course and impact of fear-avoidance beliefs in low back pain. *Spine, 31,* 682–689.

Hanvik, L. J. (1951). MMPI profiles in patients with low back pain. *Journal of Consulting Psychology, 15,* 350–353.

Hawthorne, G., Osborne, R. H., Taylor, A., & Sansoni, J. (2007). The SF36 Version 2: Critical analyses of population weights, scoring algorithms and population norms. *Quality of Life Research, 16,* 661–673.

Hedlund, J. L., & Vieweg, B. W. (1979). The Hamilton Rating Scale for Depression. *Journal of Operational Psychiatry, 10,* 149–165.

Helliwell, P., Moll, J., & Wright, V. (1992). Measurement of spinal movements. In M. I. V. Jayson (Ed.), *Measurement of spinal movements* (pp. 173–205). Edinburgh, UK: Churchill Livingstone.

Hooten, W. M., Shi, Y., Gazelka, H. M., & Warner, D. O. (2011). The effects of depression and smoking on pain severity and opioid use in patients with chronic pain. *Pain, 152,* 223–229.

Jensen, M. P., Turner, J. A., & Romano, J. M. (1994). What is the maximum number of levels needed in pain intensity measurement? *Pain, 58,* 387–392.

Karlin, B. E., Creech, S. K., Grimes, J. S., Clark, T. S., Meagher, M. W., & Morey, L. C. (2005). The Personality Assessment Inventory with chronic pain patients: Psychometric properties and clinical utility. *Journal of Clinical Psychology, 61,* 1571–1585.

Kast, E. C., & Collins, V. J. (1966). A theory of human pathological pain and its measurement: The analgesic activity of methotrimeprazine. *Journal of New Drugs, 6,* 142–148.

Keller, L. S., & Butcher, J. N. (1991). *Assessment of chronic pain patients with the MMPI-2.* Minneapolis: University of Minnesota Press.

Kelsey, J. L., Mundt, D. J., & Golden, A. I. (1992). Epidemiology of low back pain. In M. I. V. Jayson (Ed.), *The lumbar spine and back pain* (4th ed.). London: Churchill Livingstone.

Kerns, R. D., Turk, D. C., & Rudy, T. E. (1985). The West Haven–Yale Multidimensional Pain Inventory (WHYMPI). *Pain, 23,* 345–356.

Kori, S. H., Miller, R. P., & Todd, D. D. (1990). Kinesiophobia: A new view of chronic pain behavior. *Pain Management, 3,* 35–43.

Krishnan, K. R., France, R. D., Pelton, S., McCann, U. D., Davidson, J., & Urban, B. J. (1985). Chronic pain and depression: I. Classification of depression in chronic low back pain patients. *Pain, 22,* 279–287.

Kuch, K., Cox, B. J., Woszczyna, C. B., Swinson, R. P., & Shulman, I. (1991). Chronic pain in panic disorder. *Journal of Behavioral Therapy and Experimental Psychiatry, 22,* 255–229.

Lewandowski, A., Palermo, T., De la Motte, S., & Fu, R. (2010). Temporal daily associations between pain and sleep in adolescents with chronic pain versus healthy adolescents. *Pain, 151,* 220–225.

Lorenz, K. A., Sherbourne, C. D., Shugarman, L. R., Rubenstein, L. V., Wen, L., et al. (2009). How reliable is pain as the fifth vital sign?

Journal of the American Board of Family Medicine, 22, 291–298.

Lynch-Jordan, A. M., Kashikar-Zuck, S., & Goldschneider, K. R. (2010). Parent perceptions of adolescent pain expression: The Adolescent Pain Behavior Questionnaire. *Pain, 151,* 834–842.

Main, C., & Waddell, G. (1998). Behavioral responses to examination: A reappraisal of the interpretation on nonorganic signs. *Spine, 23,* 2367–2371.

Martin, B. I., Deyo, R. A., Mirza, S. K. Turner, J. A., Comstock, B. A., Hollingsworth, W., et al. (2008). Expenditures and health status among adults with back and neck problems. *Journal of the American Medical Association, 299,* 656–664.

McCarron, R. M. (2013). The DSM-5 and the art of medicine: Certainly uncertain. *Annals of Internal Medicine, 159*(5), 360–361.

McCracken, L. M., Vowles, K. E., & Eccleston, C. (2004). Acceptance of chronic pain: Component analysis and a revised assessment method. *Pain, 107,* 159–166.

McCracken, L. M., Zayfert, C., & Gross, R. T. (1992). The Pain Anxiety Symptoms Scale: Development and validation of a scale to measure fear of pain. *Pain, 50,* 67–73.

McGeary, D. D., Mayer, T. G., & Gatchel, R. J. (2006). High pain ratings predict treatment failure in chronic occupational musculoskeletal disorders. *Journal of Bone and Joint Surgery, 88,* 317–325.

McKillop, J. M., & Nielson, W. R. (2011). Improving the usefulness of the Multidimensional Pain Inventory. *Pain Research and Management: Journal of the Canadian Pain Society, 16,* 300.

McMahon, M., Gatchel, R. J., Polatin, P. B., & Mayer, T. G. (1997). Early childhood abuse in chronic spinal disorder patients: A major barrier to treatment success. *Spine, 22,* 2408–2415.

Mehra, A., Baker, D., Disney, S., & Pynsent, P. B. (2008). Oswestry scoring made easy. *Annals of the Royal College of Surgeons of England, 90,* 497–499.

Melzack, R., & Torgerson, W. S. (1971). On the language of pain. *Anesthesiology, 34,* 50–59.

Melzack, R., & Wall, P. D. (1965). Pain mechanisms: A new theory. *Science, 150,* 971–979.

Million, R., Hall, R., Nilsen, K. H., & Baker, R. D. (1982). Assessment of the progress of the back pain patient. *Spine, 7,* 204–212.

Monsen, K., & Havik, O. E. (2001). Psychological functioning and bodily conditions in patients with pain disorder associated with psychological factors. *British Journal of Medical Psychology, 74,* 183–195.

Mooney, V. (1984). Evaluating pain in the primary care office. *Journal of Musculoskeletal Medicine, 2,* 16–26.

National Institute of Arthritis and Musculoskeletal and Skin Diseases. (2010). Back pain. Retrieved from *www.niams.nih.gov/Health_Info/Back_Pain/default.asp.*

National Research Council. (2001). *Musculoskeletal disorders and the workplace: Low back and upper extremities.* Washington, DC: National Academy Press.

Ohlund, C., Eek, C., Palmblad, S., Areskoug, B., & Nachemson, A. (1996). Quantified pain drawing in subacute low back pain: Validation in nonselected outpatient industrial sample. *Spine, 21,* 1021–1031.

Ohnhaus, E. E., & Adler, R. (1975). Methodological problems in the measurement of pain: A comparison between the verbal rating scale and the visual analogue scale. *Pain, 1,* 379–384.

Ohnmeiss, D. D. (2000). Repeatability of pain drawings in a low back pain population. *Spine, 25,* 980–988.

Paolo, A. M., Ryan, J. J., & Smith, A. J. (1991). Reading difficulty of MMPI-2 subscales. *Journal of Clinical Psychology, 47,* 529–532.

Perquin, C. W., Hazebroek-Kampschreur, A. A., Hunfeld, J. A., Bohnen, A. M., van Suijlekom-Smit, L. W., Passchier, J., et al. (2000). Pain in children and adolescents: A common experience. *Pain, 87,* 51–58.

Picavet, H. S., Vlaeyen, J. W., & Shouten, J. S. (2002). Pain catastrophizing and kinesiophobia: Predictors of chronic low back pain. *Spine Journal, 2,* 402–407.

Poiraudeau, S., Rannou, F., Henanff, L. E., Coudeyre, E., Rozenberg, S., Huas, D., et al. (2006). Outcome of subacute low back pain: Influence of patients' and rheumatologists' characteristics. *Rheumatology, 45,* 718–723.

Polatin, P. B. (1991). Affective disorders in back pain. In T. G. Mayer, V. Mooney, & R. J. Gatchel (Eds.), *Contemporary conservative care for painful spinal disorders* (pp. 149–154). Philadelphia: Lea & Febiger.

Poleshuck, E. L., Gamble, S. A., Cort, N., Hoffman-King, D., Cerrito, B., Rosario-McCabe, L., et al. (2010). Interpersonal psychotherapy for co-occurring depression and chronic pain. *Professional Psychology: Research and Practice, 41,* 312–318.

Poleshuck, E. L., Talbot, N. E., Zlotnick, C., Gamble, S. A., Liu, X., Tu, X., et al. (2010). Interpersonal psychotherapy for women with comorbid depression and chronic pain. *Journal of Nervous Mental Disorders, 198,* 597–600.

Poole, H., Bramwell, R., & Murphy, P. (2009). The utility of the Beck Depression Inventory Fast Screen (BDS-FS) in a pain clinic population. *European Journal of Pain, 13,* 865–869.

Price, D. D., McGrath, P. A., Rafii, A., & Buckingham, B. (1983). The validation of visual analog scales as ratio scale measures for chronic and experimental pain. *Pain, 17,* 45–56.

Radloff, L. S. (1977). The CES-D scale: A self-report depression scale for research in the general population. *Applied Psychological Measurement, 1,* 385–401.

Rush, A. J., Polatin, P. B., & Gatchel, R. J. (2000). Depression and chronic low back pain. *Spine, 25,* 2566–2571.

Scott, J., & Huskisson, E. C. (1976). Graphic representation of pain. *Pain, 2,* 175–184.

Snook, S. H. (1987). The costs of back pain in industry. *Spine State of the Art Reviews, 2,* 1–5.

Sorkin, B. A., Rudy, T. E., Hanlon, R. B., Turk, D. C., & Stieg, R. L. (1990). Chronic pain in old and young patients: Differences appear less important than similarities. *Journal of Gerontology: Psychological Sciences, 45,* 63–68.

Stahmer, S. A., Shofer, F. S., Marino, A., Shepherd, S., & Abbuhl, S. (1998). Do quantitative changes in pain intensity correlate with pain relief and satisfaction? *Academic Emergency Medicine, 5,* 851–857.

Stanos, S. P., McLean, J., & Rader, L. (2007). Physical medicine rehabilitation approach to pain. *Medical Clinics of North America, 91,* 57–95.

Sullivan, M. J. L., Bishop, S. R., & Pivik, J. (1995). The Pain Catastrophizing Scale: Development and validation. *Psychological Assessment, 7,* 524–532.

Sullivan, M. J. L., Thorn, B., Haythornthwaite, J. A., Keefe, F. J., Martin, M., Bradley, L. A., et al. (2001). Theoretical perspectives on the relation between catastrophizing and pain. *Clinical Journal of Pain, 17,* 52–64.

Sullivan, M. J. L., Thorn, B., Rodgers, W., & Ward, C. (2004). A path model of psychological antecedents of pain experience: Clinical and experimental findings. *Clinical Journal of Pain, 20,* 164–173.

Tucker, C., & Mayer, T. (2000). Functional restoration of the patient with chronic spine pain. *Continuum, 7,* 153–178.

Turk, D. C., & Melzack, R. (Eds.). (2011). *Handbook of pain assessment* (3rd ed.). New York: Guilford Press.

Turk, D. C., & Rudy, T. E. (1988). Toward an empirically derived taxonomy of chronic pain patients: Integration of psychological assessment data. *Journal of Consulting and Clinical Psychology, 56,* 233–238.

U.S. Department of Labor. (2000). *Lost worktime injuries and illnesses: Characteristics and resulting time away from work, 1998* (Publication No. USDL 00-115). Washington, DC: Author.

Vendrig, A. A. (2000). The Minnesota Multiphasic Personality Inventory and chronic pain: A conceptual analysis of a long-standing but complicated relationship. *Clinical Psychology Review, 20,* 533–559.

Vlaeyen, J. W., Kole-Snijders, A. M., Boeren, R. G., & van Eek, H. (1995). Fear of movement/(re)injury in chronic low back pain and its relation to behavioral performance. *Pain, 62,* 363–372.

Vowles, K. E., McCracken, L. M., & Eccleston, C. (2008). Patient functioning and catastrophizing in chronic pain: The mediating effects of acceptance. *Health Psychology, 27*(Suppl. 2), S136–S143.

Waddell, G., Gordon, J. M., Kummel, E., & Venner, R. (1980). Non-organic physical signs in low back pain. *Spine, 5,* 117–125.

Waddell, G., Mewton, M., Henderson, I., Somerville, D., & Main, C. J. (1993). A Fear-Avoidance Beliefs Questionnaire (FABQ) and the role of fear-avoidance beliefs in chronic low back pain and disability. *Pain, 52,* 157–168.

Walsh, T. L., Homa, K., Hanscom, B., Lurie, J., Sepulveda, M. G., & Abdu, W. (2006). Screening for depressive symptoms in patients with chronic spinal pain using the SF-36 Health Survey. *Spine Journal, 6,* 316–320.

Ware, J. E., & Sherbourne, C. D. (1992). The MOS 36-Item Short-Form Health Survey (SF-36). *Medical Care, 30,* 473–483.

Wesley, A. L., Gatchel, R. J., Garofalo, J. P., & Polatin, P. B. (1999). Toward more accurate use of the Beck Depression Inventory with chronic back pain patients. *Clinical Journal of Pain, 15,* 117–121.

Wijnhoven, H. A., de Vet, H. C., & Picavet, H. S. (2006). Prevalence of musculoskeletal disorders is systematically higher in women than in men. *Clinical Journal of Pain, 22,* 717–724.

Wittink, H. M., & Carr, D. B. (Eds.). (2008). *Pain management: Evidence, outcomes, and quality of life: A sourcebook.* New York: Elsevier.

Worzer, W., Theodore, B. R., Rogerson, M., & Gatchel, R. J. (2008). Interpreting clinical significance: A comparison of effect sizes of commonly used patient self-report pain instruments. *Practical Pain Management, 8,* 16–29.

Wright, A., & Gatchel, R. J. (2002). Occupational rehabilitation: Interdisciplinary management of work-related musculoskeletal pain and disability. In D. C. Turk & R. J. Gatchel (Eds.), *Psychological approaches to pain management: A practitioner's handbook* (2nd ed.). New York: Guilford Press.

Zanoli, G., Stromqvist, B., & Jonsson, B. (2001). Visual analog scales for interpretation of back and leg pain intensity in patients operated for degenerative lumbar spine disorders. *Spine, 26,* 2375–2380.

Zigmond, A. S., & Snaith, R. P. (1983). The Hospital Anxiety and Depression Scale. *Acta Psychiatrica Scandinavica, 67,* 361–370.

CHAPTER 15

Headaches

Dawn C. Buse
Frank Andrasik
C. Mark Sollars

Headache is an extremely common condition that affects the majority of individuals at some point during their lifetimes (Rasmussen, 1995; Rasmussen, Jensen, Schroll, & Olesen, 1991). Although most headaches are benign, headache disorders can have a significant negative impact on occupational and educational performance, quality of life, and emotional well-being for sufferers. It is for this and many other reasons that headache disorders are best conceptualized and assessed within a biopsychosocial framework (Andrasik, Flor, & Turk, 2005) and managed with a coordinated multimodal approach (Lemstra, Stewart, & Olszynski, 2002). The biopsychosocial model assumes that the experience and expression of headache (like all chronic illnesses) is a complex interaction among biological, psychological, and social variables and that their interactions all play significant roles in the experience and outcomes of headache disorders (Andrasik et al., 2005). Within this framework, assessment of headache requires a thorough evaluation and understanding of the headache disorder in the context of the patient's life. From this perspective, one needs to conceptualize the individual experience of headache disorders (e.g., age of onset, severity and duration of attacks, triggers, prodromal and postdromal features, and response to treatments), as well as the

effect of headache on the individual's functioning, level of disability, quality of life, cognitive and emotional responses, coping styles, and psychological ramifications.

An extensive array of effective pharmacological and nonpharmacological treatments are available for headache; however, research has demonstrated that headache is commonly assessed using the traditional biomedical perspective that conceptualizes disease in terms of more narrowly defined neurophysiological dimensions (Hahn et al., 2008; Holmes, MacGregor, Sawyer, & Lipton, 2001). This approach leads to lack of understanding of the illness and the individual experiencing the illness, incorrect diagnoses, lack of agreement between patient and physician, and inadequate treatment plans (Hahn et al., 2008; Lipton et al., 2008). Gathering information about headache-related disability leads to a more accurate recognition of the severity of the effect of migraine on the patient's life and results in more aggressive, comprehensive, and effective treatment plans (Hahn et al, 2008; Holmes et al., 2001). For a review of effective medical communication strategies as applied to headache treatment, see Buse and Lipton (2008) and Hahn (2008).

The importance of utilizing a comprehensive approach to assessment is exemplified in the diagnosis and treatment of headache disorders. Diagnosis is almost entirely based on patient-reported symptoms and resulting impairment. Treatment success is largely dependent on a patient's treatment adherence to both medication use and behavioral interventions. The biopsychosocial model of headache proposes that the individual experience is based on complex interrelationships among biological factors, psychological characteristics, and the social and cultural context. In the case of headache, biological and pathophysiological predispositions and mechanisms may be "triggered" by the interplay of the individual's physiological status (e.g., level of autonomic arousal), environmental factors (e.g., stressful circumstances, certain foods, alcohol, toxins, hormonal fluctuations), the individual's ability to cope with these factors (both cognitively and behaviorally), and consequential factors (i.e., attention from family or reduction in household responsibilities) that may serve to reinforce, and thus increase, the person's chances of reporting head pain (Waggoner & Andrasik, 1990). Psychological factors do not play a causal role per se. Rather, psychological factors contribute to headache as (1) triggering factors, (2) maintaining factors, (3) exacerbating factors (to illustrate, ask the patient what is worse, onset of a headache when the patient is refreshed and rested or when work and family frustrations are at a peak), or (4) as sequelae to continued head pain and subsequent life disruption.

In applying the biopsychosocial approach to assessment of the headache patient, the core tenets of the humanistic approach to counseling (i.e., genuineness/congruence, unconditional positive regard, and empathetic understanding; Rogers, 1967) should be applied to the assessment process. Attention should be given equally to both the patient's physical and psychological well-being. It is important to involve and empower the patient in decision making, to emphasize the patient's responsibility for participation in and success of the treatment plan, and to place attention and value on the relationship and interactions between the health care provider and the patient.

In this chapter we address the biopsychosocial factors to consider when assessing patients with headache disorders. These factors include headache classification and diagnosis, identification of targets for treatment, evaluation of medical and psychological comorbidities, and the measurement of pain, headache-related disability, and quality of life. Although it is impossible to separate the biological, psychological, and social components of this disorder, we provide a brief review and identify selected instruments in the various domains. These instruments can be roughly divided into the following categories:

Bio-psychosocial

1. Headache diagnosis and symptomatology.
2. Treatment planning, optimization, and satisfaction.
3. Medication dependence, abuse, or misuse.

Bio-psycho-social

4. Psychiatric comorbidities.
5. Cognitive and psychological aspects of headache.

Biopsycho-social

6. Headache-related functional impairment, burden, and disability.
7. Health-related quality of life.

The majority of instruments we discuss were developed and validated for adults; however, we briefly discuss instruments appropriate for assessment of children and adolescents with headache or migraine. This chapter does not provide an exhaustive list but rather an overview of the most psychometrically sound and clinically useful instruments. Additional instruments for use in assessment and clinical management of headache are reviewed in Holroyd (2002).

Headache Classification, Diagnosis, and Epidemiology

Headache is a common medical condition affecting 91% of males and 96% of females at some point during their lifetimes (Rasmussen, 1995). The majority of headaches are benign, and less than 0.1% of the lifetime prevalence of headache is associated with life-threatening conditions (Silberstein & Lipton, 1993). The International Classification of Headache Diagnoses (ICHD) criteria were established to standardize headache diagnosis in clinical practice and research (Headache Classification Committee of the International Headache Society, 1988). The criteria are endorsed by all major headache societies, including the International Headache Society, and are included in the *International Classification of Diseases* (ICD), the international standard diagnostic classification for epidemiological, health management purposes, and clinical use. In 2004, the ICHD system was updated and revised (ICHD-II; Silberstein et al., 2004).

In 2013 the Headache Classification Committee of the International Headache Society (IHS) (2013) released a new "beta" version of the third edition of the International Classification of Headache Disorders (ICHD-3). The ICHD-3 beta was issued because of the marked advances in headache understanding. This version is more evidence-based, whereas prior versions were admittedly based as much on opinion as evidence. This version also reflects international efforts to "synchronize" with the World Health Organization's next revision (11th edition) of the International Classification of Diseases, or ICD-11. The ICD-11 is currently undergoing field trials and the Headache Classification Committee recommends that similar trials be conducted for the ICHD-3 beta criteria (hence, the "beta" label). It may require several years before each version is finalized. By making the ICHD-3 beta compatible with ICD-11, members of the Classification Committee believe this will greatly facilitate communication among clinicians and researchers and reimbursement as well. The ICHD-3beta version seeks to be much more precise by incorporating a hierarchical classification system permitting up to five levels of specification for many headache types; requiring a diagnosis for each specific type (prior versions have handled this variably), listed in their judged order of importance; incorporating minimal attack frequency as necessary; recommending that detailed headache diaries be utilized when precise classification is unclear; and providing an Appendix to facilitate future research and gain clarity with respect to certain headache types (new headache types, alternative proposed criteria, and old or former entities that still lack validity).

The ICHD classification system is divided into three sections. Part 1, primary headache disorders (i.e., headaches not attributable to another medical condition), Part 2, secondary headaches (i.e., headaches attributable to another medical condition), and Part 3 includes painful cranial neuropathies, other facial pains, and other headaches.

Primary headache disorders can be subdivided into migraine, tension-type headache (TTH), cluster headache and other trigeminal autonomic cephalalgias, and other primary headaches. TTH is the most common type of primary headache in the general population, with a 1-year-period prevalence ranging from 31 to 73% (Schwartz, Stewart, Simon, & Lipton, 1998). TTH can be subdivided into (1) infrequent episodic (headaches occurring less frequently than 1 day per month); (2) frequent episodic (headaches on 1–14 days per month); and (3) chronic daily (headaches on 15 or more days per month). In a large, population-based study, the 1-year-period prevalence of episodic TTH (ETTH) was 38.3%, and that of chronic TTH (CTTH) was 2.2% (Schwartz et al., 1998). The primary features of TTH are bilateral location (pain on both sides of the head), nonpulsating quality, and mild-to-moderate pain intensity, although features may vary by individual. It typically remains unchanged or improves with physical activity. Stress is cited as the most common trigger.

Schwartz et al. (1998) reported that prevalence of ETTH peaked in the fourth decade of life in both men and women and then declined thereafter. Women experience ETTH at greater rates across the life span (sex prevalence ratio of female to male = 1.16.) The prevalence of ETTH increases with higher levels of education, whereas CTTH prevalence is inversely related to education. The majority of persons with ETTH (71.8%) experience headaches 30 or fewer times per year; the rate was found to be significantly higher in European Americans than in African Americans in both men (40.1% vs. 22.8%) and women (46.8% vs. 30.9%; Schwartz et al., 1998). Due to its limited rates of disability, ETTH rarely is the basis for consultation in primary care or specialty settings.

The pathophysiology of TTH is not completely understood; however, it is agreed that the source of pain is myofascial tension

(Lenaerts & Newman, 2008). Myofascial or muscular pain tends to be dull and achy, poorly localized, and radiating, as opposed to pain signals emitting from neurological or cutaneous sources, which tend to be sharper, localized, and nonradiating. Current theories and areas of research include exploration of excessive pericranial myofascial resting muscle tension, excessive tenderness and sensitization, lowered pain thresholds, reduced blood flow in pericranial muscles, and genetic factors. It is not uncommon for migraine and TTH to coexist within the same individual and to warrant separate diagnoses (which in the past had been termed, variously, "mixed headache," "tension-vascular headache," or "combination headache").

Migraine is a common condition that affects 12–28% of people at some point in their lives and one out of four U.S. households (Lipton & Stewart, 1993). Several epidemiological studies indicate that the 1-year prevalence of migraine ranges from 6 to 15% in adult men and from 14 to 35% in adult women (Lipton & Stewart, 1993; Stovner, Zwart, Hagen, Terwindt, & Pascual, 2006). Rates vary substantially over the life cycle: approximately 4–5% of children younger than 12 experience migraine, with no significant difference between genders (Mortimer, Kay, & Jaron, 1992). Following puberty, migraine is much more common in women (Linet, Stewart, Celentano, Ziegler, & Sprecher, 1989). By early middle age, around 25% of women experience a migraine at least once a year, compared with fewer than 10% of men. After menopause, attacks in women tend to decline dramatically. After age 70 the ratio between men and women is approximately equal again, with prevalence lowering to approximately 5% (Lipton & Stewart, 1993).

Migraine attacks are usually accompanied by moderate-to-severe pain that lasts at least 4 hours. The pain is often unilateral (i.e., one-sided), may have a pulsating quality, and may be aggravated by movement and activity. People with migraine may experience nausea or vomiting, photophobia (sensitivity to light), phonophobia (sensitivity to sound), and osmophobia (sensitivity to smell). Approximately 20% of people with migraine experience aura, which is characterized by focal neurological features that usually occur in the hour preceding the headache. Migraine has five major subtypes and may occur with aura (MA) or without it (MO). Aura symptoms may include seeing flickering lights, spots or lines, loss of vision, feelings of "pins and needles" or numbness, and other symptoms. Individuals with a diagnosis of MA may also have attacks without aura.

Migraine is currently conceptualized as a neurovascular disorder (May & Goadsby, 1999) with a biological or genetic predisposition. Current understanding of the pathophysiology of migraine is based on a theory of neuronal hyperexcitability in the cerebral cortex in which a migraine attack is preceded by a complex series of neural and vascular events. Migraine is a chronic disorder with episodic attacks (Haut, Bigal, & Lipton, 2006). For purposes of diagnosis, migraine is subdivided by frequency into episodic migraine (EM; headaches occur on 14 or fewer days per month) and chronic migraine (CM; headaches occur on 15 or more days per month, of which at least eight are migraine attacks; Olesen et al., 2006). CM has been associated with more severe headache-related disability, health care costs and resource utilization, occupational and academic consequences, and psychological comorbidities (Bigal, Rapoport, Lipton, Tepper, & Sheftell, 2003; Bigal, Serrano, Reed, & Lipton, 2008; Buse, Manack, Serrano, Turkel, & Lipton, 2010).

Cluster headache (CH) is a group of headache disorders characterized by trigeminal nerve and parasympathetic nervous system activation. CH is often described as an excruciating, sharp pain in or around the eye. Cluster headaches last on average 1 hour and most often occur in "clusters" of multiple episodes over 2 weeks to 3 months; however, it is possible to experience more chronic forms of CH. CH is much less common than migraine but extremely debilitating and is experienced by men between four to seven times more often than by women (Finkel, 2003). The limited epidemiological studies have suggested prevalence rates of between 56 and 326 people per 100,000 (Torelli et al., 2006). This type of headache typically does not respond well to nonpharmacological treatments alone (Blanchard, Andrasik, Jurish, & Teders, 1982).

All headache subtypes, but especially migraine, are associated with increased rates of comorbidity with many common medical and psychiatric disorders (Buse et al., 2010; Scher, Bigal, & Lipton, 2005). Medical comorbidities with migraine include neurological disorders (e.g., stroke and epilepsy; Dayno, Silberstein, & Lipton, 1996; Ottman & Lipton, 1994), chronic pain disorders (Scher, Stewart, & Lipton, 2006), asthma (Aamodt, Stovner, Langhammer, Hagen, & Zwart, 2007), and coronary heart disease (Cook et al., 2002). Psychiatric comorbidities of migraine include depression, anxiety, panic disorder, bipolar disorder, obsessive–compulsive disorder, and suicide attempts (Buse et al., 2010; Hamelsky & Lipton, 2006; Jette, Patten, Williams, Becker, & Wiebe, 2008). The relation between migraine and depression is bidirectional, meaning that an individual who experiences one has a higher rate of risk for the other (Breslau & Davis, 1993). Anxiety and depression are correlated with greater impairment in functional ability and health-related quality of life (HRQoL) in people with migraine, and lowered HRQoL is associated with increased migraine-related disability (Lanteri-Minet, Radat, Chautard, & Lucas, 2005).

Headaches that are more chronic in nature and that are accompanied by excessive use of medication can be more difficult to treat. The diagnostic criteria for medication overuse headache (MOH) are as follows: (1) Headache occurring on ≥ 15 days per month in a person with a pre-existing headache disorder; (2) Regular overuse for > 3 months of one or more deugs that can be taken for acute and/or symptomatic treatment of headache; and (3) Not better accounted for by another ICHD-3 beta diagnosis (Headache Classification Committee of the International Headache Society, 2013; Silberstein et al., 2005). MOH tends to be unresponsive to conventional treatments and contributes to an increase in headache frequency. Thus medication overuse further complicates an already complex chronic headache picture (Andrasik, Grazzi, Usai, Buse, & Bussone, 2009; Grazzi, Andrasik, Usai, & Bussone, 2009; Silberstein, 2005).

Bio-psychosocial Assessment

Several established instruments assist health care providers in the assessment of biological factors that contribute to the occurrence and maintenance of headache disorders. These instruments facilitate screening and diagnosis, ascertain patient functioning, monitor medication consumption, and aid in treatment plan development and evaluation.

Medical and Neurological Evaluation

Assessment of headache should start with a thorough medical evaluation to rule out an acute medical condition, disease state, or structural abnormality and to evaluate the patient for appropriate medical and pharmacological treatment of headache. This includes performing a thorough neurological and general physical examination and taking a complete medical and social history. Important elements of the headache history include onset and progression, intensity, location, duration of pain, exacerbating factors, relieving factors, associated features, and current and previous treatments and provider information. Triggers, prodromal symptoms, and medical and psychological comorbidities should be assessed. Lifestyle habits, sleep, psychosocial stressors, exercise/physical activity, eating habits, substance use (e.g., caffeine, nicotine, alcohol, illicit drugs), and medication use (including prescribed, over-the-counter, and alternative medications) should also be assessed. The effect of headache on the patient's occupational and social functioning; psychological status; medical and psychiatric comorbidities; headache-related disability, including both ictal and interictal burden; HRQoL; and attitudes, beliefs, and preferences are also necessary elements of evaluation.

Once an acute medical condition is ruled out, a primary headache disorder can be diagnosed using ICHD-II criteria. Even after a primary headache disorder diagnosis is assigned, health care providers should remain vigilant for any "red flags" that may indicate severe underlying pathology (Dodick, 2003). These include the presence of systemic symptoms of illness (such as fever, frequent vomiting, stiff neck), signs and/or symptoms of certain neurological conditions (seizures, altered mental state), onset that is new and/or sudden, other associated conditions (such as headache on awakening, onset following trauma), and a headache history that is now markedly different (as regards pattern or progression in terms of severity or frequency).

Headache Screen, Diagnosis, Symptomatology

A number of instruments have been developed to facilitate initial screening and diagnosis. Selected items are reviewed in this section and in Table 15.1. The ID–Migraine helps to screen for migraines (Lipton, Dodick, et al., 2003). It contains a total of nine diagnostic questions with a three-item subset addressing the migraine-defining symptoms of disability, nausea, and photophobia. The three-item measure can stand alone as a screener with a sensitivity of 0.81 and specificity of 0.75 or be used in the longer form for applying additional diagnostic criteria.

The Brief Headache Screen (BHS) is a four-item screener that uses frequency of headaches (any and severe/disabling) and medication use to distinguish migraine, daily headache syndromes, and MOH. The BHS has demonstrated 82.6% agreement with migraine diagnoses made with the ID–Migraine (Maizels & Houle, 2008). It is the only brief screener that attempts to identify chronic migraine and daily headache syndromes.

The Migraine Severity (MIGSEV) scale is a seven-item scale designed for measuring migraine severity (El Hasnaoui et al., 2003). Questions include items on pain, tolerability, disability in daily activities, presence of nausea or vomiting, resistance to treatment, duration of attacks, and frequency of attacks and can be categorized into three dimensions: intensity of attacks, resistance to treatment, and frequency of attacks.

In addition to paper-and-pencil diagnostic instruments, there are computerized aids, such as the Computerized Headache Assessment Tool (CHAT), which is a computer-administered, branching screen assessment developed for diagnosing primary headache disorders (Maizels & Wolfe, 2008). The CHAT distinguishes between episodic, chronic, and daily disorders and can recognize medication overuse.

Headache Pain Rating and Description

Headaches, like many other pain disorders, are multifactorial and subjective, without reliable objective markers. Headache and pain are private events, and no method exists that can reliably quantify headache parameters. Simply asking the patient to rate his or her head pain on a scale of 0 (*no pain*) to 10 (*worst pain imaginable*) can be extremely useful. The question and rating scale should be kept uniform so that ratings can be compared across time and across attacks. Patients should also be asked to describe the quality of their pain, and it may be helpful to provide suggestions for them to choose from, such as "dull," "throbbing," "stabbing," and so forth. Patients may use metaphors, which may provide valuable clues to headache subtype and etiology (e.g., "it feels like my head is in a vise" or "it feels like birds are pecking at my eyes"). Some patients (especially children and adolescents) can best express their pain experience through drawing, in which case a simple instruction "Please draw your headache or pain" may yield useful information (Stafstrom, Rostasy, & Minster, 2002; Wojaczynska-Stanek, Koprowski, Wróbel, & Gola, 2008).

Headache Diary

One simple, effective way to gather data and monitor treatment is to have patients keep a "headache diary." Headache diaries can be maintained for 1–2 months to gain a more complete and accurate picture of a patient's health, functioning, and quality of life (Andrasik, Lipchik, McCrory, & Wittrock, 2005). Diaries may include virtually any data of interest, including headache frequency; severity (typically rated on a scale of 0–10); duration; medications taken; presence of aura or focal neurological symptoms; associated features; hormonal factors and menstrual cycle; mood ratings; information about sleep, diet, including meals, caffeine, alcohol, and nicotine use; weather (with a focus on barometric change); life events; and other potential triggers or exacerbators. Throughout treatment, diaries may be used to record medication use and habits, sleep, mood, "homework" and relaxation practice, analysis of dysfunctional cognitions, and other relevant data. Diaries may be kept on paper, computer, or a handheld electronic device (such as an application on a cellular phone) and may also be completed by individuals other than the patient, such

TABLE 15.1. Measures for Assessing Headache Screening and Initial Diagnosis

Name	Purpose	Brief description	No. of items, subscales, and scoring information	Psychometric properties	Reference
ID–Migraine	Headache diagnosis and symptomology	Brief screening instrument for migraine	Self-administered questionnaire with nine items. A three-item subset (screener) addressing the migraine-defining symptoms of disability, nausea, and photophobia may also stand alone.	Nine-item or three-item screen—sensitivity of .81 and specificity is .75, good test–retest reliability (kappa = .68) and a positive predictive value of .93.	Lipton, Dodick, et al. (2003)
Brief Headache Screen (BHS)	Headache diagnosis and symptomology	Screening tool designed to identify migraine and other daily headache syndromes	Four-item questionnaire. Respondents indicate the frequency of symptoms and medication use on a 5-point scale ranging from *daily or near daily* to *almost never*. In addition, two of the items require dichotomous *yes–no* responses.	82.6% agreement with migraine diagnoses made with the ID–Migraine.	Maizels & Houle (2008); Maizels & Burchette (2003)

as spouses, significant others, or parents of children with headaches (Andrasik, Burke, Attanasio, & Rosenblum, 1985; Blanchard, Andrasik, Neff, Jurish, & O'Keefe, 1981). Diaries are available for use free of charge on several headache society websites, including those of the American Headache Society (*www.americanheadachesociety.org*) and the National Headache Foundation (*www.headaches.org*).

Medication Consumption

Medication consumption can be monitored for several purposes, including checking for adherence, tapering, and watching for dependence and abuse. A patient's headache diary may be customized to facilitate this documentation. Excessive use or misuse of medication may trigger "rebound headache" or MOH (Andrasik et al., 2009; Grazzi et al., 2009; Silberstein, 2005). Timing is also important. Some classes of medications for acute headaches (e.g., triptans) are most effective when taken early in the onset of a headache (Holroyd et al., 1988); however, many patients wait to take their medication until they are sure about the type and severity of headache that they are experiencing, which can diminish effectiveness. Some patients present with a desire or need to reduce or eliminate medication use (e.g., because of pregnancy or prepregnancy planning). When tapering medications, daily logs can be useful to track headache pain, symptomatology, and side effects.

Special attention should be paid to narcotic or opioid medication use to monitor for signs of overuse, misuse, dependence, or abuse. Several instruments have been developed for monitoring opioid use with patients with chronic pain and are also suited for use with patients with headache. The Screener and Opioid Assessment for Patients with Pain (SOAPP) helps clinicians assess the suitability of long-term opioid therapy for chronic pain patients (Akbik et al., 2006). The Current Opioid Misuse Measure (COMM) can be used to help identify patients with pain who are misusing their opioid medications (Butler et al., 2007). The Medication Dependence Questionnaire in Headache (MDQ-H) was developed for use specifically with headache patients based on the fourth edition of the *Diagnostic and Statistical Manual of Mental Disorders* (DSM)-IV criteria (American Psychiatric Association, 2000) for dependence (to date, it has not been revised to accommodate the latest revision of DSM, [DSM-5; American Psychiatric Association, 2013]). Originally developed in French, it has since been translated into English (Radat et al., 2006; see Table 15.2 for more information).

Treatment Planning, Optimization, and Satisfaction

A number of scales help health care providers efficiently assess treatment needs, develop pharmacological and nonpharmacological treatment plans, monitor progress once started, and provide suggestions for ways to adjust treatment in order to maximize benefits. Several instruments have been developed for this purpose in headache and migraine care. We discuss these measures here and provide additional psychometric data in Table 15.3.

The Migraine–Assessment of Current Therapy (Migraine-ACT; Dowson et al., 2004) is a four-item self-response questionnaire that was originally developed for use in the primary care setting to assess the efficacy of acute migraine treatment and evaluate the need for change. It contains questions regarding consistency of response, global assessment of relief, headache impact, and emotional response.

The Patient Perception of Migraine Questionnaire—Revised version (PPMQ-R; Revicki et al., 2006) is a 29-item questionnaire that was designed to evaluate patient satisfaction with acute migraine treatment in five domains: efficacy, functionality, ease of use, cost, and bothersomeness of side effects. Total scores can range from 0 to 100, with higher levels of satisfaction indicated by higher scores.

The Migraine Treatment Optimization Questionnaire (MTOQ-5) assesses efficacy and patient satisfaction with current treatment based on five domains: functioning, consistency of relief, rapid relief, recurrence, and side effects (Lipton et al., 2009). The MTOQ-5 is intended to help health care providers assess the adequacy of acute headache treatment and to identify areas in which improvements can be made. Strategies are suggested based on the area(s) of deficiency

TABLE 15.2. Measures for Assessing Medication Consumption

Name	Purpose	Brief description	No. of items, subscales, and scoring information	Psychometric properties	Reference
Screener and Opioid Assessment for Patients with Pain—Revised (SOAPP-R)	Medication use/misuse/abuse	Helps assess the suitability of long-term opioid therapy for patients with chronic pain	24 items with 5 Likert-type response options, self-administered questionnaire. A subscale of 14 items can be used as a short screening instrument.	Internal consistency (coefficient alpha) of the 14 item short screener was .74. Test–retest reliability (Pearson product moment correlation between the SOAPP prediction score at baseline and at 6-month follow-up) was .71. To evaluate validity of the SOAPP, scores were compared against clinical identification of patients exhibiting aberrant drug-related behavior through any of the following: positive score on the Prescription Drug Use Questionnaire interview, positive urine toxicology screen, and/or ratings by staff as to whether patients had a serious drug problem. Of the original 24 items, 14 appeared to predict subsequent aberrant behaviors. Receiver operating characteristics curve analysis yielded an area under the curve of .881 ($p < .001$), suggesting adequate sensitivity and specificity for a screening device.	Akbik et al. (2006)
Current Opioid Misuse Measure (COMM)	Medication use/misuse/abuse	Helps identify patients with pain on opioid therapies who are misusing opioid medications	17 items with 5 Likert-type response options, self-administered questionnaire.	An initial item pool with six primary concepts was developed with input from 26 pain management and addiction specialists. One-week test–retest reliability was examined with 55 patients taking opioids for chronic, noncancer pain. Validity was examined comparing COMM scores to participant scores on the following: the Prescription Drug Use Questionnaire interview, a urine sample for toxicology screening, and clinical expert ratings of patient aberrant behaviors. Of the 40 items, 17 items appeared to adequately measure aberrant behavior, demonstrating excellent internal consistency and test–retest reliability. Cutoff scores were determined using ROC curve analysis, and reasonable sensitivity and specificity were established. 86 patients were assessed at baseline and 3 months using the COMM to evaluate the COMM's ability to assess change in patient status.	Butler et al. (2007)
Medication Dependence Questionnaire in Headache (MDQ-H)	Medication use/misuse/abuse	Developed for use specifically with patients with headache based on DSM-IV criteria for dependence	21 items with 7 response options, self-administered questionnaire.	Confirmatory structural analysis confirmed a model composed of 21 items grouped into seven factors corresponding to the seven DSM-IV diagnostic criteria for dependence. The internal consistency for factors range from "acceptable" to "satisfactory" (alpha = 0.50–0.89). A second order factor grouping the seven main factors may be taken as a general factor of dependence and has an excellent internal consistency (alpha = 0.87). Regression analysis showed that the global MDQ-H score predicted 37% of the variance in the number of days of taking medications ($p < .000$), 27% of the variance in the number of galenic units taken per week ($p < .000$), 39% of the variance in the number of days of headache ($p < .000$). Construct validity was demonstrated in that MDQ-H scores were significantly higher ($F = 41.9$; $p < .000$ for MDQ-H; $F = 10.6$) for patients with a headache associated with chronic substance use than for those without.	Radatet al. (2006)

Note. ROC,

272

and include both pharmacological and non-pharmacological treatment strategies.

The Migraine Therapy Assessment Questionnaire (MTAQ; Chatterton et al., 2002) is a nine-item questionnaire that was developed for migraine sufferers in a primary care setting. Items are defined to identify suboptimal treatment in three domains: migraine control, knowledge/behavior/treatment satisfaction, and economic burden. Higher scores indicate deficits in current treatment.

The Migraine Prevention Questionnaire (MPQ-5) was developed to facilitate the clinical implementation of the U.S. Headache Consortium Treatment Consensus Guidelines for the use of preventive pharmacotherapy for migraine treatment in clinical practice, to identify suboptimal clinical treatment of migraine, and to offer suggestions for improving therapeutic regimens (Lipton, Serrano, et al. 2007). The MPQ-5 assesses headache frequency, acute medication use, headache-related impairment in several domains, and headache-related anxiety. Responses are summed into a total score, which falls into three categories: (1) preventive treatment not indicated, (2) consider preventive treatment, and (3) offer preventive treatment. In addition to a total score, each of the five questions has individual cutoff scores, which may raise a "yellow flag" or "red flag" in one or more of the specific areas. This information should be used as an indicator that the health care professional needs to gather additional information and consider appropriate treatment and/or referral in that specific area. Recommendations include both pharmacological and nonpharmacological therapies.

Bio-*psycho*-social Assessment

Several established instruments assist health care providers in the assessment of psychological factors that contribute to the occurrence, maintenance, and worsening of headache disorders. These instruments perform important functions, which include screening for comorbid conditions, identifying disruptive thought patterns, and determining cognitive styles that can both trigger headache and affect patients' response to treatment.

Psychiatric and Cognitive Assessment

Headaches, especially migraines, are associated with increased rates of comorbidity with many common medical and psychiatric disorders (Buse et al., 2010; Scher et al., 2005). Assessment of, education about, and treatment/referral for common psychiatric comorbidities are essential components of headache assessment and care. The consequences of not assessing and treating psychiatric comorbidities may include poor treatment outcomes, problems with adherence and motivation, reduced quality of life, and potentially life-threatening consequences, such as suicidal behaviors (Breslau, Davis, & Andreski, 1991). Patients displaying even minor depressive symptoms demonstrate a poorer response to both behavioral (Blanchard et al., 1985; Jacob, Turner, Szekely, & Eidelman, 1983) and pharmacological treatments (Holroyd et al., 1988).

Psychiatric screening instruments can be used to assess for and monitor psychological functioning and comorbid conditions. Several validated instruments are available for screening and monitoring DSM-IV Axis I psychiatric disorders (again, none have been revised for DSM-5, which no longer includes a multiaxial approach). The Patient Health Questionnaire (PHQ) is a brief, self-administered questionnaire that screens for several Axis I psychological disorders based on DSM-IV criteria (Spitzer, Kroenke, Williams, & the Patient Health Questionnaire Primary Care Study Group, 1999). The PHQ-9 is the depression subscale of the Primary Care Evaluation of Mental Disorders (PRIME-MD) and can be used independently to screen for depression (Kroenke, Spitzer, & Williams, 2001). Clinically significant anxiety can be evaluated using the Generalized Anxiety Disorder–7 (GAD-7), a seven-item, self-administered questionnaire (Spitzer, Kroenke, Williams, & Lowe, 2006). Some personality disorders have been linked to poorer outcomes. Specifically, elevations on scales 1, 2, and 3 of the Minnesota Multiphasic Personality Inventory (MMPI) have been demonstrated to predict poor response to behavioral treatment for migraine (Blanchard et al., 1985; Werder, Sargent, & Coyne, 1981). (See Saper & Lake, 2002, for a review of personality disorder screening in headache care.)

TABLE 15.3. Measures for Assisting with Treatment Planning

Name	Purpose	Brief description	No. of items, subscales and scoring information	Psychometric properties	Reference
Migraine–Assessment of Current Therapy (Migraine–ACT)	Treatment satisfaction and optimization	Designed for use in the primary care setting to assess the efficacy of acute migraine treatment and evaluate the need for change. Contains questions regarding consistency of response, global assessment of relief, headache impact, and emotional response.	Four-item, self-response questionnaire with dichotomous response options (yes–no). "Yes" responses are summed (range: 0–4). "No" responses indicate a possible need to change treatment.	One-week, test–retest reliability (Pearson correlation coefficient) was high ($r = .82$) and good correlation with items from the SF-36 and MIDAS.	Dowson, Tepper, Baos, Baudet, D'Amico, & Kilminster (2004); Kilminster et al. (2006)
Patient Perception of Migraine Questionnaire—Revised (PPMQ-R)	Treatment satisfaction and optimization	A migraine-specific, self-administered questionnaire designed to evaluate patient satisfaction with acute migraine treatment.	29 items; the questionnaire has five domains measuring satisfaction with efficacy, functionality, ease of use, medication cost, and bothersomeness of medication side effects. The total score is the average of efficacy, functionality, and ease of use scores and is reported on a 0–100 scale, with higher scores indicating higher satisfaction.	Scale scores and total scores have demonstrated internal consistency reliability (Cronbach's alpha = 0.80–0.98) at baseline and following the first migraine attack. Test–retest reliability as determined by intraclass correlation coefficient at an average of 8 weeks was .79 to .91. PPMQ-R scores showed statistically significant negative correlations between migraine pain severity levels and levels of impairment in ability to work and perform usual activities.	Revicki et al. (2006)
Migraine Treatment Optimization Questionnaire (M-TOQ-5)	Treatment satisfaction and optimization	The M-TOQ-5 was designed for assessing efficacy and patient satisfaction with current acute treatment. It was intended to help HCPs assess the adequacy of current acute headache treatment and identify areas for improvement. Items include five domains: functioning, consistency	Five-item, self-response questionnaire. If all five questions are answered "yes," treatment is satisfactory; an answer of "no" to a single question suggests that a change in treatment should be considered. The change should address the specific limitation of current acute treatment. Strategies	Cronbach's alpha was 0.66 for the M-TOQ-5. Test–retest reliability based on intraclass correlations was over .80. Convergent validity among TOQ forms ranged from .89 to .96. Convergent validity with other instruments, including MIDAS, HIT-6, and MSQOL, ranged from .35 to .44.	Lipton et al. (2009)

		of relief, rapid relief, recurrence, and side effects.		
Migraine Therapy Assessment Questionnaire (MTAQ)	Treatment satisfaction and optimization	A self-administered questionnaire developed to detect impediments to optimal treatment in a primary care setting and improve patient satisfaction.	Nine items. Three domains: migraine control, knowledge/behavior/treatment satisfaction, and economic burden. Responses are scored based on a dichotomous scale (yes = 1, no = 0). A higher total score indicates problems in current treatment.	Test–retest reliability at 2 weeks for all MTAQ questions had a Cohen's kappa of at least .5 and an average Pearson's r of .72. There were significant negative correlations between MTAQ items and SF-36 scores and satisfaction. There were significant positive correlations between MTAQ items and work loss, disability, and health-care resource use.	Chatterton et al. (2002)
Migraine Prevention Questionnaire (MPQ-5)	Treatment satisfaction and optimization	Developed to facilitate the clinical implementation of U.S. Headache Consortium Treatment Consensus Guidelines and address the treatment gap for preventive pharmacotherapy in clinical practice.	Five-item, self-administered, questionnaire that assesses five areas: headache frequency, acute medication use, headache-related impairment in several domains, and worry and anxiety related to headache. Responses are summed into a total score, which falls into 1 of 3 categories: preventive treatment not indicated, consider preventive treatment, and offer preventive treatment. Each item has individual cutoff scores, which may raise a "yellow" or "red flag." This information should be used as an indicator that the health care professional should gather additional information and consider appropriate treatments.	The MPQ-5 demonstrates strong test–retest reliability (rho = .8). The MPQ-5 correlates in the predicted direction with external validators such as ictal disability (MIDAS rho = .7; HIT-6 rho = .5), interictal burden (rho = .43), health-related quality of life (rho = −.51), depression (rho = .36), and lost productive time (rho = .36).	Lipton, Serrano, Buse, Rupnow, Reed, & Bigal (2007); Lipton, Serrano, Buse, Bigal, Rupnow, & Biondi (2008)

Note. HCP, healthcare professional.

The cognitive status of the patient requires special attention in order to identify conditions (e.g., formal thought disorder) that might interfere with treatment and that need to be handled prior to treatment of the headache per se or that may otherwise compromise treatment. When significant cognitive deficits or diminished cognitive capacities are observed or suspected (such as in the case of posttraumatic headache), it may be helpful to obtain a thorough neuropsychological assessment. Penzien, Rains, and Holroyd (1993) recommend use of the Cognitive Capacities Screening Examination (Jacobs, Bernhard, Delgado, & Strain, 1977) or the Mini-Mental State Examination (MMSE; Folstein, Folstein, & McHugh, 1975) to screen for this purpose. However, it is generally not necessary to utilize these assessments once a primary headache disorder has been diagnosed unless a specific situation warrants such testing. A survey of a headache practice showed that only 2 of 88 patients diagnosed with a primary headache disorder scored in the range suggesting significant organic involvement (Lawson et al., 1988).

Cognitive Processes

In the biopsychosocial model of headache management, cognitive processes, including thoughts, beliefs, attributions, and attitudes, play a key role in the conceptualization and treatment for each patient with headache. Although numerous cognitive processes can influence headache and disability, three areas that have been empirically demonstrated to be especially important include locus of control (LOC), self-efficacy, and catastrophizing (see Nicholson, Houle, Rhudy, & Norton, 2007, for a thorough review). These constructs have been demonstrated to be related to headache-related disability, quality of life, and adherence and response to treatment. Specific cognitive goals of cognitive-behavioral therapy (CBT) for headache management include helping patients gain an internal LOC (i.e., a belief that the mechanism for change lies within oneself) as opposed to an external LOC (i.e., the belief that only the physician, medication, or medical procedures have the power to help), self-efficacy (i.e., the patient's belief in his or her ability to succeed or accomplish a certain task), and replacing catastrophizing with more realistic and positive ways of thinking (Andrasik, 2003; Buse & Andrasik, 2009).

Locus of Control. Locus of control refers to the degree to which an individual perceives that an event is under his or her personal control. These beliefs range from a completely internal LOC (in which the individual perceives the event as totally under his or her control) to a completely external LOC (in which the event is perceived as totally outside the individual's realm of influence). In most cases an individual's perception will fall in between those two extremes. Research has demonstrated that an external LOC (e.g., "The doctor is the only one who can manage my headaches," "Only medication can cure my headaches," or "Nothing that I do matters") is related to poor outcome, passive coping, less active participation in treatment, and physiological responses that include depletion of norepinephrine and increased 5-hydroxytryptamine receptor sensitization (Heath, Saliba, Mahmassani, Major, & Khoury, 2008; Scharff, Turk, & Marcus, 1995; Weiss et al., 1981). To facilitate measuring and monitoring perceived LOC among headache sufferers, Martin, Holroyd, and Penzien (1990) developed the Headache Specific Locus of Control Questionnaire (HSLC; see Table 15.4 for more information).

Self-Efficacy. Self-efficacy refers to an individual's belief that he or she can successfully accomplish an action or behavior to produce a desired outcome (Bandura, 1986). Poor self-efficacy is related to poor treatment outcome and decreased quality of life in headache management (French et al., 2000; Marlowe, 1986; Nicholson, Hursey, & Nash, 2005). Self-efficacy predicts differential response to combined pharmacological and behavioral treatment (Smith & Nicholson, 2006), and changes in self-efficacy correlate with changes in headache frequency (Bond, Dirge, Rubingh, Durrant, & Baggaley, 2004; Nicholson, Nash, & Andrasik, 2005). French et al. (2000) developed the Headache Management Self-Efficacy (HMSE) scale to assess patients' level of self-efficacy in regard to headache prevention and management (see Table 15.4 for more information).

TABLE 15.4. Measures for Assessing Locus of Control and Related Concepts

Name	Purpose	Brief description	No. of items, subscales, and scoring information	Psychometric properties	Reference
Headache Specific Locus of Control Questionnaire (HSLC)	Cognitive and psychological aspects of headache	Assesses perceived locus of control among headache sufferers.	33-item, self-response questionnaire with Likert-type options ranging from 1 (*strongly disagree*) to 5 (*strongly agree*). Consists of 3 subscales with 11 items each: Health Care Professionals Locus of Control, Internal Locus of Control, and Chance Locus of Control. A total sum score can be derived as well as scores on the three subscales.	Good internal consistency (alpha coefficient ranging from 0.84 to 0.88 between the 3 subscales), and test–retest reliability over a 3-week interval ranging from $r = .72$ to $r = .78$ among the three subscales.	Martin, Holroyd, & Penzien (1990)
Headache Management Self-Efficacy Scale (HMSE)	Cognitive and psychological aspects of headache	Used to assess patient's level of self-efficacy in regard to headache prevention and management.	25-item questionnaire. 25 headache management statements are rated by respondents on a Likert-type scale from 1, *strongly disagree*, to 7, *strongly agree*. Responses are summed to produce a total score, with higher scores reflecting greater perceived self-efficacy.	Good internal consistency (Cronbach's alpha = 0.90) and construct validity (i.e., scores were positively associated with the use of positive psychological coping strategies to both prevent and manage headache episodes and negatively associated with anxiety).	French et al. (2000)
The Pain Catastrophizing Scale (PCS) and Headache Catastrophizing Scale (HCS)	Cognitive and psychological aspects of pain/headache	Designed to assess tendency of patients with chronic pain toward catastrophizing as a cognitive style. More specifically, it assesses rumination, magnification, and helplessness. Holroyd et al. (2007) modified the PCS for use with a headache population (substituting "headache" for "pain").	13-item, self-administered questionnaire. Maintaining the original PCS scoring system, HCS items are rated on a 5-point scale from 0 (*not at all*) to 4 (*all the time*) and summed for a total score ranging from 0 to 52, with higher scores reflecting a greater likelihood of engaging in catastrophizing.	The PCS demonstrated good reliability (alpha = 0.87) and construct validity (i.e., catastrophizers, as determined by scores on the PCS, reported significantly more pain and emotional distress relative to noncatastrophizers in response to procedures inducing physical discomfort).	The Pain Catastrophizing Scale (PCS): Sullivan, Bishop, & Pivik (1995); Headache Catastrophizing Scale: Holroyd et al. (2007)

(continued)

TABLE 15.4. *(continued)*

Name	Purpose	Brief description	No. of items, subscales, and scoring information	Psychometric properties	Reference
Survey of Pain Attitudes (SOPA)	Cognitive and psychological aspects of pain	A self-response instrument, which assesses patient attitudes in seven areas: pain control, solicitude (solicitous responses from others in response to one's pain), medication (as appropriate treatment for pain), pain-related disability, pain and emotions (the interaction between emotions and pain), medical cures for pain, and pain-related harm (pain as an indicator of physical damage or harm). The Survey of Pain Attitudes—Brief Version (SOPA-B; Tait & Chibnall, 1997) is a 30-item version of the original.	A 57-item self-report questionnaire on which respondents indicate their level of agreement using a 5-point Likert scale.	The SOPA has been validated in several languages, including Chinese, Portuguese, and French Canadian. Test–retest reliability ranges from .67 to .79. Internal consistency for the seven scales ranges from .65 to .82.[a]	Jensen, Karoly, & Huger (1987); Wong, Jensen, Mak, & Fielding (2011); Pimenta, & da Cruz (2006); Duquette, McKinley, & Litowski (2005)
Chronic Pain Coping Inventory (CPCI)	Cognitive and psychological aspects of pain/ headache	A measure of strategies used by patients to cope with chronic pain. It is validated for use with adults ages 21–80 and takes approximately 10–15 minutes to complete.	The CPCI is a 70-item self-report instrument on which the individual is asked to indicate the number of days during the past week he or she employed specific coping strategies to deal with pain. The CPCI consists of nine scales that are divided into two domains: the illness-focused coping domain and the wellness-focused coping domain.	The internal consistency for the nine scales of the CPCI range from .70 to .84. Test–retest stability for the nine scales range from .55 to .84. Eight scales revealed moderate to strong associations between a patient version of the CPCI and a version completed by spouses that assesses observable behaviors (significant-other version), supporting the instruments's validity.[a]	Jensen, Turner, Romano, & Strom (1995; Hadjistavropoulos, MacLeod, & Asmundson, 1999)
Patient Health Questionnaire (PRIME-MD)	Psychiatric comorbidities	A brief, self-administered questionnaire that screens for several Axis I psychological disorders based on DSM-IV criteria.	16 items with both Likert and dichotomous (yes–no) response types, the PHQ (PRIME-MD) screens for depressive, anxiety, somatoform, alcohol, and eating disorders. Diagnostic algorithms are applied based on positive responses.	Good agreement between PHQ diagnoses and those of independent mental health professionals (kappa = .65; overall accuracy, 85%; sensitivity, 75%; specificity, 90%).	Spitzer, Kroenke, Williams, & the Patient Health Questionnaire Primary Care Study Group (1999)

278

PHQ-9	Psychiatric comorbidities	The PHQ-9 is the depression subscale of the PHQ (PRIME-MD) and can be used independently to screen for depression.	9-item self-report questionnaire based on the nine criteria for DSM-IV depression diagnoses. Items assess the frequency of symptoms over the previous 2-week period and consist of Likert-type options ranging from 0 (*not at all*) to 3 (*nearly every day*). A major depression diagnosis is warranted if at least five of the nine symptoms were present at least "more than half the days" and one of the symptoms is depressed mood or anhedonia. Severity of depression ranges from 0 to 27, with scores of 5, 10, 15, and 20 representing cutpoints for mild, moderate, moderately severe, and severe depression. An additional item asks patients to report the degree to which indicated problems have interfered with work, home life, and interpersonal interactions.	Demonstrates good internal reliability (Cronbach's alpha = 0.89) and test–retest reliability (the correlation between the self- administered PHQ-9 and the PHQ-9 administered by a mental health professional within 48 hours was .84). Receiver operating characteristics curve analysis yielded an area under the curve of .995, suggesting adequate capability in discriminating between those with and without major depression. In addition, likelihood ratios revealed a relationship between rising PHQ-9 scores and the likelihood of major depression. Good construct validity as evidenced by a strong relationship between PHQ-9 scores and functional status, disability days, and symptom-related difficulty.	Kroenke, Spitzer, & Williams (2001)
Generalized Anxiety Disorder–7 (GAD-7)	Psychiatric comorbidities	A self-administered questionnaire used for evaluating clinically significant anxiety.	7-item self-report questionnaire. Items assess the frequency of symptoms over the previous 2-week period and consist of Likert-type options ranging from 0 (*not at all*) to 3 (*nearly every day*). Items are summed with scores of 5, 10, and 15, representing mild, moderate, and severe levels of anxiety respectively. An additional item asks patients to report the degree to which indicated problems have interfered with work, home life, and interpersonal interactions.	Good internal consistency (Cronbach's alpha = 0.92) and test–retest reliability (intraclass correlation = .83). Good construct validity as evidenced by increasing GAD-7 scores associated with worsening scores on all 6 of the SF-20 functional status scales. Higher GAD-7 scores were also associated with increases in disability days, physician visits, and symptom- related difficulty. In addition, the GAD-7 was correlated with the Beck Anxiety Inventory (r = .72) and the anxiety subscale of the Symptom Checklist (r = .74).	Spitzer, Kroenke, Williams, & Lowe (2006)

aMore information is available in the instrument manual, which is available for purchase at *www4.parinc.com/Products/Product.aspx?*

Catastrophizing. "Catastrophizing" is a hopeless and overwhelming thinking pattern characterized by rumination, magnification, and helplessness. Catastrophizing is associated with poor outcomes, increased impairment, and reduced quality of life across many chronic pain conditions, including headache (Burns, Kubilus, Bruehl, Harden, & Lofland, 2003; Holroyd, Drew, Cottrell, Romanek, & Heh, 2007; Sullivan et al., 2001). Holroyd et al. (2007) examined catastrophizing, comorbid anxiety, depression, quality of life, and headache characteristics among 232 migraine sufferers. They found that catastrophizing and severity of associated symptoms (photophobia, phonophobia, and nausea) independently predicted quality of life, demonstrating that it is not just headache severity and frequency that predict quality of life but that patient perception is also directly related to quality of life. The Pain Catastrophizing Scale (PCS) was designed to assess chronic pain patients' tendency toward catastrophizing as a cognitive style (i.e., rumination, magnification, and helplessness; Sullivan, Bishop, & Pivik, 1995). Holroyd et al. (2007) modified the PCS for use with a headache population (substituting "headache" for "pain" in the Headache Catastrophizing Scale [HCS]; see Table 15.4 for more information).

Coping Style and Attitudes

Two pain-specific measures, which can be especially useful in headache assessment and management, include the Chronic Pain Coping Inventory (CPCI; Hadjistavropoulos, MacLeod, & Asmundson, 1999; Jensen, Turner, Romano, & Strom, 1995) and the Survey of Pain Attitudes (SOPA; Jensen, Karoly, & Huger, 1987). The CPCI is a measure of strategies used by patients to cope with chronic pain. The CPCI consists of nine scales that are divided into two domains: an illness-focused coping domain and a wellness-focused coping domain. The SOPA assesses patient attitudes in seven areas: pain control, solicitude (solicitous responses from others in response to one's pain), medication (as appropriate treatment for pain), pain-related disability, pain and emotions (the interaction between emotions and pain), medical cures for pain, and pain-related harm (pain as an indicator of physi-

cal damage). Both of these instruments can be useful adjuncts to cognitive-behavioral therapy for headache management in identifying targets for intervention.

Stress

The relationship between stress and headache has long been noted in the literature (Henryk-Gutt & Rees, 1973; Howarth, 1965). Stress-related migraine may occur either at the peak of stress or during a period of relaxation immediately following stress (i.e., "letdown headache"), such as the first day of spring break following a stressful week of final exams. Stress likely interacts with other precipitants to increase vulnerability to migraine without necessarily precipitating any particular migraine episode (Andrasik, 1990). It is important to realize that a patient's stress experience is idiosyncratic; stress rests within the individual's cognitive interpretive framework. That is, what determines whether any given event is stressful is more a function of how the patient appraises the event. Lazarus and Folkman (1984) distinguish between two types of appraisal: primary, that is, whether a given event is judged to be significant to the patient's well-being; and secondary, that is, whether the patient possesses the available resources or options to respond successfully to the event. What is appraised as significant by one individual may not be by another.

For any given person with headaches, stress is likely operating in one or more ways and in concert with other various biological influences (Andrasik, 1990). Take, as an example, the person with headaches who is able to drink red wine and escape headaches when feeling "on top of the world" but is not able to do so when she has not had enough sleep or is under multiple deadlines at work. Health care providers need to recognize that major stressful life events are not always the main culprit. Everyday "ups and downs" or "hassles" are sufficient to engage biological headache mechanisms (Andrasik, Wittrock, & Passchier, 2006; De Benedittis & Lorenzetti, 1992; Holm, Holroyd, Hursey, & Penzien, 1986; Levor, Cohen, Naliboff, MacArthur, & Heuser, 1986). The prolonged presence of headache or chronic pain itself exerts a psychological toll on the patient over time, such that the patient becomes "sick and tired of feeling sick and tired." The negative thoughts and emotions associated with repeated headaches can become stressors or triggers in and of themselves (referred to as "headache-related distress"), serving at that point both to help maintain the disorder and to increase the severity and likelihood of future attacks.

Biopsycho-*social* Assessment

Several established instruments assist health care providers in the assessment of social factors that contribute to the impact and maintenance of headache disorders. These instruments aid in the assessment of headache-related disability, severity of headache impact, including experienced burden between attacks, and overall quality of life.

Headache Related-Disability, Burden, and Quality of Life

Primary headaches can have a significant impact on all aspects of life, including daily functioning, productivity, and HRQoL (e.g., Andrasik, 2001, 2006; Buse, Rupnow, & Lipton, 2009). In fact, the Global Burden of Disease study conducted by the World Health Organization (WHO) identified migraine as a top-20 cause of disability worldwide (of the 135 health conditions included; Leonardi, Steiner, Scher, & Lipton, 2005). People with migraine have significantly lower SF-36 scores than people without migraine, and migraine adversely affects functioning at least as much as do depression, diabetes, and recent myocardial infarction (Bussone et al., 2004; Solomon, Skobieranda, & Gragg, 1993). Lipton, Liberman, and colleagues (2003) compared HRQoL between 200 people with migraine and 200 controls in a population-based, case-control study in England and found that people with migraine scored significantly worse in eight of the nine HRQoL domains and the two summary scores of the SF-36. They also found that migraine-related disability was inversely correlated with HRQoL. Dueland, Leira, Burke, Hillyer, and Bolge (2004) studied the impact of migraine on work, family, and leisure activi-

ties among 1,810 women ages 18 to 35 years living in Israel and eight European countries. The majority of respondents reported an inability to function fully at work or school during the prior 6 months because of migraine (74%), one or more instances of being unable to spend time with family or friends because of migraine (62%), and one or more instances of being unable to enjoy recreational or leisure activities because of migraine (67%). The presence of anxiety and depression in migraine sufferers further exacerbates the relationship and is correlated with greater impairment in functional ability and HRQoL in people with migraine, and lowered HRQoL is associated with increased migraine-related disability (Lanteri-Minet et al., 2005).

The impact of headache disorders increases as the frequency and severity of attacks increase (Bigal et al., 2003, 2008; Buse et al., 2010). Forms of chronic daily headache such as CM have been found to be associated with even greater levels of functional impairment, health service utilization, and psychiatric and medical comorbidities than episodic and lower frequency headaches (Bigal et al., 2008; Buse et al., 2010; Juang, Wang, Fuh, Lu, & Su, 2000; Lipton, Bigal, et al., 2007; Zwart et al., 2003).

Migraine can place a significant burden on individuals' lives, both during attacks (ictally) and in between attacks (interictally; Buse et al., 2009; Dahlof & Dimenäs, 1995). Interictal burden may include worry about the next attack and change or avoidance of commitments in the occupational, social, and personal arenas. Patients with high levels of interictal headache-related burden experience higher rates of psychological comorbidities. In a population-based study of interictal headache burden, 44% of respondents with "severe" levels of interictal burden met criteria for an anxiety disorder, 47% for panic disorder, and 46% for a depressive disorder, compared with 20%, 23%, and 25%, respectively, of headache sufferers with low or no interictal burden (Buse et al., 2007). These results were controlled for frequency and severity of headache, demonstrating that interictal burden is not solely related to the severity of the disease but rather to a more complex interaction of disease severity with other factors (such as cognitions and behaviors.)

Headache-Related Functional Impairment, Burden, and Disability

Over the past 15 years, headache-related burden has begun to be recognized as an immense public health problem. Because headache is not associated with premature death, traditional measures of burden (e.g., incidence/prevalence and mortality) are not applicable. To accurately measure the burden of migraine and other primary headache disorders, it is imperative that disease-specific outcome measures consistently address all dimensions of disability—physical, emotional, social, and economic. Measuring headache-related disability is challenging due to the episodic nature of the disease and variation in severity and features of attacks, both within and between individuals. Most headache instruments use a 1- or 3-month recall period in order to capture a representative period of time, whereas others use a single day. Measures may focus on the ictal or interictal burden of migraine, or both. The choice of instrument should be guided by the purposes of the assessment (e.g., research vs. clinical use) and nature of the specific headache subtype (e.g., EM vs. CM or chronic daily headache [CDH]). The most commonly used and psychometrically strongest instruments are discussed next, with additional psychometric data included in Table 15.5.

The Migraine Disability Assessment Scale (MIDAS) assesses headache-related disability or impairment. It is the most frequently used disability instrument in migraine research and clinical practice (Stewart, Lipton, Dowson, & Sawyer, 2001). This self-administered questionnaire consists of five items assessing days of missed activity or substantially reduced activity due to headache in three domains: schoolwork or paid employment, household work or chores, and nonwork (family, social, and leisure) activities, plus two optional items: headache frequency in number of days over the preceding 3 months, and an average pain rating on a scale of 0 (*no pain*) to 10 (*worst pain ever*) for the same time period. Responses to the first five items are summed, with these scores falling into one of four grades of headache-related disability: none, mild, moderate, and severe. The MIDAS has been validated for adults ages 18 and older and has been translated into and validated in multiple lan-

guages. The MIDAS is available for use free of charge and may be accessed on the American Headache Society website at *www.achenet.org/tools/migraine/index.asp.*

The Headache Needs Assessment Survey (HANA) is a questionnaire assessing two dimensions of the impact of migraine: frequency and bothersomeness. Specifically, patients provide data on these two dimensions in response to seven items with the following subscales: Anxiety/Worry, Depression/Discouragement, Self-Control, Energy, Function/Work, Family/Social Activities, and Overall Impact (Cramer, Silberstein, & Winner, 2001).

The Headache Impact Test (HIT), which assesses the impact of headache on functional health and well-being, is available in paper-and-pencil (HIT-6) and computerized (DYNHA Headache Impact Test) formats. The HIT-6 is a six-item questionnaire that measures lost time in three domains and other areas of impact (e.g., pain severity, fatigue, and mood; Kosinski et al., 2003). It is valid for adults ages 18 and older and has been translated and validated in multiple languages. (It is available in 28 languages at *www.headachetest.com/HIT6translations.html.*)

The Headache Impact Questionnaire (HImQ) combines measures of pain and disability into a single-scaled measure of severity (Stewart, Lipton, Simon, Von Korff, & Liberman, 1998). The HImQ measures the cumulative impact of headache on an individual over a 3-month period.

The Functional Assessment in Migraine (FAIM) questionnaire is derived from the World Health Organization International Classification of Impairments, Disabilities, and Handicaps Version 2 (ICIDH-2) classification system (Pathak, Chisolm, & Weis, 2005). The ICIDH-2 model includes three dimensions: (1) body structure and function, including mental functioning, (2) activity, and (3) participation.

The Migraine Interictal Burden Scale (MIBS-4; Buse et al., 2007) measures interictal burden (i.e., burden related to headache in the time between attacks) across four domains: disruption at work and school, diminished family and social life, difficulty planning, and emotional difficulty. MIBS-4 scores fall into one of the following levels of interictal burden: none, mild, moderate, or

TABLE 15.5. Measures for Assessing Headache-Related Disability and Burden

Name	Purpose	Brief description	No. of items, subscales and scoring information	Psychometric properties	Reference
Migraine severity (MIGSEV) Scale	Headache-related functional impairment, disease-related burden and disability	Measure of migraine severity; items include pain, tolerability, disability in daily activities, presence of nausea or vomiting, resistance to treatment, duration of attacks, and frequency of attacks. Items can be categorized into three dimensions: intensity of attacks, resistance to treatment, and frequency of attacks.	7 items	Seven items reflective of severity were created through literature review, expert neurologist consensus, and patient interviews. Principal components analysis identified 3 dimensions accounting for 65% of the overall variance (intensity of attacks, resistance to treatment, and frequency of attacks). Internal consistency and the reproducibility of the items was satisfactory. Test–retest at 15 days was good. The sensitivity of the severity questionnaire to differences in patients' quality of life suggested a good correlation between the items of severity and quality of life of migraineur participants. Finally, a rating system was empirically derived.	El Hasnaoui et al. (2003)
Migraine Disability Assessment Scale (MIDAS)	Headache-related functional impairment, disease-related burden and disability	Assesses headache-related disability and categorizes responses into four grades of severity.	Self-administered, five-item questionnaire. Assess days of missed activity or substantially reduced activity due to headache in three domains: schoolwork/paid employment, household work or chores, and nonwork (family, social, and leisure) activities, plus two optional items: headache frequency in number of days over the preceding 3 months and an average pain rating on a scale of 0 (*no pain*) to 10 (*worst pain ever*) for the same time period. Responses to the first five items are summed. Scores are ranked into one of four grades of headache-related disability: none, mild, moderate, and severe.	The MIDAS Questionnaire has been shown to be internally consistent, highly reliable, and valid and to correlate with physicians' clinical judgment. Test–retest reliability coefficients ranging from .59 to .80 have been reported, and internal consistency, as measured by Cronbach's alpha, was 0.83. Convergent validity with diary-based measures was .66. The MIDAS has been validated for adults ages 18 and older and has been translated and validated in multiple languages. There is also a version developed for use with pediatric and adolescent patients (PEDS-MIDAS).	Stewart, Lipton, Dowson, & Sawyer (2001)

(continued)

TABLE 15.5. *(continued)*

Name	Purpose	Brief description	No. of items, subscales and scoring information	Psychometric properties	Reference
Headache Needs Assessment Survey (HANA)	Headache-related functional impairment, disease-related burden and disability	A brief, self-administered questionnaire which assesses two dimensions of the impact of migraine: frequency and bothersomeness.	This instrument has seven questions (with the corresponding subscales of Anxiety/Worry, Depression/Discouragement, Self-Control, Energy, Function/Work, Family/Social Activities, and Overall Impact). For each item the respondent provides data on both frequency and "bothersomeness."	The HANA has good test–retest reliability (.77) and internal consistency (.92). There is a statistically significant correlation between HANA and Headache Disability Inventory total scores (.73, $p < .0001$) and high correlations with disease and treatment characteristics.	Cramer, Silberstein, & Winner (2001)
Headache Impact Questionnaire (HImQ)	Headache-related functional impairment, disease-related burden and disability	A self-administered instrument that measures the cumulative impact of headache on an individual over a 3-month period. Combines measures of pain and disability into a single scaled measure of severity.	16-item questionnaire. Items include total number of headaches, headache duration, last headache, pain intensity, need for bed rest, disability in specific domains of activity, and symptoms. The HImQ score is derived from eight items and is the sum of average pain intensity (on a scale from 0 to 10) and total lost days in all three defined domains of activity (work for pay, housework, and nonwork activities). Reduced effectiveness day equivalents are also considered. Score calculation involves both addition and multiplication.	Good internal consistency (Cronbach's alpha = 0.83) and test–retest correlation at an average of 6 weeks (.77). There is moderate convergent validity (.49) with a 90-day daily headache diary and moderate to high convergent validity with the expert physician judgment of disability.	Stewart, Lipton, Simon, Von Korff, & Liberman (1998)
Functional Assessment in Migraine	Headache-related functional impairment,	A migraine-specific self-administered instrument derived from the World Health	Items include nine mental functioning items measuring the dimensions of attention/thought	Construct validity analysis of FAIM dimensions found significant positive correlations with self-reported	Pathak, Chisolm, & Weis (2005)

(FAIM) Questionnaire	disease-related burden and disability	Organization International Classification of Impairments, Disabilities, and Handicaps: Version 2 (ICIDH-2) classification system. The ICIDH-2 model includes three dimensions: (1) body structure and function, including mental functioning, (2) activity, and (3) participation.	(five items) and perception (four items), and a list of 28 activity and participation items from which respondents choose the five items most relevant to their lifestyles.	symptom severity and significant negative correlations with functional status. Internal consistency (Cronbach's alpha) values were greater than 0.70 for all mental functioning items. Validity included moderately significant positive correlations with dimensions of the Migraine- Specific Quality of Life (MSQoL) questionnaire. The lowest correlations were seen between FAIM and the emotional dimension of the MSQoL questionnaire and the Short Form Health Survey (SF-12) component scores.	
Headache Impact Test (HIT)	Headache-related functional impairment, disease-related burden and disability	A brief, self-administered questionnaire developed to assess impact of headache on functional health and well-being. It is available in paper–pencil (HIT-6) and computerized (DYNHA Headache Impact Test) formats. The HIT-6 measures lost time in three domains and other areas of impact (e.g., pain severity, fatigue, and mood). It is valid for adults ages 18 and older and has been translated and validated in multiple languages. (It is available in 28 languages at *www.headachetest.com/ HIT6translations.html*.)	HIT-6: six-item, self-administered questionnaire with a 4-week recall period and response options ranging from *never* (6 points) to *always* (13 points), with a range of 36–78. Responses are summed and fall into the following categories: 49 or less, no impact; 50–55, some impact; 56–59, substantial impact; 60 or greater, severe impact.	The HIT-6 has demonstrated good discriminatory validity (migraine vs. nonmigraine headache and mild vs. moderate vs. severe headache) and external validity. Cronbach's alpha was 0.79. Test–retest reliability at 21 days was moderate for episodic headache and good for chronic headache.	Kosinski et al. (2003)

(continued)

TABLE 15.5. (continued)

Name	Purpose	Brief description	No. of items, subscales and scoring information	Psychometric properties	Reference
Migraine Interictal Burden Scale (MIBS-4)	Headache-related functional impairment, disease-related burden and disability	Measures interictal burden (i.e., burden related to headache between attacks) across four domains: disruption at work and school, diminished family and social life, difficulty planning, and emotional difficulty.	Four-item, self-administered questionnaire for clinical or research use. Response options range from *Don't know/NA* to *Most or all of the time*. In each column the number of responses is multiplied by an assigned value. The products are summed for a total score, which falls into one of the four levels of interictal burden: none, mild, moderate, or severe. Each category provides treatment recommendations.	This instrument was developed and validated in a large survey-based study with 30 candidate items identified from existing outcome measures and focus groups. Test–retest reliability was high across all retest intervals (rho = .69). Moderate positive correlations were seen between the MIBS-4, MIDAS, and PHQ-9, and moderate negative correlations were seen between the MIBS-4 and MSQoL (total score and subscales), which would be expected; as interictal burden increases, quality of life decreases. The correlation between ictal burden as measured by MIDAS and the MIBS-4 was .35, which demonstrated that the burden of migraine during attacks only partially predicts the burden between attacks.	Buse et al. (2007); Buse, Rupnow, & Lipton (2009)
Henry Ford Headache Disability Inventory (HDI)	Headache-related functional impairment, disease-related burden and disability	Designed as a treatment outcome measure to quantify the impact of recurrent headache on activities of daily living. Assesses both ictal and interictal burden of headache.	25-item, self-administered questionniare with two subscales: Functional (12 items) and Emotional Impairment (13 items), and reponse options *yes* (4 points), *sometimes* (2 points), or *no* (0 points). The total score is the sum of the responses with a maximum score of 100, which correlates with the highest level of disability.	Good internal consistency (.94), 6-week test–retest reliability (.83), and 1-week test–retest reliability (.76). High convergent validity with both migraine severity and spouse's perceptions of headache-related QoL.	Jacobson, Ramadan, Norris, & Newman (1995); Jacobson, Ramadan, Aggarwal, & Newman (1994)

severe. Each level provides corresponding treatment recommendations.

The Henry Ford Headache Disability Inventory (HDI) assesses both the ictal and interictal burden of headache (Jacobson, Ramadan, Aggarwal, & Newman, 1994). The HDI comprises 25 items and is designed to determine the functional and emotional impact of recurrent headache.

Quality of Life

Previous quality of life measures were largely based on chronic disease with mortality as the major end point. However, recently there has been a trend toward looking at HRQoL in diseases that do not negatively influence life expectancy, including primary headache. Quality of life (QoL) is the quantification of global well-being. HRQoL is QoL as it pertains to health status, as well as physical and mental functional status (Fayers & Machin, 2000; Guyatt, Feeny, & Patrick, 1993). HRQoL can be measured by general instruments such as the Medical Outcomes Study Health Survey–36 and Medical Outcomes Study—Short Form–12 (Ware, Kosinski, & Keller, 1996; Ware & Sherbourne, 1992) or disease-specific instruments.

Several headache-specific instruments have been developed to assess HRQoL (Andrasik, 2001; Solomon, 1997). The Migraine-Specific Quality of Life measure (MSQoL; Wagner, Patrick, Galer, & Berzon, 1996) consists of three domains: avoidance, social relationships, and feelings. The Migraine-Specific Quality of Life Questionnaire, version 2.1 (MSQoLQ v. 2.1; Martin et al., 2000) measures functional limitations and restrictions related to migraine through three dimensions: role function-restriction, role function-preventive, and emotional function. The 24-Hour Migraine Quality of Life Questionnaire (24-hr-MQoLQ; Santanello, Hartmaier, Epstein, & Silberstein, 1995) has five domains: work functioning, social functioning, energy/vitality, feelings/concerns, and migraine symptoms, each with three items. More detailed psychometric data are presented in Table 15.6.

Pediatric and Adolescent Headache

Although assessment and treatment of headache in children and adolescents is similar to adults in many ways, children and adolescents with headache may have qualitatively different medical, psychological, family, and educational presentations and needs (Andrasik & Schwartz, 2006; Powers & Andrasik, 2005; White & Farrell, 2006; Winner, Hershey, & Li, 2008). Therefore, children and adolescents with headache should be treated by health care providers with training and experience with this specific population. The basic tenets of the biopsychosocial model of assessment should be applied when working with children and adolescents, including attention to all aspects of the disease and the individual, which in the case of children and adolescents should include a focus on educational, social, and developmental factors.

Several headache-specific outcome measures have been developed and validated for use with patients below the age of 18. The pediatric MIDAS was developed to assess functional impairment and burden caused by migraine (Hershey et al., 2001). It functions similar to the adult version, except that the focus is switched from the occupational to the educational domain. Grazzi (2004) describes a second variation of the adult MIDAS, the MIDAS–Junior. Quality of Life Headache in Youth (QLH-Y) is a self-administered questionnaire developed by Langeveld, Koot, Loonen, Hazebroek-Kampschreur, and Passchier (1996) to assess psychological, physical, and social functioning and functional status in patients ages 12–18. Hartmaier, DeMuro-Mercon, Linder, Winner, and Santanello (2001) also developed a brief migraine-specific outcome measure to determine quality of life and functioning in adolescent patients with headache. Readers interested in incorporating these measures are referred to these articles and Table 15.7 for further information.

Summary

The biopsychosocial model provides an ideal framework to guide the assessment of primary headache disorders in which biological factors, environmental factors, behavioral factors, and beliefs are interwoven with the development, maintenance, progression, and remission of headache disorders (Andrasik, Flor, & Turk, 2005). Proper assessment is not only essential during an initial assess-

TABLE 15.6. Measures for Assessing Quality of Life

Name	Purpose	Brief description	No. of items, subscales and scoring information	Psychometric properties	Reference
Migraine Specific Quality of Life Questionnaire, Version 2.1 (MSQ v. 2.1)	Health-related quality of life	Measures functional limitations and restrictions related to migraine in three dimensions, role function-preventive, and emotional function, over a 4-week period.	14-item, self-adminstered questionnaire. Reponses are scored on a 0–100 scale with higher scores correlating with better quality of life.	Internal consistency (Cronbach's alpha) from 0.86 to 0.96 across dimensions. The intraclass correlation of the dimensions ranged from .57 to .63 as measured by the test–retest reliability at 4 weeks. The Pearson correlation coefficients between baseline and 4 weeks ranged from .62 to .65. There was a low to moderate correlation with SF-36 scores.	Martin et al. (2000)
Migraine-Specific Quality-of-Life (MSQoL) Measure	Health-related quality of life	Assesses the long term effects of migraine on HRQoL. It consists of three domains: avoidance, social relationships, and feelings.	20-item, self-administered questionnaire. Each of the 20 items is rated from 1 (*very much*) to 4 (*not at all*). Total scores range from 20 to 80; a transformed scale is achieved by subtraction, division, and multiplication, with a transformed score of 100 indicating maximum (best) QoL.	Internal consistency (Cronbach's alpha) = 0.90. Test–retest validity = .90 (at 24 days). High convergent validity with migraine symptom severity and moderate convergent validity with the MOS SF-36. There was a negative correlation with QoL and more migraine symptoms, medical appointments per year for migraine, and annual frequency of migraine.	Wagner, Patrick, Galer, & Berzon (1996); Patrick, Hurst, & Hughes (2000)
24-Hour Migraine Quality of Life Questionnaire (24-hr-MQoLQ)	Health-related quality of life	Measures 24-hour quality of life changes associated with an acute migriane attack. Developed for use in clinical trials of acute migraine treatment and can be used clinically to measure the impact of migraine treatment on HRQoL.	15-item, self-administered questionnaire with three items in each of five domains: work functioning, social functioning, energy/vitality, feelings/concerns, and migraine symptoms. Respondents are asked to rate each item on a 7-point scale: 1 (*maximum impairment*) to 7 (*no impairment*) over a 24-hour recall period.	Good internal consistency (Cronbach's alpha ranging from 0.74 to 0.91). Low to moderate convergent validity was seen with a migraine diary. Good construct validity in that there was an overall negative correlation between an acute migraine attack and QoL. Longer duration of migraine and the presence of nausea and/or vomiting negatively correlated with 24-hr-MQoLQ scores.	Santanello, Hartmaier, Epstein, & Silberstein (1995)

TABLE 15.7. Measures for Assessing Headache in Pediatrics

Name	Purpose	Brief description	No. of items, subscales and scoring information	Psychometric properties	Reference
PEDS-MIDAS	Pediatric and adolescent headache instruments	Used to assess functional impairment and burden caused by migraine.	Six-items in the areas of direct school-related issues, home activities, including chores and homework, and play, sports, or social activities.	2-week test–retest reliability assessment had a Pearson coefficient of .80. The correlation of the PedMIDAS score with frequency, severity, and duration had Pearson's coefficient values of .58, .27, and .23.	Hershey et al. (2001)
Quality of Life Headache in Youth (QoL-Y)	Pediatric and adolescent headache instruments	Assesses psychological, physical functioning, social functioning, and functional status in patients ages 12–18.	71-item (69 multiple choice items and 2 visual analogue scales) self-administered questionnaire. Thirteen subscales were developed to cover four subdomains: psychological functioning, functional status; physical status and social functioning. Satisfaction with life in general and satisfaction with health have visual analogue scale response options.	Indications for parent–youth agreement, construct validity, and sensitivity for headache and migraine were obtained. Stability coefficients were between .47 and .72 for the 1-week interval and between .31 and .60 for the 6-month interval. Nearly all of the QLH-Y subscales appeared to be more sensitive to differences between subjects with headaches and headache-free subjects, whereas the QL subdomain functional status was most sensitive for subjects who had suffered from a recent headache.	Langeveld, Koot, Loonen, Hazebroek-Kampschreur, & Passchier (1996)
Brief 24-hour Adolescent Migraine Functioning Questionnaire	Pediatric and adolescent headache instruments	Assesses quality of life and functioning in adolescent patients with headache in the 24 hours following a migraine attack.	18-item questionnaire. Items are rated on a 5-point scale from *not very important to extremely important*. Five domains: (1) activities, (2) social functioning, (3) cognitive functioning, (4) migraine headache symptoms, and (5) emotional functioning.	The correlation between the five domains as measured by the Spearman correlation coefficient ranged from .17 to .49, suggesting some, but minimal, overlap. Cronbach alpha for individual domains ranged from 0.50 to 0.84.	Hartmaier, DeMuro-Mercon, Linder, Winner, & Santanello (2001)

ment of a headache disorder but must also be continued as an ongoing method to track changes over time. Assessment may take the form of a physical exam, laboratory tests and imaging, observation, interview, questionnaires, and patient logs and record keeping (e.g., diaries). The clinician must always be mindful of the biopsychosocial model, as well as the tenets of effective medical communication and psychotherapy. The assessor also needs to remember the importance of providing information, understanding, and reassurance. Patient education and information exchange become an important part of the assessment process early on. Assessment also offers an opportunity to strengthen the therapeutic relationship and reinforce a patient's sense of self-efficacy and internal locus of control, as well as to build hope.

Assessment begins with a thorough physical and neurological evaluation to rule out acute medical conditions or structural defects other than a primary headache disorder. Clinicians should always remain vigilant for signs or "red flags" suggesting an acute medical issue in need of attention and maintain close medical collaboration throughout treatment to monitor such problems and to obtain assistance with medication management and modification as needed. Identification and diagnosis of specific headache subtype(s) is necessary to determine the proper treatment, to identify patients whose headaches may be occurring in part to medication abuse, to identify headache types that have been found to be resilient to nonpharmacological approaches alone (cluster and chronic daily headache), and to decide when a comprehensive, multidisciplinary approach (posttraumatic headache) or even hospitalization is most needed.

In addition to completing a thorough medical and headache history and assigning an ICHD-II (or ICHD-Beta 3) diagnosis when possible, the practitioner also needs to obtain a thorough qualitative understanding of the patient's experience and beliefs, headache-related disability and impairment in all areas of life, quality of life, level of self-efficacy, and information about related comorbidities. This information leads to a more accurate recognition of the severity of the effect of headache on the patient's life, which in turn tends to result in more effective and comprehensive treatment plans. Additional important areas of assessment

include cognitive status, psychological status, functioning in important areas of life, quality of life, and well-being. Assessment and education about common psychiatric comorbidities should be included in routine headache care, and treatment or referral should be imitated whenever appropriate. A minority of patients may require specialized neuropsychological assessment.

Headache is also common in children and adolescents. Similar to the assessment of adults with headache, it is important to assess the child or teen with headache through the biopsychosocial lens and to assess not only medical and physical but also academic, family, social, and personal variables. Children and adolescents with headache should be treated by health care providers with specialty training and knowledge of their unique medical, psychological, family, and educational needs and issues.

REFERENCES

Aamodt, A. H., Stovner, L. J., Langhammer, A., Hagen, K., & Zwart, J. A. (2007). Is headache related to asthma, hay fever, and chronic bronchitis?: The Head-HUNT Study. *Headache, 47*(2), 204–212.

Akbik, H., Butler, S. F., Budman, S. H., Fernandez, K., Katz, N. P., & Jamison, R. N. (2006). Validation and clinical application of the Screener and Opioid Assessment for Patients with Pain (SOAPP). *Journal of Pain and Symptom Management, 32*(3), 287–293.

American Psychiatric Association. (2000). *Diagnostic and statistical manual of mental disorders* (4th ed., text rev.). Washington, DC: Author.

American Psychiatric Association. (2013). *Diagnostic and statistical manual of mental disorders* (5th ed.). Arlington, VA: Author.

Andrasik, F. (1990). Psychological and behavioral aspects of chronic headache. In N. T. Mathew (Ed.), *Advances in headache: Neurologic clinics* (Vol. 8, pp. 961–976). Philadelphia: Saunders.

Andrasik, F. (2001). Migraine and quality of life: Psychological considerations. *Journal of Headache and Pain, 2*(Suppl. 1), S1–S9.

Andrasik, F. (2003). Behavioral treatment approaches to chronic headache. *Neurological Sciences, 24*(Suppl. 2), S80–S85.

Andrasik, F. (2006). Psychophysiological disorders: Headache as a case in point. In F. Andrasik (Ed.), *Comprehensive handbook of personality and psychopathology: Vol. 2. Adult psychopathology* (pp. 409–422). Hoboken, NJ: Wiley.

Andrasik, F., Burke, E. J., Attanasio, V., & Rosenblum, E. L. (1985). Child, parent, and physician reports of a child's headache pain: Relationships prior to and following treatment. *Headache, 25*, 421–425.

Andrasik, F., Flor, H., & Turk, D. C. (2005). An expanded view of psychological aspects in head pain: The biopsychosocial model. *Neurological Sciences, 26*, S87–S91.

Andrasik, F., Grazzi, L., Usai, S., Buse, D. C., & Bussone, G. (2009). Non-pharmacological approaches to treating chronic migraine with medication overuse. *Neurological Sciences, 30*(Suppl. 1), S89–S93.

Andrasik, F., Lipchik, G. L., McCrory, D. C., & Wittrock, D. A. (2005). Outcome measurement in behavioral headache research: Headache parameters and psychosocial outcomes. *Headache, 45*, 429–437.

Andrasik, F., & Schwartz, M. S. (2006). Behavioral assessment and treatment of pediatric headache. *Behavior Modification, 30*, 93–113.

Andrasik, F., Wittrock, D. A., & Passchier, J. (2006). Psychological mechanisms of tension-type headache. In J. Olesen, P. J. Goadsby, N. M. Ramadan, P. Tfelt-Hansen, & K. M. A. Welch (Eds.), *The headaches* (3rd ed., pp. 663–667). Philadelphia: Lippincott Williams & Wilkins.

Bandura, A. (1986). *Social foundations of thought and action. A social cognitive theory.* Englewood Cliffs, NJ: Prentice Hall.

Bigal, M. E., Rapoport, A. M., Lipton, R. B., Tepper, S. J., & Sheftell, F. D. (2003). Assessment of migraine disability using the Migraine Disability Assessment (MIDAS) questionnaire: A comparison of chronic migraine with episodic migraine. *Headache, 43*, 336–342.

Bigal, M. E., Serrano, D., Reed, M., & Lipton, R. B. (2008). Chronic migraine in the population: Burden, diagnosis, and satisfaction with treatment. *Neurology, 71*(8), 559–566.

Blanchard, E. B., Andrasik, F., Evans, D. D., Neff, D. F., Appelbaum, K. A., & Rodichok, L. D. (1985). Behavioral treatment of 250 chronic headache patients: A clinical replication series. *Behavior Therapy, 16*, 308–327.

Blanchard, E. B., Andrasik, F., Jurish, S. E., & Teders, S. J. (1982). The treatment of cluster headache with relaxation and thermal biofeedback. *Biofeedback and Self-Regulation, 7*, 185–191.

Blanchard, E. B., Andrasik, F., Neff, D. F., Jurish, S. E., & O'Keefe, D. M. (1981). Social validation of the headache diary. *Behavior Therapy, 12*, 711–715.

Bond, D., Dirge, K., Rubingh, C., Durrant, L., & Baggaley, S. (2004). Impact of a self-help intervention on performance of headache management behaviors: A self-efficacy approach. *Internet Journal of Allied Health Sciences and Practice, 2(1)*. Available at *http://ijahsp.nova. edu/articles/Vol2num1/pdf/bond.pdf.*

Breslau, N., & Davis, G. C. (1993). Migraine, physical health and psychiatric disorder: A prospective epidemiologic study in young adults. *Journal of Psychiatric Research, 27*, 211–221.

Breslau, N., Davis, G. C., & Andreski, P. (1991). Migraine, psychiatric disorders, and suicide attempts: An epidemiologic study of young adults. *Psychiatry Research, 37*, 11–23.

Burns, J. W., Kubilus, A., Bruehl, S., Harden, R. N., & Lofland, K. (2003). Do changes in cognitive factors influence outcome following multidisciplinary treatment for chronic pain?: A cross-lagged panel analysis. *Journal of Consulting and Clinical Psychology, 71*, 81–91.

Buse, D. C., & Andrasik, F. (2009). Behavioral medicine for migraine. *Neurologic Clinics, 27*(2), 445–465.

Buse, D. C., Bigal, M. E., Rupnow, M. F. T., Reed, M. L., Serrano, D., Biondi, D. M., et al. (2007). The Migraine Interictal Burden Scale (MIBS): Results of a population-based validation study. *Headache, 47*(5), 778.

Buse, D. C., & Lipton, R. B. (2008). Facilitating communication with patients for improved migraine outcomes. *Current Pain and Headache Reports, 12*(3), 230–236.

Buse, D. C., Manack, A., Serrano, D., Turkel, C., & Lipton, R. B. (2010). Sociodemographic and comorbidity profiles of chronic migraine and episodic migraine sufferers. *Journal of Neurology, Neurosurgery and Psychiatry, 81*, 428–432.

Buse, D. C., Rupnow, M. F., & Lipton, R. B. (2009). Assessing and managing all aspects of migraine: Migraine attacks, migraine-related functional impairment, common comorbidities, and quality of life. *Mayo Clinic Proceedings, 84*(5), 422–435.

Bussone, G., Usai, S., Grazzi, L., Rigamonti, A., Solari, A., & D'Amico, D. (2004). Disability and quality of life in different primary headaches: Results from Italian studies. *Neurological Sciences, 25*(Suppl. 3), S105–S107.

Butler, S. F., Budman, S. H., Fernandez, K. C., Houle, B., Benoit, C., Katz, N., et al. (2007).

Development and validation of the Current Opioid Misuse Measure. *Pain, 130*(1–2), 144–156.

Chatterton, M. L., Lofland, J. H., Shechter, A., Curtice, W. S., Hu, X. H., Lenow, J., et al. (2002). Reliability and validity of the Migraine Therapy Assessment Questionnaire. *Headache, 42*(10), 1006–1015.

Cook, N. R., Bensenor, I. M., Lotufo, P. A., Lee, I. M., Skerrett, P. J., Chown, M. J., et al. (2002). Migraine and coronary heart disease in women and men. *Headache, 42*, 715–727.

Cramer, J. A., Silberstein, S. D., & Winner, P. (2001). Development and validation of the Headache Needs Assessment (HANA) survey. *Headache, 41*(4), 402–409.

Dahlof, C. G. H., & Dimenäs, E. (1995). Migraine patients experience poorer subjective well-being/quality of life even between attacks. *Cephalalgia, 15*(1), 31–36.

Dayno, J. M., Silberstein, S. D., & Lipton, R. B. (1996). Migraine comorbidity: Epilepsy and stroke. *Advances in Clinical Neurosciences, 6*, 365–385.

De Benedittis, G., & Lorenzetti, A. (1992). Minor stressful life events (daily hassles) in chronic primary headache: Relationship with MMPI personality patterns. *Headache, 32*, 330–332.

Dodick, D. W. (2003). Clinical clues and clinical rules: Primary versus secondary headache. *Advanced Studies in Medicine, 3*, S550–S555.

Dowson, A. J., Tepper, S. J., Baos, V., Baudet, F., D'Amico, D., & Kilminster, S. (2004). Identifying patients who require a change in their current acute migraine treatment: The Migraine Assessment of Current Therapy (Migraine–ACT) questionnaire. *Current Medical Research and Opinion, 20*(7), 1125–1135.

Dueland, A. N., Leira, R., Burke, T. A., Hillyer, E. V., & Bolge, S. (2004). The impact of migraine on work, family, and leisure among young women: A multinational study. *Current Medical Research and Opinion, 20*(10), 1595–1604.

Duquette, J., McKinley, P. A., & Litowski, J. (2005). Test–retest reliability and internal consistency of the Quebec–French version of the Survey of Pain Attitudes. *Archives of Physical Medicine and Rehabilitation, 86*, 782–788.

El Hasnaoui, A., Vray, M., Richard, A., Nachit-Ouinekh, F., Boureau, F., & MIGSEV Group. (2003). Assessing the severity of migraine: Development of the MIGSEV scale. *Headache, 43*(6), 628–635.

Fayers, P. M., & Machin, D. (2000). *Quality of life: Assessment, analysis and interpretation.* New York: Wiley.

Finkel, A. G. (2003). Epidemiology of cluster headache. *Current Pain and Headache Reports, 7*, 144–149.

Folstein, M. F., Folstein, S. E., & McHugh, P. R. (1975). "Mini-Mental State": A practical method for grading the cognitive state of patients for the clinician. *Journal of Psychiatric Research, 12*, 189–198.

French, D. J., Holroyd, K. A., Pinell, C., Malinoski, P. T., O'Donnell, F., & Hill, K. R. (2000). Perceived self-efficacy and headache-related disability. *Headache, 40*, 647–656.

Grazzi, L. (2004). MIDAS questionnaire modification for a new MIDAS junior questionnaire: A clinical experience at the Neurological Institute "C. Besta." *Neurological Sciences, 25*(Suppl. 3), S261–S262.

Grazzi, L., Andrasik, F., Usai, S., & Bussone, G. (2009). Treatment of chronic migraine with medication overuse: Is drug withdrawal crucial? *Neurological Sciences, 30*(Suppl. 1), S85–S88.

Guyatt, G. H., Feeny, D. H., & Patrick, D. L. (1993). Measuring health-related quality of life. *Annals of Internal Medicine, 118*(8), 622–629.

Hadjistavropoulos, H. D., MacLeod, F. K., & Asmundson, G. J. (1999). Validation of the Chronic Pain Coping Inventory. *Pain, 80*, 471–481.

Hahn, S. R. (2008). Communication in the care of the headache patient. In S. D. Silberstein, R. B. Lipton, & D. W. Dodick (Eds.), *Wolff's headache and other head pain* (8th ed., pp. 805–824). New York: Oxford University Press.

Hahn, S. R., Lipton, R. B., Sheftell, F. D., Cady, R. K., Eagan, C. A., Simons, S. E., et al. (2008). Healthcare provider–patient communication and migraine assessment: Results of the American Migraine Communication Study (AMCS) Phase II. *Current Medical Research and Opinion, 24*(6), 1711–1718.

Hamelsky, S. W., & Lipton, R. B. (2006). Psychiatric comorbidity of migraine. *Headache, 46*, 1327–1333.

Hartmaier, S. L., DeMuro-Mercon, C., Linder, S., Winner, P., & Santanello, S. C. (2001). Development of a brief 24-hour adolescent migraine functioning questionnaire. *Headache, 41*(2), 150–160.

Haut, S. R., Bigal, M. E., & Lipton, R. B. (2006). Chronic disorders with episodic manifestations: Focus on epilepsy and migraine. *Lancet Neurology, 5*,148–157.

Headache Classification Committee of the International Headache Society. (1988). Classification and diagnostic criteria for headache disorders, cranial neuralgias, and facial pain. *Cephalalgia, 8*(Suppl. 7), 1–96.

Headache Classification Committee of the International Headache Society (IHS). (2013). The international classification of headache disorders (3rd ed., beta version). *Cephalalgia, 33*(9), 629–808.

Heath, R. L., Saliba, M., Mahmassani, O., Major, S. C., & Khoury, B. A. (2008). Locus of control moderates the relationship between headache pain and depression. *Journal of Headache and Pain, 9*(5), 301–308.

Henryk-Gutt, R., & Rees, W. C. (1973). Psychological aspects of migraine. *Journal of Psychosomatic Research, 17*, 141–153.

Hershey, A. D., Powers, S. W., Vockell, A. L., LeCates, S., Kabbouche, M. A., & Maynard, M. K. (2001). PedMIDAS: Development of a questionnaire to assess disability of migraines in children. *Neurology, 57*(11), 2034–2039.

Holm, J. E., Holroyd, K. A., Hursey, K. G., & Penzien, D. (1986). The role of stress in recurrent tension headaches. *Headache, 26*, 160–167.

Holmes, W. F., MacGregor, E. A., Sawyer, J. P., & Lipton, R. B. (2001). Information about migraine disability influences physicians' perceptions of illness severity and treatment needs. *Headache, 41*, 343–350.

Holroyd, K. A. (2002). Assessment and psychological management of recurrent headache disorders. *Journal of Consulting and Clinical Psychology, 70*, 656–677.

Holroyd, K. A., Drew, J. B., Cottrell, C. K., Romanek, K. M., & Heh, V. (2007). Impaired functioning and quality of life in severe migraine: The role of catastrophizing and associated symptoms. *Cephalalgia, 27*(10), 1156–1165.

Holroyd, K. A., Holm, J. E., Hursey, K. G., Penzien, D. B., Cordingley, G. E., Theofanous, A. G., et al. (1988). Recurrent vascular headache: Home-based behavioral treatment vs. abortive pharmacological treatment. *Journal of Consulting and Clinical Psychology, 56*, 218–223.

Howarth, E. (1965). Headache, personality, and stress. *British Journal of Psychiatry, 111*, 1193–1197.

Jacob, R. G., Turner, S. M., Szekely, B. C., & Eidelman, B. H. (1983). Predicting outcome of relaxation therapy in headaches: The role of "depression." *Behavior Therapy, 14*, 457–465.

Jacobs, J. W., Bernhard, M. R., Delgado, A., & Strain, J. J. (1977). Screening for organic mental syndromes in the medically ill. *Annals of Internal Medicine, 86*, 40–46.

Jacobson, G. P., Ramadan, N. M., Aggarwal, S. K., & Newman, C. K. (1994). The Henry Ford Hospital Disability Inventory (HDI). *Neurology, 44*(5), 837–842.

Jacobson, G. P., Ramadan, N. M., Norris, L., & Newman, C. W. (1995). Headache Disability Inventory (HDI): Short-term test–retest reliability and spouse perceptions. *Headache, 35*, 534–539.

Jensen, M. P., Karoly, P., & Huger, R. (1987). The development and preliminary validation of an instrument to assess patients' attitudes toward pain. *Journal of Psychosomatic Research, 31*, 393–400.

Jensen, M. P., Turner, J. A., Romano, J. M., & Strom, S. E. (1995). The Chronic Pain Coping Inventory: Development and preliminary validation. *Pain, 60*, 203–216.

Jette, N., Patten, S., Williams, J., Becker, W., & Wiebe, S. (2008). Comorbidity of migraine and psychiatric disorders: A national population-based study. *Headache, 48*(4), 501–516.

Juang, K. D., Wang, S. J., Fuh, J. L., Lu, S. R., & Su, T. P. (2000). Comorbidity of depressive and anxiety disorders in chronic daily headache and its subtypes. *Headache, 40*, 818–823.

Kilminster, S. G., Dowson, A. J., Tepper, S. J., Baos, V., Baudet, F., & D'Amico, D. (2006). Reliability, validity, and clinical utility of the Migraine-ACT questionnaire. *Headache, 46*(4), 553–562.

Kosinski, M., Bayliss, M. S., Bjorner, J. B., Ware, J. E., Jr., Garber, W. H., Batenhorst, A., et al. (2003). A six-item short-form survey for measuring headache impact: The HIT-6. *Quality of Life Research, 12*(8), 963–974.

Kroenke, K., Spitzer, R. L., & Williams, J. B. (2001). The PHQ-9: Validity of a brief depression severity measure. *Journal of General Internal Medicine, 16*(9), 606–613.

Langeveld, J. H., Koot, H. M., Loonen, M. C., Hazebroek-Kampschreur, A. A., & Passchier, J. (1996). A quality of life instrument for adolescents with chronic headache. *Cephalalgia, 16*(3), 183–196.

Lanteri-Minet, M., Radat, F., Chautard, M. H., & Lucas, C. (2005). Anxiety and depression associated with migraine: Influence on migraine subjects' disability and quality of life, and acute migraine management. *Pain, 118*, 319–326.

Lawson, P., Kerr, K., Penzien, D. B., Hursey, K. G., Ray, S. E., Arora, R., et al. (1988, November). *Caveats in using mental status examinations: Factors that influence performance.* Paper presented at the annual meeting of the Association for Advancement of Behavior Therapy, New York.

Lazarus, R. S., & Folkman, S. (1984). Coping and adaption. In W. D. Gentry (Ed.), *Handbook of behavioral medicine* (pp. 282–325). New York: Guilford Press.

Lemstra, M., Stewart, B., & Olszynski, W. (2002). Effectiveness of multidisciplinary intervention in the treatment of migraine: A randomized clinical trial. *Headache, 42,* 845–854.

Lenaerts, M. E., & Newman, L. C. (2008). Tension-type headaches: Diagnosis, comorbidity and treatment. In S. D. Silberstein, R. B. Lipton, & D. Dodick (Eds.), *Wolff's headache and other head pain* (8th ed., pp. 293–314). New York: Oxford University Press.

Leonardi, M., Steiner, T. J., Scher, A. T., & Lipton, R. B. (2005). The global burden of migraine: Measuring disability in headache disorders with WHO's Classification of Functioning, Disability, and Health (ICF). *Journal of Headache and Pain, 6,* 429–440.

Levor, R. M., Cohen, M. J., Naliboff, B. D., MacArthur, D., & Heuser, G. (1986). Psychosocial precursors and correlates of migraine headache. *Journal of Consulting and Clinical Psychology, 54,* 347–353.

Linet, M. S., Stewart, W. F., Celentano, D. D., Ziegler, D., & Sprecher, M. (1989). An epidemiologic study of headache among adolescents and young adults. *Journal of the American Medical Association, 261*(15), 1197.

Lipton, R. B., Bigal, M. E., Diamond, M., Freitag, F., Reed, M. L., & Stewart, W. F. (2007). Migraine prevalence, disease burden, and the need for preventive therapy. *Neurology, 68*(5), 343–349.

Lipton, R. B., Dodick, D., Sadovsky, R., Kolodner, K., Endicott, J., Hettiarachi, J., et al. (2003). A self-administered screener for migraine in primary care: The ID Migraine validation study. *Neurology, 61,* 375–382.

Lipton, R. B., Hahn, S. R., Cady, R. K., Brandes, J. L., Simons, S. E., Bain, P. A., et al. (2008). In-office discussions of migraine: Results from the American Migraine Communication Study (AMCS). *Journal of General Internal Medicine, 23*(8), 1145–1151.

Lipton, R. B., Kolodner, K., Bigal, M. E., Valade, D., Láinez, M. J., Pascual, J., et al. (2009).

Validity and reliability of the Migraine Treatment Optimization Questionnaire. *Cephalalgia, 29*(7), 751–759.

Lipton, R. B., Liberman, J. N., Kolodner, K. B., Bigal, M. E., Dowson, A., & Stewart, W. F. (2003). Migraine headache disability and health-related quality-of-life: A population-based case-control study from England. *Cephalalgia, 23*(6), 441–450.

Lipton, R. B., Serrano, D., Buse, D. C., Rupnow, M. F. T., Reed, M. L., & Bigal, M. E. (2007). The Migraine Prevention Questionnaire (MPQ): Development and validation. *Headache, 47*(5), 770–771.

Lipton, R. B., Serrano, D., Buse, D. C., Bigal, M. E., Rupnow, M. F. T., & Biondi, D. M. (2008). The migraine prevention questionnaire (MPQ-5): Development, psychometric testing and validation. *Headache, 48*(Suppl. 1), S65.

Lipton, R. B., & Stewart, W. F. (1993). Migraine in the United States: A review of epidemiology and health care use. *Neurology, 43*(6, Suppl. 3), S6–S10.

Maizels, M., & Burchette, R. (2003). Rapid and sensitive paradigm for screening patients with headache in primary care settings. *Headache, 43*(5), 441–450.

Maizels, M., & Houle, T. (2008). Results of screening with the Brief Headache Screen compared with a modified IDMigraine. *Headache, 48*(3), 385–394.

Maizels, M., & Wolfe, W. J. (2008). An expert system for headache diagnosis: The Computerized Headache Assessment Tool (CHAT). *Headache, 48*(1), 72–78.

Marlowe, N. (1986). Stressful events, appraisal, coping, and recurrent headache. *Journal of Clinical Psychology, 54,* 247–256.

Martin, B. C., Pathak, D. S., Sharfman, M. I., Adelman, J. U., Taylor, F, Kwong, W. J., et al. (2000). Validity and reliability of the Migraine-Specific Quality of Life Questionnaire (MSQ Version 2.1). *Headache, 40,* 204–215.

Martin, N. J., Holroyd, K. A., & Penzien, D. B. (1990). The headache-specific locus of control scale: Adaptation to recurrent headaches. *Headache, 30,* 729–734.

May, A., & Goadsby, P. J. (1999). The trigeminovascular system in humans: Pathophysiologic implications for primary headache syndromes of the neural influences on the cerebral circulation. *Journal of Cerebral Blood Flow and Metabolism, 19*(2), 115–127.

Mortimer, M. J., Kay, J., & Jaron, A. (1992). Epidemiology of headache and childhood migraine in an urban general practice using

Ad Hoc, Vahlquist and IHS criteria. *Developmental Medicine and Child Neurology, 34*(12), 1095–1101.

Nicholson, R. A., Houle, T. T., Rhudy, J. L., & Norton, P. J. (2007). Psychological risk factors in headache. *Headache, 47*(3), 413–426.

Nicholson, R. A., Hursey, K. G., & Nash, J. (2005). Moderators and mediators of behavioral treatment for headache. *Headache, 45,* 513–519.

Nicholson, R. A., Nash, J., & Andrasik, F. (2005). A self-administered behavioral intervention using tailored messages for migraine. *Headache, 45,* 1124–1139.

Olesen, J., Bousser, M. G., Diener, H. C., Dodick, D., First, M., Goadsby, P. J., et al. (2006). New appendix criteria open for a broader concept of chronic migraine. *Cephalalgia, 26,* 742–746.

Ottman, R., & Lipton, R. B. (1994). Comorbidity of migraine and epilepsy. *Neurology, 44,* 2105–2110.

Pathak, D. S., Chisolm, D. J., & Weis, K. A. (2005). Functional Assessment in Migraine (FAIM) questionnaire: Development of an instrument based upon the WHO's International Classification of Functioning, Disability, and Health. *Value Health, 8*(5), 591–600.

Patrick, D. L., Hurst, B. C., & Hughes, J. (2000). Further development and testing of the Migraine-Specific Quality of Life (MSQOL) measure. *Headache, 40,* 550–560.

Penzien, D. B., Rains, J. C., & Holroyd, K. A. (1993). Psychological assessment of the recurrent headache sufferer. In C. D. Tollison & R. S. Kunkel (Eds.), *Headache: Diagnosis and interdisciplinary treatment* (pp. 39–49). Baltimore: Williams & Wilkins.

Pimenta, C. A., & da Cruz, D. (2006). Chronic pain beliefs: Validation of the survey of pain attitudes for the Portuguese language. *Revista da Escola de Engermagem da USP, 40,* 365–373.

Powers, S. W., & Andrasik, F. (2005). Biobehavioral treatment, disability, and psychological effects of pediatric headache. *Pediatric Annals, 34,* 461–465.

Radat, F., Irachabal, S., Lafittau, M., Creac'h, C., Dousset, V., & Henry, P. (2006). Construction of a medication dependence questionnaire in headache patients (MDQ-H) validation of the French version. *Headache, 46*(2), 233–239.

Rasmussen, B. K. (1995). Epidemiology of headache. *Cephalalgia, 15,* 45–68.

Rasmussen, B. K., Jensen, R., Schroll, M., & Olesen, J. (1991). Epidemiology of headache in the general population: A prevalence study. *Journal of Clinical Epidemiology, 44,* 1147–1157.

Revicki, D. A., Kimel, M., Beusterien, K., Kwong, J. W., Varner, J. A., Ames, M. H., et al. (2006). Validation of the revised Patient Perception of Migraine Questionnaire: Measuring satisfaction with acute migraine treatment. *Headache, 46*(2), 240–252.

Rogers, C. R. (1967). *On becoming a person: A psychotherapist's view of psychotherapy.* London: Constable.

Santanello, N. C., Hartmaier, S. L., Epstein, R. S., & Silberstein, S. D. (1995). Validation of a new quality of life questionnaire for acute migraine headache. *Headache, 35*(6), 330–337.

Saper, J. R., & Lake, A. E. (2002). Borderline personality disorder and the chronic headache patient: Review and management recommendations. *Headache, 42,* 663–674.

Scharff, L., Turk, D. C., & Marcus, D. A. (1995). The relationship of locus of control and psychosocial-behavioral response in chronic headache. *Headache, 35,* 527–533.

Scher, A. I., Bigal, M. E., & Lipton, R. B. (2005). Comorbidity of migraine. *Current Opinions in Neurology, 18,* 305–310.

Scher, A. I., Stewart, W. F., & Lipton, R. B. (2006). The comorbidity of headache with other pain syndromes. *Headache, 46,* 1416–1423.

Schwartz, B. S., Stewart, W. F., Simon, D., & Lipton, R. B. (1998). Epidemiology of tension-type headache. *Journal of the American Medical Association, 279,* 381–383.

Silberstein, S. D. (2005). Chronic daily headache. *Journal of the American Osteopathic Association, 105*(4, Suppl. 2), S23–S29.

Silberstein, S. D., & Lipton, R. B. (1993). Epidemiology of migraine. *Neuroepidemiology, 12,* 179–194.

Silberstein, S. D., Olesen, J., Bousser, M.-G., Diener, H.-C., Dodick, D., First, M., et al. (2004). The International Classification of Headache Disorders (2nd ed.). *Cephalalgia, 24*(Suppl. 1), 1–160.

Silberstein, S. D., Olesen, J., Bousser, M.-G., Diener, H.-C., Dodick, D., First, M., et al. (2005). *The International Classification of Headache Disorders,* 2nd Edition: Revision of criteria for 8.2 medication-overuse headache. *Cephalalgia, 25*(6), 460–465.

Smith, T., & Nicholson, R. (2006). Are changes in cognitive and emotional factors important in improving headache impact and quality of life? *Headache, 46,* 878.

Solomon, G. D. (1997). Evolution of the measurement of quality of life in migraine. *Neurology, 48*(3), S10–S15.

Solomon, G. D., Skobieranda, F. G., & Gragg, L. A. (1993). Quality of life and well-being of headache patients: Measurement by the medical outcomes study instrument. *Headache, 33*(7), 351–358.

Spitzer, R. L., Kroenke, K., Williams, J. B., & Lowe, B. (2006). A brief measure for assessing generalized anxiety disorder: The GAD-7. *Archives of Internal Medicine, 166*(10), 1092–1097.

Spitzer, R. L., Kroenke, K., Williams, J. B. W., and the Patient Health Questionnaire Primary Care Study Group. (1999). Validation and utility of a self-report version of PRIME-MD: The PHQ Primary Care Study. *Journal of the American Medical Association, 282*(18), 1737–1744.

Stafstrom, C. E., Rostasy, K., & Minster, A. (2002). The usefulness of children's drawings in the diagnosis of headache. *Pediatrics, 109*(3), 460–472.

Stewart, W. F., Lipton, R. B., Dowson, A. J., & Sawyer, J. (2001). Development and testing of the Migraine Disability Assessment (MIDAS) Questionnaire to assess headache-related disability. *Neurology, 56,* S20–S28.

Stewart, W. F., Lipton, R. B., Simon, D., Von Korff, M., & Liberman, J. (1998). Reliability of an illness severity measure for headache in a population sample of migraine sufferers. *Cephalalgia, 18,* 44–51.

Stovner, L. J., Zwart, J. A., Hagen, K., Terwindt, G. M., & Pascual, J. (2006). Epidemiology of headache in Europe. *European Journal of Neurology, 13*(4), 333–345.

Sullivan, M. J. L., Bishop, S. C., & Pivik, J. (1995). The Pain Catastrophizing Scale: Development and validation. *Psychological Assessment, 7,* 524–532.

Sullivan, M. J., Thorn, B., Haythornthwaite, J. A., Keefe, F., Martin, M., Bradley, L. A., et al. (2001). Theoretical perspectives on the relation between catastrophizing and pain. *Clinical Journal of Pain, 17,* 52–64.

Tait, R. C., & Chibnall, J. T. (1997). Development of a brief version of the Survey of Pain Attitudes. *Pain, 70*(2–3), 229–235.

Torelli, P., Castellini, P., Cucurachi, L., Devetak, M., Lambru, G., & Manzoni, G. (2006). Cluster headache prevalence: Methodological considerations: A review of the literature. *Acta Biomedica: Atenei Parmensis, 77*(1), 4–9.

Waggoner, C. D., & Andrasik, F. (1990). Behavioral assessment and treatment of recurrent headache. In T. W. Miller (Ed.), *Chronic pain* (Vol. 1, pp. 319–361). Madison, CT: International Universities Press.

Wagner, T. H., Patrick, D. L., Galer, B. S., & Berzon, R. A. (1996). A new instrument to assess the long-term quality of life effects from migraine: Development and psychometric testing of the MSQOL. *Headache, 36*(8), 484–492.

Ware, J., Jr., Kosinski, M., & Keller, S. D. (1996). A 12-item short-form health survey: Construction of scales and preliminary tests of reliability and validity. *Medical Care, 34*(3), 220–233.

Ware, J. E., Jr., & Sherbourne, C. D. (1992). The MOS 36-Item Short-Form Survey (SF-36): I. Conceptual framework and item selection. *Medical Care, 30*(6), 473–483.

Weiss, J., Goodman, P., Losito, B., Corrigan, S., Charry, J., & Bailery, W. (1981). Behavioral depression produced by an uncontrollable stressor: Relationship to norepinephrine, dopamine, and serotonin levels in various regions of the rat brain. *Brain Research Reviews, 3,* 167–205.

Werder, D. S., Sargent, J. D., & Coyne, L. (1981). MMPI profiles of headache patients using self-regulation to control headache activity. *Headache, 21,* 164–169.

White, K., & Farrell, A. (2006). Anxiety and psychosocial stress as predictors of headache and abdominal pain in urban early adolescents. *Journal of Pediatric Psychology, 31,* 582–596.

Winner, P., Hershey, A. D., & Li, Z. (2008). Headaches in children and adolescents. In S. D. Silberstein, R. B. Lipton, & D. W. Dodick (Eds.), *Wolff's headache and other head pain* (8th ed., pp. 665–690). New York: Oxford University Press.

Wojaczynska-Stanek, K., Koprowski, R., Wróbel, Z., & Gola, M. (2008). Headache in children's drawings. *Journal of Child Neurology, 23*(2), 184–191.

Wong, W. S., Jensen, M. P., Mak, K. H., & Fielding, R. (2011). Pain-related beliefs among Chinese patients with chronic pain: The construct and concurrent predictive validity of the Chinese version of the Survey of Pain Attitudes. *Journal of Pain and Symptom Management, 42,* 470–478.

Zwart, J. A., Dyb, G., Hagen, K., Odegard, K. J., Dahl, A. A., Bovim, G., et al. (2003). Depression and anxiety disorders associated with headache frequency: The Nord–Trondelag Health Study. *European Journal of Neurology, 10,* 147–152.

CHAPTER 16

Facial Pain

Alan G. Glaros

Temporomandibular muscle and joint disorders (TMJDs) are a heterogeneous collection of disorders characterized by orofacial pain and/or masticatory dysfunction. The terminology used to describe this disorder has changed since 1934, when it was first identified. Costen's syndrome, functional temporomandibular joint disturbances, and myofascial pain–dysfunction syndrome are among the diagnostic labels that have been used in the professional literature. The current terminology, preferred by the National Institute of Dental and Craniofacial Research, recognizes that individuals suffering from these disorders may have pain or other functional problems in the musculature and/or in the tissues of the jaw joint.

TMJDs can be productively organized into three broad diagnostic classes: (1) functional disorders of the musculature of the face, head, neck, shoulders and upper back; (2) disorders involving the soft tissues of the temporomandibular joint (TMJ); and (3) disorders involving the hard structures of the TMJ. These diagnostic classes are not mutually exclusive, and patients may receive multiple diagnoses (Table 16.1).

The pain reported by patients with TMJD is typically located in the muscles of mastication, in the preauricular area, or in the TMJ. Patients with TMJD may also report headache, other facial pains, earache, dizziness, ringing in the ears, and neck/shoulder/upper and lower back pain (Lim, Smith, Bhalang,

TABLE 16.1. RDC/TMD Diagnostic Scheme for Temporomandibular Disorders

Diagnosis	Diagnostic criteria	Additional notes
Myofascial pain	Patient reports pain when masticatory muscle sites palpated. May also be associated with difficulty opening wide.	Most common of the TMJDs and most likely to be associated with psychological distress.
Disc displacement	Articular disc temporarily or permanently displaced from its normal position atop the condyle of the mandible. May be associated with jaw noises when opening or closing or difficulty opening or closing normally.	Patients most commonly report that jaw "clicks" or "pops" when they open or close. Not typically associated with pain.
Arthralgia, arthritis, arthrosis	Patient reports pain when condyle of mandible palpated or evidence of degenerative change in the hard tissues of the TMJ.	Patients most commonly report pain to palpation, without evidence of degenerative changes.

Slade, & Maixner, 2010). TMJD patients may report a variety of TMJ problems other than pain, including locking in the open or closed position and TMJ clicking, popping, and grating sounds. Patients may report difficulty opening their jaws wide, as well as a sense that their occlusion ("bite") feels "off." This spectrum of symptoms leads patients to seek care from dentists, physicians, and other health professionals (Glaros, Glass, & Hayden, 1995).

The prevalence of TMJD varies by age and gender. Prevalence studies using signs, symptoms, and clinic samples indicate that TMJDs are more prevalent in those under age 45, an atypical age distribution for a chronic, painful disorder. The prevalence ratio for females versus males is approximately 2:1 when nonclinic populations are assessed. However, the ratio of females to males can be as high as 8:1 in patient samples. Prevalence rates of TMJD vary dramatically, depending on the definition of the condition (e.g., Carlsson & LeResche, 1995; Goncalves, Dal Fabbro, Campos, Bigal, & Speciali, 2010). Estimates suggest that 4.5% of the adult population report pain and dysfunction sufficiently severe to prompt help seeking (Drangsholt & LeResche, 1999).

The assessment of a patient with suspected TMJD typically begins with a clinical interview, followed by a physical examination and imaging as needed. The physical examination often involves palpation of the masticatory muscles and TMJ and observation and measurement of opening. The physical examination should also rule out potential dental (e.g., infection) and nondental conditions (e.g., neuralgia) that might also account for the patient's complaints.

TMJD is frequently comorbid with a number of other medical conditions, including headache, muscle soreness or pain, and fibromyalgia (Aaron, Burke, & Buchwald, 2000; Glaros, Urban, & Locke, 2007; Kuttila, Kuttila, Le Bell, Alanen, & Suonpaa, 2004; Sipila, Ylostalo, Joukamaa, & Knuuttila, 2006; Storm & Wänman, 2006; Wiesinger, Malker, Englund, & Wänman, 2007). Patients with widespread pain are more likely to have more persistent pain, accompanied by greater depression and somatization (Raphael, Marbach, & Klausner, 2000). Assessment of these other con-

ditions will allow providers to individualize their treatments to better match the needs of specific patients (Turner, Holtzman, & Mancl, 2007).

There is growing recognition that TMJDs are strongly influenced by psychological factors (e.g., Giannakopoulos, Keller, Rammelsberg, Kronmuller, & Schmitter, 2010). Historically, dental students were typically trained to examine patients with possible TMJD for problems with occlusion. The role of psychological, behavioral, and emotional factors was ignored or given scant attention, despite a strong body of evidence showing that patients with TMJD, like those with other chronic pain, reported psychological distress in association with their condition.

The importance of psychological factors received explicit recognition in the Research Diagnostic Criteria for Temporomandibular Disorders (RDC/TMD; Dworkin & LeResche, 1992). Created for the research community, the RDC/TMD, which features two axes, required assessment of patients with possible TMJD for both physical disorders and psychological distress. Patients with suspected TMJD examined according to the original and revised RDC/TMD standards receive both a diagnosis for their TMJD-related clinical disorder(s) (Axis I) and an assessment of pain-related disability and psychological factors (Axis II). Indeed, among formal nosological systems for chronic pain, the RDC/TMD may be unique in its explicit requirement that psychological factors be assessed. A further revision of the RDC/TMD intended for nonresearch diagnostic purposes, the Diagnostic Criteria for Temporomandibular Disorders (DC/TMD), is under way and also includes assessment of psychological, behavioral, and emotional factors.[1]

The psychological assessment of patients with TMJD has several components, including self-assessment of pain and distress, assessment of behaviors relevant to TMJD,

---

[1]The revised version of the RDC/TMD does not differ from the original in its requirement that both clinical and psychological/behavioral factors be assessed (e.g., Anderson et al., 2010; www.rdc-tmdinternational. org; Journal of Oral Rehabilitation, 2010, Vol. 37, No. 10). A final version of the DC/RDC was published in 2014 (Schiffman et al., 2014).

psychophysiological assessment of patients, assessment of emotional status, emerging assessment techniques, and assessment of treatment effectiveness. Psychological issues are not as prevalent in patients with TMJD with soft tissue problems (e.g., disc displacement) in which pain is not a primary complaint, and the discussion therefore focuses primarily on issues associated with pain in the masticatory muscles and TMJ (i.e., on patients who receive diagnosis of myofascial pain and/or arthralgia; Table 16.1).

Self-Report of Pain and Distress

As with other chronic pain conditions, self-report is the primary source of information about pain in TMJD. A carefully conducted interview can elicit a great deal of useful information about the patient's pain, including the timing and circumstances of its onset; the quality, duration, and variability of pain; changes in pain over time; factors that increase or decrease pain; and the effect of pain on everyday functioning. Unfortunately, very few studies have systematically examined the reliability and validity of information obtained from patients with TMJD during the course of an open-ended interview. Structured interviews similar to the Structured Clinical Interview for DSM-IV are not widely used with patients with TMJD.

Under Axis II of the RDC/TMD and the DC/TMD, patients complete the Chronic Pain Grade questionnaire (Von Korff, Ormel, Keefe, & Dworkin, 1992). This questionnaire is designed to provide a simple summary measure of pain and disability. The questionnaire contains three visual/numeric scales of pain—assessing pain now, worst pain, and typical pain in the previous 6 months. (The scales are laid out like visual analogue scales but are prelabeled from 0 to 10 just below the line.) Patients also complete three visual/numeric scales assessing the pain interference with daily activities, recreational/social/family activities, and ability to work. Finally, patients report on the number of days in the previous 6 months on which they were unable to carry out their normal activities. Mean values for the three pain and three disability scales are

calculated; the disability days are rescored on a 4-point scale, with the largest values assigned to those who report 31 or more days of interference. Both the mean pain level and the disability score are then combined into a single Graded Chronic Pain score, ranging from Grade 0 to Grade IV. Grade 0 indicates no pain or disability in the past 6 months; Grades I and II indicate increasing levels of pain, with low levels of disability; Grades III and IV indicate increasing levels of disability independent of pain levels.

Population studies indicate that the Graded Chronic Pain score has good psychometric properties (John, Hirsch, Reiber, & Dworkin, 2006; Smith et al., 1997). Cronbach's alpha in these studies ranged from 0.88 to 0.91. Item–total correlations ranged from .69 to .83 (Smith et al., 1997), and an intraclass correlation was .92 (John et al., 2006). Responses on the Chronic Pain Grade questionnaire were significantly correlated with dimensions on the Short Form-36 (SF-36; Smith et al., 1997). For the SF-36 pain dimension, the correlation was –.84 with the chronic pain grade. (High scores on the SF-36 are associated with positive well-being.) Other investigations indicate that the Graded Chronic Pain score can be used as a screening tool to identify patients with TMJD with various types of pain profiles in primary care (Forssell, Santalahti, Puukka, & Talo, 2005).

Axis II also contains measures for assessing depression, comorbid physical symptoms, jaw function (including oral parafunctions in the DC/TMD). The DC/TMD also includes measures to assess anxiety and other syndromes. The depression, anxiety, and comorbid physical symptoms components employ the Depression, Anxiety, and Somatization scales of the SCL-90-R. Patients receive scores as normal, moderately depressed, or severely depressed based on specific cutoff scores for the individual scales. A jaw disability scale is also included in the original RDC/TMD Axis II, but its reliability and validity have not been thoroughly assessed (Von Korff et al., 1992).

Under Axis I of the RDC/TMD, examiners palpate masticatory muscles and the TMJ according to procedures outlined in the original and subsequent publications. These "provoked" self-reports are combined with other measures obtained in Axis I of the RDC/TMD to apply diagnostic labels. Well-trained examiners can reach a very high level of reliability (Lenton et al., 2007) for muscle palpation, and those who do not train under a gold-standard examiner can also achieve high levels of agreement for the presence and absence of masticatory muscle pain diagnoses (Lausten, Glaros, & Williams, 2004).

Can health care professionals other than dentists effectively perform the examination techniques required by the RDC/TMD? The preliminary answer appears to be "yes." Investigators have shown that dental hygienists can perform as gold-standard examiners. Lausten and colleagues (2004) showed that both dentists and nondentists can perform the RDC/TMD examination to a satisfactory level of reliability. For example, they reported 88.9% agreement that myofascial pain was present and 79.2% agreement that it was not present in a mixed sample of participants with and without TMJD. Examiner calibration, not professional experience, appears to be the most important factor for reliable measurement of TMJD symptoms using the RDC/TMD (Leher, Graf, PhoDuc, & Rammelsberg, 2005).

Attempts to substitute electronic and mechanical devices for fingertip palpation show that the devices are generally good at discriminating between treated and non-treated groups of patients and between patient and nonpatient groups (Bendtsen, Jensen, Jensen, & Olesen, 1994; Brown et al., 2000). Reliability estimates for one device showed good results, with intraclass correlations between .73 and .96 (Bernhardt, Schiffman, & Look, 2007).

It may be possible to substitute simple self-report questions for some of the examination procedures in the RDC/TMD. Nilsson and colleagues (Nilsson, List, & Drangsholt, 2006) showed that the test–retest reliability of adolescents responding to two questions ("Do you have pain in your temples, face, temporomandibular joint [TMJ] or jaws once a week or more?", "Do you have pain when you open your mouth wide or chew once a week or more?") was excellent (kappa = .83). Sensitivity and specificity of these questions for detecting a painful TMJD the same day using RDC/TMD procedures were .96 and .83, respectively,

and these values changed little when RDC/TMD assessments were made 2–4 weeks later. A somewhat longer self-administered questionnaire also showed good reliability among a sample of 50 children and adolescents (kappa = .78 –.92; Wahlund, List, & Dworkin, 1998).

The TMJ Scale is a 97-item self-report measure used to assess temporomandibular disorders (Levitt, McKinney, & Lundeen, 1988). The TMJ Scale is computer-scored according to a proprietary algorithm. The report provides information on nine subscales and a tenth global scale for the presence of some type of TMJD. Item–scale correlations corrected for overlap showed values ranging from .51 to .66; alpha coefficients for the scales ranged from 0.81 to 0.95. Test–retest correlations performed on 25 patients, with test administrations having a mean separation of 5 days, ranged from .55 to .95. Comparisons between a national clinical sample of 10,549 individuals and a cross-validation sample of 742 individuals showed that the subscale scores between the two samples differed by 13% or less, except for the "palpation pain" subscale, on which the scores differed somewhat more (Levitt & McKinney, 1994). Three of the subscales in the TMJ Scale make up the psychosocial domain. They assess psychological factors, stress, and chronicity. The sensitivity and specificity of the Psychological Factors and Stress subscales ranged from .71 to .76 when compared against the SCL-90 and the Total Stress Score on the Derogatis Stress Profile as the gold standards (Levitt, Lundeen, & McKinney, 1987).

Additional techniques for assessing pain in TMJD patients include the IMPATH:TMJ and the temporomandibular index (TMI). The term "IMPATH" stands for Interactive Microcomputer Patient Assessment Tool for Health. The items that make up IMPATH:TMJ are similar to those of a patient history questionnaire performed before a physical examination. The psychometric properties of the IMPATH:TMJ are poorly understood.

The RDC/TMD provides a diagnosis, but not a measure of severity. In contrast, the temporomandibular index (TMI; Pehling et al., 2002) assesses the severity of a TMJD. It consists of three subindices: (1) the Function

Index (FI); (2) the Muscle Index (MI); and (3) the Joint Index (JI). In one study, examiner agreement for the TMI was excellent, with an intraclass correlation coefficient of .93. Comparisons between symptomatic and control groups were significant ($p < .001$) on the TMI, suggesting that the scale can discriminate between patient and nonpatient groups (Pehling et al., 2002).

Issues in the Use of Self-Report of TMJDs

Retrospective bias can be a significant issue with interviews, whether open-ended or semistructured. Raphael and Marbach (1997) examined the date that TMJD pain began, as recorded in the medical files of 125 women with a chronic history of TMJD, and compared this value with the date reported in a structured medical interview. The discrepancy between the two reports was nearly 4 years, with patients "forward-telescoping" onset dates (i.e., dates being recalled as occurring later than recorded in the medical record) more frequently than "backward-telescoping." The intraclass correlation was .80 for the full sample. These findings imply that a single patient's report of TMJD pain onset may lead to an underestimate of chronicity.

Visual analogue scales (VASs) and numerical rating scales (NRSs) have good psychometric properties and are very easy to administer and score. The numerical values of both scales clearly lend themselves to statistical tests that use ordinal data (i.e., the so-called nonparametric tests), and many investigators use standard parametric tests to analyze these data. However, VASs and NRSs should be interpreted with caution. Patients ascribe multiple, idiosyncratic meanings to their responses on these scales (Williams, Davies, & Chadury, 2000). Nearly all inpatients reported considering multiple elements when responding to pain rating scales. Some of these elements might include comparing their current pain with their usual pain or with their worst pain and the distress caused by pain. The distribution of these elements varied. For example, 60% of patients considered the impact of pain on their ability to carry out daily routines always or often

in responding to these scales. In contrast, slightly more than 10% percent always or often thought of pain in terms of a number when responding to the scale.

Assessment of Behavior in Patients with TMJDs

Laboratory-based studies show that mild to moderate clenching in otherwise pain-free individuals significantly increases pain and can result in a diagnosis of TMJD by a blinded examiner (e.g., Farella, Soneda, Vilmann, Thomsen, & Bakke, 2010; Glaros & Burton, 2004; Glaros, Tabacchi, & Glass, 1998). Studies using experience sampling techniques also show that individuals diagnosed with TMJD have high levels of tooth contact compared with controls without pain (Chen, Palla, Erni, Sieber, & Gallo, 2007; Glaros, Williams, & Lausten, 2005). Thus the ability to assess these parafunctional oral behaviors (i.e., oral behaviors not associated with eating, drinking, talking, or swallowing) should be helpful in diagnosing patients with TMJD and in identifying those whose high levels of parafunctions may make them good candidates for habit reversal approaches to their pain (e.g., Glaros, Kim-Weroha, Lausten, & Franklin, 2007; Townsend, Nicholson, Buenaver, Bush, & Gramling, 2001).

Experience sampling method (ESM) techniques repeatedly measure a behavior or state in an individual's natural environment. Statistical theory indicates that repeated sampling should lead to reasonably accurate estimates of the actual level of behavior. Thus ESM data should provide good estimates of oral parafunctions in the patient's natural environment. Similarly, ESM data can assess pain levels and other states. The effects of retrospective bias should be markedly reduced with ESM, and there is little reason to expect that monitoring pain and other states has a reactive effect on patients with TMJD (Aaron, Turner, Mancl, Brister, & Sawchuk, 2005; Glaros, Williams, & Lausten, 2008).

ESM can be carried out using paper forms or electronic media. For patients with TMJD using ESM, the individual is usually contacted on a semirandom schedule. Investigators typically avoid fixed, nonrandom schedules (e.g., contacts precisely every 2 hours) to avoid the biasing effect of anticipating a signal (and thereby altering behavior) to complete a questionnaire. When contacted, patients are instructed to complete a questionnaire and then return to their everyday activities.

The questions that patients answer are usually very easy to complete, typically requiring only a circled response or a tap on a screen, and the number of questions is limited to reduce the time needed to respond. Patients may be contacted a few times a day (e.g., 6–8 times during waking hours; Glaros et al., 2005) to as often as every 20 minutes (Chen et al., 2007). For patients completing paper questionnaires, the signal to fill out the questionnaire may be sent to their cell phones or to a pager. Investigators using electronic devices may lend patients a "smart phone" or tablet that is programmed to display the questionnaire, accept responses to individual questions, and, in some cases, automatically transfer the information to a database. Comparisons between standard paper diaries and electronic versions of diaries show that both provide the same information and are equally accepted by patients (Green, Rafaeli, Bolger, Shrout, & Reis, 2006).

Before ESM techniques can be used effectively, investigators must verify that patients are capable of understanding the task and are motivated to respond to prompts quickly and accurately. ESM techniques rely on technology in one form or another, and patients must be comfortable with their use. Cell-enabled and tablet devices may have some technological advantages over pagers and questionnaire cards. Among these are: (1) elimination of the need for time-consuming data entry with pager questionnaire cards; (2) the ability to "lock out" responding when too much time has passed between device signaling and patient responding; (3) the ability to randomize the order of questions, enhancing the validity of responses; (4) the ability to recharge batteries simply and easily; and (5) simple or unattended downloading of data, depending on the specific device and programming. Cell-enabled devices have their drawbacks as well; they may be sensitive to mishandling and breakage, and they can be attractive objects vulnerable to theft.

Whether investigators use paper or electronic approaches to ESM, it is important to establish a normative database so that the patient's values can be readily compared with those of a control participant without pain. In one study, the percent of time that the controls without pain engaged in tooth contact was 45% (Glaros et al., 2005), whereas another study (Chen et al., 2007) reported tooth contact 8.9% of the time in controls without pain. In every case, the proportion of time in tooth contact reported by patients diagnosed with pain was markedly higher (typically, 50% to nearly 300% higher).

The technology that underlies ESM can also be used for other assessment purposes. Aaron and colleagues (2006), for example, used electronic diaries to examine daily pain coping mechanisms in patients with TMJD and catastrophizing in these patients (Turner, Mancl, & Aaron, 2004). Similarly, the technology can be used to assess the effect of treatment with patients with TMJD (Turner, Mancl, & Aaron, 2005) and as a mechanism to facilitate treatment (Glaros et al., 2007).

Is it possible to obtain clinically useful information about oral parafunctional behaviors with a questionnaire? Ohrbach and colleagues have developed the Oral Behaviors Checklist, a self-report scale for identifying and quantifying the frequency of oral parafunctional behaviors (Markiewicz, Ohrbach, & McCall, 2006). In one study, electromyographic (EMG) data were obtained from both masticatory muscles and the biceps while various tasks, particularly those involving oral behaviors, were performed. The data showed intertrial reliability ranging from .80 to .99 for tasks involving the biceps muscles and from .87 to .75 for individuals with TMJD and controls, respectively, for tasks involving the masseter and temporalis muscles. These findings are similar to those reported by Glaros and Waghela (2006), who also showed high levels of reliability between EMG and behavior in a sample of individuals without pain. Further research will show whether a simple questionnaire such as the Oral Behaviors Checklist can validly replace data obtained from experience sampling methods.

Psychophysiological Evaluation of TMJDs

Electromyographic evaluation of TMJDs is based on the hypothesis that patients with TMJD either have characteristically and chronically high levels of muscle activity in the facial region as compared with control participants or that they are more reactive to stressors than individuals without TMJD. Studies examining this perspective have reported mixed results. The lack of consistency in these studies is probably due to methodological factors and an inappropriate assumption that the laboratory setting is an ecologically valid venue for collecting EMG data. EMG data obtained from the masticatory muscles, particularly the masseter and temporalis, show great sensitivity to jaw position. In the masseter, EMG values are least when the posterior teeth are separated by about 8–12 mm. As the temporalis and masseter muscles become more active, the teeth come closer together and eventually meet. The ratio between the EMG values at a resting baseline and the tooth-contact position can be as high as 3.5-fold (Glaros, Forbes, Shanker, & Glass, 2000; Glaros & Waghela, 2006). Jaw position can powerfully affect masticatory EMG activity, and failure to control for jaw position may be an important reason for the discrepancies in the studies.

Similarly, questions can be raised about the ecological validity of the laboratory setting. When investigators use technologies that permit collection of EMG data while individuals go about their everyday activities (Peck, Kaldenberg, de Vries, Klineberg, & Murray, 2007), the results are consistent with the findings of Glaros and colleagues (2005); viz., individuals diagnosed with the myofascial pain of TMJD show higher levels of EMG activity during the day than controls without TMJD.

As miniaturization of electronic devices proceeds, it should become easier to validate the hypothesis that patients with TMJD diagnosed with myofascial pain spend greater proportions of the day with activated masticatory muscles than their counterparts without TMJD. Under controlled laboratory conditions, it is possible to distinguish among various oral activities (including both functional and parafunctional activities) with a high degree of sensitivity and specificity (Gallo, Guerra, & Palla, 1998; Ohrbach, Markiewicz, & McCall, 2008). For patients with TMJD, it may be sufficient to detect overall levels of parafunctional activity rather than to distinguish among separate behaviors.

The relationship of TMJD to sleep-related conditions such as grinding of the teeth ("bruxism") is controversial (Janal, Raphael, Klausner, & Teaford, 2007). Some patients do not appear to engage in sleep-related grinding, whereas others do. In those with sleep-related grinding, the polysomnographic findings between grinders with orofacial pain and those without pain are similar (Camparis & Siqueira, 2006). Treatment of patients with mouth guards ("splints" or interocclusal appliances) shows no differences in wear patterns between those who reported pain reduction and those who did not (Chung, Kim, & Kim, 2000). Considering the cost of a polysomnographic evaluation, these data do not provide a strong basis for routine evaluation of sleep problems in patients with TMJD.

Assessment of Emotional Status

Like many other patients with chronic pain, patients with TMJD with pain can also suffer from emotional disorders, most typically depression and somatization (Manfredini, di Poggio, Romagnoli, Dell'Osso, & Bosco, 2004; Manfredini, Winocur, Ahlberg, Guarda-Nardini, & Lobbezoo, 2010). Whether a patient with TMJD should be formally assessed for such conditions will depend on the specific presentation of symptoms reported by an individual patient.

However, the risk of emotional distress is predictably greater in some patients with TMJD than in others. Individuals who report muscle pain (e.g., an RDC/TMD diagnosis of myofascial pain or a combination of myofascial pain and arthralgia) are much more likely to report emotional problems than patients diagnosed with jaw-related disorders (e.g., displacement of the articular disc; Bertoli, de Leeuw, Schmidt, Okeson, & Carlson, 2007; Reissmann,

John, Schierz, & Wassell, 2007). Various measures of stress, including general stress, health-related stress, and stressors related to financial and job status, are significant risk factors for myofascial pain (Akhter et al., 2007).

Psychosocial variables can successfully predict some diagnostic labels and also whether a new patient with TMJD is likely to develop a chronic problem. McCreary, Clark, Merril, Flack, and Oakley (1991) correctly identified 74% of patients diagnosed with structural problems of the joint and 46% of patients with myofascial pain. Individuals with elevated scores on the Chronic Pain Index, the Beck Depression Inventory, and scales 8 and 3 of the MMPI, along with an RDC/TMD diagnosis of myofascial pain accompanied by jaw limitations, are also those most likely to have a chronic problem (Epker & Gatchel, 2000). Individuals at high risk for a chronic condition can, fortunately, benefit from treatment. In a 1-year follow-up of high-risk patients who received either a cognitive-behavioral intervention for pain and distress or no psychosocial intervention, Gatchel, Stowell, Wildenstein, Riggs, and Ellis (2006) reported that the group receiving the cognitive-behavioral intervention reported significantly lower levels of pain, greater coping, and less emotional distress than those who received no intervention. In addition, the early intervention group also reported reduced utilization of medical services. Psychological factors contribute significantly to the prediction of chronicity, even when potential genetic contributors (e.g., catechol-O-methyltransferase [COMT] haplotype) are taken into account (Slade et al., 2007).

Patients with TMJD report more physical and sexual abuse than equivalent groups without TMJD (Campbell, Riley, Kashikar-Zuck, Gremillion, & Robinson, 2000; Curran et al., 1995; Fillingim, Maixner, Sigurdsson, & Kincaid, 1997). This literature is largely based on cross-sectional studies, and, like many cross-sectional studies, it suffers from ascertainment bias. One prospective-style study (Raphael, Widom, & Lange, 2001) examined the risk for developing a pain problem following documented physical or sexual abuse. The data showed no increased risk for a future pain problem.

Whereas generalized physical or sexual abuse has an uncertain relationship to TMJD, direct injury to the jaw or face, sustained as a result of a motor vehicle accident, for example, is a significant risk factor for TMJD (Sale & Isberg, 2007). Intubation delivered during surgery has also been identified as a risk factor for TMJD, particularly in those with some prior symptoms of TMJD (Martin, Wilson, Ross, & Souter, 2007). Reports of physical and sexual abuse should not be dismissed out of hand as unrelated to TMJD but should be explored further for evidence of direct injury to the face or jaw.

Emerging Assessment Techniques

An emerging line of evidence suggests that quantitative sensory testing (QST) may become a valuable tool in the assessment of patients with TMJD. Using QST, the function of sensory neurons is evaluated by presenting controlled thermal, tactile, and vibratory stimuli. Following stimulation, patients indicate the degree of discomfort or sensation evoked by each technique. Ideally, the pattern of results generated for each patient points to a specific deficit or problem in a sensory neuron. The technique has been used to assess patients with trigeminal neuralgia (Eliav, Gracely, Nahlieli, & Benoliel, 2004), TMJD (Eliav et al., 2003; Park, Clark, Kim, & Chung, 2010), and other disorders involving the neurological system (Zohsel, Hohmeister, Oelkers-Ax, Flor, & Hermann, 2006).

Some functional magnetic resonance imaging (fMRI) studies suggest that this technique may also be beneficial in identifying differences in pain processing between patients and nonpatient controls (Nash et al., 2010a, 2010b). These differences involve overall levels of neural activity and levels in specific brain regions and activation of cortical regions in response to applied pain stimuli. Although significant work still needs to be conducted, fMRI may be more useful in patients with myofascial pain than in those with degenerative or inflammatory conditions of the joint (Byrd, Romito, Dzemidzic, Wong, & Talavage, 2009; Koh, List, Petersson, & Rohlin, 2009).

Commercial manufacturers market a variety of devices for diagnosing TMJDs, and many have a seal of approval from the American Dental Association. Evidence suggests that these devices can measure various aspects of TMJDs safely. However, their sensitivity and specificity for stand-alone diagnosis is unacceptably low (Baba, Tsukiyama, Yamazaki, & Clark, 2001).

Measures of Treatment Effectiveness

For most patients with TMJD, relief from pain and improved function are the major goals of treatment. The same measures used to assess baseline levels of pain (e.g., VASs, NRSs) can also be used to assess treatment. The smallest detectable difference in pain for patients with TMJD responding to a VAS is 28 millimeters (Kropmans, Dijkstra, van Veen, Stegenga, & de Bont, 1999), with a range of 15 to 43 mm, depending on the number of repetitions (Kropmans, Dijkstra, Stegenga, Stewart, & de Bont, 2002). Taking within-subject variability into account, a change of 38–51% from the initial pain level can be considered clinically meaningful (Emshoff, Emshoff, & Bertram, 2010; Kropmans et al., 2002; van Grootel, van der Bilt, & van der Glas, 2007).

Quality-of-life measures can also be used to assess treatment progress. Investigators use multiple measures to rate quality of life in patients with TMJD, including the Oral Health Impact Profile (OHIP; John, Reissmann, Schierz, & Wassell, 2007; Luo, McMillan, Wong, Zheng, & Lam, 2007; Reissmann et al., 2007) and the Child Health Questionnaire–Child Form 87 (CHQ-CF87; Jedel, Carlsson, & Stener-Victorin, 2007). Oral health-related quality of life measures typically assess the degree to which patients feel comfortable engaging in typical oral behaviors (e.g., chewing and eating, talking, opening the jaw comfortably). Because pain is often associated with limitations in these activities (Dahlstrom, & Carlsson, 2010), improvement in these measures of function can be taken as indirect evidence that pain is diminishing.

Treatment of TMJD pain can affect patient beliefs and coping (Jensen, Turner, & Romano, 2007), and the use of cognitive coping strategies (along with reduced depression) can be associated with positive outcomes for patients with orofacial pain (Riley, Myers, Robinson, Bulcourf, & Gremillion, 2001). Self-care strategies practiced by patients with TMJD do not appear to be associated with initial levels of pain, but depression and sleep quality are associated with self-care frequency and efficacy (Riley et al., 2007). These studies point to the value of assessing beliefs, coping, and depression in patients with TMJD.

Conclusions and Recommendations

Patients with TMJD commonly report pain, and they report success with treatment when pain is reduced. Accordingly, techniques for measuring pain have considerable utility in the assessment of patients with TMJD. Parafunctional oral habits appear to characterize some patients with TMJD, and assessment of these behaviors can provide important insights into the mechanisms of pain in these patients. On the other hand, laboratory-based psychophysiological assessments, which originally appeared to have great value for assessing patients with TMJD, are strongly influenced by extraneous factors that make interpretation of data difficult.

Patients with TMJD may suffer from comorbid psychological conditions such as depression and anxiety, and the presence of comorbid psychological conditions can markedly affect the outcome of treatment. Furthermore, coping strategies and patient beliefs can also influence and be affected by treatment outcomes. Thus, assessing multiple psychological factors in patients with TMJD, particularly those with myofascial pain, can provide a more complete picture of each patient and encourage individualization of treatment for these patients. QST and fMRI have promising, but unknown, potential in assessing patients with TMJD.

Research in the assessment of patients with TMJD has been surprisingly active and creative. The lines between traditional psychological assessment, typically using self-report instruments of various kinds, and more "dental" or "medical" approaches can no longer be drawn with ease. For a health care provider interested in assessing patients with TMJD, a strong background in traditional psychological assessment techniques and deep knowledge of both TMJD and psychometrics will be highly beneficial.

REFERENCES

Aaron, L. A., Burke, M. M., & Buchwald, D. (2000). Overlapping conditions among patients with chronic fatigue syndrome, fibromyalgia, and temporomandibular disorder. *Archives of Internal Medicine, 160,* 221–227.

Aaron, L. A., Turner, J. A., Mancl, L., Brister, H., & Sawchuk, C. N. (2005). Electronic diary assessment of pain-related variables: Is reactivity a problem? *Journal of Pain, 6,* 107–115.

Aaron, L. A., Turner, J. A., Mancl, L. A., Sawchuk, C. N., Huggins, K. H., & Truelove, E. L. (2006). Daily pain coping among patients with chronic temporomandibular disorder pain: An electronic diary study. *Journal of Orofacial Pain, 20,* 125–137.

Akhter, R., Hassan, N. M., Aida, J., Kanehira, T., Zaman, K. U., & Morita, M. (2007). Association between experience of stressful life events and muscle-related temporomandibular disorders in patients seeking free treatment in a dental hospital. *European Journal of Medical Research, 12,* 535–540.

Anderson, G. C., Gonzalez, Y. M., Ohrbach, R., Truelove, E. L., Sommers, E., Look, J. O., et al. (2010). The Research Diagnostic Criteria for Temporomandibular Disorders: VI. Future directions. *Journal of Orofacial Pain, 24,* 79–88.

Baba, K., Tsukiyama, Y., Yamazaki, M., & Clark, G. T. (2001). A review of temporomandibular disorder diagnostic techniques. *Journal of Prosthetic Dentistry, 86,* 184–194.

Bendtsen, L., Jensen, R., Jensen, N. K., & Olesen, J. (1994). Muscle palpation with controlled finger pressure: New equipment for the study of tender myofascial tissues. *Pain, 59,* 235–239.

Bernhardt, O., Schiffman, E. L., & Look, J. O. (2007). Reliability and validity of a new fingertip-shaped pressure algometer for assessing pressure pain thresholds in the temporomandibular joint and masticatory muscles. *Journal of Orofacial Pain, 21,* 29–38.

Bertoli, E., de Leeuw, R., Schmidt, J. E., Okeson, J. P., & Carlson, C. R. (2007). Prevalence and impact of post-traumatic stress disorder symptoms in patients with masticatory muscle or temporomandibular joint pain: Differences and similarities. *Journal of Orofacial Pain, 21,* 107–119.

Brown, F. F., Robinson, M. E., Riley, J. L., Gremillion, H. A., McSolay, J., & Meyers, G.

(2000). Better palpation of pain: Reliability and validity of a new pressure pain protocol in TMD. *Cranio, 18,* 58–65.

Byrd, K. E., Romito, L. M., Dzemidzic, M., Wong, D., & Talavage, T. M. (2009). fMRI study of brain activity elicited by oral parafunctional movements. *Journal of Oral Rehabilitation. 36,* 346–361.

Camparis, C. M., & Siqueira, J. T. (2006). Sleep bruxism: Clinical aspects and characteristics in patients with and without chronic orofacial pain. *Oral Surgery, Oral Medicine, Oral Pathology, Oral Radiology, and Endodontics, 101,* 188–193.

Campbell, L. C., Riley, J. L., III, Kashikar-Zuck, S., Gremillion, H., & Robinson, M. E. (2000). Somatic, affective, and pain characteristics of chronic TMD patients with sexual versus physical abuse histories. *Journal of Orofacial Pain, 14,* 112–119.

Carlsson, G., & LeResche, L. (1995). Epidemiology of temporomandibular disorders. In B. J. Sessle, P. S. Bryant, & R. Dionne (Eds.), *Temporomandibular disorders and related pain conditions* (pp. 211–226). Seattle, WA: IASP Press.

Chen, C. Y., Palla, S., Erni, S., Sieber, M., & Gallo, L. M. (2007). Nonfunctional tooth contact in healthy controls and patients with myogenous facial pain. *Journal of Orofacial Pain, 21,* 185–193.

Chung, S. C., Kim, Y. K., & Kim, H. S. (2000). Prevalence and patterns of nocturnal bruxofacets on stabilization splints in temporomandibular disorder patients. *Cranio, 18,* 92–97.

Curran, S. L., Sherman, J. J., Cunningham, L. L., Okeson, J. P., Reid, K. I., & Carlson, C. R. (1995). Physical and sexual abuse among orofacial pain patients: Linkages with pain and psychologic distress. *Journal of Orofacial Pain, 9,* 340–346.

Dahlstrom, L., & Carlsson, G. E. (2010). Temporomandibular disorders and oral health-related quality of life: A systematic review. *Acta Odontologica Scandinavica, 68,* 80–85.

Drangsholt, M., & LeResche, L. (1999). Temporomandibular disorder pain. In I. K. Crombie, P. R. Croft, S. J. Linton, L. LeResche, & M. Von Korff (Eds.), *Epidemiology of pain: A report of the Task Force on Epidemiology of the International Association for the Study of Pain* (pp. 203–233). Seattle, WA: IASP Press.

Dworkin, S. F., & LeResche, L. (1992). Research diagnostic criteria for temporomandibular disorders: Review, criteria, examinations and specifications, critique. *Journal of Craniomandibular Disorders, 6,* 301–355.

Eliav, E., Gracely, R. H., Nahlieli, O., & Benoliel, R. (2004). Quantitative sensory testing in trigeminal nerve damage assessment. *Journal of Orofacial Pain, 18,* 339–344.

Eliav, E., Teich, S., Nitzan, D., el Raziq, D. A., Nahlieli, O., Tal, M., et al. (2003). Facial arthralgia and myalgia: Can they be differentiated by trigeminal sensory assessment? *Pain, 104,* 481–490.

Emshoff, R., Emshoff, I., & Bertram, S. (2010). Estimation of clinically important change for visual analog scales measuring chronic temporomandibular disorder pain. *Journal of Orofacial Pain. 24,* 262–269.

Epker, J., & Gatchel, R. J. (2000). Coping profile differences in the biopsychosocial functioning of patients with temporomandibular disorder. *Psychosomatic Medicine, 62,* 69–75.

Farella, M., Soneda, K., Vilmann, A., Thomsen, C. E., & Bakke, M. (2010). Jaw muscle soreness after tooth-clenching depends on force level. *Journal of Dental Research, 89,* 717–721.

Fillingim, R. B., Maixner, W., Sigurdsson, A., & Kincaid, S. (1997). Sexual and physical abuse history in subjects with temporomandibular disorders: Relationship to clinical variables, pain sensitivity, and psychologic factors. *Journal of Orofacial Pain, 11,* 48–57.

Forssell, H., Santalahti, P., Puukka, P., & Talo, S. (2005). Searching for an assessment instrument to determine temporomandibular disorder pain profiles for the purposes of primary health care. *International Journal of Rehabilitation Research, 28,* 203–209.

Gallo, L. M., Guerra, P. O., & Palla, S. (1998). Automatic on-line one-channel recognition of masseter activity. *Journal of Dental Research, 77,* 1539–1546.

Gatchel, R. J., Stowell, A. W., Wildenstein, L., Riggs, R., & Ellis, E., III. (2006). Efficacy of an early intervention for patients with acute temporomandibular disorder-related pain: A one-year outcome study. *Journal of the American Dental Association, 137,* 339–347.

Giannakopoulos, N. N., Keller, L., Rammelsberg, P., Kronmuller, K. T., & Schmitter, M. (2010). Anxiety and depression in patients with chronic temporomandibular pain and in controls. *Journal of Dentistry 38,* 369–376.

Glaros, A. G., & Burton, E. (2004). Parafunctional clenching, pain, and effort in temporomandibular disorders. *Journal of Behavioral Medicine, 27,* 91–100.

Glaros, A. G., Forbes, M., Shanker, J., & Glass, E. G. (2000). Effect of parafunctional clenching on temporomandibular disorder pain and proprioceptive awareness. *Cranio, 18,* 198–204.

Glaros, A. G., Glass, E. G., & Hayden, W. J. (1995). History of treatment received by patients with TMD: A preliminary investigation. *Journal of Orofacial Pain, 9,* 147–151.

Glaros, A. G., Kim-Weroha, N., Lausten, L., & Franklin, K.-L. (2007). Comparison of habit reversal and a behaviorally modified dental treatment for temporomandibular disorders: A pilot investigation. *Applied Psychophysiology and Biofeedback, 32,* 149–154.

Glaros, A. G., Tabacchi, K. N., & Glass, E. G. (1998). Effect of parafunctional clenching on TMD pain. *Journal of Orofacial Pain, 12,* 145–152.

Glaros, A. G., Urban, D., & Locke, J. (2007). Temporomandibular disorders and headache: Evidence for diagnostic and behavioural overlap. *Cephalalgia, 27,* 542–549.

Glaros, A. G., & Waghela, R. (2006). Psychophysiological definitions of clenching. *Cranio, 24,* 252–257.

Glaros, A. G., Williams, K., & Lausten, L. (2005). The role of parafunctions, emotions and stress in predicting facial pain. *Journal of the American Dental Association, 136,* 451–458.

Glaros, A. G., Williams, K., & Lausten, L. (2008). Diurnal variation in pain reports in temporomandibular disorder patients and non-pain controls. *Journal of Orofacial Pain, 22,* 115–121.

Goncalves, D. A., Dal Fabbro, A. L., Campos, J. A., Bigal, M. E., & Speciali, J. G. (2010). Symptoms of temporomandibular disorders in the population: An epidemiological study. *Journal of Orofacial Pain, 24,* 270–278.

Green, A. S., Rafaeli, E., Bolger, N., Shrout, P. E., & Reis, H. T. (2006). Paper or plastic?: Data equivalence in paper and electronic diaries. *Psychological Methods, 11,* 87–105.

Janal, M. N., Raphael, K. G., Klausner, J., & Teaford, M. (2007). The role of tooth-grinding in the maintenance of myofascial face pain: A test of alternate models. *Pain Medicine, 8,* 486–496.

Jedel, E., Carlsson, J., & Stener-Victorin, E.

(2007). Health-related quality of life in child patients with temporomandibular disorder pain. *European Journal of Pain, 11*, 557–563.

Jensen, M. P., Turner, J. A., & Romano, J. M. (2007). Changes after multidisciplinary pain treatment in patient pain beliefs and coping are associated with concurrent changes in patient functioning. *Pain, 131*, 38–47.

John, M. T., Hirsch, C., Reiber, T., & Dworkin, S. F. (2006). Translating the research diagnostic criteria for temporomandibular disorders into German: Evaluation of content and process. *Journal of Orofacial Pain, 20*, 43–52.

John, M. T., Reissmann, D. R., Schierz, O., & Wassell, R. W. (2007). Oral health-related quality of life in patients with temporomandibular disorders. *Journal of Orofacial Pain, 21*, 46–54.

Koh, K. J., List, T., Petersson, A., & Rohlin, M. (2009). Relationship between clinical and magnetic resonance imaging diagnoses and findings in degenerative and inflammatory temporomandibular joint diseases: A systematic literature review. *Journal of Orofacial Pain, 23*, 123–139.

Kropmans, T. J., Dijkstra, P. U., van Veen, A., Stegenga, B., & de Bont, L. G. (1999). The smallest detectable difference of mandibular function impairment in patients with a painfully restricted temporomandibular joint. *Journal of Dental Research, 78*, 1445–1449.

Kropmans, T. J. B., Dijkstra, P. U., Stegenga, B., Stewart, R., & de Bont, L. G. M. (2002). Repeated assessment of temporomandibular joint pain: Reasoned decision-making with use of unidimensional and multidimensional pain scales. *Clinical Journal of Pain, 18*, 107–115.

Kuttila, S., Kuttila, M., Le Bell, Y., Alanen, P., & Suonpaa, J. (2004). Characteristics of subjects with secondary otalgia. *Journal of Orofacial Pain, 18*, 226–234.

Lausten, L. L., Glaros, A. G., & Williams, K. (2004). Inter-examiner reliability of physical assessment methods for assessing temporomandibular disorders. *General Dentistry, 52*, 509–513.

Leher, A., Graf, K., PhoDuc, J. M., & Rammelsberg, P. (2005). Is there a difference in the reliable measurement of temporomandibular disorder signs between experienced and inexperienced examiners? *Journal of Orofacial Pain, 19*, 58–64.

Lenton, P., Garfinkel, L., Huggins, K. H., Jackson, A., Look, J., Pan, W., et al. (2007,

March). *Examiner reliability for the RDC/TMD Group-I myofascial pain diagnoses*. Paper presented at the annual meeting of the International Association for Dental Research, New Orleans, LA.

Levitt, S. R., Lundeen, T. F., & McKinney, M. W. (1987). *The TMJ Scale manual*. Durham, NC: Pain Resource Center.

Levitt, S. R., & McKinney, M. W. (1994). Validating the TMJ scale in a national sample of 10,000 patients: Demographic and epidemiologic characteristics. *Journal of Orofacial Pain, 8*, 25–35.

Levitt, S. R., McKinney, M. W., & Lundeen, T. F. (1988). The TMJ scale: Cross-validation and reliability studies. *Cranio, 6*, 17–25.

Lim, P. F., Smith, S., Bhalang, K., Slade, G. D., & Maixner, W. (2010). Development of temporomandibular disorders is associated with greater bodily pain experience. *Clinical Journal of Pain, 26*, 116–120.

Luo, Y., McMillan, A. S., Wong, M. C., Zheng, J., & Lam, C. L. (2007). Orofacial pain conditions and impact on quality of life in community-dwelling elderly people in Hong Kong. *Journal of Orofacial Pain, 21*, 63–71.

Manfredini, D., di Poggio, A. B., Romagnoli, M., Dell'Osso, L., & Bosco, M. (2004). Mood spectrum in patients with different painful temporomandibular disorders. *Cranio, 22*, 234–240.

Manfredini, D., Winocur, E., Ahlberg, J., Guarda-Nardini, L., & Lobbezoo, F. (2010). Psychosocial impairment in temporomandibular disorders patients: RDC/TMD axis II findings from a multicentre study. *Journal of Dentistry, 38*, 765–772.

Markiewicz, M. R., Ohrbach, R., & McCall, W. D., Jr. (2006). Oral Behaviors Checklist: Reliability of performance in targeted waking-state behaviors. *Journal of Orofacial Pain, 20*, 306–316.

Martin, M. D., Wilson, K. J., Ross, B. K., & Souter, K. (2007). Intubation risk factors for temporomandibular joint/facial pain. *Anesthesia Progress, 54*, 109–114.

McCreary, C. P., Clark, G. T., Merril, R. L., Flack, V., & Oakley, M. E. (1991). Psychological distress and diagnostic subgroups of temporomandibular disorder patients. *Pain, 44*, 29–34.

Nash, P. G., Macefield, V. G., Klineberg, I. J., Gustin, S. M., Murray, G. M., & Henderson, L. A. (2010a). Bilateral activation of the trigeminothalamic tract by acute orofacial cutaneous and muscle pain in humans. *Pain, 151,* 384–393.

Nash, P. G., Macefield, V. G., Klineberg, I. J., Gustin, S. M., Murray, G. M., & Henderson, L. A. (2010b). Changes in human primary motor cortex activity during acute cutaneous and muscle orofacial pain. *Journal of Orofacial Pain, 24,* 379–390.

Nilsson, I. M., List, T., & Drangsholt, M. (2006). The reliability and validity of self-reported temporomandibular disorder pain in adolescents. *Journal of Orofacial Pain, 20,* 138–144.

Ohrbach, R., Granger, C., List, T., & Dworkin, S. (2008). Preliminary development and validation of the Jaw Functional Limitation Scale. *Community Dentistry and Oral Epidemiology, 36,* 228–236.

Ohrbach, R., Markiewicz, M. R., & McCall, W. D., Jr. (2008). Waking-state oral parafunctional behaviors: Specificity and validity as assessed by electromyography. *European Journal of Oral Sciences, 116,* 438–444.

Park, J. W., Clark, G. T., Kim, Y. K., & Chung, J. W. (2010). Analysis of thermal pain sensitivity and psychological profiles in different subgroups of TMD patients. *International Journal of Oral and Maxillofacial Surgery, 39,* 968–974.

Peck, C. C., Kaldenberg, M., de Vries, S., Klineberg, I. J., & Murray, G. M. (2007, March). *Nonfunctional masseter activity in jaw muscle pain subjects.* Paper presented at the annual meeting of the International Association for Dental Research, New Orleans, LA.

Pehling, J., Schiffman, E., Look, J., Shaefer, J., Lenton, P., & Fricton, J. (2002). Interexaminer reliability and clinical validity of the Temporomandibular Index: A new outcome measure for temporomandibular disorders. *Journal of Orofacial Pain, 16,* 296–304.

Raphael, K. G., & Marbach, J. J. (1997). When did your pain start?: Reliability of self-reported age of onset of facial pain. *Clinical Journal of Pain, 13,* 352–359.

Raphael, K. G., Marbach, J. J., & Klausner, J. (2000). Myofascial face pain: Clinical characteristics of those with regional vs. widespread pain. *Journal of the American Dental Association, 131,* 161–171.

Raphael, K. G., Widom, C. S., & Lange, G. (2001). Childhood victimization and pain in adulthood: A prospective investigation. *Pain, 92,* 283–293.

Reissmann, D. R., John, M. T., Schierz, O., & Wassell, R. W. (2007). Functional and psycho-social impact related to specific temporomandibular disorder diagnoses. *Journal of Dentistry, 35,* 643–650.

Riley, J. L., III, Myers, C. D., Currie, T. P., Mayoral, O., Harris, R. G., Fisher, J. A., et al. (2007). Self-care behaviors associated with myofascial temporomandibular disorder pain. *Journal of Orofacial Pain, 21,* 194–202.

Riley, J. L., III, Myers, C. D., Robinson, M. E., Bulcourf, B., & Gremillion, H. A. (2001). Factors predicting orofacial pain patient satisfaction with improvement. *Journal of Orofacial Pain, 15,* 29–35.

Sale, H., & Isberg, A. (2007). Delayed temporomandibular joint pain and dysfunction induced by whiplash trauma: A controlled prospective study. *Journal of the American Dental Association, 138,* 1084–1091.

Schiffman, E., Ohrbach, R., Truelove, E., Look, J., Anderson, G., Goulet, J.-P., et al. (2014). Diagnostic criteria for temporomandibular disorders (DC/TMD) for clinical and research applications: Recommendations of the International RDC/TMD Consortium Network and Orofacial Pain Special Interest Group. *Journal of Facial and Oral Pain and Headache, 28,* 6–27.

Sipila, K., Ylostalo, P. V., Joukamaa, M., & Knuuttila, M. L. (2006). Comorbidity between facial pain, widespread pain, and depressive symptoms in young adults. *Journal of Orofacial Pain, 20,* 24–30.

Slade, G. D., Diatchenko, L., Bhalang, K., Sigurdsson, A., Fillingim, R. B., Belfer, I., et al. (2007). Influence of psychological factors on risk of temporomandibular disorders. *Journal of Dental Research, 86,* 1120–1125.

Smith, B. H., Penny, K. I., Purves, A. M., Munro, C., Wilson, B., Grimshaw, J., et al. (1997). The Chronic Pain Grade questionnaire: Validation and reliability in postal research. *Pain, 71,* 141–147.

Storm, C., & Wänman, A. (2006). Temporomandibular disorders, headaches, and cervical pain among females in a Sami population. *Acta Odontologica Scandinavica, 64,* 319–325.

Townsend, D., Nicholson, R. A., Buenaver, L., Bush, F., & Gramling, S. (2001). Use of a habit reversal treatment for temporomandibular pain in a minimal therapist contact format. *Journal of Behavior Therapy and Experimental Psychiatry, 32,* 221–239.

Turner, J. A., Holtzman, S., & Mancl, L. (2007). Mediators, moderators, and predictors of therapeutic change in cognitive-behavioral therapy for chronic pain. *Pain, 127,* 276–286.

Turner, J. A., Mancl, L., & Aaron, L. A. (2004). Pain-related catastrophizing: A daily process study. *Pain, 110,* 103–111.

Turner, J. A., Mancl, L., & Aaron, L. A. (2005). Brief cognitive-behavioral therapy for temporomandibular disorder pain: Effects on daily electronic outcome and process measures. *Pain, 117,* 377–387.

van Grootel, R. J., van der Bilt, A., & van der Glas, H. W. (2007). Long-term reliable change of pain scores in individual myogenous TMD patients. *European Journal of Pain, 11,* 635–643.

Von Korff, M., Ormel, J., Keefe, F. J., & Dworkin, S. F. (1992). Grading the severity of chronic pain. *Pain, 50,* 133–149.

Wahlund, K., List, T., & Dworkin, S. F. (1998).

Temporomandibular disorders in children and adolescents: Reliability of a questionnaire, clinical examination, and diagnosis. *Journal of Orofacial Pain, 12,* 42–51.

Wiesinger, B., Malker, H., Englund, E., & Wänman, A. (2007). Back pain in relation to musculoskeletal disorders in the jaw-face: A matched case-control study. *Pain, 131,* 311–319.

Williams, A. C. de C., Davies, H. T. O., & Chadury, Y. (2000). Simple pain rating scales hide complex idiosyncratic meanings. *Pain, 85,* 457–463.

Zohsel, K., Hohmeister, J., Oelkers-Ax, R., Flor, H., & Hermann, C. (2006). Quantitative sensory testing in children with migraine: Preliminary evidence for enhanced sensitivity to painful stimuli especially in girls. *Pain, 12,* 10–18.

CHAPTER 17

Diabetes

Linda Gonder-Frederick
Laura K. Campbell
Jaclyn A. Shepard

From a biopsychosocial perspective, diabetes is a complex disorder that can vary greatly across individuals in terms of its underlying pathophysiology, age and developmental stage at diagnosis, severity of symptoms, complications and comorbidities, treatment demands, and impact on quality of life. For example, Type 1 diabetes (T1D) is caused by insulin deficiency, whereas Type 2 diabetes (T2D) is caused by insulin resistance, and the two types of diabetes often require very different types of treatment. T1D can onset as early as infancy or in later adulthood, whereas T2D was traditionally regarded as an "adult-onset" disease. However, the prevalence of T2D in children and adolescents has dramatically increased in recent years due to the epidemic spread of childhood obesity (Pinhas-Hamiel & Zeitler, 2005). The demands of diabetes treatment also vary widely, ranging from oral medications to insulin injections to more complex insulin pump regimens. Severity of the disease and its health impact also vary, with some individuals at higher risk for acute complications, such as diabetic ketoacidosis (DKA) and severe hypoglycemia, or long-term complications such as retinopathy, neuropathy, nephropathy, and cardiovascular disease.

Because of these differences, clinical assessment and treatment planning in diabetes must be individually tailored based on age, type of diabetes, disease severity, regimen requirements, impact on life, and, of course, the specific presenting or referral problem. In addition to differences in disease characteristics, the clinical health psychologist working with the diabetes population needs to consider many other areas for possible assessment, including the emotional, cognitive, behavioral, and environmental aspects of diabetes. As in any psychological assessment, the clinical interview is the foundation for gathering data in the various domains, which will guide formulation and treatment recommendations. In this chapter, we provide recommendations for tailoring the traditional clinical interview to patients with diabetes, focusing on diabetes-specific information that should be obtained in most cases. This information includes a comprehensive diabetes-related medical history, as well as other data needed to understand the psychosocial impact of diabetes in different domains of the individual patient's life. The assessment must also be tailored to the presenting problem or referral issue for individual patients. Some of the most common reasons for referral to clinical psychologists include depression, adjustment disorders, obstacles to diabetes management, eating disorders, and obesity. Diabetes affects the entire family and, for this reason, family members and significant others may also be referred to clinical psychologists due to their own difficulties in coping with their loved ones' diabetes.

There are numerous assessment tools, both general and diabetes-specific, that can be useful supplements to the clinical interview. However, selection of assessment tools must also be hypothesis-driven and tailored to individual patient and clinician needs. The measures included in this chapter are those that (1) address some of the most common presenting problems and referral questions in patients with diabetes, (2) are most commonly used by clinical health psychologists working with patients with diabetes, and (3) have demonstrated adequate psychometric properties. It is important to make a distinction between instruments used in research and those used in clinical settings. There are literally hundreds of diabetes-specific questionnaires and measures frequently used as predictors and outcome measures in research, but in many cases their clinical utility is unknown. However, clinicians may still find some of these measures useful, especially for monitoring diabetes-specific treatment goals, such as improved quality of life, reduction in a specific type of diabetes-related distress, increased self-efficacy, or improved diabetes management behaviors. For this reason, clinicians are encouraged to search the research literature when diabetes-specific measures would enhance patient assessment, treatment, and/or monitoring.

This chapter begins with recommendations for tailoring the traditional clinical interview for patients with diabetes, including a detailed description of factors in the medical, psychological, behavioral, social, and environmental domains. The remainder of the chapter reviews specific instruments that can be useful in assessment for the most common presenting problems or those that screen for syndromes that should almost always be assessed in this patient population, such as depression. Some of the instruments suggested, including those for depression and eating disorders, are widely used in clinical settings, and information concern-ing administration, scoring, reliability, and validity are easily accessible. Clinical health psychologists may be less familiar with the diabetes-specific instruments, so psychometric information for these is summarized in Table 17.1.

The Diabetes-Tailored Clinical Interview

The clinical interview is designed to obtain detailed information concerning the patient's diabetes, medical history, and treatment regimen, as well as the emotional, cognitive, behavioral, social, occupational, and physical impact of diabetes on the individual's life. To understand the relationship between the individual patient's current problems and his or her diabetes, the clinician must have at least a basic understanding of the pathophysiology and medical issues relevant to diabetes, the requirements and demands of treatment, and the potential acute and long-term complications of the disease. It is also important for the clinician to have an understanding of the complex treatment regimens patients must follow for diabetes management, especially the unique challenges these burdensome self-management routines present for individuals with T1D and T2D. The extent to which different areas are explored in depth is individually tailored to the presenting problem or to pertinent information revealed in the interview. However, there are essential questions that should be asked of nearly every patient in the assessment of diabetes history and status. These include:

1. Age of diabetes onset, as well as experiences just prior to and following the diagnosis.
2. Treatment regimen/physician recommendations, including detailed information about medications/insulin regimens, blood glucose (BG) monitoring frequency, dietary requirements, and exercise plan.
3. Comorbid medical conditions, long-term diabetic complications, associated treatment demands, and their impact on physical and mental health.
4. Adherence to different aspects of treatment regimen and the most pertinent barriers to optimal diabetes care from the patient's perspective.

TABLE 17.1. Psychometric Properties of Diabetes-Specific Assessment Measures

Measure	Description	No. of items	Reliability	Validity
PAID	Self-report questionnaire measure of diabetes-related emotional distress in patients with T1D and T2D	20	Internal consistency: Total scale: alpha = 0.95 Subscales: alpha = 0.69–0.95 Test–retest (2-month): r = .83	Construct Convergent, discriminant Criterion-related Concurrent, predictive
DDS	Self-report questionnaire measure of diabetes-specific emotional distress in patients with T1D and T2D	17	Internal consistency: Total scale: alpha = 0.95 Subscales: alpha = 0.88–0.90	Construct Convergent, discriminant
HFS	Self-report questionnaire measure of fear of hypoglycemia in patients with T1D and T2D	33	Internal consistency: Total scale: alpha = 0.60–0.96 Worry subscale: alpha = 0.89–0.96 Behavior subscale: alpha = 0.54–0.84 Test–retest: r = .59–.76	Construct Convergent, discriminant Criterion-related Concurrent, predictive Content External
D-FISQ	Self-report questionnaire measure of fear of self-injecting (FSI) and self-testing (FST) in patients with T1D and T2D	30	Internal consistency: FSI subscale: alpha = 0.89 FST subscale: alpha = 0.97 Test–retest: FSI subscale: r = .66–.68 FST subscale: r = .50–.51	Construct Convergent, discriminant Criterion-related Concurrent, predictive
SCI-R	Self-report questionnaire measure of perceived adherence to diabetes self-care regimen in patients with T1D and T2D	15	Internal consistency: alpha = 0.84–0.87	Construct Convergent Criterion-related Concurrent
SDSCA	Brief self-report questionnaire measure of perceived diabetes self-management in patients with T1D and T2D	11 core items 14 supplemental/optional items	Interitem correlation: Mean r = .47 Test–retest: r = .40–.78 (except medication subscale) r = −.05	Criterion-related Predictive
CIMS	Updated and expanded version of Barriers to Self-Care Scale. Self-report questionnaire measure of perceived obstacles to optimal diabetes self-care	21	Internal consistency: Total scale: alpha = 0.95–0.98 Subscales: alpha = 0.74–0.97 Test–retest: Total scale: alpha = 0.66–0.80 Subscales: alpha = 0.43–0.75	Criterion-related Concurrent, predictive

5. Relevant lifestyle behaviors, including diet, smoking, exercise, alcohol, and drug use.
6. Potentially harmful or life-threatening self-treatment behaviors (e.g., insulin omission or overdosing, binge eating and/or purging).
7. Level of diabetes control, including the most recent glycosylated hemoglobin (HbA1c) test results (a measure of average diabetes control over the previous 6–8 weeks).
8. History of hospitalizations due to diabetes (e.g., for DKA, severe hypoglycemia, or diabetic complications).
9. Hypoglycemia history, including frequency and severity of episodes, driving problems secondary to hypoglycemia, and hypoglycemic awareness (i.e., ability to feel and recognize early warning symptoms).
10. Capacity to perform routine daily activities, to work and function physically.
11. Any traumatic experience related to diabetes or significant problems secondary to diabetes and/or its management (e.g., automobile accidents or other potentially dangerous events caused by hypoglycemia).

The diabetes-tailored clinical interview should also assess other possible diabetes-related psychological, cognitive, social, and behavioral domains, including:

1. The presence of depression and its effect on the patient's ability to manage diabetes.
2. Personal worries and concerns about diabetes (e.g., fear of hypoglycemia or complications).
3. Diabetes-related anxiety problems, such as needle phobias or fear of finger sticks.
4. Eating disorders or habits that interfere with diabetes control.
5. Adequacy of knowledge and understanding regarding diabetes and the different aspects of diabetes management, including adequacy of knowledge about nutrition.
6. The potential of neurocognitive deficits secondary to recurrent severe hypoglycemia or frequent DKA.
7. Personal attitudes toward diabetes (e.g.,

"Describe in one or two sentences what diabetes means to you").
8. Beliefs about diabetes (e.g. perceived self-efficacy).
9. Support system, including the role of significant others in diabetes management, their attitudes about diabetes, and the presence of interpersonal conflict related to diabetes.
10. Openness with others about diabetes or fear of others knowing about the disease.

If possible, gathering collateral information from spouses, significant others, or other caregivers is also highly recommended. In addition, clinical health psychologists are encouraged to contact patients' endocrinologists and other health care team members, such as nurses, dieticians, and diabetes educators, who can provide important data and assist with treatment planning and execution. When the patient with diabetes is a child or adolescent, parents and other important people in the support system involved in diabetes management should be interviewed. In addition, the role of friends and peers in the patients' diabetes self-care should also be assessed, especially in adolescent patients.

Assessment of Emotional Status

Depression

It is critical to assess symptoms of depression in patients with diabetes, including children and adolescents, because of its unique relationship with diabetes and its impact on diabetes management and control. Studies estimate that the risk for clinical depression is 2–4 times greater in patients with diabetes than in the general population (Anderson, Freedland, Clouse, & Lustman, 2001; Das-Munshi et al., 2007). Episodes of depression are longer in children and adolescents with T1D than in youth with depression but without diabetes (Kovacs, Obrosky, Goldston, & Drash, 1997). Adults with comorbid diabetes and depression are more likely than patients with diabetes but without depression to have significant functional disability and decreased work productivity and attendance due to illness or injury (Egede,

2004a, 2004b). For T1D, comorbid depression is associated with a greater number of severe hypoglycemic episodes compared with controls with T1D but without depression (Katon et al., 2013). In both T1D and T2D, depressive disorders and subclinical depression are associated with poorer diabetes self-management and treatment adherence (Ciechanowski, Katon, & Russo, 2000; Hermanns, Kulzer, Krichbaum, Kubiak, & Haak, 2006) and, as a result, hyperglycemia and poorer metabolic control (Hassan, Loar, Anderson, & Heptulla, 2006; Lustman et al., 2000) and increased diabetic complications such as neuropathy, nephropathy, and cardiovascular disease (de Groot, Anderson, Freedland, Clouse, & Lustman, 2001; Rubin et al., 2010). This unique relationship was highlighted by a recent international study that examined the degree of poor health outcomes and functional impairment associated with depression in patients with various chronic diseases. Comorbid depression and diabetes was found to be the most disabling combination (Moussavi et al., 2007).

Of note, the majority of research in this area is correlational, and the longitudinal prospective studies that are needed to establish causal relationships between diabetes, quality of life, diabetes management, and metabolic control have yet to be conducted. In a recent meta-analysis of 10 longitudinal or prospective studies on depression and diabetes, depression was found to significantly increase the risk of mortality in individuals with diabetes, underscoring the importance of early detection and treatment of depression to improve health outcomes (Park, Katon, & Wolf, 2013).

Structured interviews, such as the Structured Clinical Interview for DSM-IV Disorders (SCID; First, Spitzer, Gibbon, & Williams, 1995), are the gold standard for the assessment and diagnosis of psychiatric disorders such as major depressive disorder. However, administration is time-consuming and burdensome and typically not pragmatic in clinical settings. More commonly, self-report screening questionnaires, such as the Beck Depression Inventory, Second Edition (BDI-II; Beck, Steer, & Brown, 1996) and the Center for Epidemiologic Studies Depression Scale (CES-D; Radloff, 1977, 1991), are used to assess depressive symptoms in older

adolescents and adults with diabetes. A similar self-report questionnaire used frequently in children with diabetes is the Children's Depression Inventory (CDI; Kovacs, 1985). Normative data for the BDI-II, CES-D, and CDI are easily accessible, and all of these instruments have demonstrated excellent reliability and validity. Although self-report screening is helpful in identifying patients with depressive symptoms, a more thorough diagnostic interview will be needed to determine whether a mood disorder is present. In the case of children and adolescents, questionnaire and interview data assessing parents' perspectives regarding their children's mood should also be collected.

There has been some concern that assessment of depression in chronically ill patients, including those with diabetes, will yield inflated scores because many somatic symptoms of depression, such as fatigue and changes in appetite, overlap with nonspecific symptoms of medical illnesses. Lustman, Clouse, Griffith, Carney, and Freedland (1997) examined the sensitivity, specificity, and positive predictive value of the BDI in diabetes. BDI scores of patients who met *Diagnostic and Statistical Manual of Mental Disorders* (DSM) criteria for major depression were compared with those who did not, and scores for the group with depression were significantly higher. Items reflecting cognitive symptoms (e.g., problems concentrating) were better at discriminating patients with and without depression, but somatic symptoms were also more prevalent in patients with depression, suggesting that these symptoms were secondary to depression, not diabetes. These authors recommended a BDI cutoff score of 12 for screening purposes, based on their findings that this criterion provides the best balance of sensitivity (i.e., detects true positives) and specificity (i.e., rules out true negatives).

Eating Disorders

The prevalence of eating disorders, particularly the DSM disorder eating disorder not otherwise specified (EDNOS), and subclinical eating problems in adolescent females with T1D is estimated to be twice that in those without diabetes (Jones, Lawson, Daneman, Olmsted, & Rodin, 2000). Therefore, adolescent and young adult women with T1D should be assessed for eating disorders and/or disordered eating behaviors. Some young women with T1D and disordered eating may present with severe weight loss, as in anorexia, or purge through self-induced vomiting or laxative misuse. But more common is engaging in compensatory behavior by way of omitting or reducing insulin to lose weight, a phenomenon recently termed "diabulimia" in the popular press (Bryden et al., 1999; Fairburn, Peveler, Davies, Mann, & Mayou, 1991; Jones et al., 2000; Peveler et al., 2005). Young women whose regimen includes multiple daily insulin injections rather than insulin pump therapy (Battaglia, Alemzadeh, Katte, Hall, & Perlmuter, 2006), as well as those who are overweight or obese (Colton, Olmsted, Daneman, Rydall, & Rodin, 2007), appear to be at greater risk for insulin omission. Central issues related to emergence and improvement of insulin restriction include fear of gaining weight secondary to improved BG and problems with diabetes management (Goebel-Fabbri et al., 2011). Not surprisingly, insulin omission results in poorer glycemic control (Jones et al., 2000) and earlier onset of diabetes-related complications, including retinopathy, nephropathy, vascular problems, neuropathy, and mortality (Colas, Mathieu, & Tehobroutsky, 1991; Goebel-Fabbri et al., 2008; Peveler et al., 2005; Rydall, Rodin, Olmsted, Devenyi, & Daneman, 1997; Steel, Young, Lloyd, & Clarke, 1987). Finally, although it is rare, young women who have concurrent T1D and anorexia nervosa have a significantly higher mortality rate than women with either disorder alone (Nielsen, Emborg, & Molbak, 2002).

Binge eating disorder (BED), now recognized in DSM-5 as a diagnostically distinct eating disorder, and night-eating syndrome (NES), which is currently subsumed in the DSM diagnosis EDNOS, have been associated with T2D in the literature (Allison et al., 2007; American Psychiatric Association, 2013; Herpertz et al., 1998; Wing, Marcus, Epstein, Blair, & Burton, 1989). BED and NES are both characterized by increased caloric intake without compensatory or purging behaviors and are associated with obesity, which increases the risk of developing T2D (Allison et al., 2007). There is some evidence to suggest that binge eating signifi-

cantly affects glycemic control in patients with T2D (Mannucci et al., 2002) and is associated with an earlier onset of this disease (Kenardy et al., 2001).

The most common self-report screening measures for symptoms of eating disorders are the Eating Attitudes Test (EAT-26; Garner, Olmsted, Bohr, & Garfinkel, 1982), the Eating Disorder Inventory (EDI-3; Garner, 2004), and the Eating Disorder Examination Questionnaire (EDE-Q; Fairburn & Beglin, 1994; Mond, Hay, Rodgers, Owen, & Beumont, 2004). The Eating Disorder Examination (EDE) is also available in seminstructured diagnostic interview format (Fairburn & Cooper, 1993). There is not currently a screening questionnaire for diabulimia, but the limited research in this area suggests that critical care nurses and school health personnel play a key role in the early detection and prevention of insulin omission (Ruth-Sahd, Schneider, & Haagen, 2009; Hasken, Kresl, Nydegger, & Temme, 2010). Additionally, although any of the aforementioned instruments can be useful in assessing general eating disorder attitudes and behaviors, diabetes-specific questions should also be included as part of a clinical interview to determine whether the patient is engaging in insulin reduction/omission, binge eating, or other disordered eating behaviors. It is also important to keep in mind that, in patients with diabetes, even subclinical disordered eating may have a negative impact on diabetes management and metabolic control.

Diabetes-Related Emotional Distress and Adjustment

There is also evidence that depressive symptoms in patients with diabetes may sometimes be indicative of diabetes-related distress rather than a depressive episode and that diabetes-related distress is independently and even more strongly linked with diabetes control and management than depression (Fisher et al., 2007). For these reasons, reduction of diabetes-related distress is often an important treatment goal. This section summarizes several psychometrically sound and clinically useful measures of diabetes-related emotional distress, adjustment problems, and coping issues. Specific information regarding each instrument's psychometric properties is summarized in Table 17.1. Several interrelated instruments have been developed to help the clinician measure overall diabetes-related distress and also to identify specific aspects of living with diabetes that are most problematic for individual patients.

One commonly used assessment tool in this domain is the Problem Areas in Diabetes Scale (PAID; Polonsky et al., 1995; Snoek, Welch, Pouwer, & Polonsky, 2000; Welch, Jacobson, & Polonsky, 1997; Welch, Weinger, Anderson, & Polonsky, 2003). The PAID is a self-report screening questionnaire that measures diabetes-related distress and psychosocial adjustment in adolescents and adults. Each item reflects one of four areas of distress specific to diabetes, including emotional problems (e.g., "feeling constantly burned out by the constant effort to manage diabetes"), treatment-related problems (e.g., "feeling discouraged with your diabetes regimen"), food-related problems (e.g., "feelings of deprivation regarding food and meals"), and social support–related problems (e.g., "feeling that your friends and family are not supportive of your diabetes efforts"). Items are rated on a 5-point Likert scale and total PAID scores range from 0 to 100, with higher scores indicating more emotional distress. PAID scores have been shown to be independently associated with diabetes treatment adherence, even when controlling for the effect of general emotional distress, such as depressive symptoms, and with glycemic control (Polonsky et al., 1995). The instrument is widely used and has been translated into several languages, including Spanish, Dutch, German, and Japanese.

In order to improve the PAID by optimizing scale length, content, and readability, Polonsky and colleagues (2005) created the Diabetes Distress Scale (DDS; Polonsky et al., 2005), which combines items from the original PAID and two other instruments— the ATT39 (Dunn, Smartt, Beeney, & Turtle, 1986) and the Questionnaire on Stress in Patients with Diabetes–Revised (QSD-R; Herschbach et al., 1997). The ATT39 was originally developed to assess psychological adjustment to diabetes and has 39 items stating attitudes about various aspects of diabetes (e.g., "I do not like being told what to eat, when to eat, and how much to eat"). The items are scored on a 5-point Likert

scale ranging from "I disagree completely" to "I agree completely." A total score and scores for six subscales are computed: Diabetes Stress, Coping, Guilt, Alienation–Cooperation, Illness Conviction, and Tolerance for Ambiguity. The QSD-R was developed to assess diabetes-related psychosocial stress. It is made up of 45 items and 8 stress scales, including Leisure Time, Depression/Fear of Future, Hypoglycemia, Treatment Regimen/Diet, Physical Complaints, Work, Partner, and Doctor–Patient Relationship.

Items for the DDS (Polonsky et al., 2005) were chosen based on feedback from patients and diabetes health care professionals. The original version included 28 items reflecting four conceptually driven subscales: Emotional Burden (e.g., "feeling overwhelmed by the demands of living with diabetes"), Physician-Related Distress (e.g., "feeling that my doctor doesn't take my concerns seriously enough"), Regimen-Related Distress (e.g., "feeling that I am not sticking closely enough to a good meal plan"), and Diabetes-Related Interpersonal Distress (e.g., "feeling that my friends/family don't appreciate how difficult living with diabetes can be"). Based on recent research showing that two DDS items ("Feeling overwhelmed with the demands of living with diabetes" and "Feeling that I am often failing with my diabetes routine") have high sensitivity and specificity (.95 and .87, respectively), Fisher and colleagues (2007) recommend using these items as a stand-alone screener for diabetes-specific distress and administering the full DDS measure to patients who screen positive on these two items.

Diabetes-Specific Anxiety Problems or Syndromes

Several studies have found that individuals with diabetes have higher prevalence rates for anxiety disorders when compared with individuals without diabetes or the general population (Kruse, Schmitz, & Thefeld, 2003; Li et al., 2008). This finding appears especially true for female patients (Lloyd, Dyer, & Barnett, 2006; Shaban, Fosbury, Kerr, & Cavan, 2006). Therefore, the clinical interview with a patient diagnosed with diabetes should include screening for symptoms of anxiety disorders, which can include general screening questionnaires, such as the Beck Anxiety Inventory (BAI; Beck & Steer, 1990). In addition to symptoms of traditional anxiety disorders, individuals with diabetes may also experience diabetes-specific anxiety associated with their medical conditions or treatment regimens. Two of the most common types of diabetes-specific anxiety problems are fear of hypoglycemia and fear of needles.

The Hypoglycemia Fear Survey (HFS; Clarke, Gonder-Frederick, Snyder, & Cox, 1998; Cox, Irvine, Gonder-Frederick, Nowacek, & Butterfield, 1987; Irvine, Cox, & Gonder-Frederick, 1992) was originally designed to measure (1) degree of anxiety or worry associated with hypoglycemic episodes and (2) behaviors to avoid these episodes and their negative consequences in adults with T1D. In order to minimize risk for long-term complications of diabetes, patients need to maintain tight control of their BG levels through diet, exercise, and medications and/or insulin that lower BG levels. Intensive insulin treatment, which involves multiple daily injections or insulin pump therapy, improves diabetes control and reduces the progression or development of long-term complications related to hyperglycemia. However, intensive therapy also significantly increases the risk of hypoglycemia (DCCT Research Group, 1991), which in its mild forms is potentially unpleasant, frightening, or inconvenient and, in its more severe forms, is potentially dangerous and even life threatening. Severe hypoglycemia can result in disorientation, unconsciousness, seizures, coma, and even death. Other potential negative consequences of severe hypoglycemia include increased anxiety, social embarrassment, and physical injury to oneself or others, especially when driving or operating machinery.

Because of these negative consequences, patients with high levels of fear of hypoglycemia (FOH) may attempt to maintain higher BG levels in order to avoid episodes, putting them at increased risk for poorer metabolic control and long-term complications (Irvine et al. 1992; Gonder-Frederick, Cox & Clarke, 1997; Gonder-Frederick, 2013). Spouses, parents, and other significant others may also develop significant FOH about their loved one(s). Studies have shown that risk factors for high levels of FOH include a

history of frequent or traumatic episodes of severe hypoglycemia, experience of a recent hypoglycemia episode, and trait anxiety (Gonder-Frederick et al., 2006).

The original HFS (Irvine, Cox, & Gonder-Frederick, 1994) was a 25-item measure with two subscales. The 15-item Worry subscale describes a number of anxiety-provoking aspects of hypoglycemia (e.g., not having food or drink available for treatment), and the 10-item Behavior subscale describes behaviors aimed at avoiding hypoglycemia and its negative consequences (e.g., keeping BG higher when alone). A total score on the HFS is obtained by adding the Behavior and Worry subscale items. Adequate reliability and validity of this instrument have been demonstrated (see Table 17.1), although test–retest reliability can vary because FOH may increase after hypoglycemic episodes. The original HFS was revised in 1998 to include more avoidance items in the Behavior subscale (e.g., limiting driving) and more anxiety-provoking situations to the Worry subscale (e.g., accidentally injuring oneself or others). The current version has 15 Behavior subscale items and 18 Worry subscale items that are rated on a 0–4 Likert scale (Gonder-Frederick, Schmidt, et al., 2011). Recent studies of the factor structure of the HFS indicate that there are three factors, one of which is related to the tendency to keep BG levels higher in order to avoid hypoglycemia (Gonder-Frederick et al., 2013). The HFS has been adapted for use in children and adolescents with T1D, adults with T1D or T2D taking insulin, as well as parents and spouses or partners of patients with diabetes (Gonder-Frederick, Nyer, Shepard, Vajda, & Clarke, 2011; Hajos, Polonsky, Pouwer, Gonder-Frederick, & Snoek, 2014).

The Diabetes Fear of Injecting and Self-Testing Questionnaire (D-FISQ) is a self-report questionnaire that assesses the degree to which insulin-treated patients have a fear of self-injecting (FSI) insulin and/or a fear of self-testing (FST) BG with a lancing device (Mollema, Snoek, Ader, Heine, & van der Ploeg, 2001; Mollema, Snoek, Heine, & van der Ploeg, 2001; Mollema, Snoek, Pouwer, Heine, & van der Ploeg, 2000; Simmons et al., 2007). Mollema, Snoek, Ader, and colleagues (2001) found that high levels of FSI and FST are associated with diabetes-related distress, symptoms of anxiety and depression, poorer general well-being, and poorer diabetes treatment adherence. The D-FISQ has been used in children, adolescents, and adults with T1D, as well as older adolescents (> age 16) and adults with T2D. It consists of two 15-item subscales, FSI and FST, which were identified through exploratory factor analysis (Mollema et al., 2000). Items are rated on a 4-point Likert scale indicating the degree to which each statement presented is true about the patient. Subscale and total scores can be derived, though the authors suggest that the subscales are more clinically useful.

Treatment Adherence and Barriers to Self-Care in Patients with Diabetes

Diabetes management presents unique challenges because treatment is composed of a cluster of patient behaviors that must be performed on a daily basis, typically multiple times per day. Because of the demand and difficulty of self-treatment, problems with diabetes management are one of the most common reasons patients with diabetes are referred to clinical health psychologists. Diabetes treatment regimens, especially for T1D, are not only complex and time-consuming but also often physically intrusive and painful, and they may generate social embarrassment and stigma. These regimens typically include frequent BG monitoring, counting carbohydrates in meals and snacks, calculating and administering the correct insulin dose several times per day, and anticipating the impact of physical activity and exercise on BG. Regimens for T2D may require insulin but more commonly involve oral medications and following diet and exercise plans. Adherence in diabetes is not a unidimensional construct, and patients may demonstrate adequate self-care in one aspect of the treatment regimen but not others (Glasgow, 1994). Adherence to insulin and medication show the highest rates, whereas adherence to BG monitoring (Franciosi et al., 2001; Ruggiero et al., 1997), diet, and exercise (Vijan et al., 2005) are much lower.

Specific aspects of adherence will be more relevant to different presenting problems. For example, in patients referred for chronic severe hyperglycemia, poor metabolic control, and/or frequent episodes of DKA,

assessment of insulin adherence is a high priority. Alternatively, in patients referred due to problems associated with frequent episodes of severe hypoglycemia, such as automobile accidents or loss of consciousness, assessment of BG monitoring, exercise regimens, and adequate carbohydrate consumption would be essential. For patients presenting with frequent episodes of either severe hypo- or hyperglycemia, adherence to recommended BG monitoring is important. In addition to assessing level of adherence to different aspects of the diabetes regimen, it is also important to gain an understanding of the environmental, social, and psychological barriers to adherence from the patient's perspective. For example, adolescents may omit their insulin before lunch at school because of concerns about social stigma, and some adults may not have easy access to safe places outdoors for exercise such as walking.

The Self-Care Inventory (SCI; La Greca, 2004) and the Self-Care Inventory–Revised (SCI-R; Weinger, Butler, Welch, & La Greca, 2005) are self-report measures of adherence for use in children, adolescents, and adults with T1D and T2D. Until recently, the published psychometric properties of the SCI only pertained to children and adolescents. In 2005, Weinger and colleagues revised the SCI to reflect current diabetes treatment practices and published psychometric findings for the SCI-R for adult patients. For current clinical use, the SCI-R is recommended, because it assesses behaviors relevant to more contemporary treatment regimens. The SCI-R comprises 15 items across six domains of self-care: diet, BG monitoring, medication administration, exercise, low BG levels, and preventative/routine aspects of self-care. Items are rated on a 5-point Likert scale reflecting the degree to which patients followed treatment recommendations over the preceding month, with higher scores representing higher levels of adherence.

The Summary of Diabetes Self-Care Activities (SDSCA; Toobert & Glasgow, 1994; Toobert, Hampson, & Glasgow, 2000) is another widely used measure of self-care in adults with diabetes. It can be administered as a paper-and-pencil questionnaire or by computer or Internet. The most recent version is composed of 11 core items and 14 optional questions covering five different domains of diabetes self-care, including diet, exercise, BG testing, foot care, and smoking status. The original SDSCA included a domain about medication taking; however, the authors report that these questions demonstrated strong ceiling effects, lacked variability, and demonstrated low test–retest reliability. The revised SDSCA includes optional questions about medication adherence to be used if the domain is of interest to the clinician. Scores are computed for each domain by calculating the mean number of days per week patients engage in each activity (e.g., "How many of the last seven days have you followed a healthful eating plan?"). Because the SDSCA demonstrates low inter-item correlations for the diet subscale, individual item scores are used. Reverse scoring is necessary for some items (Toobert et al., 2000).

The Challenges to Illness Management Scale (CIMS; Glasgow, Toobert, & Gillette, 2001) is the updated and expanded version of the original Barriers to Self-Care Scale (Glasgow, 1994; Glasgow, McCaul, & Schafer, 1986), used to measure perceived obstacles to optimal diabetes self-care. The CIMS assesses a variety of potential barriers to diabetes management in adults with diabetes, including those associated with close interpersonal relationships, health care providers, work, and community. It also assesses barriers to specific aspects of self-care, such as lowering dietary fat intakes, engaging in physical activity, taking medications, and managing stress. Two versions of the measure exist. The CIMS/Difficulty version requires patients to rate, on a 5-point Likert scale, how difficult each barrier was to overcome over the previous 3 months in trying to reach their self-management goals. The CIMS/Confidence version requires patients to rate, on a 10-point Likert scale, how confident they were over the previous 3 months that they could follow their self-management plan when faced with each obstacle.

Summary

This chapter reviewed the key areas that clinical health psychologists should address in the biopsychosocial assessment of patients with diabetes, as well as specific measures that may be useful during a clinical evalua-

tion. Because of the complexity of diabetes and its treatment and because of its many potential psychological, behavioral, social, and physical effects on the patient, clinical assessment is not straightforward. Rather, an individually tailored approach is recommended that takes into consideration the numerous diabetes-specific issues that may be problematic for different patient groups. As in any clinical psychology setting, patient assessment in diabetes is an ongoing process over the course of evaluation and treatment and should be tailored and modified to address individual needs. However, certain domains are almost always relevant to treatment of patients with diabetes, regardless of age and disease type. In fact, many of the clinical problems outlined in this chapter are also quite relevant for the pediatric population, including depression, other types of general and diabetes-specific emotional distress, treatment adherence, eating disorders, and the role that significant others play in the patient's diabetes management and self-care (Silverstein et al., 2005; Wysocki, Buckloh, & Greco, 2009). Finally, these guidelines and recommendations are obviously not exhaustive, and there are a number of less common presenting problems that may be the focus of assessment. Some of these include possible surreptitious insulin dosing, questions of mental competency to manage diabetes, and refusal to reveal diabetes to others, even to those who may potentially have to deal with a medical emergency, such as friends and coworkers. Although not exhaustive, our hope is that these guidelines and recommendations will provide a starting point for clinical health psychologists facing the challenging task of biopsychosocial assessment of individuals living with diabetes.

REFERENCES

Allison, K. C., Crow, S. J., Reeves, R. R., West, D. S., Foreyt, J. P., Dilillo, V. G., et al. (2007). Binge eating disorder and night eating syndrome in adults with type 2 diabetes. *Obesity, 15*, 1287–1293.

American Psychiatric Association. (2013). *Diagnostic and statistical manual of mental disorders* (5th ed.). Arlington, VA: Author.

Anderson, R. J., Freedland, K. E., Clouse, R. E.,

& Lustman, P. J. (2001). The prevalence of comorbid depression in adults with diabetes. *Diabetes Care, 24*, 1069–1078.

Battaglia, M. R., Alemzadeh, R., Katte, H., Hall, P. L., & Perlmuter, L. C. (2006). Brief report: Disordered eating and psychosocial factors in adolescent females with type 1 diabetes mellitus. *Journal of Pediatric Psychology, 31*, 552–556.

Beck, A. T., & Steer, R. A. (1990). *Manual for the Beck Anxiety Inventory*. San Antonio, TX: Psychological Corporation.

Beck, A. T., Steer, R. A., & Brown, G. K. (1996). *Manual for the Beck Depression Inventory—II*. San Antonio, TX: Psychological Corporation.

Bryden, K. S., Neil, A., Mayou, R. A., Peveler, R. C., Fairburn, C. G., & Dunger, D. B. (1999). Eating habits, body weight, and insulin misuse. *Diabetes Care, 22*, 1956–1960.

Ciechanowski, P. S., Katon, W. J., & Russo, J. E. (2000). Depression and diabetes: Impact of depressive symptoms on adherence, function, and costs. *Archives of Internal Medicine, 160*, 3278–3285.

Clarke, W. L., Gonder-Frederick, L. A., Snyder, A. L., Cox, D. J. (1998). Maternal fear of hypoglycemia in their children with insulin dependent diabetes mellitus. *Journal of Pediatric Endocrinology and Metabolism, 11*, 189–194.

Colas, C., Mathieu, P., & Tehobroutsky, G. (1991). Eating disorders and retinal lesions in type I (insulin-dependent) diabetic women. *Diabetologia, 34*, 288.

Colton, P. A., Olmsted, M. P., Daneman, D., Rydall, A. C., & Rodin, G. M. (2007). Five-year prevalence and persistence of disturbed eating behavior and eating disorders in girls with type 1 diabetes. *Diabetes Care, 30*, 2861–2862.

Cox, D. J., Irvine, A., Gonder-Frederick, L., Nowacek, G., & Butterfield, J. (1987). Fear of hypoglycemia: Quantification, validation, and utilization. *Diabetes Care, 10*, 617–621.

Das-Munshi, J., Stewart, R., Ismail, K., Bebbington, P. E., Jenkins, R., & Prince, M. J. (2007). Diabetes, common mental disorders, and disability: Findings from the UK National Psychiatric Morbidity Survey. *Psychosomatic Medicine, 69*, 543–550.

DCCT Research Group. (1991). Epidemiology of severe hypoglycemia in the Diabetes Control and Complications Trial. *American Journal of Medicine, 90*, 450–459.

de Groot, M., Anderson, R., Freedland, K. E., Clouse, R. E., & Lustman, P. J. (2001). Association of depression and diabetes complications: A meta-analysis. *Psychosomatic Medicine, 63*, 619–630.

Dunn, S. M., Smartt, H., Beeney, L., & Turtle, J. (1986). Measurement of emotional adjustment in diabetic patients: Validity and reliability of ATT39. *Diabetes Care, 9*, 480–489.

Egede, L. E. (2004a). Diabetes, major depression, and functional disability among U.S. adults. *Diabetes Care, 27*, 421–428.

Egede, L. E. (2004b). Effects of depression on work loss and disability bed days in individuals with diabetes. *Diabetes Care, 27*, 1751–1753.

Fairburn, C. G., & Beglin, S. J. (1994). Assessment of eating disorders: Interview or self-report questionnaire? *International Journal of Eating Disorders, 16*, 363–370.

Fairburn, C. G., & Cooper, Z. (1993). The Eating Disorder Examination. In C. G. Fairburn & G. T. Wilson (Eds.), *Binge eating: Nature, assessment, and treatment* (12th ed., pp. 317–360). New York: Guilford Press.

Fairburn, C. G., Peveler, R. C., Davies, B., Mann, J. I., & Mayou, R. A. (1991). Eating disorders in young adults with insulin dependent diabetes mellitus: A controlled study. *British Journal of Medicine, 303*, 17–20.

First, M. B., Spitzer, R. L., Gibbon, M., & Williams, J. B. W. (1995). The Structured Clinical Interview for DSM-III-R Personality Disorders (SCID-II): Part I. Description. *Journal of Personality Disorders, 9*, 2–12.

Fisher, L., Skaff, M. M., Mullan, J. T., Arean, P., Mohr, D., Masharani, U., et al. (2007). Clinical depression versus distress among patients with type 2 diabetes. *Diabetes Care, 30*, 542–548.

Franciosi, M., Pellegrini, F., De Berardis, G., Belfiglio, M., Cavaliere, D., Di Nardo, B., et al. (2001). The impact of blood glucose self-monitoring on metabolic control and quality of life in type 2 diabetic patients. *Diabetes Care, 24*, 1870–1877.

Garner, D. (2004). *Eating Disorder Inventory—3: Professional manual*. Lutz, FL: Psychological Assessment Resources.

Garner, D. M., Olmsted, M. P., Bohr, Y., & Garfinkel, P. E. (1982). The Eating Attitudes Test: Psychometric features and clinical correlates. *Psychological Medicine, 12*, 871–878.

Glasgow, R. E. (1994). Social–environmental factors in diabetes: Barriers to self-care. In

C. Bradley (Ed.), *Handbook of psychology and diabetes: A guide to psychological measurement in diabetes research and practice* (pp. 335–349). Amsterdam: Harwood Academic.

Glasgow, R. E., McCaul, K. D., & Schafer, L. C. (1986). Barriers to regimen adherence among persons with insulin-dependent diabetes. *Journal of Behavioral Medicine, 9,* 65–77.

Glasgow, R. E., Toobert, D. J., & Gillette, C. D. (2001). Psychosocial barriers to diabetes self-management and quality of life. *Diabetes Spectrum, 14,* 33–41.

Goebel-Fabbri, A. E., Anderson, B. J., Fikkan, J., Franko, D. L., Pearson, K., & Weinger, K. (2011). Improvement and emergence of insulin restriction in women with type 1 diabetes. *Diabetes Care, 34,* 545–550.

Goebel-Fabbri, A. E., Fikkan, J., Franko, D. L., Pearson, K., Anderson, B. J., & Weinger, K. (2008). Insulin restriction and associated morbidity and mortality in women with type 1 diabetes. *Diabetes Care, 31,* 415–419.

Gonder-Frederick, L. (2013). Fear of hypoglycemia: A review. *Diabetic Hypoglycemia, 5,* 3–11.

Gonder-Frederick, L. A., Cox, D. J., & Clarke, W. L. (1997) The emotional, behavioral and social effects of hypoglycemia. *Seminars in Neuropsychiatry, 2,* 56–75.

Gonder-Frederick, L. A., Fisher, C. D., Ritterband, L. M., Cox, D. J., Hou, L., DasGupta, A., et al. (2006). Predictors of fear of hypoglycemia in adolescents with type 1 diabetes and their parents. *Pediatric Diabetes, 7,* 215–222.

Gonder-Frederick, L. A., Nyer, M., Shepard, J. A., Vajda, K., & Clarke, W. (2011). Assessing fear of hypoglycemia in children with type 1 diabetes and their parents. *Diabetes Management, 1,* 627–639.

Gonder-Frederick, L. A., Schmidt, K. M., Vajda, K. A., Greear, M. L., Singh, H., Shepard, J. A., et al. (2011). Psychometric properties of the Hypoglycemia Fear Survey—II for adults with type 1 diabetes. *Diabetes Care, 34,* 801–806.

Gonder-Frederick, L. A., Vajda, K. A., Schmidt, K. M., Cox, D. J., Devries, J. H., Erol, O., et al. (2013). Examining the Behavior Subscale of the Hypoglycemia Fear Survey using aggregated data from five countries. *Diabetic Medicine, 30,* 603–609.

Hajos, T. R. S., Polonsky, W. H., Pouwer, F., Gonder-Frederick, L., & Snoek, F. J. (2014). Toward defining a cutoff score for elevated fear of hypoglycemia on the Hypoglycemia

Fear Survey Worry Subscale in patients with type 2 diabetes. *Diabetes Care, 37,* 102–108.

Hasken, J., Kresl, L., Nydegger, T., & Temme, M. (2010). Diabulimia and the role of school health personnel. *Journal of School Health, 80,* 465–469.

Hassan, K., Loar, R., Anderson, B. J., & Heptulla, R. A. (2006). The role of socioeconomic status, depression, quality of life, and glycemic control in type I diabetes mellitus. *Journal of Pediatrics, 149,* 526–531.

Hermanns, N., Kulzer, B., Krichbaum, M., Kubiak, T., & Haak, T. (2006). How to screen for depression and emotional problems in patients with diabetes: Comparison of screening characteristics of depression questionnaires, measurement of diabetes-specific emotional problems and standard clinical assessment. *Diabetologia, 49,* 469–477.

Herpertz, S., Albus, C., Wagener, R., Kocnar, M., Wagner, R., Henning, A., et al. (1998). Comorbidity of diabetes and eating disorders. *Diabetes Care, 21,* 1110–1116.

Herschbach, P., Duran, G., Waadt, S., Zettler, A., Amm, C., & Marten-Miitag, B. (1997). Psychometric properties of the Questionnaire on Stress in Patients with Diabetes—Revised (QSD-R). *Health Psychology, 16,* 171–174.

Irvine, A., Cox, D., & Gonder-Frederick, L. (1992). Fear of hypoglycemia: Relationship to physical and psychological symptoms in patients with insulin-dependent diabetes mellitus. *Health Psychology, 11,* 135–138.

Irvine, A., Cox, D., & Gonder-Frederick, L. (1994). The Fear of Hypoglycemia Scale. In C. Bradley (Ed.), *Handbook of psychology and diabetes: A guide to psychological measurement in diabetes research and practice* (pp. 133–155). Amsterdam: Harwood Academic.

Jones, J. M., Lawson, M. L., Daneman, D., Olmsted, M. P., & Rodin, G. (2000). Eating disorders in adolescent females with and without type 1 diabetes: Cross-sectional study. *British Medical Journal, 320,* 1563–1566.

Katon, W. J., Young, B. A., Russo, J., Lin, E. H. B., Ciechanowski, P., Ludman, E. J., et al. (2013). Association of depression with increased risk of severe hypoglycemic episodes in patients with diabetes. *Annals of Family Medicine, 11,* 245–250.

Kenardy, J., Mensch, M., Bowen, K., Green, B., Walton, J., & Dalton, M. (2001). Disordered eating behaviors in women with type 2 diabetes mellitus. *Eating Behaviors, 2,* 183–192.

Kovacs, M. (1985). The Children's Depression

Inventory (CDI). *Psychopharmacology Bulletin, 21,* 995–998.

Kovacs, M., Obrosky, D. S., Goldston, D., & Drash, A. (1997). Major depressive disorder in youths with IDDM: A controlled prospective study of course and outcome. *Diabetes Care, 20,* 45–51.

Kruse, J., Schmitz, N., & Thefeld, W. (2003). On the association between diabetes and mental disorders in a community sample. *Diabetes Care, 26,* 1841–1846.

La Greca, A. (2004). *Manual for the Self-Care Inventory.* Miami, FL: Author.

Li, C., Barker, L., Ford, E. S., Zhang, X., Strine, T. W., & Mokdad, A. H. (2008). Diabetes and anxiety in U. S. adults: Findings from the 2006 behavioral risk factor surveillance system. *Diabetic Medicine, 25*(7), 878–881. Retrieved June 17, 2008, from *www.blackwellsynergy.com/doi/pdf/10.1111/j.1464-5491.2008.02477.x.*

Lloyd, C. E., Dyer, P. H., & Barnett, A. H. (2000). Prevalence of symptoms of depression and anxiety in a diabetes clinic population. *Diabetic Medicine, 17,* 198–202.

Lustman, P. J., Anderson, R. J., Freedland, K. E., de Groot, M., Carney, R. M., & Clouse, R. E. (2000). Depression and poor glycemic control: A meta-analytic review of the literature. *Diabetes Care, 23,* 934–942.

Lustman, P. J., Clouse, R. E., Griffith, L. S., Carney, R. M., & Freedland, K. E. (1997). Screening for depression in diabetes using the Beck Depression Inventory. *Psychosomatic Medicine, 59,* 24–31.

Mannucci, E., Tesi, F., Ricca, V., Pierazzuoli, E., Barciulli, E., Moretti, S., et al. (2002). Eating behavior in obese patients with and without type 2 diabetes mellitus. *International Journal of Obesity, 26,* 848–853.

Mollema, E. D., Snoek, F. J., Ader, H. J., Heine, R. J., & van der Ploeg, H. M. (2001). Insulin-treated diabetes patients with fear of self-injecting or fear of self-testing: Psychological comorbidity and general well-being. *Journal of Psychosomatic Research, 51,* 665–672.

Mollema, E. D., Snoek, F. J., Heine, R. J., & van der Ploeg, H. M. (2001). Phobia of self-injecting and self-testing in insulin-treated diabetes patients: Opportunities for screening. *Diabetic Medicine, 18,* 671–674.

Mollema, E. D., Snoek, F. J., Pouwer, F., Heine, R. J., & van der Ploeg, H. M. (2000). Diabetes Fear of Injecting and Self-Testing Questionnaire. *Diabetes Care, 23*(6), 765–769.

Mond, J. M., Hay, P. H., Rodgers, B., Owen, C., & Beumont, P. J. V. (2004). Validity of the Eating Disorder Examination Questionnaire (EDE-Q) in screening for eating disorders in community samples. *Behaviour Research and Therapy, 42,* 551–567.

Moussavi, S., Chatterji, S., Verdes, E., Tandon, E., Patel, V., & Ustun, B. (2007). Depression, chronic disease, and decrements in health: Results from the World Health Surveys. *Lancet, 370,* 851–858.

Nielsen, S., Emborg, C., & Molbak, A. G. (2002). Mortality in concurrent type 1 diabetes and anorexia nervosa. *Diabetes Care, 25,* 309–312.

Park, M., Katon, W. J., & Wolf, F. M. (2013). Depression and risk of mortality in individuals with diabetes: A meta-analysis and systematic review. *General Hospital Psychiatry, 35,* 217–225.

Peveler, R. C., Bryden, K. S., Neil, A. H., Fairburn, C. G., Mayou, R. A., Dunger, D. B., et al. (2005). The relationship of disordered eating habits and attitudes in clinical outcomes in young adult females with Type 1 diabetes. *Diabetes Care, 28,* 84–88.

Pinhas-Hamiel, O., & Zeitler, P. (2005). Advances in epidemiology and treatment of type 2 diabetes in children. *Advances in Pediatrics, 52,* 223–259.

Polonsky, W. H., Anderson, B. J., Lohrer, P. A., Welch, G., Jacobson, A. M., Aponte, J. E., et al. (1995). Assessment of diabetes-related distress. *Diabetes Care, 18,* 754–760.

Polonsky, W. H., Fisher, L., Earles, J., Dudl, J., Lees, J., Mullan, J., et al. (2005). Assessing psychosocial distress in diabetes. *Diabetes Care, 28*(3), 626–631.

Radloff, L. S. (1977). The CES-D Scale: A self-report depression scale for research in the general population. *Applied Psychological Measurement, 1,* 385–401.

Radloff, L. S. (1991). The use of the Center for Epidemiologic Studies Depression Scale in Adolescents and Young Adults. *Journal of Youth and Adolescence, 20,* 149–166.

Rubin, R. R., Gaussoin, S. A., Peyrot, M., DiLillo, V., Miller, K., Wadden, T. A., et al. (2010). Cardiovascular disease risk factors, depression symptoms and antidepressant medicine use in the Look AHEAD (Action for Health in Diabetes) clinical trial of weight loss and diabetes. *Diabetologia, 53,* 1581–1589.

Ruggiero, L., Glasgow, R., Dryfoos, J. M., Rossi, J. S., Prochaska, J. O., Orleans, C. T., et al. (1997). Diabetes self-management: Self-reported recommendations and patterns in a large population. *Diabetes Care, 20,* 568–576.

Ruth-Sahd, L. A., Schneider, M., & Haagen, B. (2009). Diabulimia: What is it and how to recognize it in critical care. *Dimensions of Critical Care Nursing, 28,* 147–153.

Rydall, A. C., Rodin, G. M., Olmsted, M. P., Devenyi, R. G., & Daneman, D. (1997). Disordered eating behavior and macrovascular complications in young women with insulin-dependent diabetes mellitus. *New England Journal of Medicine, 336,* 1849–1854.

Shaban, M. C., Fosbury, J., Kerr, D., & Cavan, D. A. (2006). The prevalence of depression and anxiety in adults with type 1 diabetes. *Diabetic Medicine, 23,* 1381–1384.

Silverstein, J., Klingensmith, G., Copeland, K., Plotnick, L., Kaufman, F., Laffel, L., et al. (2005). Care of children and adolescents with type 1 diabetes: A statement of the American Diabetes Association. *Diabetes Care, 28,* 186–212.

Simmons, J. H., McFann, K. K., Brown, A. C., Rewers, A., Follansbee, D., Temple-Trujillo, R. E., et al. (2007). Reliability of the Diabetes Fear of Injecting and Self-Testing Questionnaire in pediatric patients with type I diabetes. *Diabetes Care, 30,* 987–988.

Snoek, F. J., Welch, G. W., Pouwer, F., & Polonsky, W. H. (2000). Diabetes-related emotional distress in Dutch and U.S. diabetic patients. *Diabetes Care, 23,* 1305–1309.

Steel, J. M., Young, R. J., Lloyd, G. G., & Clarke, B. F. (1987). Clinically apparent eating disorders in young diabetic women: Associations with painful neuropathy and other complications. *British Medical Journal, 294,* 859–862.

Toobert, D., & Glasgow, R. (1994). Assessing diabetes self-management: The summary of diabetes self-care activities questionnaire. In C. Bradley (Ed.), *Handbook of psychology and diabetes: A guide to psychological measurement in diabetes research and practice* (pp. 351–375). Amsterdam: Harwood Academic.

Toobert, D. J., Hampson, S. E., Glasgow, R. E. (2000). The Summary of Diabetes Self-Care Activities measure: Results from 7 studies and a revised scale. *Diabetes Care, 23,* 943–950.

Vijan, S., Stuart, N. S., Fitzgerald, J. T., Ronis, D. L., Hayward, R. A., Slater, S., et al. (2005). Barriers to following dietary recommendations in type 2 diabetes. *Diabetic Medicine, 22,* 32–38.

Weinger, K., Butler, H. A., Welch, G. W., & La Greca, A. M. (2005). Measuring diabetes self-care: A psychometric analysis of the self-care inventory-revised with adults. *Diabetes Care, 28*(6), 1346–1352.

Welch, G., Weinger, K., Anderson, B., & Polonsky, W. H. (2003). Responsiveness of the Problem Areas in Diabetes (PAID) questionnaire. *Diabetic Medicine, 20,* 69–72.

Welch, G. W., Jacobson, A. M., & Polonsky, W. H. (1997). The Problem Areas in Diabetes Scale: An evaluation of its clinical utility. *Diabetes Care, 20,* 760–766.

Wing, R. R., Marcus, M. D., Epstein, L. H., Blair, E. H., & Burton, L. R. (1989). Binge eating in obese patients with type II diabetes. *International Journal of Eating Disorders, 8,* 671–689.

Wysocki, T., Buckloh, L. M., & Greco, P. (2009). The psychological context of diabetes mellitus in youths. In M. C. Roberts & R. G. Steele (Eds.), *Handbook of pediatric psychology* (pp. 287–302). New York: Guilford Press.

CHAPTER 18

Gastrointestinal Disorders

Brenda B. Toner
Iman Hussain

Research in the area of gastrointestinal (GI) diseases has mainly focused on biological and medical aspects. In general, relatively little attention has been directed toward our psychosocial understanding and assessment of GI disorders. There has been one notable exception, namely the psychosocial understanding of functional GI disorders in general and irritable bowel syndrome (IBS) in particular. This chapter focuses on the psychosocial understanding and assessment of IBS because this is where most of the theoretical and empirical work has focused. IBS is one of the most common syndromes seen by primary health care providers and gastroenterologists. It is the most common GI diagnosis seen in primary care (> 12% of primary care practice and 41% of patients seen by gastroenterologists; Mitchell & Drossman 1987; Russo, Gaynes, & Drossman, 1999). Health-related quality of life is poorer for these individuals than for healthy patients with diabetes, chronic renal disease, or functional dyspepsia (Gralnek, Hays, Kilbourne, Naliboff, & Mayer, 2000). Persons afflicted with IBS have more hospitalizations, work absenteeism, and physician visit rates than the general population (Drossman et al., 1993) and diagnosis is associated with unnecessary tests, procedures, and surgeries. Difficulties in diagnosis and treatment produce uncertainty, frustration, and dissatisfaction within the patient–doctor relationship (Drossman, 1995a, 1995b, 1997; Toner, 2005).

Biopsychosocial Model for IBS

Mounting evidence suggests that the impact of IBS is best understood within a biopsychosocial context that is not explained by symptoms alone (Drossman, Corazziari, Spiller, Thompson, & Rome III Committee, 2006). Within the past decade there has been an increasing body of evidence to support the concept that IBS is a multidetermined disorder of brain–gut function in which emotional and cognitive areas of the brain modulate bowel motility, visceral hypersensitivity, and inflammation and in which altered bowel function has psychosocial consequences (Drossman, Camilleri, Mayer, & Whitehead, 2002). The gut interacts directly with the brain, providing a bidirectional interaction along the brain–gut axis. There is reliable evidence that supports the view that social and psychological stressors and associated alterations in mood alter the function of the gut and IBS symptoms (Levy et al., 2006).

Many of the approaches used in the psychosocial assessment for IBS have been adapted from cognitive-behavioral models that were developed by investigators and clinicians working with individuals who presented to mental health professionals with depression and anxiety disorders (Toner, 2005). Although there is increasing evidence that there is an association between individuals with psychological distress (anxiety and depression) and IBS, the general consensus reveals that this is not specific to IBS but that this association occurs in a variety of illnesses. Individuals with IBS may also experience symptoms such as gynecological and urinary conditions, headaches, chronic fatigue syndrome, and fibromyalgia. It is helpful for the mental health care professional to work in collaboration with the client to identify which associations may be relevant to and interact with their IBS.

Process of Obtaining a Diagnosis of IBS

A diagnosis of IBS is usually made by a primary doctor or a gastroenterologist. Patients who have received a diagnosis of IBS are sometimes referred to or seek out a psychologist, psychiatrist, or other health care or mental health care professional for help with these chronic and painful symptoms. Before individuals with IBS finally reach the office of a health psychologist, they may have experienced frustration with the health care system looking for an explanation for their IBS.

The following is a brief description of experiences of individuals in the process of receiving a diagnosis of IBS as documented in the literature. The patient–physician relationship is challenging to navigate for both the patient and the physician. Patients seeking diagnosis and treatment often report an unsatisfactory experience. Patients often report a lack of empathy, adequate treatment, and sufficient medical explanation (Drossman, 1998). As well, clients often report the perception of not being taken seriously and feeling that their conditions are not fully recognized or appreciated.

Physicians share frustration with patients over this poorly understood illness, as well as a lack of effective treatments (Creed et al., 2006). After undergoing a series of tests to rule out structural and biochemical abnormalities, simply being told that "there is nothing organically wrong" is not helpful to the patient who is experiencing chronic and painful symptoms. Although the opportunity to make a positive diagnosis is available through the Rome diagnostic criteria, most primary care physicians and some gastroenterologists are unaware of these criteria, and only a portion of practitioners use them in clinical practice (Creed et al., 2006). Patients seeking clear explanations may encounter uncertain or even conflicting views (Creed et al., 2006). IBS is generally diagnosed with a careful history taking, a general physical examination, and routine laboratory studies. The Rome III Diagnostic Criteria for IBS include recurrent abdominal pain or discomfort at least 3 days/month in the previous 3 months associated with two or more of the following (Drossman et al., 2006):

1. Improvement with defecation
2. Onset associated with a change in frequency of stool
3. Onset associated with a change in form (appearance) of stool

Integrating the Person's Perspective into the Assessment Protocol

When the person who has received a diagnosis of IBS is referred to a mental health professional, it is essential to establish collaborative working partnerships. Health care professionals can work in partnership with individuals with IBS by eliciting their concerns and discussing them in ways that are individually relevant and affirming (Toner et al., 2006; Kennedy, Robinson, & Rogers, 2003).

The illness experience of individuals living with IBS has not been formally integrated into our assessment protocols. In a recent quantitative survey that focused on the patient's perspective, most sufferers reported living for years with IBS, experiencing frequent, episodic symptoms that caused major interferences in daily life (Bertram, Kurland, Lydick, Locke, & Yawn, 2001; International Foundation for Functional Gastrointestinal Disorders, 2002). Symptoms were most often experienced as severe. Anticipation and worry over when and where the next symptom would occur resulted in limiting planning and engaging in many daily activities. Frustration, isolation, and lack of validation for their IBS were identified as major problems. As summarized in recent reviews (Toner et al., 2006; Chang et al., 2006), people felt frustrated due to the lack of understanding and validation from family, coworkers, and health providers and a sense of isolation from the embarrassing nature of their symptoms and feeling alone with the disorder (Bertram et al., 2001). As reported by Toner (2005), there is only one scale that has been specifically designed to assess concerns or cognitions of people who have a diagnosis of IBS. (This scale is discussed later in the chapter in the section on self-report instruments.) Further work needs to be conducted to identify and integrate the patient's perspective into the development and refinement of assessment and outcome measures. One concern that has been repeatedly voiced by patients with IBS has been the stigma of living with a chronic and debilitating condition that has been trivialized by society in general and often misunderstood by health care professionals (Toner et al., 2006). One possible challenge in developing a strong working partnership with clients with IBS is the social stigma associated with the disorder. Often individuals who have received a diagnosis of IBS come in to see health care or mental health care professionals feeling demoralized and thinking that their illness is not taken seriously. This is not a distortion or an error in thinking but more than likely an accurate reflection of the stigma associated with the so-called functional somatic disorders.

It is important to highlight that some of the language and labels used in the health and mental health profession may serve to further trivialize or invalidate the experience of people who are living with a disorder that is often not taken seriously. For example, certain cognitive concepts or labels, such as "distortion," "irrationality," and "erroneous or faulty thinking" are especially unhelpful because they infer that individual pathology or idiosyncratic cognitions are a primary cause of the person's problem, while placing minimal emphasis on other social and biological determinants of health (Toner, Segal, Emmott, & Myran, 2000). In particular, it is important to test the hypothesis that the client's perceptions and cognitions do match the realities of their life situations. The following section highlights what is published about the realities of individuals who live with this chronic and painful illness that is often misunderstood and stigmatized (Toner, 1994).

Identifying and Challenging Societal Cognitions, Stigma, and Myths

As discussed by Nancy Norton (Toner et al., 2006), president and founder of the International Foundation for Functional Gastrointestinal Disorders (IFFGD), living with IBS means living with a debilitating chronic condition that is invisible to others, embarrassing to talk about, misunderstood by the public at large, and often equated with psychological problems or psychiatric disorders. It is not surprising that patients find IBS embarrassing or difficult to talk about. The following example serves to highlight the degree of stigma in our society, reflected by the media. In 1999, the IFFGD produced an educational public service announcement about IBS for television. Prior to distribution, 50% of the major media outlets surveyed stated that they would not air the production if the word "bowel" were used. The shame and trivialization associated with IBS is part of a larger issue for so-called functional disorders in other medical conditions. These syndromes have been traditionally defined by physical symptoms that do not have identified underlying structural or biochemical abnormalities. Functional disorders are often contrasted with organic disease and thought to be less legitimate or real (Fabrege, 1991). In Western societies, there is a moral and pejorative connotation attributed to a functional disorder. As discussed by Kirmayer and Robbins (1991), illness in our Western society is sometimes attributed to impersonal causes and viewed as an accident that befalls the patient as victim (e.g., cancer, stroke) or is viewed as psychologically caused, mediated, and potentially under the person's voluntary control (e.g., depression, addictions, functional somatic disorders). This may leave patients with disorders such as IBS feeling that their problems are perceived as a moral weakness or defect. Validating their symptoms and challenging society's view of the artificial dualism of organic/

functional components of illness and the associated legitimacy of some illnesses over others enhances the therapeutic alliance and increases the likelihood of a more valid and reliable assessment (Toner, 1994). Women are especially attentive to the possibility that their symptoms are not being taken seriously because research has shown that disorders that are more common in women than men are more likely to be trivialized or not taken as seriously (Lips, 1997). In spite of a growing understanding of IBS as a disorder of brain–gut function, there are several societal myths that are alive and well today and that serve to further demoralize the person who has received a diagnosis of IBS. A sampling of these myths includes that symptoms are trivial; that if the pain is severe, there must be an organic cause; that patients with IBS benefit from the sick role; and that people with IBS are difficult patients. For a discussion on challenging these myths in partnership with IBS patients, the interested reader is referred to an article by Toner and Casati (2002). Some individuals with IBS have developed what Toner and colleagues in 2000 termed "bowel performance anxiety." This is a frequent and distressing apprehension about bowel symptoms in a public context, leading to the avoidance of such situations or a heightened state of physiological arousal both in anticipation of and during such public events. This is often very distressing to individuals because their symptoms severely limit their daily activities and impede their enjoyment and quality of life (QoL). The general goal of working with individuals with bowel performance anxiety is to decrease avoidance of such public situations and to help them cope with the associated anxiety, shame, and embarrassment associated with symptoms. In addition to eliciting individual cognitions and behaviors, it is helpful to identify, acknowledge, and challenge societal cognitions about IBS symptoms as previously discussed. Doing this serves to acknowledge that their sense of anxiety, shame, and embarrassment are understandable in the light of the stigma associated with discussing bowel functions in our society. This is similar to acknowledging to a young woman with an eating disorder that, yes, big business is preoccupied with selling the image of young, beautiful, and slim women as a commodity. The challenge is to understand the internalization of these destructive social cognitions and to be helpful to the individual client by discussing his or her cognitions and behaviors within a larger sociopolitical context (Toner, 2005).

Social Factors

It is important to acknowledge that health and illness, including IBS, occur within a larger social context. The meaning and expression of illness occur against a complex backdrop of a multitude of social determinants of health. Although there have been many studies evaluating the role of stress and sexual abuse in IBS, there has been relatively little effort to date directed toward identifying other social factors that have been associated with IBS. Several social determinants of health need to be incorporated into our understanding of health and health-related illnesses. These include the social gradient (including socioeconomic status), stress, early life, social exclusion, work, unemployment, social support, addiction, food, and transportation. The few social determinants that have been investigated in IBS include life stressors, such as history of sexual, physical and emotional abuse; early life experiences, including gender role socialization; social support; and social factors that have been assessed by quality-of-life scales. This section focuses on the association between women and social factors, as little focus has been directed on social factors in men with IBS.

Life Stress

As summarized by Levy et al. (2006), several studies found that patients with IBS report more lifetime and daily stressors compared with medical control groups or healthy controls. Although stress affects the gut in most people, patients with IBS appear to experience greater reactivity to a variety of stressors, including social stressors. Stress has been found to be associated with both symptom onset and severity in patients with IBS. Moreover, as reviewed by Creed et al. (2006) and Levy et al. (2006), stressful life events and chronic social stress have been shown to adversely affect health status and clinical outcome in patients with IBS. However, no studies to date have assessed gender differences in life stress related to functional gastrointestinal disorders (FGIDs; Toner et al., 2006). Although the data support a significant role for life stress in IBS, future studies will need to determine whether there are similarities and differences in the relationship between stress and FGIDs in women and men.

History of Sexual, Physical, and Emotional Abuse

One form of social stress or oppression that has received increased attention in the past decade in the study of FGIDs is sexual, physical, and emotional abuse. However, most work in this area has included only female samples. In the few studies investigating abuse histories that have included men, significant differences are either not statistically reported or quantified due to insufficient numbers of men in the sample. Talley, Boyce, and Owen (1995) found no differences between male and female patients with IBS with regard to a history of sexual, physical, emotional, or verbal abuse. In contrast, Walker, Katon, Roy-Byrne, Jemelka, and Russo (1993) found that all of the IBS patients who reported a history of sexual abuse were female. In a primary care sample, Longstreth and Wolde-Tsadik (1993) found that a history of sexual abuse was more common in women than in men, but the authors did not differentiate between patients with or without IBS. Moreover, a review of literature has shown strong and consistent relationships of sexual and physical abuse history and interpersonal violence with FGID symptoms and disorders (Leserman & Drossman, 2007). Clearly, further research is needed to determine whether there are gender differences in the history of abuse in FGIDs.

Gender Role Socialization

Gender role socialization, beginning in early life and continuing throughout life, is one important social factor that affects health and well-being. The literature suggests that many of the physical and mental health concerns experienced by women are influenced by socialization into the female gender role. Prominent concerns voiced by women diag-

nosed with IBS include shame about bodily functions, pleasing others, bloating and physical appearance, assertion, and anger. Gender role themes need to be taken into account to help shape the formation of presenting issues during assessment and treatment sessions. There is a clear interconnectedness between the health and well-being of the physical body and its ability to reflect the mental and emotional terrain of the individual. Under stress, the body responds with less attention to digestive processes in preparation for fight or flight, sending energy to different areas of the body. Gender role themes can contribute to this stress response and chronically affect digestion. As well, the state of the physical body can influence the mental and emotional health of an individual. The surrounding environment, bringing the importance of gender role analysis into the forefront of assessment and treatment, also influences the physical and psychological experiences of IBS. It is important to be aware that the prominent gender role associations expressed by women with IBS are not specific to IBS. Rather, they are common throughout clinical and nonclinical populations in their experience of gender roles. In an extensive review of the literature, there is much support for the idea that gender role socialization is related to depression, relationship problems, agoraphobia, chronic fatigue syndrome, eating disorders, and irritable bowel syndrome. Until sufficient numbers of men are included in study samples, the gender role themes and concerns for men with IBS will remain unknown (Toner & Akman, 2000).

Despite postulated links between health problems, such as eating disorders, depression, anxiety disorders, and functional somatic disorders, including IBS, there have been few empirical investigations. Toner and her colleagues (2000) identified several common gender role concerns or themes that have been highly salient and meaningful to women with functional bowel disorders. These themes have been incorporated into a cognitive-behavioral assessment and treatment protocol for women. Results from a randomized trial indicated that women in the CBT condition improved compared with an educational control group at the end of treatment on a composite outcome score that included ratings of satisfaction, QoL, global well-being, and pain (Drossman et al., 2003).

Although further research will need to dismantle which components in the cognitive-behavioral therapy (CBT) treatment protocol were responsible for improvement at the end of treatment, the gender role themes discussed in this section were identified and integrated into a manualized cognitive assessment and treatment protocol (Toner et al., 2000). Toner and her colleagues (2012) identified and integrated gender role themes into a Gender Role Socialization Scale (GRSS), a scale developed to address the internalization of gender role messages for women that may influence their well-being. This scale can be used to examine the relationship between internalized gender role messages and the various types of health concerns that women experience, which will lead to the facilitation of development of prevention and treatment protocols. Moreover, the GRSS exhibits cross-cultural applicability and high validity. Rather than focusing on specific symptoms or diagnostic categories, the GRSS is applicable to female clients who present a varying range of symptoms (Toner et al., 2012). Examples of items found in this scale are "I am to blame if I have low self-esteem"; "No matter how I feel I must always try to look my best"; "In a relationship, I feel I must always put my partner's needs before my own."

Shame and Bodily Functions

One central theme that women with IBS commonly report is feelings of shame associated with losing control of bodily functions. Women receive different social messages than men. Women are taught that bodily functions are something to be kept private and secret as compared with men. One important implication of such teachings is that for women, bowel functioning becomes a source of shame and embarrassment more so than it does for men. The sanction against public admission and/or display of bodily functioning in women can be seen as part of the socialization process that encourages girls and women to be always clean, neat, fresh, and in control (Toner et al., 2012). This same socialization process permits boys and men to be more unrestrained, messy, and dirty and even to view their bodily functions as a source of amusement and pleasure.

For example, while belching and passing gas are not usually desirable in public for either sex, girls and women are socialized into believing that they are especially not ladylike. Belching and passing gas contests are traditionally less frequent among female than male adolescents.

Bloating and Physical Appearance

The finding that women often score higher on indices of bloating and constipation can also be viewed as a gender-related theme. Society's focus on how women look and its perpetuation of thinness as a necessary standard of attractiveness (Toner & Akman, 2012; Lips, 1997), may lead women to experience bloating not only as a source of physical discomfort but of psychological distress as well. For many women, the sensation of being overweight, with or without an increase in the size of their abdomens, may evoke worry and shame about their bodies and therefore about themselves. To the degree that women are subjected to being valued and/or devalued for their physical attractiveness (e.g., thinness), they will be attentive to and concerned by those IBS symptoms that have an impact on how they experience their bodies. The physical and psychological distress that women may experience with abdominal discomfort, coupled with the perception that their pain is being minimized or trivialized by health care professionals, may lead women to respond by becoming more hypervigilant to any sign of pain or discomfort. This increased attention to bodily symptoms may lead to increased pain in some with women with IBS.

Pleasing Others, Assertion and Anger

Women, as compared with men, are socialized to please others, often at the expense of their own needs (Bepko & Krestan, 1990; Jack, 1999). To some degree, this may contribute to women's higher rates of doctor visits and multiple consultations: Patients who believe that their physicians do not understand their experience may seek help elsewhere rather than show displeasure with their current physicians. This would hold true as well for those patients who feel unable to be assertive or angry with their physicians because of the socialized ideal of women as compliant, understanding, and never overtly angry. Women who express anger, make demands, or question authority are often given the label "hysteric," have their complaints dismissed, or have their femininity called into question (Bepko & Krestan, 1990). These potential repercussions for women who express their own wants and needs are often sufficient to keep women silent. Self-silencing is a helpful construct developed by Jack (1999) to describe this socially constructed experience. According to Jack, women are socialized to behave in certain ways to maintain safe, intimate relationships. These social expectations of women can lead to the silencing of certain thoughts, feelings, and behaviors rather than jeopardizing relationships that are in place. A study by Ali et al. (2000) points to the relevance of this construct for IBS patients. These authors compared female patients with IBS with female patients with inflammatory bowel disease (IBD) and found that patients with IBS scored higher on measures of self-silencing than patients with IBD. Future research will need to identify themes that are salient for men with IBS to determine similarities and differences between women and men with IBS.

Health-Related Quality of Life

Several studies have found that patients with IBS and functional dyspepsia have impaired health-related quality of life (HRQoL) compared with patients with other chronic conditions. Few studies have investigated whether women and men with FGIDs differ on HRQoL measures. In a study of referral center and primary care patients, Simrén, Abrahamsson, Svedlund, and Björnsson (2001) found that women with IBS reported a lower QoL compared with men with IBS. In another study, Lee, Mayer, Schmulson, Chang, and Naliboff (2001) also found that women with IBS reported lower scores on an HRQoL measure. However, after these authors controlled for gender differences in the general population, most of the gender effects disappeared. The only remaining gender effect was greater bodily pain scores in female patients with IBS.

Dancey, Hutton-Young, Moyle, and Devins (2002) found that men and women with IBS reported similar HRQoL scores, as well as similar levels of symptom severity,

perceived stigma, and illness intrusiveness. However, these authors also found significant gender differences in the relationship among these variables. For example, among women, IBS symptom severity exerted a significant impact on QoL. For men, the psychosocial impact of illness intrusiveness was greater in every domain except sexual relations. The authors suggest that these results have implications for how gender socialization shapes sex differences in the wider experience of IBS.

Self-Report Questionnaires and Structured Psychiatric Interviews

There are several self-report measures and structured interviews that have been used to assess various psychological and social factors in individuals who have received a diagnosis of IBS. The following section gives a brief summary of measures that have established validity and reliability in this population.

Anxiety, Depression and Somatic Symptoms

A major problem with most measures of anxiety and depression that are administered to individuals with a variety of somatic or bodily symptoms is that the scales include items that focus on somatic symptoms. Accordingly, individuals with bodily symptoms may receive a high score that inappropriately suggests anxiety or depression. The Hospital Anxiety and Depression Scale has overcome this methodological issue by omitting bodily symptoms (Zigmond & Snaith, 1983). This scale has been widely used in this population. The Symptom Checklist (SCL-90) includes a subscale for Somatization (Derogatis, Lipman, & Covi, 1973). Many investigators in the field have used it. Again, the main problem with this scale is that it contains several gut-related symptoms that are related to bowel symptoms. Accordingly, individuals with IBS may receive an elevated score, inappropriately suggesting a somatization disorder.

Several structured psychiatric interviews have been used in this population. The two most frequently cited are the Structured Clinical Interview for DSM-IV (SCID) and the Diagnostic Interview Schedule (DIS). The DIS is a highly structured interview that requires special training. The SCID-I is a diagnostic semistructured interview used to diagnose major DSM-IV Axis I disorders, and the SCID-II is a semistructured interview used to diagnose DSM-IV Axis II personality disorder. Often, the SCID supplements the DIS with additional data (First, Spitzer, Gibbon, & Williams, 1997).

Cognitions and Concerns

According to Toner (2005), only one scale has been specifically designed to assess concerns or cognitions of people who have a diagnosis of IBS. Briefly, items for this scale were initially generated from diaries of thought records from participants with a diagnosis of functional bowel disorders, the majority of whom had a diagnosis of IBS. The Cognitive Scale for Functional Bowel Disorders (Toner et al., 1998) is a valid and reliable measure that can serve as an assessment, as well as a treatment outcome measure. Examples of items include: "I am constantly frustrated by my bowel symptoms"; "My bowel symptoms make me feel out of control"; "I cannot function normally when I have bowel symptoms"; "I often worry about passing gas in public"; "I often feel that this abdominal pain will never go away." Cognitions and concerns such as these may be identified and incorporated into specific cognitive and behavioral strategies and techniques in order to reduce IBS symptoms and the impact of the symptoms on QoL. Further work needs to be done to identify and integrate the patient's perspective into the development and refinement of assessment and outcome measures. The Cognitive Scale for Functional Bowel Disorders exhibits high reliability, high content and face validity, and minimal social desirability contamination (Toner et al., 1998).

Life Experiences

The Life Experience Survey and the Life Events and Difficulties Schedule (LEDS) are two scales that are helpful. In addition, the LEDS is a detailed interview-based method that has been used successfully in this population. Research using these measures has found that stressful events predict the onset of IBS, symptom exacerbation, and IBS symptom intensity.

Health-Related Quality of Life

Generic measures and illness-specific QoL measures have been useful in IBS. The most widely used generic measure is the Medical Outcomes Survey, Short Form (SF-36) (Ware & Sherbourne, 1992). This self-report measure and the shorter version, the SF-12, are both good assessment measures for generic QoL in IBS. The Irritable Bowel Syndrome Quality of Life (IBS-QoL) is a 34-item self-report measure with good psychometric and methodological properties that is widely used as an IBS QoL-specific measure. It has eight subscales; Dysphoria, Interference with Activity, Body Image, Health Worry, Food Avoidance, Social Reaction, Sexual, and Relationship.

Sexual and Physical Abuse

Several studies have found that sexual and physical abuse are higher in women receiving a diagnosis of IBS compared with nonclinical control groups. This finding may not be specific to women with IBS but comparable to women in a variety of clinical groups. Patients with abuse histories report more severe pain, greater psychological distress, greater functional impairment, and more frequent visits to the doctor relative to patients with IBS without a history of abuse. The most frequently used assessment of abuse is the measure developed by Drossman, Li, Leserman, Toome, and Hu (1996). This structured interview was developed to assess the presence of sexual and physical abuse histories, as well as the details concerning the abuse. The interview includes questions regarding the suffering of serious physical injuries during the sexual abuse, the fear of being killed or seriously injured during the abuse, and number of perpetrators of sexual abuse (Leserman et al., 1997).

Summary

It is important to acknowledge that the meaning and expression of illness occurs within a complex network of biological, psychological, and social determinants of health. This chapter has reviewed the limited theoretical and empirical work that has been published in order to better understand and assess the biopsychosocial factors in IBS. These include brain–gut interactions, stigma, cognitions and concerns, depression and anxiety, other bodily symptoms, life stress, history of sexual, physical, and emotional abuse, gender role socialization, and HRQoL. In general, these factors are thought to or have been demonstrated to influence the experience of IBS. Most of the work in this area, however, has included women-only samples or did not test for gender effects due to small numbers of men in the study. Little is empirically known about our understanding and assessment of men with IBS (Toner et al., 2006).

REFERENCES

Ali, A., Toner, B. B., Stuckless, N., Gallop, R., Diamant, N. E., Gould, M. I., et al. (2000). Emotional abuse, self-blame, self-silencing in women with irritable bowel syndrome. *Psychosomatic Medicine, 62,* 76–82.

Bepko, C., & Krestan, J. (1990). *Too good for her own good.* New York: Harper & Row.

Bertram, S., Kurland, M., Lydick, E., Locke, G. R., & Yawn, B. P. (2001). The patient's perspective of irritable bowel syndrome. *Journal of Family Practice, 50,* 521–525.

Chang, L., Toner, B. B., Fukudo, S., Guthrie, E., Locke, G. R., Norton, N. J., et al. (2006). Gender, age, society, culture and the patient's perspective in the disorders of gastrointestinal function. *Gastroenterology, 130,* 1435–1446.

Creed, F., Bradley, L., Francisconi, C., Drossman, D. A., Naliboff, B., & Olden, K. (2006). Psychosocial aspects of functional gastrointestinal disorders. In D. A. Drossman, E. Corazziari, N. J. Talley, W. G. Thompson, & W. E. Whitehead (Eds.), *Encyclopedia of gastroenterology* (pp. 295–368). McLean, VA: Degnon Associates.

Dancey, C. P., Hutton-Young, A., Moyle, S., & Devins, G. M. (2002). Perceived stigma, illness intrusiveness and quality of life in men and women with irritable bowel syndrome. *Psychology, Health, and Medicine, 17,* 381–395.

Derogatis, L. R., Lipman, R. S., & Covi, L. (1973). SCL-90: An outpatient psychiatric rating scale: Preliminary report. *Psychopharmacology Bulletin, 9,* 13–28.

Drossman, D. A. (1995a). Diagnosing and treating patients with refractory functional gastrointestinal disorders. *Annals of Internal Medicine, 123*(9), 688–697.

Drossman, D. A. (1995b). Psychosocial factors in the care of patients with gastrointestinal disorders. In T. Yamada (Ed.), *Textbook of gastroenterology* (pp. 620–637). Philadelphia: Lippincott.

Drossman, D. A. (1997). Psychosocial sound bites: Exercises in the patient–doctor relationship. *American Journal of Gastroenterology, 92*(9), 1418–1423.

Drossman, D. A. (1998). Presidential Address: Gastrointestinal illness and the biopsychosocial model. *Psychosomatic Medical Journal, 60*(3), 258–267.

Drossman, D. A., Camilleri, M., Mayer, E. A., & Whitehead, W. E. (2002). AGA technical review on irritable bowel syndrome. *Gastroenterology, 123,* 2108–2131.

Drossman, D. A., Corazziari, E., Spiller, R. C., Thompson, W. G., & Rome III Committee. (2006). *ROME III: The functional gastrointestinal disorders* (3rd ed.). McLean, VA: Degnon Associates.

Drossman, D. A., Li, Z., Andruzzi, E., Temple, R., Talley, N. J., Thompson, W. G., et al. (1993). U.S. Householder Survey of Functional Gastrointestinal Disorders: Prevalence, Sociodemography and Health Impact. *Digestive Diseases and Sciences, 38,* 1569–1580.

Drossman, D. A., Li, Z., Leserman, J., Toome, T. C., & Hu, Y. J. (1996). Health status by gastrointestinal diagnosis and abuse history. *Gastroenterology, 110,* 999–1007.

Drossman, D. A., Toner, B. B., Whitehead, W. E., Diamant, N. E., Dalton, C. B., Duncan, S., et al. (2003). Cognitive-behavioral therapy versus education and desipramine versus placebo for moderate to severe functional bowel disorders. *Gastroenterology, 125,* 19–31.

Fabrege, H., Jr. (1991). Somatization in cultural–historical perspective. In L. J. Kirmayer & J. M. Robbins (Eds.), *Current concepts of somatization: Research and clinical perspectives* (pp. 181–199). Washington, DC: American Psychiatric Press.

First, M. B., Spitzer, R. L., Gibbon, M., & Williams, J. B. W. (1997). *User's guide for the Structured Clinical Interview for DSM-IV Axis I Disorders: SCID-I Clinician Version.* Washington, DC: American Psychiatric Press.

Gralnek, I. M., Hays, R. D., Kilbourne, A., Naliboff, B., & Mayer, E. (2000). The impact of irritable bowel syndrome on health-related quality of life. *Gastroenterology, 119*(3), 655–660.

International Foundation for Functional Gastrointestinal Disorders. (2002). *IBS in the real world survey* [Pamphlet]. Milwaukee, WI: International Foundation for Functional Gastrointestinal Disorders.

Jack, D. C. (1999). Silencing the self: Inner dialogues and outer realities. In T. Joiner & J. Coyne (Eds.), *The interactional nature of depression* (pp. 221–246). Washington, DC: American Psychological Association.

Kennedy, A., Robinson, A., & Rogers, A. (2003). Incorporating patients' views and experiences of life with IBS in the development of an evidence based self-help guidebook. *Patient Education and Counseling, 50,* 303–310.

Kirmayer, L. J., & Robbins, J. M. (1991). Functional somatic syndromes. In L. J. Kirmayber & J. M. Robbins (Eds.), *Current concepts of somatization* (pp. 79–105). Washington, DC: American Psychiatric Association.

Lee, O. Y., Mayer, E. A., Schmulson, M., Chang, L., & Naliboff, B. (2001). Gender-related differences in IBS symptoms. *American Journal of Gastroenterology, 96,* 2184–2193.

Leserman, J., & Drossman, D. A. (2007). Relationship of abuse history to functional and gastrointestinal disorders and symptoms: Some possible mediating mechanisms. *Trauma, Violence and Abuse, 8*(3), 331–343.

Leserman, J., Li, Z., Drossman, D. A., Toomey, T. C. Nachman, G., & Glogau, L. (1997). Impact of sexual and physical abuse dimensions on health status: Development of an abuse severity measure. *Psychosomatic Medicine, 59,* 152–160.

Levy, R. L., Olden, K. W., Naliboff, B. D., Bradley, L. A., Francisconi, C., Drossman, D. A., et al. (2006). Psychosocial aspects of the functional gastrointestinal disorders. *Gastroenterology, 130*(5), 1447–1458

Lips, H. (1997). *Sex and gender.* Mountain View, CA: Mayfield.

Longstreth, G. F., & Wolde-Tsadik, G. (1993). Irritable bowel-type symptoms in HMO examinees. *Digestive Diseases and Sciences, 38,* 1581–1589.

Mitchell, C. M., & Drossman, D. A. (1987). Survey of the AGA membership relating to patients with functional gastrointestinal disorders. *Gastroenterology, 92,* 1282–1284.

Patrick, D. L., Drossman, D. A., Fredrick, I. O., DiCesare, J., & Puder, K. L. (1998). Quality of life in persons with irritable bowel syndrome: Development of a new measure. *Digestive Diseases and Sciences, 43,* 400–411.

Pinhas, L., Toner, B. B., Ali, A., Garfinkel, P. E., & Stuckless, N. (1999). The effects of the ideal of female beauty on mood and body satisfaction. *International Journal of Eating Disorders, 25,* 223.

Russo, M. W., Gaynes, B. N., & Drossman, D. A. (1999). A national survey of practice patterns of gastroenterologists with comparison to the past two decades. *Journal of Clinical Gastroenterology, 29*(4), 339–343.

Simrén, M., Abrahamsson, H., Svedlund, J., & Björnsson, E. S. (2001). Quality of life in patients with irritable bowel syndrome seen in referral centers versus primary care: The impact of gender and predominant bowel pattern. *Scandinavian Journal of Gastroenterology, 36*(5), 545–552.

Sperber, A. D., Carmel, S., Atzmon, Y., Weisberg, I., Shalit, Y., Neumann, L., et al. (2000). Use of the Functional Bowel Disorder Severity Index (FBDSI) in a study of patients with the irritable bowel syndrome and fibromyalgia. *American Journal of Gastroenterology, 95,* 995–998.

Talley, N. J., Boyce, P., & Owen, B. K. (1995). Psychological distress and seasonal symptom changes in irritable bowel syndrome. *American Journal of Gastroenterology, 90*(12), 2115–2119.

Toner, B. B. (1994). Cognitive-behavioural treatment of functional somatic syndromes: Integrating gender issues. *Cognitive Behavioural Practice, 11,* 157–178.

Toner, B. (2005). Cognitive-behavioral treatment of irritable bowel syndrome. *CNS Spectrums, 10*(11), 883–890.

Toner, B. B., & Akman, D. (2000). Gender role and irritable bowel syndrome: Literature review and hypothesis. *American Journal of Gastroenterology, 95,* 11–16.

Toner, B. B., & Akman, D. (2012). Using a feminist- and trauma-informed approach in research and therapy with women. In L. Greaves & N. Poole (Eds.), *Becoming trauma informed* (pp. 37–46). Toronto, Ontario, Canada: Centre for Addiction and Mental Health Press.

Toner, B. B., & Casati, J. (2002). Diseases of the digestive system. In T. J. Boll, S. B. Johnson, N. Perry, & R. H. Rozensky (Eds.), *Handbook of clinical health psychology: Vol. 1. Medical disorders and behavioral applications* (pp. 283–305). Washington, DC: American Psychological Association.

Toner, B. B., Chang, L., Fukudo, S., et al. (2006). Gender, age, society, culture and the patient's perspective in functional gastrointestinal disorders. In D. A. Drossman, E. Corazziari, N. J. Talley, W. G. Thompson, & W. E. Whitehead (Eds.), *Encyclopedia of gastroenterology: The functional gastrointestinal disorders* (Rome III; 3rd ed., pp. 231–294). McLean, VA: Degnon Associates.

Toner, B. B., Segal, Z., Emmott, S., & Myran, D. (2000). *Cognitive-behavioral treatment of irritable bowel syndrome: The brain–gut connection.* New York: Guilford Press.

Toner, B. B., Stuckless, N., Ali, A., Downie, F., Shelagh, E., & Akman, D. (1998). The development of a Cognitive Scale for Functional Bowel Disorders. *American Psychosomatic Society, 60,* 492–497.

Toner, B., Tang, T., Ali, A., Akman, D., Stuckless, N., Rolin-Gilman, C., et al., (2012), Developing a gender role socialization scale. In J. L Oliffe & L. Greaves (Eds.), *Designing and conducting gender, sex and health research.* Thousand Oaks, CA: Sage.

Walker, E. A., Katon, W. J., Roy-Byrne, P. P., Jemelka, R. P., & Russo, J. (1993). Histories of sexual victimization in patients with irritable bowel syndrome or inflammatory bowel disease. *American Journal of Psychiatry, 150*(10), 1502–1506.

Ware, J. E., & Sherbourne, C. D. (1992). The MOS 36-Item Short Form Health Survey (SF-36): I. Conceptual framework and item selection. *Medical Care, 30,* 473–483.

Zigmond, A. S., & Snaith, R. P. (1983). The Hospital Anxiety Depression Scale. *Scandinavian Journal of Psychiatry, 67*(6), 361–370.

CHAPTER 19

Insomnia

Daniel J. Taylor
Christina S. McCrae
Kenneth L. Lichstein
Adam D. Bramoweth

Chronic insomnia affects about 9–15% of the general population, depending on the definition (for a review, see Ohayon, 2002), and up to 50% of primary care clinic patients (Katz & McHorney, 1998; Simon & VonKorff, 1997). Insomnia is also a risk factor for a number of medical and mental disorders (for a review, see Taylor, Lichstein, & Durrence, 2003). The annual direct cost of insomnia is estimated to be $13.9 billion, with total costs of $30–35 billion per year (Walsh & Engelhardt, 1999).

Clinically, the diagnosis of primary insomnia requires a complaint of difficulty falling asleep, staying asleep, or nonrestorative sleep, lasting at least 3 nights per week for at least 3 months, which causes difficulty with daytime functioning (American Psychiatric Association, 2013). However, a large proportion of insomnia is comorbid with other medical and mental disorders (Taylor, Lichstein, Durrence, Riedel, & Bush, 2005; Taylor, Mallory, et al., 2007). This complicates the process of assessing and diagnosing insomnia. Part of the art of assessing comorbid insomnia is to clinically determine what portion of the insomnia is being caused by the precipitating event, what is being caused by perpetuating behaviors, and where to intervene first (Spielman, Saskin, & Thorpy, 1987). A precise assessment of insomnia can greatly aid treatment planning, ensuring the best possible outcome.

There are several important areas that must be assessed in an insomnia intake interview. These include sleep history (including insomnia course), psychosocial issues, comorbid medical and psychiatric disorders, and current medications and substances used. The clinician has a variety of tools to accomplish this goal, such as semistructured interviews, self-report questionnaires, and physiological measures. This chapter discusses common instruments used to assess insomnia and comorbid medical, psychiatric, and sleep disorders. The purpose of each assessment is given, as well as a description of the content assessed, the number and types of items, aspects of the biopsychosocial model assessed (see Table 19.1), appropriate populations, and validity and reliability data (only coefficients with ranges below .7 are reported).

Buysse, Ancoli-Israel, Edinger, Lichstein, and Morin (2006) recently performed an excellent review of this area, making recommendations for a standard *research* assessment of insomnia. This chapter, however, is focused more on the *clinical* assessment of insomnia, although many of the measures reviewed here are in line with the Buysse et al. (2006) recommendations.

TABLE 19.1. Recommended Clinical Measures for Insomnia

Measure	Purpose	Biopsychosocial content
Semistructured interview		
Sleep/insomnia Duke SIS IIS SCISD-5	Diagnosis, treatment planning	Physical, behavioral, cognitive, emotional, environmental
Psychiatric SCID-I and SCID-II MINI PDSQ	Diagnosis, treatment planning	Physical, behavioral, cognitive, emotional, environmental
Self-report		
Sleep/insomnia Sleep diary	Diagnosis, treatment, outcome	Behavioral (optional = emotional, physical, environmental)
PSQI		Physical, behavioral, emotional, environmental
ISI		Physical, behavioral, emotional
Fatigue MFI FSS	Outcome	Behavioral, physical, cognitive
Depression/anxiety IDS-SR BDI II STAI	Diagnosis, treatment, outcome	Emotional, physical, behavioral, cognitive
Quality of life SF 36 Q-LES-Q	Outcome assessment	Physical, behavioral, emotional Physical, behavioral, cognitive, emotional
Neuropsychological	Outcome assessment	Cognitive, behavioral, emotional
Biological	Diagnosis, treatment planning	
PSG		Physical, behavioral
Actigraphy		Physical, behavioral, environmental (models equipped with light sensor)

Areas of Assessment

Semistructured Interviews

Insomnia/Sleep History

Properly done, the insomnia and sleep history, supplemented with sleep diaries, is *clinically* sufficient for adequate assessment. The overarching goal is to determine what predispositions the patient may have (e.g., family history, hyperarousal, short sleeper, evening type), what precipitated the original and/or current episode (e.g., job stress, death in family, illness, marital problems), and what behaviors and cognitions are perpetuating the illness (e.g., excessive time in bed, worrying about sleep). The interview should include questions that not only evaluate sleep–wake functioning but also

common comorbidities (medical, psychiatric, or substance-related; discussed later). Specifically, the nature of the primary sleep complaint should be explored, as well as presleep conditions and routines; sleep–wake schedules and patterns; nocturnal symptoms; daytime activities and function; and current and past medical and psychiatric histories. Semistructured or structured interviews, although sometimes awkward, help ensure that practitioners with varying levels of training in sleep will obtain similar, and hopefully adequate, details of the areas listed here.

Insomnia Interview Schedule. The Insomnia Interview Schedule (IIS) is a semistructured interview designed to facilitate the collection of a detailed sleep history (Morin,

1993). The interview provides a thorough evaluation and diagnosis of insomnia according to DSM-IV (American Psychiatric Association, 1994), the International Classification of Sleep Disorders (American Sleep Disorders Association, 1997), and commonly used research criteria (Morin, 1993). The IIS gathers a wide variety of information, including nature and severity of the insomnia complaint (e.g., problems falling asleep or staying asleep, waking up too early in the morning); sleep–wake schedule (usual bed- and waking times, final arising time); frequency and duration of napping; frequency of problems and time required to fall asleep; frequency and duration of nighttime awakenings; total sleep duration; use of prescription and over-the-counter sleep medications/aids (including alcohol); history of sleep difficulties; bedroom environment (bed partner, noise, temperature); diet and exercise habits; sleep habits (watching television in bed or bedroom); symptoms of other sleep disorders (e.g., apnea); medical/psychiatric history and medication use; and current or past psychopathology. The IIS contains 95–100 questions, requires about 20–30 minutes to administer, and is designed for administration by a clinician or mental health professional capable of making clinical judgments. Some knowledge of sleep disorders is needed, so training is required for individuals unfamiliar with sleep disorders. The IIS is appropriate for administration to English-speaking adults who are able to participate in the interview. The reliability and validity of the IIS remain to be demonstrated.

Duke Structured Interview Schedule for DSM-IV-TR and International Classification of Sleep Disorders, Second Edition, Sleep Disorders Diagnoses. The Duke Structured Interview Schedule (SIS) is a structured interview designed to obtain a sleep history, to screen for sleep disorders, and to gauge the relative contribution of psychological, behavioral, environmental, and medical factors (Edinger et al., 2006). This measure was developed by Edinger and colleagues to provide sleep disorder diagnoses that meet criteria for both DSM-IV-TR (American Psychiatric Association, 2000) and the International Classification of Sleep Disorders, Second Edition (American Acad-

emy of Sleep Medicine, 2005). Most important, insomnia diagnoses obtained from this interview will meet the research diagnostic criteria recommended for insomnia research studies by an expert panel from the American Academy of Sleep Medicine (Edinger et al., 2004). The interview includes approximately 150 questions, but many are skipped because of rule-out questions (e.g., use a checklist for parasomnias, only ask questions if checked). The interview is approximately 93 pages long and takes 30–90 minutes to complete depending on how many sleep problems the patient endorses. It includes checklists of "emotional symptoms," "medical conditions and symptoms," and "medication, drugs, and other substances." These are not in-depth interviews of these areas and appear to be mainly used for categorizing insomnia type (e.g., primary insomnia, psychophysiological insomnia, idiopathic insomnia). Appropriate populations for this assessment include English-speaking adults capable of participating in the interview. Currently, reliability and validity data for the Duke SIS remain to be demonstrated.

Structured Clinical Interview for DSM-5 Sleep Disorders. The Structured Clinical Interview for DSM-5 Sleep Disorders (SCISD-5) is a new measure designed by the first author's lab, which was an extension of the Duke SIS but was made considerably shorter (i.e., 8 pages) by including only sleep disorders as defined by DSM-5 (American Psychiatric Association, 2013). This measure was specifically designed to allow an independent evaluator with a master's degree or higher and minimal training in sleep disorders (i.e., 3 hours didactics) and administration (i.e., 3–4 supervised interviews) to obtain a reliable sleep disorder diagnosis in adults only. As with the other interviews, the SCISD-5 has yet to be validated, but these studies are under way. (A copy of the measure can be obtained by contacting Daniel J. Taylor.)

Psychiatric Disorders

Sleep and psychiatric disorders are highly comorbid, and it is important to attempt to determine the relative impact insomnia and comorbid psychiatric disorders have on each other. The sleep interviews listed previously provide a fair coverage of this area; the IIS somewhat more than the Duke SIS. However, a structured interview specifically geared toward mental disorders may make this task easier and more consistent. Several structured and semistructured psychiatric interviews exist. We discuss a few of the more commonly used instruments here.

Structured Clinical Interview for DSM-IV. The Structured Clinical Interview for DSM-IV (SCID) is the most commonly used semistructured psychiatric interview. It has two parts—Axis I Disorders (SCID-I; First, Spitzer, Gibbon, & Williams, 1996) and Personality Disorders (SCID-II; First, Gibbon, Spitzer, Williams, & Benjamin, 1997). The SCID-I is a semistructured interview designed to facilitate the diagnosis of the major DSM-IV disorders. It is divided into six modules assessing broad categories of psychiatric disturbance (i.e., mood disorders, psychotic disorders, alcohol use disorders, other substance use disorders, anxiety disorders, and other disorders). It is worth noting that the SCID-I does not cover any sleep disorders, including insomnia. The SCID-II is similar to the SCID-I, but it assesses the 11 personality disorders within DSM-IV-TR and the two personality disorders found in the appendix (depressive and passive–aggressive). It has the added benefit of a 119-item yes–no screening personality questionnaire that takes the patient about 20 minutes to complete. The clinician then asks the patient about only affirmative answers to determine a diagnosis. Both versions of the SCID are designed for administration by a clinician or trained mental health professional, but they are frequently used in research studies by well-trained and supervised nonclinician research assistants. Appropriate populations for assessment include both adult patients and nonpatients who are capable of completing the interview. The SCID-I generally produces interrater reliability scores (kappa) in the .60 range, with scores in the .8 range for major depression and generalized anxiety disorders (Segal, Hersen, & Van Hasselt, 1994). Kappa scores for the most recent version of the SCID-II were > .80 for all disorders except depressive personality disorder (kappa = .65), with most being > .90 (Maffei et al., 1997). (Computer-assisted versions

are available from Multi-Health Systems, Toronto, Ontario, Canada.)

Mini-International Neuropsychiatric Interview. The Mini-International Neuropsychiatric Interview (MINI) is a short, structured clinical interview developed to make 17 DSM-IV and ICD-10 Axis I psychiatric diagnoses (Sheehan et al., 1998). Administration time is approximately 10–25 minutes, depending on the number of diagnoses present, and the interview can be administered by both clinicians and well-trained nonclinician research assistants. The MINI can be used in both patient and nonpatient populations and is appropriate for adults capable of completing the interview. The psychometrics of the MINI (reliability, sensitivity, specificity) have been explored in a clinical population and compared against the Composite International Diagnostic Interview (CIDI; Lecrubier et al., 1997) and the SCID-I (Sheehan et al., 1997). The performance of the MINI was equivalent to these longer interviews. In the clinical population studied, concordance rates for the three most frequent diagnoses were .68 for major depressive disorder, .62 for generalized anxiety disorder, and .66 for social phobia. The MINI demonstrated predictive values > .70 and negative predictive values > .90. Few false positives are likely to be generated using the MINI.

Psychiatric Diagnostic Screening Questionnaire. The Psychiatric Diagnostic Screening Questionnaire (PDSQ) is a self-report measure designed to screen for psychiatric symptoms and can be used as both a diagnostic tool and an outcome measure (Zimmerman & Mattia, 2001). The PDSQ screens for symptoms in 13 DSM-IV Axis I disorders in five areas (eating, mood, anxiety, substance abuse, and somatoform disorders). This measure has 126 yes–no items and takes approximately 10–15 minutes to complete. The PDSQ also includes six items that screen for the presence of psychosis. Follow-up interview materials are provided for use with patients who score above cutoffs for multiple disorders. The PDSQ is appropriate to use with adult patients and nonpatients who are capable of completing the measure. Although a relatively new instrument, the PDSQ has extensive reliability and validity data. All 13 subscales of the PDSQ demonstrate good to excellent levels of internal consistency. Test–retest reliability less than 2 weeks apart was good on nine subscales with an overall mean test–retest reliability of .83. The PDSQ also has excellent sensitivity and high negative predictive values. Using cutoff scores that result in a sensitivity of 90%, the mean negative predictive value of the subscales is 97%.

Self-Report Instruments

Sleep

As mentioned in the preceding section on interviews, several self-report instruments can enhance the quality of data obtained and used in the treatment of insomnia. One of those measures, the sleep diary, is essential. However, there are many circumstances (e.g., with acute inpatients) in which this is not possible. Therefore, we review the sleep diary, along with other single time-point retrospective estimates, next.

Sleep Diary. Sleep diaries are the most commonly used clinical measure of subjective sleep patterns in patients reporting insomnia, and, combined with a thorough sleep, medical, and psychiatric history, they represent a minimally sufficient assessment procedure in clinical practice. Sleep diaries ask participants to give an estimate of their sleep the previous night and generally include information on bedtime and waking time, sleep onset latency, nighttime awakenings, waking after sleep onset, sleep efficiency ([total sleep time ÷ time in bed] × 100), and sleep quality. Information from sleep diaries is generally collected for 1–2 weeks. Typically, overnight sleep studies are considered the gold standard for assessment of sleep disorders (Carskadon et al., 1976; Coursey, Frankel, Gaarder, & Mott, 1980). Although researchers have found that people with insomnia consistently underestimate total sleep time and overestimate sleep onset latencies in comparison with polysomnography (PSG), they also found that the correlations between sleep diaries and PSG are high ($r = .63–.87$), especially given that the range of scores was restricted to the worst sleepers. Further, sleep diaries are better than single-point retrospective estimates of typical sleep

(Coursey et al., 1980; Lichstein et al., 2006). Although sleep diaries are not objective measures of sleep, they are the cheapest and most efficient way to measure sleep and thus the mostly likely to be utilized in clinical practice. They are also favored over PSG (Buysse et al., 2006) because they focally address the self-report of insomnia, the key diagnostic factor. Numerous versions of sleep diaries have been published, and recently a "consensus" diary was developed by several leaders in the field of sleep medicine in an attempt to standardize the data collected from these instruments (Carney et al., 2012).

Pittsburgh Sleep Quality Index. The Pittsburgh Sleep Quality Index (PSQI) is a self-report questionnaire that takes about 5 minutes to complete and is used to assess sleep quality and disturbance retrospectively for the preceding 30 days (Buysse, Reynolds, Monk, Berman, & Kupfer, 1989). The 19 self-reported items assess several sleep-related factors and are used to obtain seven component scores: subjective sleep quality, sleep latency, sleep duration, habitual sleep efficiency, sleep disturbances, use of sleeping medication, and daytime dysfunction. It also includes five other-reported (i.e., bed partner or roommate) questions that are for clinical information purposes only. Regardless of the form of the original data, each component is placed on an ordinal scale (0 = *no difficulty* to 3 = *severe difficulty*). The seven component scores are then summed to yield a global PSQI score, which has a range of 0–21, with higher scores representing worse sleep quality. Global scores > 5 distinguish good versus poor sleepers with acceptable levels of sensitivity (89.6%) and specificity (86.5%).

It is important to note here that the term "poor sleepers" is not equivalent to insomnia, as people with sleep apnea and narcolepsy are also considered "poor sleepers," and in fact these disorders are assessed within the PSQI. Therefore, this instrument is useful mainly as a screen for the presence of significant sleep disturbance in patients in general medical and psychiatric practice and provides information to guide the clinician in specific areas requiring further evaluation, but it can also be used as an outcome measure. Appropriate populations for assessment include English-speaking adult patients and nonpatients. Reliability and validity were originally assessed over 18 months in good sleepers and poor sleepers (including both patients with depression and with sleep disorders). Internal consistency and test–retest validity were good.

Insomnia Severity Index. The Insomnia Severity Index (ISI) is a self-report questionnaire designed to evaluate the perceived severity of insomnia over the previous 2 weeks (Morin, 1993) that can be used to assist in diagnosis, in treatment planning, and as an outcome measure. The ISI assesses severity of difficulties in falling asleep and maintaining sleep, early morning awakenings, dissatisfaction with current sleep pattern, extent to which sleep difficulties interfere with daytime functioning, how noticeable the sleep problem is to others and its negative impact on quality of life, and the level of distress or worry caused by the sleep difficulties. The questionnaire takes about 1–2 minutes to complete and contains seven items, each rated on a 5-point Likert-type scale, and item scores are summed to obtain a total score, ranging from 0 to 28. The following guidelines are recommended for clinical interpretation: 0–7, absence of clinically significant insomnia; 8–14, subthreshold insomnia; 15–21, moderate insomnia; and 22–28, severe insomnia. Although originally designed to screen for insomnia in the general population, the ISI is also useful for patient populations. The ISI was originally written in English, and an equivalent version (Blais, Gendron, Mimeault, & Morin, 1997) is also available in Canadian French (Morin, 1993). Internal consistency is good, and test–retest reliability (r = .65) is adequate (Bastien, Vallieres, & Morin, 2001). Convergent validity with other sleep measures is also reasonably good (PSQI r = .67; sleep diary r's = .32–.91). When used to screen for primary insomnia, a cutoff score of 14 has been shown to optimize sensitivity and specificity (Bastien et al., 2001).

Comorbid Medical Disorders

Although a medical *examination* is not necessary when evaluating insomnia, a thorough medical *history* is. A number of medical conditions and medications can impair sleep, making it important to try to identify the interrelationship between insomnia and comorbid medical factors so that a proper treatment course can be chosen. A structured interview can make this task easier and more consistent, and all of the sleep interviews listed herein provide some form of this information. The Cornell Medical Index, described next, might facilitate a more thorough evaluation of medical status.

Cornell Medical Index. The Cornell Medical Index (CMI) is a self-report questionnaire written in informal language (i.e., no medical terminology) that is designed to approximate a comprehensive medical examination (Brodman, Erdmann, Lorge, Wolff, & Broadbent, 1951). The CMI has 223 items. Each question allows a "yes" or "no" answer and pertains to four different areas of functioning: (1) bodily symptoms, (2) previous illnesses, (3) family history of illness, and (4) psychological symptoms. The CMI takes about 10–15 minutes to complete and is appropriate for adult patients and nonpatients who are capable of completing the measure. The CMI has been shown to correspond closely with hospital records based on physician examinations (Brodman, Erdmann, Lorge, & Wolff, 1949).

Medications. Drugs and alcohol can have significant effects on sleep, making it essential that they be inquired about at each intake, and preferably throughout treatment. The simplest way to accomplish this is to ask patients to fill out a form that asks what substances they have taken in the past week or take regularly, when they traditionally take them, and the frequency, duration, and amount of substances. No uniform version of this exists, but the insomnia interviews listed earlier in the chapter provide questions or checklists that inquire about substance/medication usage.

Comorbid Mental Disorders

There are no self-report measures that adequately assess all mental disorders. Because insomnia is frequently comorbid with depression and anxiety (Taylor et al., 2005), it is often useful to specifically assess anxiety and depression levels with self-report instruments during the initial intake and throughout treatment. Some of the most commonly used ones are discussed here.

Beck Depression Inventory. The Beck Depression Inventory (BDI-II) is the most frequently used self-report measure of depression (Beck, Steer, Ball, & Ranieri, 1996). It can be used to assist in diagnosis, in treatment planning, and as an outcome measure. The content assessed includes sadness, pessimism, past failure, loss of pleasure, guilt feelings, punishment feelings, self-dislike, self-criticalness, suicidal thoughts or wishes, crying, agitation, loss of interest, indecisiveness, worthlessness, loss of energy, changes in sleep patterns, irritability, changes in appetite, concentration difficulty, tiredness or fatigue, and loss of interest in sex. The BDI-II is a 21-item self-report measure that takes about 5 minutes to complete, is appropriate for both adolescents and adults (Beck & Steer, 1993) and asks participants to indicate the statement in each item that best describes how they felt during the previous 2 weeks. Beck, Steer, and Garbin (1988) found good reliability estimates for 15 nonpsychiatric samples. The BDI-II has also been shown to differentiate psychiatric patients from nonpatients and dysthymic patients from patients with major depressive disorders (Steer, Beck, Brown, & Berchick, 1987).

Inventory of Depressive Symptomatology—Self-Report. The Inventory of Depressive Symptomatology—Self-Report (ISD-SR) is a self-report alternative to the BDI-II that assesses both neurovegetative symptomatology and cognitive-affective disturbance (Bagby, Ryder, Schuller, & Marshall, 2004; Rush et al., 1986; Rush, Guillon, Basco, Jarrett, & Trivedi, 1996; Rush et al., 2005). It can be used to assist in diagnosis, in treatment planning, and as an outcome measure in adult patients and nonpatients. The 30 items take about 6–8 minutes to complete and ask participants to rate on a 0–3 scale how each item describes them over the preceding 2 weeks. The IDS-SR is sensitive to symptom change associated with medications or psychotherapy (Rush et al., 1996). The IDS-SR has a good internal consistency—Cronbach's alpha ranges from 0.67 to 0.94—and the clinician-rated version of the IDS had an excellent interrater reliability. The IDS-SR is highly correlated with the BDI-II.

State–Trait Anxiety Inventory. The State–Trait Anxiety Inventory (STAI) is made up of two scales: State and Trait (Spielberger, Gorsuch, Lushene, & Jacobs, 1983). The State scale consists of statements that ask people to describe how they feel at a particular moment in time (e.g., calm, tense), and the Trait scale consists of statements describing how people generally feel (e.g., confident). Each of the scales contains 20 items and takes about 2–3 minutes to complete; each item uses a 4-point Likert-type scale. The measure is appropriate to use with adult patients and nonpatients. The internal consistency for the State scale ranged from .65–.96, and the test–retest reliability ranged from .34–.96. The internal consistency of the Trait scale ranged from .72–.96, and the test–retest reliability range from .82–.94 (Barnes, Harp, & Jung, 2002).

Fatigue

Sleepiness and fatigue are actually two different constructs, which insomnia patients tend to confuse. By their nature, people with insomnia tend not to have a great deal of sleepiness during the day, but they do often report greater levels of fatigue than people without insomnia, making fatigue a useful outcome to monitor. Two fatigue inventories have been recommended for use in research on insomnia, and either of these should suffice if clinicians want to provide an added level of assessment to their practice.

Multidimensional Fatigue Inventory. The Multidimensional Fatigue Inventory (MFI) is a self-report questionnaire designed to measure fatigue (Smets, Garssen, Bonke, & De Haes, 1995). It can be used to assist in diagnosis, in treatment planning, and as an outcome measure. It covers the dimensions of general fatigue, physical fatigue, mental fatigue, reduced motivation, and reduced activity. The MFI takes about 20 minutes to complete, and each of the 20 items uses a 5-item Likert-type scale ranging from *yes, that is true* to *no, that is not true.* The MFI is appropriate to use in both patient and nonpatient populations. The MFI has an internal consistency range of from .65–.80.

Convergent validity between the MFI and visual analogue scale fatigue scores range from .23–.77 (Smets et al., 1995).

Fatigue Severity Scale. The Fatigue Severity Scale (FSS) is a self-report questionnaire used to measure subjective severity of fatigue (Krupp, LaRocca, Muir-Nash, & Steinberg, 1989). It can be used to assist in diagnosis, in treatment planning, and as an outcome measure. The FSS appears to measure multiple dimensions of fatigue, including estimates of general fatigue (Schwartz, Jandorf, & Krupp, 1993), and is able to differentiate fatigue from daytime sleepiness (Lichstein, Means, Noe, & Aguillard, 1997). The nine items take about 1 minute to complete and are placed on a 7-point scale and then averaged, yielding a total score range of 1–7, with higher scores representing higher severity. It is appropriate to use in both patient and nonpatient populations. The FSS has high internal consistency, clearly differentiates patients from controls, and exhibits excellent test–retest reliability (Schwartz et al., 1993).

Quality of Life

Ultimately, clinicians treat patients in hopes of improving their quality of life. This is done by directly treating the disorder, in this case insomnia, that is impairing quality of life. Clinicians typically measure the disorder of interest (i.e., insomnia) to see whether treatment is working, but they rarely track the ultimate outcome variable, quality of life. Next we review two measures of quality of life that have been approved for use by Buysse et al. (2006) and that will be useful in clinical practice.

Medical Outcomes Study 36-Item Short-Form Health Survey. The Medical Outcomes Study 36-Item Short-Form Health Survey (SF-36) is a self-report questionnaire used primarily as an outcome measure. It assesses bodily pain, general mental health, vitality (energy and fatigue), general health perceptions, and limitations in social or role activities because of physical or emotional problems and in physical activities because of health problems (McHorney, Ware, Lu, & Sherbourne, 1994; McHorney, Ware, & Raczek, 1993). It is appropriate to use in adult patients and nonpatients and takes about 5 minutes to complete. The SF-36 has good reliability and construct validity, being able to distinguish between groups with expected health differences (McHorney et al., 1993). There are shorter versions of this quality-of-life measure that appear to also have adequate reliability and validity (i.e., SF-12, SF-8).

Quality of Life Enjoyment and Satisfaction Questionnaire. The Quality of Life Enjoyment and Satisfaction Questionnaire (Q-LES-Q) is self-report measure designed to assess the degree of enjoyment and satisfaction experienced by individuals in multiple areas of daily functioning (Endicott, Nee, Harrison, & Blumenthal, 1993). The Q-LES-Q is primarily used as an outcome measure. Responses are grouped into eight areas of functioning, which include physical health, subjective feelings, leisure time activities, social relationships, general activities, work, household duties, and school/coursework. Each of the 93 items is scored on a 5-point Likert-type scale that indicates the degree of enjoyment or satisfaction achieved during the preceding week. It can be used with adult patients and nonpatients and takes about 10 minutes to complete. Endicott and colleagues report good test–retest reliability and strong internal consistency across eight subscales (Endicott et al., 1993). In addition, the authors found that the Q-LES-Q was sensitive to changes in symptom severity of depression and that it measured important dimensions of the illness that were not reflected in severity measures.

Psychomotor and Cognitive Performance

Clinically, psychomotor and cognitive performance assessment is somewhat less important than it is in research. To date, the widest use of neuropsychological measures in insomnia research has been to assess for negative daytime residual effects of sleep medications. Additionally, a few studies have used similar measures to examine post-treatment improvements in the "hallmark" daytime complaints of patients (e.g., difficulties with concentration, memory, and ability to function) following behavioral treatment for insomnia, but the results have been mixed. Appropriate populations for assessment vary depending on the specific neuropsychological measure in question, but generally include English-speaking adults who are capable of completing the instruments. Most neuropsychological instruments are designed for administration by clinicians and researchers with special training in neuropsychological assessment. Unfortunately, validity and reliability information for the use of these instruments with patients with insomnia and other sleep disorders is not available.

Physiological Measures

Insomnia is often comorbid with other sleep disorders, such as sleep apnea (i.e., repeated cessation of breathing during sleep), and may actually be caused by them (e.g., sleep maintenance insomnia occurs when a patient is awakened by an apnea episode). These other sleep disorders often have significant consequences, such as excessive daytime sleepiness and decreased physical health. Therefore, clinicians should always assess for other sleep disorders when assessing insomnia. The insomnia interviews described earlier do assess for symptoms of sleep disorders, but sometimes more objective assessments may be in order, and these are described in this section.

Polysomnography.

Polysomnography (PSG) is a physiological assessment of sleep, which is generally considered the gold standard for diagnosing sleep disorders other than insomnia, such as obstructive sleep apnea (OSA) and periodic limb movement disorder (PLMD). A comprehensive PSG will record central and frontal electroencephalograph (EEG) sites (C3 and C4, Fz), two eye lead channels (right and left outer canthus), mental/submental electromyogram (EMG), one channel electrocardiogram (EKG; modified lead ll), anterior tibialis by EMG, snore sounds recorded by microphone placed on neck, air flow measured by nasal thermistor, indirect respiratory effort (thoracic and abdominal movement by electropiezo transducer) and SaO_2 (i.e., blood oxygen saturation) by pulse oximetry. All of the above electrodes are necessary to rule out occult sleep disorders.

Actigraphy

An actigraph contains an accelerometer encased in a wristwatch-like device that is typically worn on the dominant wrist and provides objective information about sleep–wake patterns and circadian rhythms based on behavior (i.e., motor activity). Some newer models come equipped with event markers or integral ambient light sensors. The premise of actigraphy is that a lack of movement is associated with sleep. An actigraph is capable of long-term monitoring for 24 hours a day (a minimum of 3 days; 1 week is recommended). The completion of a daily sleep diary concurrent with actigraphic measurement is recommended to verify daily bedtimes and waking times. Actigraphy is appropriate for use with both child, adolescent, and adult populations, and in particular may be useful for several special populations (e.g., elderly/nursing home patients, infants, psychiatric patients, and individuals in inaccessible situations, such as space; Littner, Kushida, et al., 2003). Actigraphy gives a valid and reliable estimate of sleep in normal, healthy adult populations but may be less reliable as sleep becomes more disturbed (Ancoli-Israel et al., 2003). Older algorithms found that actigraphy overestimated sleep (by 25–49 minutes) in people with insomnia, because they would lie awake in bed motionless, which was scored as sleep (Hauri & Wisbey, 1992; Jean-Louis, Zizi, Von Gizycki, & Hauri, 1999). However, newer, more sensitive algorithms have found that actigraphy provides a satisfactory measure of four out of five sleep variables (number of awakenings, wake after sleep onset, total sleep time, and sleep efficiency) compared with PSG (Lichstein et al., 2006).

Recommendations

The recommendations to follow are for clinical purposes only. Readers interested in research assessment of insomnia are directed to Buysse et al.'s (2006) recommendations, which were specifically developed for those purposes. The breadth of areas that need assessment during an insomnia intake (sleep, medical, and mental) are significant enough that it is probably unwise to do such an assessment without some form of structured or semistructured interview. These interviews provide significant benefits, such as increased consistency and accuracy, the importance of which cannot be overstated. Any of the insomnia interviews reviewed, *when combined with sleep diaries*, should give sufficient data for the correct diagnosis and treatment of insomnia. The IIS appears to be the best choice because it provides enough data to determine diagnosis for billing purposes, appears to perform an adequate review of medical systems, and comes in the very useful text written by Morin (1993), which gives an excellent description of the assessment and cognitive-behavioral treatment of insomnia. Use of a self-report sleep diary is essential in the assessment of insomnia, and nearly so during treatment. Numerous versions of sleep diaries are currently available, none of which shows superior utility.

The self-report measures described herein can provide the clinician with a much richer picture of his or her patients and would allow the clinician to publish case studies should the opportunity arise. We generally suggest using only one of the measures listed under each general category (e.g., fatigue, depression). However, we cannot recommend one over another within the categories. When alternatives exist within a category, they generally have similar reliability and validity data.

In terms of biological assessments, neither PSG nor actigraphy is generally recommended for the routine assessment of insomnia (Littner, Hirshkowitz, et al., 2003; Littner, Kushida, et al., 2003; Littner et al., 2004). PSG may be indicated when the sleep history reveals symptoms or signs indicative of an occult sleep disorder (e.g., apnea, PLMD) or when treatment of insomnia has failed. Actigraphy can serve as a convenient objective measure of sleep over longer periods of time, which may be preferable to sleep diaries or single time-point estimates in many situations (i.e., residential populations or individuals with low intelligence).

In the era of managed care, in which most clinicians may not have time to perform an extensive battery when assessing insomnia, a 15-minute algorithm can be used. Combined with sleep diaries (preferably completed beforehand), the clinician should perform a brief history of the sleep complaint (e.g., precipitants, duration, intensity, and daytime consequences) and then assess for comorbid disorders (mental, physical, and sleep) or substances that may be causing the insomnia. Thus equipped, the clinician can hopefully determine whether immediate treatment is advisable, whether a more detailed assessment is necessary, or whether a referral is warranted.

Differential Diagnosis

To this point we have only made allusions to differential diagnosis because it is such a complex topic, with varying opinions regarding importance for treatment. Insomnia can be a sign that another severe mental, physical, or sleep disorder is present that deserves immediate treatment. It is beyond the scope of this chapter to go into details about all of the disorders that are important to consider within the differential diagnosis of insomnia, but following are some of the most common differential diagnoses that should be considered. It is important to note that several studies have now shown that even when insomnia is comorbid with another disorder, it is still treatable with behavioral approaches specifically targeting only the insomnia (Stepanski & Rybarczyk, 2006) and that the comorbid disorder sometimes improves as well (Taylor, Lichstein, Weinstock, Sanford, & Temple, 2007).

Insomnia is an associated criterion in most psychiatric disorders, making this a common area that needs to be considered in differential diagnosis. The five categories of psychiatric disorders most commonly seen in patients presenting with sleep complaints are psychoses, mood disorders, anxiety disorders, panic disorder, and alcoholism. It is important to assess for all of these, as well as for other psychiatric disorders, during the first interview, with an attempt to determine sequencing when evaluating insomnia within the context of other psychiatric disorders. If insomnia follows the onset of one of these disorders, it is likely more important to treat the other psychiatric disorder first and see whether insomnia subsequently improves. However, if the two disorders only covary some of the time, it is probably safe to conclude that the insomnia is a separate entity requiring separate treatment.

There are also several medical disorders and medications commonly associated with insomnia, and these also should be considered in differential diagnosis. The medical disorders most commonly comorbid with insomnia include chronic pain, hypertension, gastrointestinal problems, and breathing problems. These should all be assessed while taking the medical history. Hyperthyroidism is another medical disorder that can result in significant insomnia, and patients should generally be referred to their primary care physicians to be tested for this during their first evaluation. The classes of medications that can cause insomnia include selective serotonin reuptake inhibitors and beta adrenoreceptor agonists (i.e., beta blockers). When assessing insomnia it is always important to review what medications a patient is taking, what the side effects of those medications are, and, finally, when he or she is taking them (i.e., late afternoon administration of alerting medications is worse than early morning administration).

Finally, other sleep disorders, such as circadian rhythm disorders, sleep apnea, PLMD, and restless-legs syndrome, can all be misconstrued as insomnia, so particular attention should also be paid to these disorders within differential diagnosis. Circadian rhythm disorders are often overlooked in the differential diagnosis of insomnia. Circadian rhythms incompatible with societal sleep–wake schedule demands can lead to difficulties initiating or maintaining sleep. Perhaps the quickest method to determine a patient's endogenous circadian rhythm is to ask him or her what he or she thinks the ideal biological bed- and wake times would be if he or she did not have to go to work or other obligations. If the times are more than 2–3 hours off of a reasonable bedtime (9–11 P.M.), then it is likely that he or she has a circadian rhythm disorder. The use of sleep diaries can provide a more detailed picture of the patient's sleep cycle; patients with circadian rhythm disorders will often show a 2–3 hour shift in bedtime and waking time (often with an increase in total sleep time to reverse sleep debt) on the weekends, when they are not forced into the sleep schedule required by work and other obligations. Patients with delayed sleep phase will describe very late bedtimes and waking times, whereas those with advanced sleep phase will describe very early times. Another self-report measure that may be helpful in determining circadian phase is the Morningness–Eveningness Scale (Horne & Ostberg, 1976).

Sleep apnea is characterized by multiple breathing stoppages during sleep that last at least 10 seconds, and patients with this disorder sometimes report heavy snoring, daytime sleepiness, and waking up gasping or choking during the night. Risk factors for sleep apnea include: age over 30 years, being male or a postmenopausal female, obesity, having a large neck (i.e., > 17 inches for men and > 16 inches for women), and craniofacial abnormalities (Guilleminault & Abad, 2004; Malhotra & White, 2002). PLMD is characterized by frequent involuntary limb movements that occur during sleep and result in awakenings. Relatedly, restless-legs syndrome, which is sometimes concurrent with PLMD, is characterized by complaints of itchy, tingling legs at night, which can be misconstrued as sleep-onset insomnia. In the case of apnea and PLMD, the patient frequently is unaware of what is happening while he or she is asleep, and all he or she reports is frequent awakenings during the night, which can be misconstrued as insomnia. PSG is the best way to diagnose these two disorders, but current guidelines suggest using PSG in insomnia assessment only if there is a strong suspicion of other sleep disorders (Sateia, Doghramji, Hauri, & Morin, 2000).

REFERENCES

American Academy of Sleep Medicine. (2005). *International classification of sleep disorders: Diagnostic and coding manual* (2nd ed.). Westchester, IL: Author.

American Psychiatric Association. (2000). *Diagnostic and statistical manual of mental disorders* (4th ed., text rev.). Washington, DC: Author.

American Psychiatric Association. (2013). *Diagnostic and statistical manual of mental disorders* (5th ed.). Arlington, VA: Author.

American Sleep Disorders Association. (1997). *International classification of sleep disorders—revised: Diagnostic and coding manual*. Rochester, MN: Author.

Ancoli-Israel, S., Cole, R., Alessi, C., Chambers, M., Moorcroft, W., & Pollak, C. P. (2003).

The role of actigraphy in the study of sleep and circadian rhythms. *Sleep, 26*(3), 342–392.

Bagby, R. M., Ryder, A. G., Schuller, D. R., & Marshall, M. B. (2004). The Hamilton Depression Rating Scale: Has the gold standard become a lead weight? *American Journal of Psychiatry, 161*(12), 2163–2177.

Barnes, L. L. B., Harp, D., & Jung, W. S. (2002). Reliability generalization of scores on the Spielberger State–Trait Anxiety Inventory. *Educational and Psychological Measurement, 62*(4), 603–618.

Bastien, C., Vallieres, A., & Morin, C. (2001). Validation of the Insomnia Severity Index as an outcome measure for insomnia research. *Sleep Medicine, 2,* 297–307.

Beck, A. T., & Steer, R. A. (1993). *Beck Depression Inventory: Manual.* San Antonio, TX: Psychological Corporation.

Beck, A. T., Steer, R. A., Ball, R., & Ranieri, W. F. (1996). Comparison of Beck Depression Inventories–IA and II in psychiatric outpatients. *Journal of Personality Assessment, 67*(3), 588–597.

Beck, A. T., Steer, R. A., & Garbin, M. G. (1988). Psychometric properties of the Beck Depression Inventory: Twenty-five years of evaluation. *Clinical Psychology Review, 8,* 77–100.

Blais, F. C., Gendron, L., Mimeault, V., & Morin, C. M. (1997). Evaluation de l'insomnie: Validation de trois questionnaires. *L'Encephale, 23*(6), 447–453.

Brodman, K., Erdmann, A. J., Lorge, I., & Wolff, H. G. (1949). The Cornell Medical Index: An adjunct to medical interview. *Journal of the American Medical Association, 140,* 530–534.

Brodman, K., Erdmann, A. J., Jr., Lorge, I., Wolff, H. G., & Broadbent, T. H. (1951). The Cornell Medical Index–Health Questionnaire: II. As a diagnostic instrument. *Journal of the American Medical Association, 145*(3), 152–157.

Buysse, D. J., Ancoli-Israel, S., Edinger, J. D., Lichstein, K. L., & Morin, C. M. (2006). Recommendations for a standard research assessment of insomnia. *Sleep, 29*(9), 1155–1173.

Buysse, D. J., Reynolds, C. F., III, Monk, T. H., Berman, S. R., & Kupfer, D. J. (1989). The Pittsburgh Sleep Quality Index: A new instrument for psychiatric practice and research. *Psychiatry Research, 28*(2), 193–213.

Carney, C. E., Buysse, D. J., Ancoli-Israel, S., Edinger, J. D., Krystal, A. D., Lichstein, K. L., et al. (2012). The Consensus Sleep Diary: Standardizing prospective sleep self-monitoring. *Sleep, 35*(2), 287–302.

Carskadon, M. A., Dement, W. C., Mitler, M. M., Guilleminault, C., Zarcone, V. P., & Spiegel, R. (1976). Self-reports versus sleep laboratory findings in 122 drug-free subjects with complaints of chronic insomnia. *American Journal of Psychiatry, 133*(12), 1382–1388.

Coursey, R. D., Frankel, B. L., Gaarder, K. R., & Mott, D. E. (1980). A comparison of relaxation techniques with electrosleep therapy for chronic, sleep-onset insomnia: A sleep-EEG study. *Biofeedback and Self Regulation, 5*(1), 57–73.

Edinger, J. D., Bonnet, M. H., Bootzin, R. R., Doghramji, K., Dorsey, C. M., Espie, C. A., et al. (2004). Derivation of research diagnostic criteria for insomnia: Report of an American Academy of Sleep Medicine Work Group. *Sleep, 27*(8), 1567–1596.

Edinger, J. D., Kirby, A. C., Lineberger, M. D., Loiselle, M. M., Wohlgemuth, W. K., & Means, M. K. (2006). *Duke Structured Interview Schedule for DSM-IV-TR and International Classification of Sleep Disorders (ICSD-2): Sleep disorder diagnoses.* Unpublished manual.

Endicott, J., Nee, J., Harrison, W., & Blumenthal, R. (1993). Quality Of Life Enjoyment And Satisfaction Questionnaire: A new measure. *Psychopharmacology Bulletin, 29*(2), 321.

First, M. B., Gibbon, M., Spitzer, R. L., Williams, J. B. W., & Benjamin, L. S. (1997). *Structured Clinical Interview for DSM-IV Axis II Personality Disorders (SCID-II).* Washington, DC: American Psychiatric Press.

First, M. B., Spitzer, R. L., Gibbon, M., & Williams, J. B. W. (1996). *Structured Clinical Interview for DSM-IV Axis I Disorders, Clinician Version (SCID-CV).* Washington, DC: American Psychiatric Press.

Guilleminault, C., & Abad, V. C. (2004). Obstructive sleep apnea syndromes. *Medical Clinics of North America, 88*(3), 611–630, viii.

Hauri, P. J., & Wisbey, J. (1992). Wrist actigraphy in insomnia. *Sleep, 15*(4), 293–301.

Horne, J. A., & Ostberg, O. (1976). A self-assessment questionnaire to determine morningness–eveningness in human circadian rhythms. *International Journal of Chronobiology, 4*(2), 97–110.

Jean-Louis, G., Zizi, F., Von Gizycki, H., & Hauri, P. (1999). Actigraphic assessment of sleep in insomnia: Application of the Acti-graph Data Analysis Software (ADAS). *Physiology and Behavior, 65*(4–5), 659–663.

Katz, D. A., & McHorney, C. A. (1998). Clinical correlates of insomnia in patients with chronic illness. *Archives of Internal Medicine, 158*(10), 1099–1107.

Krupp, L. B., LaRocca, N. G., Muir-Nash, J., & Steinberg, A. D. (1989). The Fatigue Severity Scale: Application to patients with multiple sclerosis and systemic lupus erythematosus. *Archives of Neurology, 46*(10), 1121–1123.

Lecrubier, Y., Sheehan, D. V., Weiller, E., Amorim, P., Bonora, I., Sheehan, K. H., et al. (1997). The Mini International Neuropsychiatric Interview (MINI): A short diagnostic structured interview: Reliability and validity according to the CIDI. *European Psychiatry, 12*(5), 224–231.

Lichstein, K. L., Means, M. K., Noe, S. L., & Aguillard, R. N. (1997). Fatigue and sleep disorders. *Behaviour Research and Therapy,* 733–740.

Lichstein, K. L., Stone, K. C., Donaldson, J., Nau, S. D., Soeffing, J. P., Murray, D., et al. (2006). Actigraphy validation with insomnia. *Sleep, 29*(2), 232–239.

Littner, M., Hirshkowitz, M., Kramer, M., Kapen, S., Anderson, W. M., Bailey, D., et al. (2003). Practice parameters for using polysomnography to evaluate insomnia: An update. *Sleep, 26*(6), 754–760.

Littner, M., Kushida, C. A., Anderson, W. M., Bailey, D., Berry, R. B., Davila, D. G., et al. (2003). Practice parameters for the role of actigraphy in the study of sleep and circadian rhythms: An update for 2002. *Sleep, 26*(3), 337–341.

Littner, M. R., Kushida, C., Anderson, W. M., Bailey, D., Berry, R. B., Hirshkowitz, M., et al. (2004). Practice parameters for the dopaminergic treatment of restless legs syndrome and periodic limb movement disorder. *Sleep, 27*(3), 557–559.

Maffei, C., Fossati, A., Agostoni, I., Barraco, A., Bagnato, M., Donati, D., et al. (1997). Interrater reliability and internal consistency of the Structured Clinical Interview for DSM-IV Axis II Personality Disorders (SCID-II), version 2.0. *Journal of Personality Disorders, 11*(3), 279–284.

Malhotra, A., & White, D. P. (2002). Obstructive sleep apnoea. *Lancet, 360*(9328), 237–245.

McHorney, C. A., Ware, J. E., Jr., Lu, J. F., & Sherbourne, C. D. (1994). The MOS 36-Item Short-Form Health Survey (SF-36): III. Tests of data quality, scaling assumptions, and reliability across diverse patient groups. *Medical Care, 32*(1), 40–66.

McHorney, C. A., Ware, J. E., Jr., & Raczek, A. E. (1993). The MOS 36-Item Short-Form Health Survey (SF-36): II. Psychometric and clinical tests of validity in measuring physical and mental health constructs. *Medical Care, 31*(3), 247–263.

Morin, C. M. (1993). *Insomnia: Psychological assessment and management.* New York: Guilford Press.

Ohayon, M. M. (2002). Epidemiology of insomnia: What we know and what we still need to learn. *Sleep Medicine Reviews, 6*(2), 97–111.

Rush, A. J., Giles, D. E., Schlesser, M. A., Fulton, C. L., Weissenburger, J., & Burns, C. (1986). The Inventory for Depressive Symptomatology (IDS): Preliminary findings. *Psychiatry Research, 18*(1), 65–87.

Rush, A. J., Guillon, C. M., Basco, M. R., Jarrett, R. B., & Trivedi, M. H. (1996). The Inventory of Depressive Symptomology (IDS): Psychometric properties. *Psychological Medicine, 26,* 477–486.

Rush, A. J., Trivedi, M. H., Carmody, T. J., Ibrahim, H. M., Markowitz, J. C., Keitner, G. I., et al. (2005). Self-reported depressive symptom measures: Sensitivity to detecting change in a randomized, controlled trial of chronically depressed, nonpsychotic outpatients. *Neuropsychopharmacology, 30*(2), 405–416.

Sateia, M., Doghramji, K., Hauri, P., & Morin, C. (2000). Evaluation of chronic insomnia. *Sleep, 23*(2), 1–24.

Schwartz, J. E., Jandorf, L., & Krupp, L. B. (1993). The measurement of fatigue: A new instrument. *Journal of Psychosomatic Research, 37*(7), 753–762.

Segal, D. L., Hersen, M., & Van Hasselt, V. B. (1994). Reliability of the Structured Clinical Interview for DSM-III-R: An evaluative review. *Comprehensive Psychiatry, 35*(4), 316–327.

Sheehan, D. V., Lecrubier, Y., Sheehan, K. H., Amorim, P., Janavs, J., Weiller, E., et al. (1998). The Mini-International Neuropsychiatric Interview (M.I.N.I): The development and validation of a structured diagnostic psychiatric interview for DSM-IV and ICD-10. *Journal of Clinical Psychiatry, 59*(Suppl. 20), 22–33.

Sheehan, D. V., Lecrubier, Y., Sheehan, K. H., Janavs, J., Weiller, E., Keskiner, A., et al.

(1997). The validity of the Mini International Neuropsychiatric Interview (MINI) according to the SCID-P and its reliability. *European Psychiatry, 12*(5), 232–241.

Simon, G. E., & VonKorff, M. (1997). Prevalence, burden, and treatment of insomnia in primary care. *American Journal of Psychiatry, 154*(10), 1417–1423.

Smets, E. M., Garssen, B., Bonke, B., & De Haes, J. C. (1995). The Multidimensional Fatigue Inventory (MFI): Psychometric qualities of an instrument to assess fatigue. *Journal of Psychosomatic Research, 39*(3), 315–325.

Spielberger, C. D., Gorsuch, R. L., Lushene, P. R., & Jacobs, G. A. (1983). *Manual for the State–Trait Anxiety Inventory: STAI (Form Y).* Palo Alto, CA: Consulting Psychologists Press.

Spielman, A. J., Saskin, P., & Thorpy, M. J. (1987). Treatment of chronic insomnia by restriction of time in bed. *Sleep, 10*, 45–55.

Steer, R. A., Beck, A. T., Brown, G., & Berchick, R. J. (1987). Self-reported depressive symptoms that differentiate recurrent-episode major depression from dysthymic disorders. *Journal of Clinical Psychology, 43*(2), 246.

Stepanski, E. J., & Rybarczyk, B. (2006). Emerging research on the treatment and etiology of secondary or comorbid insomnia. *Sleep Medicine Reviews, 10*(1), 7–18.

Taylor, D. J., Lichstein, K. L., & Durrence, H. H. (2003). Insomnia as a health risk factor. *Behavioral Sleep Medicine, 1*(4), 227.

Taylor, D. J., Lichstein, K. L., Durrence, H. H., Riedel, B. W., & Bush, A. J. (2005). Epidemiology of insomnia, depression, and anxiety. *Sleep, 28*(11), 1457–1464.

Taylor, D. J., Lichstein, K. L., Weinstock, J., Sanford, S., & Temple, J. (2007). A pilot study of cognitive-behavioral therapy of insomnia in people with mild depression. *Behavior Therapy, 38*(1), 49–57.

Taylor, D. J., Mallory, L. J., Lichstein, K. L., Durrence, H. H., Riedel, B. W., & Bush, A. J. (2007). Comorbidity of chronic insomnia with medical problems. *Sleep, 30*(2), 213–218.

Walsh, J. K., & Engelhardt, C. L. (1999). The direct economic costs of insomnia in the United States for 1995. *Sleep, 22*(Suppl. 2), S386–S393.

Zimmerman, M., & Mattia, J. I. (2001). The Psychiatric Diagnostic Screening Questionnaire: Development, reliability and validity. *Comprehensive Psychiatry, 42*(3), 175–189.

CHAPTER 20

HIV and AIDS

Anne-Lise C. Smith
Dean G. Cruess
Seth C. Kalichman

Recent estimates indicate that 1.2 million adolescents and adults were living with HIV infection in the United States at the end of 2006, with about one in five (21%) believed to be unaware of their diagnosis. An estimated 56,300 adolescents and adults were newly diagnosed with HIV infection in the United States in 2006 (Centers for Disease Control and Prevention [CDC], 2008; Hall et al., 2008). With the introduction of highly active antiretroviral therapy (HAART), people living with HIV/AIDS (PLWHA) show both improved disease prognosis and increased long-term survival; however, HIV/AIDS has now come to be viewed as a chronic, life-threatening illness with many challenges. Ample research demonstrates that biological and psychosocial factors are associated with quality of life, disease progression, and mortality among PLWHA (e.g., Leserman et al., 2007). Individuals with HIV disease are confronted with a host of psychosocial stressors in addition to the progressive loss of physical functioning. Some major transitions that HIV-positive individuals are confronted with include serostatus notification, viral load changes, and the transition from HIV to AIDS, each of which may elicit a variety of strong psy-

chological reactions. Moreover, prevalence rates of psychiatric and substance use disorders are disproportionately higher among PLWHA as compared with the general population (Bing et al., 2001). Thus a thorough biopsychosocial assessment is central to effective disease management.

This chapter discusses the assessment of psychological and neurocognitive disorders and other factors that commonly occur among PLWHA. The psychological assessment of PLWHA does not differ greatly from the assessment of individuals with other medical and psychiatric conditions; however, emphasis is placed on specific areas of the evaluation that are highlighted in this chapter. For example, we advocate that attention should be given to the presence of personal and familial psychiatric history, adjustment disorders, neurocognitive impairment, substance use, HIV risk behaviors, and adherence to treatment. Within the domain of psychiatric disorders, we believe that special attention should also be given to the assessment of trauma and abuse histories, which are shown to be associated with behaviors that place people at initial risk for HIV infection and also perhaps disease progression. Trained mental health professionals can assist with the differential diagnosis of psychiatric and neurocognitive disorders. Moreover, thorough biopsychosocial assessment may lead to effective treatment of disorders, which may subsequently aid in the efficacy of and adherence to HAART as well.

Mood Disorders among PLWHA

Mood disorders are associated with emotional distress, maladaptive coping strategies, substance use, poor adherence to HAART, and risk behaviors associated with the spread of HIV (Boarts, Sledjeski, Bogart, & Delahanty, 2006; Meade, Graff, Griffin, & Weiss, 2008; Treisman, Fishman, Schwartz, Hutton, & Lyketsos, 1998). Due to space limitations, we focus our attention on depression and bipolar disorder among PLWHA.

Depression

Depression is one of the most common presenting mental health problems among PLWHA, but it is frequently underdiagnosed and undertreated (Asch et al., 2003). Estimates of depression in individuals who are HIV positive range from 5 to 36%, depending on demographic characteristics, disease stage, and diagnostic methods employed (Bing et al., 2001; Cruess et al., 2003). A meta-analysis of 10 studies indicated that PLWHA are not at higher risk of depression by virtue of their health status (Ciesla & Roberts, 2001). Rather, epidemiological evidence suggests that depression rates among PLWHA are consistent with respective subpopulations at risk for HIV/AIDS. For instance, gay men who are HIV positive show similar rates of depression to those of gay men who are HIV negative; both groups have higher rates of depression than the general population (Cruess, 2003; Evans & Perkins, 1990). Similar rates of depression have also been found among injection drug users who are HIV positive and their uninfected counterparts (Lipsitz et al., 1994). Because depression is known to have an impact on immune functioning, it is especially important to assess and treat depressive symptoms among PLWHA.

Depression has been linked to decrements in specific indicators of immune functioning relevant to persons with HIV/AIDS. Studies have found that increased levels of depressive symptoms are associated with decreased numbers and also decline of CD4 cell counts (white blood cells that help fight infection) over time (Burack et al., 1993; Ickovics et al., 2001; Ironson et al., 1994; Leserman et al., 2000; Lyketsos, Hoover, et al., 1993). In a recent study, higher levels of depressive symptoms were associated with lower number of CD4 cells among HIV-positive individuals in rural Uganda (Kaharuza et al., 2006). Other studies have also found that depressive symptoms adversely affect the number and function of killer lymphocytes (Alciati, Gallo, Monforte, Brambilla, & Mellado, 2007; Leserman et al., 1997; Evans et al., 2002), which are a vital part of the innate immune system with the functional capacity to destroy HIV-infected cells and inhibit HIV infection of cells by suppressing HIV entry and replication. There is also evidence that reductions in depressive symptoms can enhance natural killer (NK) cell activity in patients with HIV. For example, Cruess and colleagues (2005) evaluated 57 women with HIV-positive diagnoses and found an association between a resolution of major depression and increased NK cell activity over a 2-year period. Because depression affects elements of the immune system vital to the health and well-being of individuals who are HIV positive, it is important to assess for depression among all persons with HIV/AIDS.

In a longitudinal study of gay men with HIV-positive diagnoses, Leserman, Petitto, and Gu (2002) found that depressive symptoms were associated with more rapid disease progression. Specifically, over the course of 9 years, depressive symptoms predicted faster onset of AIDS-defining conditions. The reverse was not true, in that disease progression did not predict subsequent depression. Also, individuals who reported having depression prior to the study were 5 times more likely to develop a recurrent depressive episode over the course of the study (Leserman et al., 2002). Similarly, in the San Francisco Men's Health Study, researchers found that depression was associated with faster progression to AIDS over 9 years of the study. Men with HIV-positive diagnoses who met depression cutoff scores on the Center for Epidemiologic

Studies Depression Scale (CES-D; Radloff, 1977) at baseline progressed to AIDS more quickly compared with participants who reported fewer depressive symptoms at baseline (Page-Shafer, Delorenze, Satariano, & Winkelstein, 1996). For many individuals, it appears that developing depression in HIV is related to having a personal history of depression. There is also evidence that depression may accelerate HIV disease progression; thus depression warrants thorough evaluation and treatment.

Other pertinent issues must be considered when conducting assessments among PLWHA. As discussed earlier, major depression is not caused by the HIV infection per se but may result from the demands placed on the individual (Leserman et al., 2002). It is also the case that a history of depression may precede the onset of HIV. Another important facet of depression in PLWHA is the experience of AIDS-related stigmas. Studies in the United States and in Africa show a close association between depressive symptoms and internalized stigma beliefs (Lee, Kochman, & Sikkema, 2002; Simbayi et al., 2007). People with HIV who endorse beliefs regarding self-blame, self-degradation, and being contaminated are more likely to be depressed than their counterparts. In fact, internalized AIDS stigmas predict depressive symptoms over and above other common correlates of depression, including health status.

Consequently, levels of depressive symptoms should be evaluated in PLWHA. It is not necessary for symptoms to reach diagnostic criteria for major depressive disorder in order to affect the health and health-related behaviors of PLWHA. It should be noted that HIV and some medications can cause physical and vegetative symptoms that mimic depression. Somatic symptoms secondary to HIV, such as fatigue and weight loss, can overlap with symptoms of depression and artificially inflate scores on depression inventories, thus confounding the assessment of depression among PLWHA. Accordingly, depression should be assessed among PLWHA by employing instruments that emphasize cognitive–affective symptoms of depression. The Beck Depression Inventory (BDI; Beck, Ward, Mendelson, Mock, & Erbaugh, 1961), the CES-D (Radloff, 1977), and the Hamilton Depression

Rating Scale (HDRS; Hamilton, 1960; Williams, 1988) are all widely used self-report scales that can be modified so that cognitive and affective items are emphasized. For example, the first 12 items of the 21-item BDI can be used as a cognitive–affective depression subscale (Kalichman, Sikkema, & Somlai, 1995), and somatic symptoms can also be excluded from the CES-D (Burack et al., 1993; Moore et al., 1999). Eleven items of the 17-item HDRS reflect cognitive–affective symptoms (Leserman et al., 1997; Morrison, Petitto, & Have, 2002) and have been used effectively to evaluate depression among PLWHA. Interviewers should be mindful of specific symptom endorsements on standard depression inventories and semistructured interviews, rather than relying on standard cutoff scores, in order to distinguish between cognitive–affective depression and somatic symptoms due to HIV disease.

Although revised versions are now available for the BDI and the CES-D (i.e., the BDI-II; Beck, Steer, & Brown, 1996; and the CES-D-R; Eaton, Muntaner, & Smith, 1998), the original versions, mentioned before, continue to be the most widely used and cited measures in studies of PLWHA. As such, the original versions are included in this chapter. Even though the BDI, the CES-D, and the HRSD (see Table 20.1) are very helpful screening instruments, they are not sufficient for establishing a diagnosis of depression. A diagnosis of major depression requires an interview that includes personal and familial history and exclusion of other causes of altered mental status, such as cognitive impairment or side effects of treatment.

In sum, a thorough assessment helps to differentiate between overlapping symptoms of depression and HIV and also to determine whether current complaints of depression preceded or are secondary to HIV. Depression should not be considered an inevitable response to living with HIV/AIDS. Rather, providers must carefully assess for depressive symptoms and also communicate to their patients that depression is a treatable disorder that responds well to both psychotherapy and medication. Treatment of depression may alleviate symptoms, improve treatment adherence, and also improve health status.

TABLE 20.1. Diagnostic and Screening Measures for the Biopsychosocial Assessment of PLWHA

Name of measure	Construct measured	Format	Reference
	Mood disorders		
Beck Depression Inventory (BDI)	Depressive symptoms	Self-report measure, 21 items, takes about 5–10 minutes.	Beck et al. (1961)
Center for Epidemiologic Studies Depression Scale (CES-D)	Depressive symptoms	Self-report measure, 20 items, takes about 5 minutes.	Radloff (1977)
Hamilton Depression Rating Scale (HDRS)	Depressive symptoms	Clinician-administered scale, 17 items, takes about 15–20 minutes.	Hamilton (1960); Williams (1988)
Mood Disorder Questionnaire (MDQ)	Bipolar disorder; lifetime history of mania or hypomania symptoms	Self-report screening instrument, 13 items, takes about 10 minutes.	Hirschfeld et al. (2000)
	Posttraumatic stress disorder		
Structured Clinical Interview for DSM-IV (SCID; PTSD module)	Diagnosis of PTSD	Clinician-administered diagnostic interview, 21 items, takes about 15–45 minutes.	Spitzer et al. (1990)
Posttraumatic Stress Diagnostic Scale (PDS)	PTSD symptoms	Self-report screening measure, 49 items, takes about 10–15 minutes.	Foa (1995)
Impact of Event Scale— Revised (IES-R)	Subjective distress caused by traumatic or stressful life events. Yields Intrusion, Avoidance, and Hyperarousal subscales.	Self-report screening measure, 22 items, takes about 5–10 minutes.	Weiss et al. (1997)
	Neurocognitive disorders		
Modified HIV dementia scale (M-HDS)	HIV-associated dementia (HAD)	Patient-completed screening instrument, 4 areas, takes about 5–7 minutes.	Davis et al. (2002)
	Substance and alcohol use disorders		
CAGE Questionnaire	Alcohol abuse or dependence	Clinician-administered or self-report screening instrument, 4 questions, takes about 1 minute.	Ewing (1984)
Alcohol Use Disorders Identification Test (AUDIT)	Hazardous or harmful alcohol consumption	Clinician-administered or self-report, 10 items, takes about 2–3 minutes.	Babor et al. (2001)
Drug Abuse Screening Test (DAST)	Abuse of or dependence on substances other than alcohol	Structured interview or self-report, available in 28-, 20-, or 10-item versions.	Skinner (1982)
	HIV risk behaviors		
Risk Assessment Battery (RAB)	Sexual and drug risk behaviors associated with HIV transmission	Self-report questionnaire, 45 items, takes less than 15 minutes.	Metzger et al. (2001)

(continued)

TABLE 20.1. *(continued)*

Name of measure	Construct measured	Format	Reference
	Adherence to HAART		
AIDS Clinical Trials Group (ACTG) Adherence Interview	Adherence to combination antiretroviral therapy	Self-report measure, 5 areas, takes about 5–10 minutes.	Chesney et al. (2000)
Unannounced telephone-based pill counts	Adherence to medications	Telephone contact is made unannounced once every 21–28 days, and patients count their pills in their homes.	Kalichman et al. (2007, 2008)
Millon Behavioral Medicine Diagnostic (MBMD)	Psychosocial factors that affect medical treatment. Can be used to predict problems with adherence.	Self-report measure, 165 items, takes about 20–25 minutes.	Millon et al. (2001)
Medication Adherence Training Instrument (MATI)	Assesses medication adherence, provides education, and enhances patient motivation	Structured clinician-administered protocol. Initial interview takes about 60 minutes. Two follow-up visits take about 10–20 minutes each.	McPherson-Baker et al. (2005)
	HIV/AIDS-related quality of life		
Revised Functional Assessment of HIV Infection Quality of Life Instrument (FAHI)	HIV-related quality of life	Self-report measure, 44 items, takes about 10–15 minutes.	Peterman et al. (1997)
Medical Outcomes Study HIV Health Survey (MOS-HIV)	HIV-related quality of life	Self-report measure, 35 items, takes about 5–10 minutes.	Wu et al. (1997)

Bipolar Disorder/Mania

Bipolar disorder is a type of serious mental illness that is characterized by manic, hypomanic, or mixed episodes that alternate with depressive episodes (American Psychiatric Association, 2013). When individuals are manic, they may demonstrate extremely elated or irritable mood, racing thoughts, and decreased need for sleep and may engage in impulsive and high-risk behaviors. Evidence suggests that comorbid bipolar and substance use disorders are common. For instance, in an epidemiological study, more than half (56%) of individuals with bipolar disorders also reported lifetime substance use disorders (Regier et al., 1990). Concurrent mania and substance abuse may place individuals at greater risk for HIV. In a recent study of individuals with comorbid

bipolar and substance use disorders, recent manic episode and severity of drug use (e.g., cocaine, stimulants) predicted increased risk of engaging in sexual behaviors associated with HIV, including sex with multiple partners, paying to have sex with prostitutes, and sex trading (Meade et al., 2008). Symptoms of mania, such as hypersexuality and disinhibition, may be amplified by substance use and thus hinder safer-sex practices. It is important to refer individuals with bipolar disorder for treatment, so as to improve their functioning and prevent symptoms from progressing.

Although there are multiple causes for mania, it is typically associated with a personal or familial history of bipolar disorder. In a retrospective chart review of 162 patients with HIV, Lyketsos, Hanson, and Fishman (1993) identified 14 patients who had experienced mania either early or late in the course of HIV. Individuals who experienced a manic episode in the early, asymptomatic stages of HIV infection were more likely to have a personal or familial history of mood disorder and thus likely had a genetic predisposition to mania. In contrast, individuals who experienced their first manic episode in the later stages of immunosuppression, after the onset of AIDS, were less likely to have a personal or familial history of mood disorder; these individuals were also more likely to have dementia. Accordingly, late-onset or "AIDS mania" is likely due to primary effects of the virus on the central nervous system and is associated with a more severe presentation (Lyketsos, Hanson, & Fishman, 1993; Treisman et al., 1998).

Given that primary and secondary mania appear to have different symptom profiles, clinicians need to conduct a comprehensive interview to assess for these mood-related symptoms and need to be sure to inquire about family history and any prior episodes of these events. The Mood Disorders Questionnaire (MDQ; Hirschfeld et al., 2000) is a brief screening instrument that can be used to detect a lifetime history of manic or hypomanic symptoms (see Table 20.1). The MDQ is not intended to replace a clinical evaluation and does not establish a bipolar diagnosis. Questions appear face valid and simply assist in gathering information about manic and hypomanic symptoms. Individuals whose symptom endorsements are suggestive of a possible bipolar disorder should be referred for a thorough evaluation and treatment. The MDQ can also assist providers in identifying individuals for whom antidepressant medications may be contraindicated.

Trauma and Stress-Related Disorders among PLWHA

A considerable body of literature demonstrates that a history of childhood sexual abuse is highly prevalent among PLWHA. In studies of HIV-positive individuals, rates of childhood sexual abuse range between 15 and 68% across studies (Allers & Benjack, 1991; Kalichman, Gore-Felton, Ben-

otsch, Cage, & Rompa, 2004; Liebschutz, Feinman, Sullivan, Stein, & Samet, 2000; O'Leary, Purcell, Remien, & Gomez, 2003). In a study of men and women diagnosed HIV positive, Kalichman, Sikkema, DiFonzo, Luke, and Austin (2002) found that 68% of women and 35% of men reported sexual assault after the age of 15, approximately half of whom (51% of women and 46% of men) also reported sexual abuse in childhood. These studies indicate that rates of childhood sexual abuse are much higher among PLWHA than in the general population (24.7% for women and 16% for men; Felitti, Anda, & Nordenberg, 1998).

Childhood sexual abuse has long-term effects on later psychological functioning, including poorer self-esteem, increased depression, maladaptive coping strategies, and the tendency to experience revictimization in adulthood (Ehlers & Clark, 2000; Johnson & Harlow, 1996; Jumper, 1995). Early abuse experiences (including sexual, physical, and emotional abuse) are also associated with major public health problems, including but not limited to illicit drug use, alcoholism, and sexually transmitted diseases (Edwards et al., 2005; Felitti et al., 1998). Among both men and women, increased severity of childhood emotional, physical, or sexual abuse was found to be positively correlated with lifetime prevalence of sexually transmitted diseases (STDs; Medrano & Hatch, 2005). In another study, individuals who reported moderate to severe trauma symptoms, such as intrusions and avoidance, were more likely to report recent unprotected sexual intercourse (Gore-Felton & Koopman, 2002). Across studies, the experience of sexual abuse, whether as a child or as an adult, has been shown to be associated with increased sexual risk taking, having a greater number of lifetime partners, and substance use and dependence, all of which are risk factors for HIV infection (Gore-Felton & Koopman, 2002; Greenberg, 2001; Lodico & DiClemente, 1994; Rotheram-Borus, Mahler, & Koopman, 1996; Thompson, Kao, & Thomas, 2005; Wilsnack, Wilsnack, & Kristjanson, 2004). Thus the general consensus of these studies is that a history of trauma, and perhaps sexual abuse in particular, can have long-term emotional and behavioral consequences that may place the victim at risk for psychiatric disorders, high-risk sexual behaviors, and substance abuse, all of which have profound health implications for PLWHA. Trauma experiences are therefore a significant risk factor for HIV infection and subsequently a complicating factor for managing HIV/AIDS.

Recent research indicates that trauma severity also predicts mortality among patients with HIV disease. Leserman and colleagues (2007) found that lifetime trauma was associated with both all-cause and AIDS-related deaths in a sample of 611 individuals with HIV positive diagnoses studied over the course of 41 months. Participants who endorsed three or more categories of lifetime traumas (e.g., sexual abuse, physical abuse, childhood physical neglect, childhood emotional neglect; presence of other types of traumas that occurred before age 18, such as the death of an immediate family member [mother, father, or sibling]; or other lifetime traumas, such as the death of a spouse/partner) were about 3 times more likely to die of all-cause or AIDS-related deaths as compared with those who reported less than three trauma categories (Leserman et al., 2007). Evidence also suggests that trauma histories and posttraumatic stress symptoms are associated with poorer medication adherence among PLWHA (Boarts et al., 2006). If not assessed or if left untreated, trauma exposure can pose significant psychosocial, medical, and public health concerns, especially among PLWHA.

Some individuals who experience traumatic events may go on to develop posttraumatic stress disorder (PTSD; American Psychiatric Association, 2013). Criteria for a diagnosis of PTSD require direct or vicarious exposure to an extreme stressor that engenders a reaction of intense fear, horror, or helplessness. Characteristics of the event and the individual's perception of threat are subsumed under Criterion A in DSM-5 and must be present for a diagnosis of PTSD. People must also evidence one reexperiencing symptom (Criterion B), one avoidance symptom (Criterion C), two negative alterations in cognitions and mood (Criterion D), and two hyperarousal symptoms (Criterion E). Disturbance must persist for more than 1 month (Criterion F) and interfere with role functioning (Criteria G; 2013).

A thorough screening and assessment of trauma history, PTSD symptoms, and maladaptive coping strategies that may interfere with disease management are vital for PLWHA. Methods of assessment range from structured clinical interviews that yield specific diagnoses to standardized paper-and-pencil measures that quantify symptom severity. The Structured Clinical Interview for DSM-IV (SCID) is the most widely used and researched diagnostic interview (Spitzer, Williams, Gibbon, & First, 1990). However, the SCID requires special training and often an extensive clinical background to administer. Validated self-report measures include the Posttraumatic Stress Diagnostic Scale (PDS; Foa, 1995; Foa, Cashman, Jaycox, & Perry, 1997) and the Impact of Event Scale—Revised (IES-R; Weiss & Marmar, 1996). The PDS quantifies the severity of PTSD symptoms and has been used widely across a variety of traumatized populations. The IES-R assesses psychological responses to traumatic or stressful life events and has also been used widely across a variety of traumatized populations, including among them PLWHA (Sikkema et al., 2007). The PDS and the IES-R (see Table 20.1) are brief screening instruments and are not intended to replace structured diagnostic interviews. If PLWHA meet criteria for PTSD, a referral should be made to a licensed professional for appropriate evaluation and treatment.

It is not necessary for symptoms to meet all diagnostic criteria for PTSD in order to affect health and health-related behavior of PLWHA. Evidence suggests that partial PTSD, defined as having at least one symptom in each DSM criterion category, can be associated with significant functional impairment (Stein, Walker, Hazen, & Forde, 1997). That being said, it is of note that many people exposed to trauma do not go on to develop diagnosable PTSD or even show long-term impairments in physical or psychological well-being (Kessler, Sonnega, & Bromet, 1995; Ozer, Best, Lipsey, & Weiss, 2001). Furthermore, research shows that some individuals report growth from trauma (Tedeschi & Calhoun, 1995), so it is important to understand during the assessment process that traumatic events and individuals' reactions to trauma vary widely and do not necessarily lead to poor mental and physical outcomes.

Adjustment Disorder

Major depressive disorder and PTSD should be distinguished from adjustment disorder (AD), which is characterized by excessive and prolonged distress in response to stressful life circumstances. Symptoms should not meet criteria for another mental disorder (American Psychiatric Association, 2013). Whereas normative stress reactions tend to subside within a reasonable time frame, AD entails sufficient, and sometimes chronic, distress as to justify clinical attention. As mentioned previously, individuals with HIV disease are confronted with a host of psychosocial stressors in addition to the progressive loss of physical functioning (e.g., serostatus notification, the transition from HIV to AIDS, stigmas associated with health and lifestyle status). At each of these events, it is not uncommon for individuals to have a variety of strong psychological reactions, including overwhelming grief and suicidal thoughts (Treisman & Angelino, 2004). Thus it is important that PLWHA receive supportive counseling at the time of HIV testing and at subsequent changes in health status. Clinicians should refer to DSM-5 (American Psychiatric Association, 2013) to diagnose AD.

HIV-Associated Neurocognitive Disorders

Neurocognitive impairment occurs frequently across the HIV disease spectrum. The virus enters the central nervous system (CNS) in the early stages of infection, which can result in numerous cognitive, motor, and behavioral changes (Ferrando, 2000). Data indicate that HIV-associated mild neurocognitive disorder (MND), previously termed minor cognitive motor disorder (MCMD), and HIV-associated dementia (HAD) result from primary effects of the virus on the brain. Diagnostic criteria for these disorders were originally developed by the American Academy of Neurology AIDS Task Force in 1991. Recently, a working group sponsored by the National Institute of Mental Health and the National Institute of Neurological Diseases and Stroke revised the existing categories and diagnostic criteria and also proposed asymptomatic neurocognitive

impairment (ANI) as a third HIV-induced neurocognitive disorder (Antinori et al., 2007). These conditions range in degree from mild to severe neurocognitive impairment. Given that even mild decrements in neurocognitive functioning are found to be associated with increased mortality among PLWHA (Mayeux et al., 1993; Wilkie et al., 1998), it is important to assess neurocognitive symptoms in the early stages of the disease, so as to establish a baseline and also to observe changes in impairment over time.

Asymptomatic Neurocognitive Impairment

Asymptomatic neurocognitive impairment (ANI) is characterized by mild neurocognitive impairment without evidence of associated functional impairment. A diagnosis of ANI requires acquired impairment in at least two cognitive domains, as determined by neuropsychological testing. Impairment must not meet criteria for delirium or dementia, interfere with activities of daily living, nor be due to other etiology (Antinori et al., 2007). Antinori and colleagues (2007) provide recommendations for the assessment and diagnosis of ANI, MND, and HAD.

Mild Neurocognitive Disorder

Mild neurocognitive disorder (MND) results in mild to moderate neurocognitive impairment that interferes with work and activities of daily living. MND is characterized by milder symptom expression and functional impairment as compared with HAD and does not necessarily lead to HAD. Both MND and HAD are diagnoses of exclusion (Ferrando, 2000); other causes of neurocognitive impairment must be ruled out before establishing either diagnosis. Criteria for MND involve acquired mild to moderate impairment in at least two cognitive domains, as determined by neuropsychological testing. In addition, neurocognitive impairment must cause mild functional impairment, patients should not meet criteria for delirium or dementia, and symptoms should not be due to other etiology (Antinori et al., 2007). A patient who meets criteria for MND should be referred for a clinical neurological consultation or neuropsychological testing. Goodkin and colleagues (2001) report that MND may be more responsive to treatment, as it does not exhibit levels of neuronal cell death observed in HIV-associated dementia.

HIV-Associated Dementia

Moderate to severe impairments of neurocognitive functioning, including HAD, are common in the advanced stages of immunosuppression. HAD is a subcortical dementia that is characterized by progressive cognitive and functional impairment. Criteria for HAD require marked impairment in at least two cognitive domains, as determined by neuropsychological testing. Disturbance must cause moderate to severe impairment in work or activities of daily living and should not be due to other etiology (Antinori et al., 2007).

It is important to evaluate levels of neurocognitive impairment in PLWHA. Brief screening instruments can assist with the detection of possible impairment and help determine whether patients should be referred for more comprehensive neuropsychological testing and evaluation. The Mini-Mental State Examination (MMSE; Folstein, Folstein, & McHugh, 1975) has been widely used to screen for suspected cases of dementia. However, the MMSE is more sensitive to cortical deficits and does not adequately assess subcortical impairments associated with HAD (McArthur, 1994). The HIV Dementia Scale (HDS; Power, Selnes, Grim, & McArthur, 1995) is a more sensitive instrument than the MMSE in detecting HAD, and it has been found to distinguish between individuals with frank dementia and those who are cognitively unimpaired (Power et al., 1995). The HDS does not, however, demonstrate adequate sensitivity in detecting subtle neurocognitive impairments (Bottiggi et al., 2007). It should be noted that the HDS includes a subtest on attention that involves measuring antisaccadic eye movements, which has been challenging for non-neurologists to administer (Davis, Skolasky, Selnes, Burgess, & McArthur, 2002). A modified HIV dementia scale (M-HDS; Davis et al., 2002) excludes the item on attention and thus is simpler for non-neurologists to administer (see Table 20.1). Scores of ≤ 10 on the original HDS and of ≤ 7.5 on the M-HDS are indicative of possible HAD. Individuals who score at or below the cutoffs should be referred for neuropsychological evaluation. A diagnosis of HAD requires a history and neurological exam, exclusion of other causes of altered mental status, and neuropsychological testing.

It is important to note that symptoms of HAD (e.g., impaired concentration, apathy, irritability, social withdrawal) can be mistaken for depression. Neuropsychological testing is helpful in differentiating between HIV-related neurological impairments and other psychiatric symptoms. Ultimately, advanced neuropsychological testing is critically important in detecting HIV-related cognitive and neurological change. In particular, early sensitive and reliable diagnosis, including differential diagnosis between neurocognitive disorders and confounding conditions, remains a central focus in the future assessment and treatment of PLWHA.

Comorbidity

High rates of comorbid conditions are observed among PLWHA (Disney, Kidorf, & Kolodner, 2006; Israelski et al., 2007; Pence, Miller, & Whetten, 2006). It is particularly important to assess co-occurring mood disorders, ADs, posttraumatic stress, neurocognitive impairment, substance and alcohol abuse, and HIV risk behaviors. When present, consideration needs to be given to treating these co-occurring disorders concurrently. It is also important to assess levels of adherence to treatment recommendations. Routine use of screening and assessment tools can help to identify and diagnose psychiatric and neurocognitive syndromes and other factors that commonly co-occur in HIV (see Table 20.1). Careful assessment and diagnosis can lead to appropriate treatment referrals, which may lead to symptom relief, improved adherence, and improved health outcomes for PLWHA.

Behavioral Factors among PLWHA

Substance Use and Abuse

Substance use has been a major factor in the spread of HIV infection since the beginning of the AIDS epidemic, as HIV can be spread directly through the sharing of contaminated needles used for injection. Noninjection drugs and alcohol are also associated with the spread of HIV, due to the disinhibiting effects of substance use on decision making and sexual risk taking. In one study, researchers found that HIV incidence rates were higher among recently infected individuals who reported amphetamine use within the past year (6.3% per year) as compared with nonusers (2.1% per year; Buchacz et al., 2005). Amphetamine and its derivative methamphetamine, in particular, are associated with HIV and other sexually transmitted diseases (Mimiaga et al., 2008; Schwarcz et al., 2007; Urbina & Jones, 2004) and with high-risk sexual behaviors, including unprotected anal sex and having multiple sexual partners (Halkitis, Green, & Carragher, 2006; Halkitis, Shrem, & Martin, 2005). Research demonstrates that the probability of spreading or contracting HIV infection increases as the number of sexual partners increases, particularly when sex partners are concurrent, that is, overlapping in time (Morris & Kretzschmar, 1997). It is of note that methamphetamine use has increased among gay and bisexual men, particularly in urban areas, and is prevalent in circuit parties and commercial sex environments (Halkitis, Green, & Mourgues, 2005). It is also common for methamphetamine users to engage in other substance abuse, thereby creating the complicated pattern of polydrug abuse.

In addition to facilitating high-risk sexual activity, substance use can also be dangerous for people who are taking antiretroviral medications. Illicit substances may have dangerous interactions with some medications included in HAART regimens. In particular, some protease inhibitors are metabolized through the same hepatic pathway as recreational drugs, with the potential for hazardous interactions. Substance abusers are also at risk for nonadherence to medication regimens, which can increase the chances of treatment failure, especially with regard to antiretroviral resistance, which can develop with even minimal nonadherence.

Alcohol abuse is commonly assessed among PLWHA using standardized instruments such as the CAGE Questionnaire (Ewing, 1984) and the Alcohol Use Disorders Identification Test (AUDIT; Babor, Higgins-Biddle, Saunders, & Monteiro,

2001). Other substance use is commonly assessed using the Drug Abuse Screening Test (DAST; Skinner, 1982). These measures are well established and provide useful screening information that should be followed up with clinical diagnostic evaluations (Maisto, Carey, Carey, Gordon, & Gleason, 2000). See Table 20.1 for alcohol and substance-related screening tools.

HIV Risk Behaviors

The Risk Assessment Battery (RAB; Metzger, Nalvaline, & Woody, 2001) is a valid and reliable screening instrument that assesses HIV risk behaviors in the preceding month. It was designed for use in substance-using populations. The RAB (see Table 20.1) comprises two subscales that assess HIV-related sexual and drug risk behaviors. The subscales are summed to generate a total risk score (0–64). Individuals who endorse risk behaviors should be encouraged to seek HIV testing if they are unaware of their disease status. Additionally, both individuals who are HIV positive and those who are uninfected who express interest in modifying risk behaviors should be provided with referrals to HIV risk-reduction services (e.g., drug treatment, STD/HIV prevention counseling; CDC, 2006).

Treatment Adherence

Antiretroviral therapies effectively suppress HIV replication and improve the health of people living with HIV/AIDS. Although pharmacological profiles vary, most antiretroviral (ARV) regimens demand at least 85% adherence to achieve optimal clinical outcomes and to avoid development of resistant viral strains (Bangsberg, Kroetz, & Deeks, 2007). Studies have shown that PTSD and depressive symptoms predict lower adherence to HIV medications, with depression also predicting the poor medical outcomes that stem from failed HIV treatments, namely lower CD4 cell counts and elevated HIV in the blood (e.g., viral load; Boarts et al., 2006). Other research demonstrates that patients who receive antidepressive medication are more adherent to HAART than those who do not receive antidepressant medication (Barton, Kobayashi, Maravi, & Yun, 2005). These findings underscore the importance of assessing mental health disorders that affect disease progression and medication adherence. Assessment and treatment of psychiatric disorders among PLWHA may lead to improvements in both medication adherence and disease course.

The most common means of monitoring medication adherence relies on self-report, often relying on adapted versions of the AIDS Clinical Trials Group (ACTG) Adherence Interview (Chesney et al., 2000). This instrument asks individuals to think back over the previous week and recall whether medications were missed, followed by a day-by-day assessment for the previous 3 days. Recall over the previous week is emphasized in addition to the previous 3 days to ensure including weekend doses. In a comprehensive literature review of self-reported HIV treatment adherence instruments, Simoni and colleagues (2006) indicated that the ACTG Interview has demonstrated evidence for reliability and predictive validity. Reynolds and colleagues (2007) offer recommendations for administering the ACTG Interview in clinical settings. Self-reported adherence can also be assessed using a single item that asks patients to estimate the percentage of their medications that they took in the past week, using a visual analogue scale with anchors for 0, 50, and 100% of doses taken. The single-item visual analogue scale corresponds well with other measures of adherence, as well as HIV viral load (Giordano, Guzman, Clark, Charlebois, & Bangsberg, 2004).

The Millon Behavioral Medicine Diagnostic (MBMD; Millon, Antoni, Millon, Meagher, & Grossman, 2001) can be used to identify patients who may be at increased risk for poor adherence and who may thus benefit from adherence counseling (Cruess, Minor, Antoni, & Millon, 2007). The MBMD is a measure of psychosocial factors that influence individuals' responses to medical treatment. In particular, the MBMD Medication Abuse scale, which measures facets of medication noncompliance, has been used successfully to predict adherence problems in a sample of patients with HIV-positive diagnoses (Cruess et al., 2007). With regard to interventions aimed at improving adherence, the Medication Adherence Training Instrument (MATI; McPherson-Baker, Jones, Durán, Klimas, & Schneiderman, 2005) is a manualized protocol that assesses adherence to HAART, provides education about HIV disease and its treatment, and empowers patients to improve their adherence.

An objective approach to clinically monitoring medication adherence involves the use of pill counts. Unfortunately, office-based pill counts are often suspect because patients will not always bring all of their medications to be counted and because some patients may avoid bringing all of their medications to avoid revealing their nonadherence (e.g., pill dumping). Office-based pill counts are unfortunately among the least reliable means of measuring adherence, achieving only 75% sensitivity for detecting nonadherence to ARV regimens (Giordano et al., 2004). The primary sources of error in office-based pill counts stem from patients failing to have all of their pills with them at the time of the count. To resolve the limitations posed by office-based pill counts, Bangsberg, Hecht, Charlebois, Chesney, and Moss (2001) developed a home-based pill-counting procedure. Unannounced home-based pill counts have demonstrated a high degree of correspondence with other objective measures of medication adherence, including significantly corresponding with plasma viral load. However, unannounced home-based pill counts are typically not feasible for use in clinical care.

A recent adaptation of the unannounced pill count uses the telephone to conduct unannounced pill counts in the patient's home. Kalichman and colleagues (Kalichman et al., 2007, 2008) developed an unannounced telephone-based pill count and observed high degrees of concordance with pill counts conducted during unannounced home visits. In addition, telephone-based unannounced pill counts correspond to patient viral load in expected directions. Although unannounced telephone-based pill counts have not yet been tested for use in clinical care settings, this approach may hold considerable promise for use in medication adherence monitoring. See Table 20.1 for adherence-related instruments.

HIV-Related Quality of Life

Quality of life refers to individuals' perceived emotional, social, and physical functioning and well-being. Global measures of quality of life assess the impacts of illness and treatment on patients' day-to-day functioning and well-being over time. Quality of life among PLWHA can be assessed using the revised Functional Assessment of Human Immunodeficiency Virus Infection (FAHI; Peterman, Cella, Mo, & McCain, 1997) and the Medical Outcomes Study HIV Health Survey (MOS-HIV; Wu, Revicki, Jacobson, & Malitz, 1997). Both measures have demonstrated reliability and validity in numerous clinical trials and are also appropriate for use in clinical settings (see Table 20.1).

Conclusion

In conclusion, a comprehensive approach to assessment of HIV and AIDS addresses biological, neurocognitive, and psychosocial factors associated with disease progression and quality of life among PLWHA. A thorough biopsychosocial assessment can help to differentiate between separate but overlapping disorders that commonly occur among PLWHA. Accurate diagnosis ultimately guides patients toward appropriate treatments that can help to alleviate symptoms of psychological distress, decrease HIV risk behaviors, and improve treatment adherence. Early intervention may also help to slow disease progression and lead to better treatment outcomes.

REFERENCES

Alciati, A., Gallo, L., Monforte, A. D., Brambilla, F., & Mellado, C. (2007). Major depression-related immunological changes and combination antiretroviral therapy in HIV-seropositive patients. *Human Psychopharmacology, 22*(1), 33–40.

Allers, C. T., & Benjack, K. J. (1991). Connections between childhood abuse and HIV infection. *Journal of Counseling and Development, 70,* 309–313.

American Academy of Neurology AIDS Task Force. (1991). Nomenclature and research case definitions for neurologic manifestations of human immunodeficiency virus-type 1 (HIV-1) infection: Report of a working group of the American Academy of Neurology AIDS Task Force. *Neurology, 41,* 778–785.

American Psychiatric Association. (2013). *Diagnostic and statistical manual of mental disorders* (5th ed.). Arlington, VA: Author.

Antinori, A., Arendt, G., Becker, J. T., Brew, J. T., Byrd, D. A., Cherner, M., et al. (2007). Updated research nosology for HIV-associated neurocognitive disorders. *Neurology, 69,* 1789–1799.

Asch, S. M., Kilbourne, A. M., Gifford, A. L., Burnam, M. A., Turner, B., Shapiro, M. F., et al. (2003). Underdiagnosis of depression in HIV: Who are we missing? *Journal of General Internal Medicine, 18*(6), 450–460.

Babor, T. F., Higgins-Biddle, J. C., Saunders, J. B. & Monteiro, M. G. (2001). *AUDIT—The Alcohol Use Disorders Identification Test: Guidelines for use in primary care* (2nd ed.). Geneva, Switzerland: World Health Organization.

Bangsberg, D. R., Hecht, F. M., Charlebois, E. D., Chesney, M., & Moss, A. (2001). Comparing objective measures of adherence to HIV antiretroviral therapy: Electronic medication monitors and unannounced pill counts. *AIDS and Behavior, 5,* 275–281.

Bangsberg, D. R., Kroetz, D. L., & Deeks, S. G. (2007). Adherence-resistance relationships to combination HIV antiretroviral therapy. *Current HIV/AIDS Reports, 4,* 65–72.

Barton, P. L., Kobayashi, J. S., Maravi, M., & Yun, L. W. II. (2005). Antidepressant treatment improves adherence to antiretroviral therapy among depressed HIV-infected patients. *Journal of Acquired Immune Deficiency Syndrome, 38,* 432–438.

Beck, A. T., Steer, R. A., & Brown, G. K. (1996). *Manual for Beck Depression Inventory—II (BDI-II).* San Antonio, TX: Psychological Corporation.

Beck, A. T., Ward, C. H., Mendelson, M., Mock, J., & Erbaugh, J. (1961). An inventory for measuring depression. *Archives of General Psychiatry, 4,* 53–63.

Bing, E., Burnam, M., Longshore, D., Fleishman, J., Sherbourne, C., London, A., et al. (2001). Psychiatric disorders and drug use among human immunodeficiency virus-infected adults in the United States. *Archives of General Psychiatry, 58,* 721–728.

Boarts, J. M., Sledjeski, E. M., Bogart, L. M., & Delahanty, D. L. (2006). The differential impact of PTSD and depression on HIV disease markers and adherence to HAART in people living with HIV. *AIDS and Behavior, 10*(3), 253–261.

Bottiggi, K. A., Chang, J. J., Schmitt, F. A, Avison, M. J., Mootoor, Y., Nath, A., et al. (2007). The HIV Dementia Scale: Predictive power in mild dementia and HAART. *Journal of Neurological Sciences, 260*(1–2), 11–15.

Buchacz, K., McFarland, W., Kellogg, T. A., Loeb, L., Holmberg, S. D., Dilley, J., et al. (2005). Amphetamine use is associated with increased HIV incidence among men who have sex with men in San Francisco. *AIDS, 19*(13), 1423–1424.

Burack, J. H., Barrett, D. C., Stall, R. D., Chesney, M. A., Ekstrand, M. L., & Coates, T. J. (1993). Depressive symptoms and CD4 lymphocyte decline among HIV-infected men. *Journal of the American Medical Association, 270*(21), 2568–2573.

Centers for Disease Control and Prevention. (2006). Revised recommendations for HIV testing of adults, adolescents, and pregnant women in health-care settings. *Morbidity and Mortality Weekly Report, 55*(RR14), 1–17.

Centers for Disease Control and Prevention. (2008). HIV prevalence estimates—United States, 2006. *Morbidity and Mortality Weekly Report, 57*(39), 1073–1076.

Chesney, M. A., Ickovics, J. R., Chambers, D. B., Gifford, A. L., Neidig, J., Zwickl, B., et al. (2000). Self-reported adherence to antiretroviral medications among participants in HIV clinical trials: The AACTG adherence instruments. Patient Care Committee and Adherence Working Group of the Outcomes Committee of the Adult AIDS Clinical Trials Group (AACTG). *AIDS Care, 12*(3), 255–266.

Ciesla, J. A., & Roberts, J. E. (2001). Meta-analysis of the relationship between HIV infection and risk for depressive disorders. *American Journal of Psychiatry, 58*(5), 725–730.

Cruess, D. G., Douglas, S. D., Petitto, J. M., Ten Have, T., Gettes, D., Dubé, B., et al. (2005). Association of resolution of major depression with increased natural killer cell activity among HIV-seropositive women. *American Journal of Psychiatry, 162*(11), 2125–2130.

Cruess, D. G., Evans, D. L., Repetto, M. J., Gettes, D., Douglas, S. D., & Petitto, J. M. (2003). Prevalence, diagnosis, and pharmacological treatment of mood disorders in HIV disease. *Biological Psychiatry, 54*(3), 307–316.

Cruess, D. G., Minor, S., Antoni, M. H., & Millon, T. (2007). Utility of the Millon Behavioral Medicine Diagnostic (MBMD) to predict adherence to highly active antiretroviral therapy (HAART) medication regimens among HIV-positive men and women. *Journal of Personality Assessment, 89*(3), 277–290.

Davis, H. F., Skolasky, R. L., Selnes, O. A., Burgess, D. M., & McArthur, J. C. (2002). Assessing HIV-associated dementia: Modified HIV dementia scale versus the grooved pegboard. *AIDS Read, 12*(1), 29–38.

Disney, E., Kidorf, M., & Kolodner, K. (2006). Psychiatric comorbidity is associated with drug use and HIV risk in syringe exchange participants. *Journal of Nervous and Mental Disease, 194*(8), 577–583.

Eaton, W., Muntaner, C., & Smith, C. (1998). *Revision of the Center for Epidemiologic Studies Depression (CES-D) Scale.* Baltimore: Johns Hopkins University Prevention Center.

Edwards, V. J., Anda, R. F., Dube, S. R., Dong, M., Chapman, D. F., & Felitti, V. J. (2005). The wide-ranging health consequences of adverse childhood experiences. In K. Kendall-Tackett & S. Giacomoni (Eds.), *Child victimization: Maltreatment, bullying, and dating violence prevention and intervention* (pp. 8–12). Kingston, NJ: Civic Research Institute.

Ehlers, A., & Clark, D. M. (2000). A cognitive model of posttraumatic stress disorder. *Behaviour Research and Therapy, 38*(4), 319–345.

Ewing, J. A. (1984). Detecting alcoholism: The CAGE Questionnaire. *Journal of the American Medical Association, 252,* 1905–1907.

Evans, D. L., & Perkins, D. O. (1990). The clinical psychology of AIDS. *Current Opinions in Psychiatry, 3,* 96–102.

Evans, D. L., Ten Have, T. R., Douglas, S. D., Gettes, D. R., Morrison, M., Chiappini, M. S., et al. (2002). Association of depression with viral load, CD8 T lymphocytes, and natural killer cells in women with HIV infection. *American Journal of Psychiatry, 159*(10), 1752–1759.

Felitti, V. J., Anda, R. F., & Nordenberg, D. (1998). Relationship of childhood abuse and household dysfunction to many of the leading causes of death in adults: The Adverse Childhood Experiences (ACE) Study. *American Journal of Preventive Medicine, 14*(4), 245–258.

Ferrando, S. J. (2000). Diagnosis and treatment of HIV-associated neurocognitive disorders. *New Directions for Mental Health Services, 87,* 25–35.

Foa, E. B. (1995). *Posttraumatic Stress Diagnostic Scale: Manual.* Minneapolis, MN: National Computer Systems.

Foa, E. B., Cashman, L., Jaycox, L., & Perry, K. (1997). The validation of a self-report measure of posttraumatic stress disorder: The Posttraumatic Diagnostic Scale. *Psychological Assessment, 9*(4), 445–451.

Folstein, M. F., Folstein, S. E., & McHugh, P. R. (1975). Mini-Mental State: A practical method for grading the cognitive state of patients for the clinician. *Journal of Psychiatric Research, 12,* 189–198.

Giordano, T. P., Guzman, D., Clark, R., Charlebois, E. D., & Bangsberg, D. (2004). Measuring adherence to antiretroviral therapy in a diverse population using a visual analogue scale. *HIV Clinical Trials, 5,* 74–79.

Goodkin, K., Wilkie, F. L., Concha, M., Hinkin, C. H., Symes, S., Baldewicz, T. T., et al. (2001). Aging and neuro-AIDS conditions and the changing spectrum of HIV-1-associated morbidity and mortality. *Journal of Clinical Epidemiology, 54*(12, Suppl. 1), S35–S43.

Gore-Felton, C., & Koopman, C. (2002). Traumatic experiences: Harbinger of risk behavior among HIV-positive adults. *Journal of Trauma and Dissociation, 3*(4), 121–135.

Greenberg, J. B. (2001). Childhood sexual abuse and sexually transmitted diseases in adults: A review of implications for STD/HIV programs. *International Journal of STD and AIDS, 12,* 778–783.

Halkitis, P. N., Green, K. A., & Carragher, D. J. (2006). Methamphetamine use, sexual behavior, and HIV seroconversion. *Journal of Gay and Lesbian Psychotherapy, 10*(3/4), 95–109.

Halkitis, P. N., Green, K. A., & Mourgues, P. (2005). Longitudinal investigation of methamphetamine use among gay and bisexual men in New York City: Findings from Project BUMPS. *Journal of Urban Health, 82*(Suppl. 1), 18–25.

Halkitis, P. N., Shrem, M. T., & Martin, F. W. (2005). Sexual behavior patterns of methamphetamine-using gay and bisexual men. *Substance Use and Misuse, 40,* 703–709.

Hall, H. I., Song, R., Rhodes, P., Prejean, J., An, Q., Lee, L. M., et al. (2008). Estimation of HIV incidence in the United States. *Journal of the American Medical Association, 300*(5), 520–529.

Hamilton, M. (1960). A rating scale for depression. *Journal of Neurology, Neurosurgery and Psychiatry, 23,* 56–62.

Hirschfeld, R. M., Williams, J. B., Spitzer, R. L., Calabrese, J. R., Flynn, L., Keck, P. E., Jr., et al. (2000). Development and validation of a screening instrument for bipolar spectrum disorder: The Mood Disorder Questionnaire. *American Journal of Psychiatry, 157*(11), 1873–1875.

Ickovics, J. R., Hamburger, M. E., Vlahov, D., Schoenbaum, E. E., Schuman, P., Boland, R. J., et al. (2001). Mortality, CD4 cell count decline, and depressive symptoms among HIV-seropositive women: Longitudinal analysis from the HIV Epidemiology Research Study. *Journal of the American Medical Association, 285*(11), 1466–1474.

Ironson, G., Friedman, A., Klimas, N., Antoni, M., Fletcher, M. A., Laperriere, A., et al. (1994). Distress, denial, and low adherence to behavioral interventions predict faster disease progression in gay men infected with human immunodeficiency virus. *International Journal of Behavioral Medicine, 1*(1), 90–105.

Israelski, D. M., Prentiss, D. E., Lubega, S., Balmas, G., Garcia, P., Muhammad, M., et al. (2007). Psychiatric co-morbidity in vulnerable populations receiving primary care for HIV/AIDS. *AIDS Care, 19*(2), 220–225.

Johnson, L., & Harlow, L. (1996). Childhood sexual abuse linked with adult substance use, victimization, and AIDS risk. *AIDS Education and Prevention, 8,* 44–57.

Jumper, S. A. (1995). A meta-analysis of the relationship of child sexual abuse to adult psychological adjustment. *Child Abuse and Neglect, 19,* 715–728.

Kaharuza, F. M., Bunnell, R., Moss, S., Purcell, D. W., Bikaako-Kajura, W., Wamai, N., et al. (2006). Depression and CD4 cell count among persons with HIV infection in Uganda. *AIDS and Behavior, 10*(Suppl. 1), S105–S111.

Kalichman, S. C., Amaral, C., Cherry, C., Flanagan, J., Pope, H., Eaton, L., et al. (2008). Monitoring antiretroviral adherence by unannounced pill counts conducted by telephone: Reliability and criterion-related validity. *HIV Clinical Trials, 9,* 298–308.

Kalichman, S. C., Amaral, C. M., Stearns, H., White, D., Flanagan, J., Pope, H., et al. (2007). Adherence to antiretroviral therapy assessed by unannounced pill counts conducted by telephone. *Journal of General Internal Medicine, 22,* 1003–1006.

Kalichman, S. C., Gore-Felton, C., Benotsch, E., Cage, M., & Rompa, D. (2004). Trauma symptoms, sexual behaviors, and substance abuse: Correlates of childhood sexual abuse and HIV risks among men who have sex with men. *Journal of Child Sexual Abuse, 13*(1), 1–15.

Kalichman, S. C., Sikkema, K. J., DiFonzo, K., Luke, W., & Austin, J. (2002). Emotional adjustment in survivors of sexual assault living with HIV-AIDS. *Journal of Traumatic Stress, 15,* 189–296.

Kalichman, S. C., Sikkema, K. J., & Somlai, A. (1995). Assessing persons with human immunodeficiency virus (HIV) infection using the Beck Depression Inventory: Disease processes and other potential confounds. *Journal of Personality Assessment, 64*(1), 86–100.

Kessler, R. C., Sonnega, A., & Bromet, E. (1995). Posttraumatic stress disorder in the National Comorbidity Survey. *Archives of General Psychiatry, 52*(12), 1048–1060.

Lee, R., Kochman, A., & Sikkema, K. (2002). Internalized stigma among people living with HIV/AIDS. *AIDS and Behavior, 6,* 309–319.

Leserman, J., Pence, B. W., Whetten, K., Mugavero, M. J., Thielman, N. M., Swartz, M. S., et al. (2007). Relation of lifetime trauma and depressive symptoms to mortality in HIV. *American Journal of Psychiatry, 164*(11), 1707–1713.

Leserman, J., Petitto, J. M., Golden, R. N., Gaynes, B. N., Gu, H., Perkins, D. O., et al. (2000). Impact of stressful life events, depression, social support, coping, and cortisol on progression to AIDS. *American Journal of Psychiatry, 157*(8), 1221–1228.

Leserman, J., Petitto, J. M., & Gu, H. (2002). Progression to AIDS, a clinical AIDS condition and mortality: Psychosocial and physiological predictors. *Psychological Medicine, 32*(6), 1059–1073.

Leserman, J., Petitto, J. M., Perkins, D. O., Folds, J. D., Golden, R. N., & Evans, D. L. (1997). Severe stress, depressive symptoms, and changes in lymphocyte subsets in human immunodeficiency virus-infected men: A 2-year follow-up study. *Archives of General Psychiatry, 54*(3), 279–285.

Liebschutz, J. M., Feinman, G., Sullivan, L., Stein, M., & Samet, J. (2000). Physical and sexual abuse in women infected with the human immunodeficiency virus: Increased illness and health care utilization. *Archives of Internal Medicine, 160,* 1659–1664.

Lipsitz, J. D., Williams, J. B., Rabkin, J. G., Remien, R. H., Bradbury, M., el Sadr, W., et al. (1994). Psychopathology in male and female intravenous drug users with and with-

out HIV infection. *American Journal of Psychiatry, 151*(11), 1662–1668.

Lodico, M. A., & DiClemente, R. J. (1994). The association between childhood sexual abuse and prevalence of HIV-related risk behaviors. *Clinical Pediatrics, 33,* 498–502.

Lyketsos, C. G., Hanson, A. L., & Fishman, M. (1993). Manic syndrome early and late in the course of HIV. *American Journal of Psychiatry, 150*(2), 326–327.

Lyketsos, C. G., Hoover, D. R., Guccione, M., Senterfitt, W., Dew, M. A., Wesch, J., et al. (1993). Depressive symptoms as predictors of medical outcomes in HIV infection: Multicenter AIDS Cohort Study. *Journal of the American Medical Association, 270*(21), 2563–2567.

Maisto, S., Carey, M., Carey, K., Gordon, C., & Gleason, J. (2000). Use of the AUDIT and the DAST-10 to identify alcohol and drug use disorders among adults with a severe and persistent mental illness. *Psychological Assessment, 12,* 186–192.

Mayeux, R., Stern, Y., Tang, M. X., Todak, G., Marder, K., & Sano, M. (1993). Mortality risks in gay men with human immunodeficiency virus infection and cognitive impairment. *Neurology, 43*(1), 176–182.

McArthur, J. C. (1994). Neurological and neuropathological manifestations of HIV infection. In I. Grant & A. Martin (Eds.), *Neuropsychology of HIV infection* (pp. 56–107). New York: Oxford University Press.

McPherson-Baker, S., Jones, D., Durán, R. E., Klimas, N., & Schneiderman, N. (2005). Development and implementation of a medication adherence training instrument for persons living with HIV: The MATI. *Behavior Modification, 29*(2), 286–317.

Meade, C. S., Graff, F. S., Griffin, M. L., & Weiss, R. D. (2008). HIV risk behavior among patients with co-occurring bipolar and substance use disorders: Associations with mania and drug abuse. *Drug and Alcohol Dependence, 92,* 296–300.

Medrano, M. A., & Hatch, J. P. (2005). Childhood trauma, sexually transmitted diseases and the perceived risk of contracting HIV in a drug using population. *American Journal of Drug and Alcohol Abuse, 31*(3), 403–416.

Metzger, D. S., Nalvaline, H. A., & Woody, G. E. (2001). Assessment of substance abuse: HIV Risk Assessment Battery. In R. Carson-Dewitt (Ed.), *Encyclopedia of drugs, alcohol, and addictive behavior* (pp. 148–150). Framington Hills, MI: Macmillan Reference Books.

Millon, T., Antoni, M., Millon, C., Meagher, S., & Grossman, S., (2001). *Millon Behavioral Medicine Diagnostic.* Minneapolis, MN: NCS Assessments.

Mimiaga, M. J., Reisner, S. L., Vanderwarker, R., Gaucher, M. J., O'Connor, C. A., Medeiros, M. S., et al. (2008). Polysubstance use and HIV/STD risk behavior among Massachusetts men who have sex with men accessing Department of Public Health mobile van services: Implications for intervention development. *AIDS Patient Care and STDs, 22*(9), 745–751.

Moore, J., Schuman, P., Schoenbaum, E., Boland, B., Solomon, L., & Smith, D. (1999). Severe adverse life events and depressive symptoms among women with, or at risk for, HIV infection in four cities in the United States of America. *AIDS, 13,* 2459–2468.

Morris, M., & Kretzschmar, M. (1997). Concurrent partnerships and the spread of HIV. *AIDS, 11,* 641–648.

Morrison, M. F., Petitto, J. M., & Have, T. T. (2002). Depressive and anxiety disorders in women with HIV infection. *American Journal of Psychiatry, 159*(5), 789–796.

O'Leary, A., Purcell, D., Remien, R. H., & Gomez, C. (2003). Childhood sexual abuse and sexual transmission risk behaviour among HIV-positive men who have sex with men. *AIDS Care, 15*(1), 17–26.

Ozer, E. J., Best, S. R., Lipsey, T. L., & Weiss, D. S. (2001). Predictors of posttraumatic stress disorder and symptoms in adults: A meta-analysis. *Psychological Bulletin, 129,* 52–73.

Page-Shafer, K., Delorenze, G. N., Satariano, W. A., & Winkelstein, W. (1996). Comorbidity and survival in HIV-infected men in the San Francisco Men's Health Survey. *Annals of Epidemiology, 6*(5), 420–430.

Pence, B. W., Miller, W. C., & Whetten, K. (2006). Prevalence of DSM-IV-defined mood, anxiety, and substance use disorders in an HIV clinic in the southeastern United States. *Journal of Acquired Immune Deficiency Syndromes, 42*(3), 298–306.

Peterman, A. H., Cella, D., Mo, F., & McCain, N. (1997). Psychometric validation of the revised Functional Assessment of Human Immunodeficiency Virus Infection (FAHI) quality of life instrument. *Quality of Life Research, 6,* 572–584.

Power, C., Selnes, O. A., Grim, J. A., & McAr-
thur, J. C. (1995). HIV dementia scale: A rapid screening test. *Journal of Acquired Immune Deficiency Syndromes and Human Retrovirology, 8*(3), 273–278.

Radloff, L. (1977). The CES-D Scale: A self-report depression scale for research in the general population. *Applied Psychological Measurement, 1*(3), 85–401.

Regier, D. A., Farmer, M. E., Rae, D. S., Locke, B. Z., Keith, S. J., Judd, L. L., et al. (1990). Comorbidity of mental disorders with alcohol and other drug abuse: Results from the Epidemiologic Catchment Area (ECA) Study. *Journal of the American Medical Association, 264*(19), 2511–2518.

Reynolds, N. R., Sun, J., Nagaraja, H. N., Gifford, A. L., Wu, A. W., & Chesney, M. A. (2007). Optimizing measurement of self-reported adherence with the ACTG Adherence Questionnaire: A cross-protocol analysis. *Journal of Acquired Immune Deficiency Syndromes, 46*(4), 402–409.

Rotheram-Borus, M., Mahler, K. A., & Koopman, C. (1996). Sexual abuse history and associated multiple risk behavior in adolescent runaways. *American Journal of Orthopsychiatry, 66*(3), 390–400.

Schwarcz, S., Scheer, S., McFarland, W., Katz, M., Valleroy, L., Chen, S., et al. (2007). Prevalence of HIV infection and predictors of high-transmission sexual risk behaviors among men who have sex with men. *American Journal of Public Health, 97*(6), 1067–1075.

Sikkema, K. J., Hansen, N. B., Kochman, A., Tarakeshwar, N., Neufeld, S., Meade, C. S., et al. (2007). Outcomes from a group intervention for coping with HIV/AIDS and childhood sexual abuse: Reductions in traumatic stress. *AIDS and Behavior, 11*(1), 49–60.

Simbayi, L. C., Kalichman, S. C., Strebel, A., Cloete, A., Henda, N., & Mqeketo, A. (2007). Internalized stigma, discrimination, and depression among men and women living with HIV/AIDS in Cape Town, South Africa. *Social Science and Medicine, 64*(9), 1823–1831.

Simoni, J. M., Kurth, A. E., Pearson, C. R., Pantalone, D. W., Merrill, J. O., & Frick, P. A. (2006). Self-report measures of antiretroviral therapy adherence: A review with recommendations for HIV research and clinical management. *AIDS and Behavior, 10*(3), 227–245.

Skinner, H. (1982). The Drug Abuse Screening Test. *Addictive Behaviors, 7,* 363–371.

Spitzer, R. L., Williams, J. B. W., Gibbon, M., &

First, M. B. (1990). *Structured Clinical Interview for DSM-III-R—Patient edition* (SCID-P). Washington, DC: American Psychiatric Press.

Stein, M. B., Walker, J. R., Hazen, A. L., & Forde, D. R. (1997). Full and partial posttraumatic stress disorder: Findings from a community survey. *American Journal of Psychiatry, 154*, 1114–1119.

Tedeschi, R. G., & Calhoun, L. G. (1995). *Trauma and transformation: Growing in the aftermath of suffering.* Thousand Oaks, CA: Sage.

Thompson, J. C., Kao, T., & Thomas, R. J. (2005). The relationship between alcohol use and risk-taking sexual behaviors in a large behavioral study. *Preventive Medicine: An International Journal Devoted to Practice and Theory, 41*(1), 247–252.

Treisman, G., Fishman, M., Schwartz, J., Hutton, H., & Lyketsos, C. (1998). Mood disorders in HIV infection. *Depression and Anxiety, 7*(4), 178–187.

Treisman, G. J., & Angelino, A. F. (2004). *The psychiatry of AIDS: A guide to diagnosis and treatment.* Baltimore: Johns Hopkins University Press.

Urbina, A., & Jones, K. (2004). Crystal methamphetamine, its analogues, and HIV infection: Medical and psychiatric aspects of a new epidemic. *Clinical Infectious Diseases, 38*(6), 890–894.

Weiss, D., & Marmar, C. (1997). The Impact of Event Scale—Revised. In J. Wilson & T. Keane (Eds.), *Assessing psychological trauma and PTSD* (pp. 399–411). New York: Guilford Press.

Wilkie, F. L., Goodkin, K., Eisdorfer, C., Feaster, D., Morgan, R., Fletcher, M. A., et al. (1998). Mild cognitive impairment and risk of mortality in HIV-1 infection. *Journal of Neuropsychiatry, 10*(2), 125–132.

Williams, J. B. W. (1988). A structured interview guide for the Hamilton Depression Rating Scale. *Archives of General Psychiatry, 45*, 742–747.

Wilsnack, S. C., Wilsnack, R. W., & Kristjanson, A. F. (2004). Child sexual abuse and alcohol use among women: Setting the stage for risky sexual behavior. In L. J. Koenig, L. S. Doll, A. O'Leary, & W. Pequegnat (Eds.), *From child sexual abuse to adult sexual risk: Trauma, revictimization, and intervention* (pp. 181–200). Washington, DC: American Psychological Association.

Wu, A. W., Revicki, D. A., Jacobson, D., & Malitz, F. E. (1997). Evidence for reliability, validity and usefulness of the Medical Outcomes Study HIV Health Survey (MOS-HIV). *Quality of Life Research, 6*, 481–493.

PART IV

Assessment
of Special
Populations

CHAPTER 21

Cultural Concerns

Luz Garcini
Kate Murray
Jessica Barnack-Tavlaris
Elizabeth A. Klonoff

The existence, persistence, and negative impact of health disparities are now so well known and documented across so many indices (e.g., Klonoff, 2009; Smedley, Stith, & Nelson, 2002) that in 2010, as part of the Patient Protection and Affordable Care Act (Public Law 111-148), the National Center on Minority Health and Health Disparities was redesignated as an institute in itself, the National Institute on Minority Health and Health Disparities (U.S. Department of Health and Human Services, 2011). In the 2002 Institute of Medicine (IOM) report (Smedley et al., 2002), a number of sources for these disparities were identified. Although the IOM concluded that some of these sources are related to the way health care is administered in the United States, others appeared to be related to aspects of the clinical encounter itself. Because issues associated with the clinical encounter are more amenable to change, we focus primarily on those. These issues primarily center on clinical uncertainty when interacting with minority patients and clinician beliefs and stereotypes about the behavior or health of minorities. The IOM report went on to note that how patients respond to actual or perceived discriminatory behaviors from the

health care system can affect the extent to which patients display medical mistrust or refuse to comply with physician directives.

Essential to best addressing the needs of minority populations is the development and implementation of culture- and context-sensitive assessments. The use of culturally competent methods facilitates understanding of specific barriers and resources that are likely to influence treatment decisions and dynamics of the clinical encounter. Minority and culturally diverse populations are not exclusively ethnic and racial groups but also include people with disabilities and individuals who may be treated differently because of factors such as age, socioeconomic status, or sexual orientation. Nevertheless, this chapter focuses primarily on a discussion of cultural considerations in the assessment of ethnic and racial minorities with the caveat that the need for context-sensitive assessments among other minority groups is equally relevant.

Culture- and context-sensitive assessments of ethnic and racial minorities extend beyond categorization of groups to encompass the development of a deeper understanding of a group's shared values, beliefs, attitudes, experiences, and expectations

(Yali & Revenson, 2004). Thus this chapter presents an overview of the assessment of specific culturally relevant constructs, including ethnicity, discrimination, cultural concepts of disease and illness, and acculturation, that are important to the appropriate and effective treatment of ethnic/racial minorities. Although there are numerous other topics relevant to cross-cultural health psychology, such as the role of interpersonal dynamics, communication styles, and coping strategies, a more detailed analysis is outside the scope of this chapter. Although compilations of many measures across an array of ethnic groups are available (e.g., Davis & Engle, 2011), we have elected to identify those measures most often used in health-related research, as these are most likely to be relevant in clinical health psychology contexts.

An Overview of the Implications of Proxies in This Area

There is no a priori reason to believe that race or ethnicity alone actually accounts for the variance in health outcomes across groups. The search for biological differences across groups has long been a focus of medicine in the United States, rooted in arguments supporting slavery centuries ago and continuing up through the present day (Kawachi, Daniels, & Robinson, 2005). Yet the numbers of illnesses with clear genetic links (e.g., Tay–Sachs disease or sickle-cell anemia) are small (Adler & Rehkopf, 2008), and efforts to mitigate risk among genetically susceptible groups aim to reduce environmental conditions that trigger disease (Kawachi et al., 2005). Therefore, even in the limited instances in which biological differences are identified, the most salient point of intervention is with the social and environmental factors that can mitigate risk and improve health outcomes.

Instead of focusing on biological differences, many researchers focus on the degree to which race/ethnicity is a proxy for other factors. Socioeconomic status (SES) has been one of the most prominently identified confounders (Freeman, 1989, 2004; Kawachi et al., 2005). Racial and ethnic minority groups are much more likely to live in poverty in the United States, with approximately twice as many Blacks and Hispanics living below the poverty level as Whites in 2009 (U.S. Census Bureau, 2012). Living in poverty means that people do not have the financial resources to obtain adequate health care and experience a wide range of environmental hazards and daily living challenges. In fact, many studies have demonstrated that SES is a stronger predictor of health disparities than is race/ethnicity (Kawachi et al., 2005; Link & McKinlay, 2009; Ward et al., 2004). However, Kawachi and colleagues (2005) warn against viewing SES as a confounder of race because "race, as an ascriptive characteristic, is antecedent to class—that is, it is race that influences class position in the U.S. society, not the other way around" (p. 146). This is an important distinction that is explored in greater detail later in the chapter.

Educational attainment is another factor often included in measures of SES. Lower levels of educational attainment are linked to worse health outcomes and life expectancy across racial/ethnic groups (Braveman, Cubbin, Egerter, Williams, & Pamuk, 2010). Individuals with limited health literacy may not recognize symptoms or the need to have symptoms evaluated and may end up presenting for treatment at later stages of disease progression. Community education and patient navigator programs have arisen based on the need to assist individuals with lower health literacy to ensure appropriate awareness of and treatment for medical concerns. Although low health literacy is not unique to racial and ethnic minority groups, it is an additional factor that needs to be simultaneously assessed by health service providers.

Powers, Trinh, and Bosworth (2010) conducted a comprehensive computerized search of the literature from 1969 to 2010 in an effort to identify measures of health literacy that could quickly and easily be used by clinicians. Two somewhat time-intensive instruments were used as external criteria: the Test of Functional Health Literacy in Adults (TOFHLA; Parker, Baker, Williams, & Nurss, 1995), which has both an English and a Spanish version, and the Rapid Estimate of Adult Literacy in Medicine (REALM; Davis et al., 1993). The TOFHLA takes about 22 minutes to administer and involves answering 50 reading comprehension questions about three medically related prose passages; the REALM consists of 66 medical words that are read out loud, with points given for correct pronunciation. For brief multi-item assessments, Powers et al. (2010) suggest using either the Newest Vital Sign (Weiss et al., 2005) or the Medical Term Recognition Test (METER; Rawson et al., 2010). The Newest Vital Sign consists of reading and applying information from the nutritional label on a pint of ice cream, whereas the METER requires patients to discriminate medical words in a list that includes 40 medical and 40 nonmedical words. When there is time to ask only a single question, Powers et al. (2010) recommend "asking patients how confident they are filling out medical forms, how often they have someone help them read health information, or to rate their own reading ability" (p. 83) as a rough measure of health literacy.

Many members of underrepresented groups live in racially/ethnically segregated neighborhoods; recently there has been increased interest in the role that living in those neighborhoods may play in health disparities, particularly as it relates to health behaviors (e.g., Do et al., 2008). A full review of this area is beyond the scope of this chapter. However, the effects of living in a segregated neighborhood may have serious consequences for our understanding of health disparities. For example, Morland, Wing, Diez Roux, and Poole (2002) demonstrated that there were three times fewer places to consume alcohol in wealthy versus poor neighborhoods and four times as many supermarkets in White versus Black neighborhoods; these factors likely contribute to the differences in availability of fresh produce as a function of neighborhood racial characteristics (Morland & Filomena, 2007). Data also suggest that segregated neighborhoods have more fast-food outlets both overall (Block, Scribner, & DeSalvo, 2004) and as a proportion of the total number of available restaurants (Powell, Chaloupka, & Bao, 2007). Similarly, there are fewer recreational facilities in minority neighborhoods (Moore, Diez Roux, Evenson, McGinn, & Brines, 2008; Powell, Slater, Chaloupka, & Harper, 2006). There also are data to suggest that cancer risks associated with ambient air toxins are greater in extremely/highly segregated neighborhoods versus low/moderately segregated ones, and that this effect is greatest in Latino neighborhoods but is present in White, Black, and Asian neighborhoods as well (Morello-Frosch & Jesdale, 2006). Whereas the link between segregation and health outcomes appears to be fairly robust for Blacks, results for Latinos are much more inconsistent (e.g., Lee & Ferraro, 2007).

Segregation can affect the quality of medical care as well. Popescu, Cram, and Vaughan-Sarrazin (2011) looked at racial differences in the quality of hospitals and distance to the hospital for Medicare patients admitted with acute myocardial infarction. After accounting for distance, African Americans were less likely to be admitted to high-quality hospitals and more likely to be admitted to low-quality ones; however, when analyses matched patients by home ZIP code, these differences were no longer significant, suggesting that the differences were due, in part, to residential ZIP code characteristics. Similarly, Hao et al. (2011) demonstrated that health-related quality of life in cancer survivors was poorer for those living in highly segregated African American communities and that when segregation was included in the equation, racial differences were no longer significant.

Taken together, these results suggest that, when trying to plan for a health-related intervention, clinicians must ask about the nature of the neighborhood in which patients from underrepresented groups reside. Access to fresh fruits and vegetables, a safe environment in which to exercise, and other, similar constraints that may be present in segregated neighborhoods may require specific plans if an intervention is to be successful. Moreover, it is important to assess the various confounders and proxies detailed here within clinical settings. Additional information on assessment of these constructs is provided next.

Measures of Ethnicity

Part of initiating a diagnostic or treatment process involves having the patient share information about him- or herself. Typically this begins with demographic information, such as age, gender, occupation, disease/medical history, and race/ethnicity. Not surprisingly, each of these variables can have a profound impact on diagnosis and treatment. For example, certain medications end up being more potent for the elderly on a dose-for-dose basis, because of the increased time it takes for medication to clear the kidneys with age. Similarly, some medications approved for use by a man cannot safely be taken by a woman if there is any chance she might become pregnant while taking it. However, these same constraints may also apply to issues of race/ethnicity. For example, in 2005 the Food and Drug Administration approved BiDil, a fixed-dose combination of isosorbide dinitrate and hydralazine hydrochloride (i–h) used in the treatment of heart failure, only for those individuals who self-identify as "Black." This is the first drug ever approved for use only by one racial group. As personalized medicine becomes more of a reality, the development of other drugs (or even of various health psychology interventions) that appear to be effective with one racial/ethnic group versus another needs to be addressed.

Clearly, before one can begin to implement an intervention or even measure characteristics associated with different cultural, ethnic, or racial groups, one must first determine to which group a participant belongs. This is not as trivial a question as it may seem. For example, Moscou, Anderson, Kaplan, and Valencia (2003) found that 33% of 81 participants from one clinic and 22% of 59 participants from another clinic viewed their own race/ethnicity differently from how they were categorized in the clinics' databases, and one-quarter of all participants expressed a preference for being able to select more than one category versus being limited to a single one. Similar contradictory results have been reported for births in North Carolina (Buescher, Gizlice, & Jones-Vessey, 2005). Investigators have shown that how ethnicity questions are asked affects obtained responses (e.g., Harris-Kojetin & Mathiowetz, 1998); specifically, different question ordering has been shown to affect responses to race questions and racial identification.

The assessment of race and ethnicity has largely been based on the Office of Management and Budget (OMB) classification system established in 1977 and subsequently updated. Although information about race has been collected in the United States as early as the 1790 census, the 1977 directive established four major racial groups (White; Black; American Indian/Alaska Native; and Asian and Pacific Islander) and one ethnicity distinction (Hispanic or not Hispanic; Mays, Ponce, Washington, & Cochran, 2003). Although the assessment of these categories has expanded over the last 35 years, many highlight the limitations of this approach, including the lack of specificity within groups and confusion over the differentiation between race and ethnicity when individuals self-report. In addition, it was only with the 2000 Census that individuals were able to mark more than one racial category when self-identifying. In their detailed review of the evolution of race/ethnicity assessment, Mays et al. (2003) highlight the convoluted way race/ethnicity assessment in the United States has changed over this time and the ongoing limitations of the ways in which this information is collected.

Specific Recommendations for Assessing Race/Ethnicity

Race/ethnicity is often assessed using a single variable employing a categorical response format that compels patients to select a single, predetermined group that may not adequately represent the heterogeneity of a patient's background (Comstock, Castillo, & Lindsay, 2004). Given that racial/ethnic identification is a complex and multidimensional construct, when providing categories one must allow for multiple responses, as well as a write-in option in addition to the commonly used ethnic/racial checklist. Providing patients with an additional opportunity to detail information on their ethnic/racial background would add incremental validity to the assessment of a patient's identity. Smith, Woo, and Austin (2010) recommend that when providing ethnic/racial checklists, providers ensure these are representative of current immigrant and population trends, as well as inclusive of subgroups commonly seeking services at preidentified health centers. When providing patients with ethnic/racial categories, providers must remember to be sensitive to selecting and using terms that are widely recognizable and inoffensive to respondents.

Another relevant recommendation in the assessment of race/ethnicity within clinical settings is to ask patients to report on multigenerational ethnic and/or racial backgrounds in addition to self-identification (Maradiegue & Edwards, 2006; Phinney & Ong, 2007). Learning about the ethnic/racial background of a patient's family may be particularly useful in identifying patients with mixed or multiethnic identities, which may present unique challenges to clinical treatment. Lea and Monsen (2003) recommend that providers collect background information on a minimum of three family generations (i.e., parents and grandparents) in order to maximize the value of family history for clinical purposes. This increased detail in assessment acknowledges the growing diversity and complexities associated with self-identified race and ethnicity in the United States.

Finally, it is important to emphasize that information on ethnicity and/or race must be supplemented with information on a patient's cultural and contextual background (e.g., SES, acculturation, discrimination, country of birth, educational attainment, and health literacy) to better understand the patient's identity and potential background experiences that may influence the approach to treatment.

Discrimination

Researchers in the area of discrimination and racism have described different "levels" at which racism occurs (Brondolo, 2011). Each of these levels potentially has a different health effect. *Cultural racism* reflects societal customs, beliefs, attitudes, and practices that promote one culture as superior over others. This level typically is evident in societies in which there is widespread agreement about stereotypes associated with certain groups. Cultural racism is often communicated through stereotyped mass media representations of groups. *Institutional racism* refers to the policies, practices, and procedures that consistently result in unequal treatment for particular groups. Although many of the more obvious laws and policies have been outlawed (e.g., the "Jim Crow" laws), there still exist outcomes that are assumed to reflect these policies. Some of the clearest examples are residential segregation and racial/ethnic differences

in interactions with the criminal justice system. *Interpersonal racism* refers to individual interactions that are perceived to be discriminatory. Incidences of interpersonal racism range from everyday experiences of racist actions involving stigmatizing and/or prejudicial attitudes to threats and harassment. Finally, *internalized racism* occurs when an individual accepts the negative stereotypes the society promulgates about the individual's group.

The level of racism that has received the most attention in health-related research is perceived interpersonal racism. There have been a number of reviews in the literature that have demonstrated the negative impact perceived discrimination can have on an individual's physical and mental health (e.g., Mays, Cochran, & Barnes, 2007; Paradies, 2006; Williams & Mohammed, 2009). For example, Pascoe and Richman (2009) utilized a meta-analytic strategy, first to demonstrate the degree to which discrimination was related to physical and mental health outcomes and then to see if it was possible to determine some of the mechanisms through which this occurs. They concluded that perceived discrimination indeed was associated with negative health outcomes and that this may be related to increased physiological and psychological stress responses, as well as to more unhealthy lifestyle behaviors and fewer health-promoting ones, even after controlling for important demographic factors. They also concluded that active coping, social support, and group identification all may serve important protective functions. Most of the assessment instruments that have been developed to date focus on this concept of interpersonal racism.

Recently there has been increased attention to the possibility that at least some of the known health disparities are the result of interpersonal racism on the part of health care providers (e.g. Klonoff, 2009). As a result, investigators have begun to look more carefully at the behavior of health care providers using paradigms that have been well established in social psychology to identify prejudice and racism in ways that do not rely on asking the participant. These include methods such as the Implicit Association Test, which has been used to demonstrate that implicit racial bias could be related to physician decisions (e.g., Green et al.,

2007). In addition, investigators are looking at the nature of communication between physicians and diverse patients to assess the degree to which aspects of the communication process itself results in discriminatory behavior (e.g., Street, Gordon, & Haidet, 2007). Lyles et al. (2011) found in a sample of Kaiser diabetes patients that minorities were more likely to report both general and medical discrimination; medical discrimination was related to poorer health literacy, limited English proficiency, and depression.

However, institutional racism also plays a role, either directly or indirectly. Many of the now well-established health disparities (e.g., Klonoff, 2009; Smedley et al., 2002) can be thought of as outcomes of institutional racism. In this context, "institutional racism" refers not only to issues of access to care but also to issues of access to inferior care. In Klonoff's (2009) review, for example, most of the studies reviewed controlled for SES, patient population, or at least some measure of health care quality; nonetheless, disparities across an array of procedures and diseases were still present. Many of the studies reviewed noted that at least some of the variance in the obtained disparities could be accounted for by the hospitals in which minorities tend to receive their care. For example, differences in postsurgical mortality rates were partially explained by the mortality rates of the hospitals in which the surgery occurred (Lucas, Stukel, Morris, Siewers, & Birkmeyer, 2006). For late mortality rates following cancer surgery, hospital factors accounted for 36 and 54% of the excess mortality for African Americans with breast and colon cancer, respectively; for both kinds of cancers, hospitals that served large minority populations had higher late mortality rates for both European American and minority patients (Breslin et al., 2009). Disparities exist even in systems in which, presumably, individuals from all groups have equal access, such as the Veterans Health Administration (VHA). Trivedi, Grebla, Wright, and Washington (2011) looked at changes in the VHA system between 2000 and 2009 and found improvements in quality of care indicators over this time period and minimal levels of disparities in process-of-care measures (e.g., rates of cholesterol screening). However, disparities remained for many important outcomes

(e.g., blood pressure control, blood glucose, cholesterol); these were primarily within-facility differences (i.e., different results for patients of different races within the same facility) rather than differences between facilities (such as a concentration of African American patients at VHA centers that perform poorly for all patients). Similar racial/ethnic differences in blood pressure control in a population of veterans with Type 2 diabetes mellitus also have been reported (Axon, Gebregziabher, Echols, Gilbert, & Egede, 2011).

Medical Mistrust

Discrimination in the health care setting, disparate health outcomes, and known institutional actions that evidenced harm against members of minority groups led to the idea that medical mistrust may be a factor in differences in medical compliance. Many believe this mistrust is the legacy of Tuskegee and other organized efforts to conduct research or provide "treatment" to members of minority groups that not only was without adequate consent but in fact was harmful to participants. The Centers for Disease Control and Prevention (CDC; n.d.) has a website devoted to the Tuskegee study (*www.cdc.gov/tuskegee/index.html*); that website not only describes the study itself but also includes the apology offered to the African American community by then President William Jefferson Clinton in 1997 for the fact that "your federal government orchestrated a study so clearly racist" (*www.cdc.gov/tuskegee/clintonp.htm*). There also are reports of African Americans failing to be compensated for biological and other materials that resulted in significant profits for other, European American individuals and institutions (e.g., Henrietta Lacks, as described by Skloot, 2010). One of the first patient groups for whom this mistrust was identified were AIDS patients (e.g., Klonoff & Landrine, 1999a); what has come to be called "HIV/AIDS conspiracy beliefs" have been shown to be related to risky sexual behavior (Bogart, Galvan, Wagner, & Klein, 2011) and to lower antiretroviral medication adherence (Bogart, Wagner, Galvan, & Banks, 2010).

Although a number of measures of aspects of mistrust have been developed (e.g., the Group-Based Medical Mistrust Scale [Thompson, Valdimarsdottir, Winkel, Jandorf, & Redd, 2004]; Patient Trust in Medical Researchers [Mainous, Smith, Geesey, & Tilley, 2006]; the Health Care System Distrust Scale [Shea et al., 2008]), none has been used with sufficient frequency that one could be recommended over another. Table 21.1 provides additional detail on each of these measures. Nonetheless, when working with a patient from an underrepresented group who does not appear to be complying with treatment recommendations, medical mistrust should be considered as one possible explanation.

Specific Recommendations for Assessing the Experience of Perceived Discrimination

Several scales have been developed to measure the experience of racial discrimination, and we consider many to be appropriate for use in the clinical setting (Brondolo et al., 2005; Klonoff & Landrine, 1999b; Krieger, 1990; Krieger, Smith, Naishad-

ham, Hartman, & Barbeau, 2005; Kwok et al., 2011; Landrine & Klonoff, 1996; Landrine, Klonoff, Corral, Fernandez, & Roesch, 2006; Malcarne, Chavira, Fernandez, & Liu, 2006; Shariff-Marco et al., 2011; Shariff-Marco et al., 2009; Utsey, 1999; Utsey & Ponterotto, 1996; Williams, Yan, Jackson, & Anderson, 1997; see Table 21.2). Bastos, Celeste, Faerstein, and Barros (2010) provide a recent review of the psychometric properties of these and other racial discrimination scales. In selecting a scale for clinical use, special attention should be paid to the population on which the scale was been validated, because the circumstances in which racial discrimination is experienced can vary by racial/ethnic group. Measures that assess an individual's appraisal of the discriminatory events (e.g., Landrine & Klonoff, 1996; Landrine et al., 2006; Utsey & Ponterotto, 1996; Utsey, 1999) also can be useful to help clinicians to identify whether the discrimination is being perceived as a threat, which could further affect physical and psychological well-being.

TABLE 21.1. Measures of Medical Mistrust

Instrument	Factors measured	No. of items	Validity	Reliability	Population
Group-Based Medical Mistrust Scale (Thompson, Valdimarsdottir, Winkel, Jandorf, & Redd, 2004)	1. Suspicion 2. Group disparities in health care 3. Lack of support from health care providers	12	Regressions relating measures for cancer screening pros and cons	Alpha for total = 0.83; for factor 1 = 0.80, 2 = 0.76, and 3 = 0.55; split-half r = 0.75	79 African American and 89 Latina women with no previous diagnosis of cancer
Trust in Medical Researchers Scale (Mainous, Smith, Geesey, & Tilley, 2006)	1. Participant deception 2. Researcher honesty	12	Individuals with higher scores more likely to volunteer to participate in future; correlates with Health Insurance Trust Scales and Trust in Physicians Scales	Alpha for entire scale = 0.84; factor 1 = 0.78, factor 2 = 0.75	512 telephone respondents (400 complete), 71.4% White, 23.4% African American, 3.8% other, and 1.4% unknown
Revised Health Care System Distrust Scale (Shea et al., 2008)	1. Values distrust 2. Competence distrust	9	Correlations with Physician Trust subscale of the Primary Care Assessment Survey −.42 and −.55; and a global item assessing general social trust −.35 and −.27	Total alpha = 0.83, values = 0.73, competence = 0.77	Final group: total 255; 56% Black; 36% White; 8% other

TABLE 21.2. Adult Discrimination Measures

Instrument	Factors measured	No. of items	Evidence of validity	Reliability	Population
Everyday Discrimination Scale (Williams et al., 1997)	Frequency of experiences in day-to-day life	9	N/A	Internal: Cronbach's alpha = 0.88	African American adults Use with African American adolescents (Clark et al., 2004)
Experiences of Discrimination (Krieger, 1990; Krieger et al., 2005)	Self-reported discrimination in different situations and frequency of occurrence	9	Construct validity; concordance between self-report and key informant reports	Internal: Cronbach's alpha ≥ 0.74 Interitem: $r = .14–.53$ Test–retest: $r \geq .69$	African American and Latino adults
Racial/Ethnic Discrimination (Shariff-Marco et al., 2009, 2011)	Adapted Everyday Discrimination Scale and added question about language discrimination; evaluated "one-stage" and "two-stage" approaches	8	Construct validity	One-stage approach: Cronbach's alpha = 0.88 Two-stage approach: Cronbach's alpha = 0.81	Found to be useful with multiple racial/ethnic groups
Schedule of Racist Events (Landrine & Klonoff, 1996; Klonoff & Landrine, 1999b)	Recent, Lifetime, and appraisal	18	External and construct validity	Internal: Cronbach's alpha = 0.94–0.95 Test–retest: $r = .95–.96$	African American adults
General Ethnic Discrimination Scale (Landrine et al., 2006)	Modeled on Schedule of Racist Events (Recent, Lifetime, and Appraisal)	18	Construct validity	Internal: Cronbach's alpha = Whites (0.91–0.92), Blacks (0.93–0.95), Latinos (0.93–0.94), Asian Americans (0.91–0.94)	African American, Latino, Asian American

Measure	Description	Number of Items	Validity	Reliability	Population
Index of Race-Related Stress (Utsey & Ponterotto, 1996) Brief version also available (Utsey, 1999)	Experience with racist or discriminatory events and reactions to the event Subscales: 1. Cultural 2. Institutional 3. Individual 4. Collective Racism	46	Construct, concurrent, and criterion-related validity	Internal: Cronbach's alpha: Cultural = 0.89, Institutional = 0.82, Individual = 0.84, Collective = 0.74 Test-retest (collected from 2 samples): Cultural: .58–.77, Institutional = .69–.71 Individual = .54–.61, Collective = .75–.79	African American, Mexican, and Filipino adults
Scale of Ethnic Experience (Malcarne et al., 2006)	Ethnicity-related cognitive constructs across multiple ethnic groups. Subscales: 1. Ethnic Identity 2. Perceived Discrimination 3. Mainstream Comfort 4. Social Affiliation	32 (9 items for Perceived Discrimination)	Criterion and construct validity	Internal consistency: Perceived Discrimination: Cronbach's alpha = 0.76–0.91 Test-retest: Perceived Discrimination = .46–.82	
Perceived Ethnic Discrimination Scale—Community Version (Brondolo et al., 2005)	Lifetime experiences of ethnic discrimination. Subscales: 1. Lifetime Exposure 2. Discrimination in the Media 3. Discrimination against Family Members 4. Discrimination in Different Settings 5. Past Week Discrimination	70	Construct validity	Internal consistency: All Cronbach's alpha > 0.76	African American and Latino adults Validated in multiethnic Asian sample (Kwok et al., 2011)

Cultural Concepts of Disease and Illness

Another area that has received a fair amount of attention is culture-specific concepts of disease and illness. Again, much of this has entered into mainstream medicine. The National Center for Complementary and Alternative Medicine (NCCAM) was formally established by Congress under Title VI, Section 601of the Omnibus Appropriations Act of 1999 (Public Law 105-277; *www.nih.gov/about/almanac/organization/ NCCAM.htm*). The goal of NCCAM is to provide scientific evaluation of the usefulness and safety of interventions that are considered to be complementary and alternative; this includes practices, products, disciplines, and interventions that are not generally considered part of conventional Western medicine. Examples may be practices and products that come from various ethnic/racial groups.

Failure to understand and account for culturally specific disease concepts and beliefs can have devastating and even fatal consequences (for an example, see Fadiman, 1997). Often what appears to be noncompliance is, rather, the serious divide between one culture's view of the etiology and treatment of a disease or set of symptoms and that of another culture. Similarly, the failure to understand, and if necessary to incorporate into treatment, culturally specific understandings of disease genesis can lead to poor outcomes. For example, if a patient believes that cancer is a punishment for some previous wrongdoing, trying to persuade him or her to obtain treatment, continue with follow-up, and, where appropriate, engage in additional preventive care is unlikely to be successful because none of these activities relates to the act for which the individual is being punished. As a result, it is crucial that one gain an understanding of some of the beliefs and attitudes that individuals have about the cause and treatment of their particular illness.

Specific Recommendations for Assessing Beliefs about Illness Causes

Despite considerable literature on the importance of culture-specific beliefs and behaviors surrounding a disease, there has been less research on the development and vali-

dation of measures for cross-cultural use, particularly in clinical settings. Among the most widely discussed and easily integrated into clinical practice are assessments outlined in the work of Kleinman, Eisenberg, and Good (1978). They argue the importance of understanding patient's perceptions of their *illness* ("experiences of disvalued changes in states of being and in social function; the human experience of sickness") versus medical models of *disease* ("abnormalities in the structure and function of body organs and systems") in order to provide effective treatment (p. 251). They proposed eight open-ended questions to be asked in the clinical interview setting that provide an opportunity for the patient to share his or her definition of the problem and beliefs about the causes and treatments for their presenting problem. Table 21.3 provides a list of these eight questions. By understanding the patient's model of illness, clinicians can openly address differences in the two approaches and mitigate conflicting beliefs and values that may interfere with treatment. Frequently referred to as "Kleinman's Eight Questions," this approach has been widely used in cross-cultural medicine and can be quickly and efficiently incorporated into clinical practice.

Other measures have been developed to assess illness attributions more specifically across cultural groups (Landrine & Klonoff, 1994b; Murguia, Zea, Reisen, & Peterson, 2000). The measures developed by these two

---

TABLE 21.3. Kleinman's Eight Questions for Cross-Cultural Clinical Assessments

1. What do you think caused the problem?

2. Why do you think it happened when it did?

3. What do you think your sickness does to you? How does it work?

4. How severe is your sickness? Will it have a short course?

5. What kind of treatment do you think you should receive?

6. What are the most important results you hope to receive from this treatment?

7. What are the chief problems your sickness has caused for you?

8. What do you fear most about your sickness?

Note. Based on Kleinman, Eisenberg, and Good (1978).

groups of investigators differentiate between behavioral and environmental attributions of illness (e.g., hygiene, exposure to toxins, and lifestyle attributions) versus more supernatural causes (e.g., God's punishment, fate, and voodoo/hexes). Although these measures assess important cultural differences in illness attributions in a quantitative format, one of them (Landrine & Klonoff, 1994b) provides little information on scale validation, and the other (Murguia et al., 2000) would be challenging to implement in a clinical setting.

Other measures of illness attributions have been widely used to examine health behaviors and outcomes with diverse clinical populations; however, they have not been implemented and evaluated with cross-cultural populations. The Illness Perceptions Questionnaire (IPQ; Weinman, Petrie, Moss-Morris, & Horne, 1996), the revised version of the scale (IPQ-R; Moss-Morris et al., 2002), and the abbreviated version of the scale (Brief IPQ; Broadbent, Petrie, Main, & Weinman, 2006) have all been extensively linked to differences in treatment/medication adherence, illness behaviors, and somatoform symptoms, among others. The measures focus on different components of illness attributions, including the patient's identification of the illness (e.g., name and symptoms associated with the illness), perceived timeline and consequences, and the causes and cures of the illness based on Leventhal's self-regulatory model (Moss-Morris et al., 2002). The Brief IPQ contains only nine items and provides a useful, brief assessment of illness perceptions; however, additional research is needed to determine whether the measures perform equally well across cultures when relating perceptions of illness to health outcomes.

Acculturation

Background on Acculturation and Health

Acculturation has been frequently defined as the changes in cultural beliefs, attitudes, values, and behaviors that occur when individuals enter and interact with a new culture. As acculturation incorporates beliefs about the causes and nature of illnesses, it also incorporates other cultural values, beliefs, behaviors, and attitudes that may

contribute to health disparities and differential utilization and effectiveness of health interventions. In the United States, research has underscored the fact that, following migration, individuals vary not only in the degree to which they adapt to U.S. culture but also in the degree to which they maintain their native culture. Therefore, acculturation is seen as a bidimensional process involving acculturation to a new culture, as well as enculturation to the culture of origin (Cuellar, Arnold, & Maldonado, 1995; Marin & Gamba, 1996). Berry's (1997) model of acculturation outlines four categories of acculturation: integration (high identification with both U.S. and native cultures), assimilation (low identification with native culture and high identification with U.S. culture), separation (high identification with native culture and low identification with U.S. culture), and marginalization (low identification with both native and U.S. cultures). Immigration research and policy have consistently emphasized integration as the preferred form of acculturation (Ager & Strang, 2008); however, most measures of acculturation are not constructed to differentiate across the four groups.

Acculturation has frequently been cited as an important factor when working with migrant communities in contributing to health differences seen between immigrant and U.S.-born groups. Many immigrants report better health outcomes than their U.S. counterparts, an effect known as the *healthy migrant effect*. However, the health-protective factors evident at arrival tend to disappear quickly, with second-generation family members experiencing similar health profiles as their U.S.-born counterparts (Kagawa-Singer, Dadia, Yu, & Surbone, 2010). Changing lifestyles, including dramatic changes to food systems and neighborhood conditions following migration to the United States, are leading contributors to the shifting disease profiles evident among immigrant community members (Omran, 1971; Popkin, 2006). The changing cultural lifestyle patterns have been underscored as important points for assessment and intervention in health promotion programs, for example, in supporting the maintenance of healthy native cultural behaviors or minimizing the adoption of unhealthy U.S. cultural practices. Moreover, the role of acculturation in the acceptability and effectiveness of health interventions is an important focus of adapting evidence-based interventions and evaluating treatment outcomes (Barrera, Toobert, Strycker, & Osuna, 2011; Castro, Barrera, & Holleran Steiker, 2010).

Numerous measures of acculturation have been proposed for general use, as well as for specific cultural groups. However, acculturation has been a challenging construct to assess, with many researchers highlighting the limitations of commonly used measures and methodologies (Hunt, Schneider, & Comer, 2004) and little consensus over how best to operationalize acculturation. Limitations include the lack of longitudinal data that examine the process of acculturation over time and how these changes in cultural beliefs, values, and lifestyles are causally linked to health outcomes. Therefore, most research examining acculturation and health employ cross-sectional designs to see differences in health behaviors and outcomes across levels of acculturation. Moreover, most of this work is atheoretical and descriptive.

Most measures of acculturation have placed a heavy emphasis on language preference, ability, and use in measuring level of acculturation (Lara, Gamboa, Kahramanian, Morales, & Bautista, 2005). Language has been shown to account for the largest amount of the variance in acculturation scales, yet most scales do not fully capture the complexities of language use (Lara et al., 2005), and acculturation remains a robust construct even for those cultures for which English is the native language (Landrine & Klonoff, 1994a). Above and beyond whether one can communicate directly with one's health care provider or not, it is obvious that the specific language one speaks would not in and of itself account for the myriad differences as a function of acculturation.

Instead, language use and acculturation may be a proxy for other factors, such as immersion (or lack thereof) in one's own ethnic enclave and limited exposure to customs and ways of life within the broader community and culture. The maintenance of traditional lifestyles or the adoption of new cultural habits may indicate the degree of residential segregation or experiences of discrimination and persecution by majority cultures that influence these lifestyle decisions. Therefore, it is the broader context of acculturation, such as SES, neighborhood environment, or legal status, and not necessarily the measured components of acculturation, that drive the relation between acculturation and health.

This is further supported by the fact that the correlation between measured acculturation and health behaviors holds up even when language is not a factor, such as with African Americans. Hooper, Baker, de Ybarra, McNutt, and Ahluwalia (2011) demonstrated that level of acculturation predicted smoking abstinence at the end of the intervention and at 3 and 6 months, with more traditional African Americans being less likely to quit smoking. Cultural superstitions were most consistently related to decreased likelihood of abstinence, as in previous studies (e.g., Klonoff & Landrine, 1996, 1999a); however, more acculturated religious beliefs and practices and interracial attitudes reflecting more distrust of European Americans were associated with an increased likelihood of cessation at 6 months. Similar results for smoking were obtained by Guevarra et al. (2005); however, they also demonstrated that women who underperformed breast self-examinations (BSEs) were more acculturated, whereas women who overperformed BSE were more traditional. These BSE data appeared to be related to preferences for African American newspapers, music, activities, people, and so forth. Finally, Ard, Skinner, Chen, Aickin, and Svetkey (2005) found that African American acculturation was related to dietary intake; traditional African Americans had lower intakes of fruits and vegetables and milk and dairy and higher intakes of meat, nuts, and fat than more acculturated African Americans. Therefore, the significance of acculturation remains, even among groups in which language differences are not a concern.

Specific Recommendations for Assessing Acculturation

It is important for all health data to include information on the patient's native and preferred language, country of birth, and years lived in the United States (if not born in the United States). These basic demographic characteristics provide important information that can influence access and utilization of health care services and the need for additional resources, such as translated materials and interpreter services when interacting with the health care setting. It is not appropriate for children or family members to interpret in clinical settings, and there are state and national guidelines for ensuring that patients receive the translation services they need (e.g., California Health Interpreters Association, 2002). Obtaining information on the country of birth and years lived in the United States can trigger the need for more in-depth assessment of acculturation and the values, beliefs, and behaviors that may influence treatment outcomes.

Although the association between acculturation and specific health outcomes is well documented, the assessment of acculturation in health research has not always involved the use of well-established scales. As previously mentioned, the use of proxy measures, most of which focus on language acculturation, is widespread. The use of well-validated multiple-item measures of acculturation is necessary to facilitate understanding of how specific aspects of this construct may be associated to particular health outcomes. In addition, measures should assess the degree of acculturation and affiliation both with U.S. culture and native culture in two separable dimensions, although many older measures do not do this. Tables 21.4 and 21.5 provide a summary of the characteristics and psychometric properties of multiple-item measures of acculturation that have been used in health research with Latinos and other racial groups, respectively. For Latinos, two scales, the Short Acculturation Scale for Hispanics (SASH; Marin, Sabogal, Marin, Otero-Sabogal, & Perez-Stable, 1987) and the Acculturation Rating Scale for Mexican Americans (ARSMA; Dawson, Crano, & Burgoon, 1996), have been shown to be associated with health outcomes amenable for intervention. Specifically, the SASH was found to be effective in predicting specific metabolic syndrome risk factors (e.g., body mass index [BMI], body fat percentage, diastolic blood pressure; Vella, Ontiveros, Zubia, & Bader, 2011), whereas the ARSMA-Short Form was found to be valuable to predict healthy eating, substance use, and sexual behavior among Latinos (Kasirye et al., 2005). Other well-established

measures also have been found to predict health outcomes among Asian Americans (e.g., Chen, Juon, & Lee, 2011; Dodani & Dong, 2011; Brotto, Chou, Singh, & Woo, 2008) and African Americans (e.g., Baker, 2011; Ard et al., 2005; Guevarra et al., 2005). Note that we intentionally omitted the Suinn–Lew Asian Self-Identity Acculturation Scale (Suinn, Rickard-Figueroa, Lew, & Vigil, 1987) from Table 21.5, even though it has often been used in research, because it includes the use of terms that are now considered to be offensive. Although primarily developed for use in research, the scales presented here may be amenable for adaptation and use in clinical contexts.

When evaluating clinical health interventions it is important to assess acculturation to ensure that a program works for individuals at all stages of acculturation (Barrera et al., 2011). However, many measures of acculturation may not provide the specificity needed for the health concern or intervention at hand. Most measures of acculturation include only a few items related to health behaviors, such as food preferences. Therefore, individuals designing health interventions targeting specific health behaviors may want to incorporate a more detailed assessment of the corresponding domains. For example, nutrition interventions should assess cultural attitudes toward food and daily consumption of traditional versus U.S.-style foods, whereas cancer-screening programs will want to address indigenous beliefs about the causes and treatments for cancer. Although not tested empirically thus far, the assessment of intervention-specific cultural health beliefs and behaviors across the acculturation continuum has great promise to advance health and acculturation science, both conceptually and theoretically.

Summary and Conclusions

As should be evident, there are multiple variables that need to be assessed when clinicians begin to work with individuals (and families) from ethnic/racial minority groups. Included among these variables are: demographics, including age, SES, language, education, health literacy, and a measure of ethnicity/race that affords the maximum information about how the individual perceives him- or

TABLE 21.4. Latino Adult Acculturation Measures

Instrument	Factors measured	No. of items	Validity	Reliability	Population
Abbreviated Multidimensional Acculturation Scale (Zea et al., 2003)	1. Nativity 2. Length of time in United States 3. Language proficiency 4. Cultural Competence	42	Validated with community and college students	Internal consistency: alpha = 0.83–0.97	Latino adults
ARSMA-II (Cuellar et al., 1980, 1995)	1. Language use and preference 2. Ethnic identity and classification 3. Cultural heritage and ethnic behaviors 4. Ethnic interaction Two orientation scales: Anglo orientation and Mexican orientation	30	Correlation with ARSMA r = .89	Test–retest: Scale 1 r = .96 Scale 2 r = .94	Latino adults
Bidimensional Acculturation Scale for Hispanics (Marin & Gamba, 1996)	1. Language use 2. Media preference 3. Generation	24	Subscale validation for seven criteria (e.g., length of time in the United States, age at arrival, ethnic self-identification)	Internal consistency: alpha = 0.80–0.90	Latino adults
Brief Acculturation Scale for Hispanics (Norris et al., 1996)	1. Language use 2. Generation	4	Consistently measures validity for acculturation, generation, length of time in the United States	Internal consistency: alpha = 0.80–0.90	Latino adults
Language-Based Acculturation Scale (LAS; Deyo et al., 1985)	Language	4	Construct (natality and generation)	Coefficient of scalability (Guttman) = 0.81 Coefficient of reproducibility = 0.96	Latino adults
ARSMA Short Form (Dawson et al., 1996)	Single factor for acculturation	10	Correlated with ARSMA r = .98	Internal consistency: alpha = 0.96	Latino adults
Short Acculturation Scale for Hispanics (SASH; Marin et al., 1987)	1. Language use 2. Media preferences 3. Ethnic social relations	12	r = .65 (with similar measures) criterion, construct (generation, length of residence, self-evaluation, age of arrival)	Internal consistency: alpha = 0.92 total sample; Internal consistency: alpha = 0.78–0.90 subscales	Latino adults

TABLE 21.5. Acculturation Measures for African American, Asian, and Multiple Groups

Instrument	Factors measured	No. of items	Validity	Reliability	Population
African American adult acculturation measures					
African American Acculturation Scale—Revised (Klonoff & Landrine, 2000)	1. Religious Beliefs and Practices 2. Preference for Things African American 3. Interracial Attitudes 4. Family Practices 5. Health Beliefs and Practices 6. Cultural Superstitions 7. Segregation 8. Family Values	47	Significant differences on all subscales based on level of residential segregation	Alpha for entire scale = 0.93; for each factor: 1 = 0.89; 2 = 0.89; 3 = 0.87; 4 = 0.79; 5 = 0.77; 6 = 0.76; 7 = 0.76; 8 = 0.67 Split half r = .79	520 African American adults (277 women and 243 men)
Scale to Assess African American Acculturation (Snowden & Hines, 1999)		10	Difference in acculturation levels by importance of religion	Alpha = 0.75	923 African Americans in individual face-to-face interviews
Two-Dimensional Black Acculturation Scale (Cole & Jacob Arriola, 2007)	1. Culture, Heritage, and Identity (CHI) 2. Out-Group Comfort (OC)	42 items, 26 on CHI and 16 on OC	Correlations with the Black Racial Identity Attitudes Scale	Alpha CHI = 0.82—0.90, OC = 0.84—0.89	3 groups of African American college students
Asian Acculturation measures					
Vancouver Index of Acculturation (Ryder, Alden, & Paulhus, 2000)	1. Heritage subscale 2. Mainstream subscale	20	Correlations among subscales and time lived and educated in West, Western identification and SL-ASIA mean score	Alphas for Heritage range from 0.91 to 0.92 for different groups; alphas for Mainstream range from 0.85 to 0.89 for different groups	Originally developed to assess bidimensional acculturation in Chinese Canadians; version can be generalized to other locations and groups
Asian American Multidimensional Acculturation Scale (Gim Chung, Kim, & Abreu, 2004)	1. AAMAS—Culture of Origin (CO) 2. AAMAS—Asian American (AA) 3. AAMAS—European American (EA)	15 items for each subscale; 10 measuring cultural behavior, 3 cultural identity, and 2 cultural knowledge	Correlation with SL-ASIA	Alphas: CO = 0.87–0.91, AA = 0.78–0.83, EA = 0.76–0.81; test-retest reliability: CO = .98, AA = .75, EA = .78	Populations of Chinese, Korean, Japanese, Filipino, Vietnamese, and "other" (Singaporean, Cambodian, Indonesian, Thai)
Multiple-group acculturation measures					
Stephenson Multigroup Acculturation Scales (SMAS; Stephenson, 2000)	1. Dominant Society Immersion (DSI) 2. Ethnic Society Immersion (ESI)	32 (15 DSI, 17 ESI)	Correlations with modified versions of the ARSMA-II and the BAS to make them more generalizable	Alpha for entire scale 0.86; for ESI = 0.97; and for DSI = 0.90	436 participants from 5 ethnic groups. 62% nonstudent community members

herself; perceived discrimination, including medical mistrust if necessary; health beliefs and concepts; and acculturation. This was a very cursory overview, and practitioners should not assume that this overview alone would allow one to be culturally competent. Instead, readers are referred to established professional guidelines for greater detail on cross-cultural competencies, such as those proposed by the American Psychological Association (*www.apa.org/pi/oema/resources/policy/multicultural-guidelines.aspx*). However, in combination with specific training in working with ethnic/racial groups, instruments such as those presented here can be very helpful in determining alternative and hopefully more successful intervention strategies.

REFERENCES

Adler, N. E., & Rehkopf, D. H. (2008). U.S. disparities in health: Descriptions, causes, and mechanisms. *Annual Review of Public Health, 29,* 235–252.

Ager, A., & Strang, A. (2008). Understanding integration: A conceptual framework. *Journal of Refugee Studies, 21,* 166–191.

Ard, J. D., Skinner, C. S., Chen, C., Aickin, M., & Svetkey, L. P. (2005). Informing cancer prevention strategies for African Americans: The relationship of African American acculturation to fruit, vegetable, and fat intake. *Journal of Behavioral Medicine, 28,* 239–247.

Axon, R. N., Gebregziabher, M., Echols, C., Gilbert, G., & Egede, L. E. (2011). Racial and ethnic differences in longitudinal blood pressure control in veterans with Type 2 diabetes mellitus. *Journal of General Internal Medicine, 26,* 1278–1283.

Baker, J. R. (2011). Cultural influences on health promoting behaviors of older African American women. *Journal of National Black Nurses Association, 22,* 53–58.

Barrera, M., Jr., Toobert, D., Strycker, L., & Osuna, D. (2011). Effects of acculturation on a culturally adapted diabetes intervention for Latinas. *Health Psychology, 31*(1), 51–54.

Bastos, J. L., Celeste, R. K., Faerstein, E., & Barros, A. J. D. (2010). Racial discrimination and health: A systematic review of scales with a focus on their psychometric properties. *Social Science and Medicine, 70,* 1091–1099.

Berry, J. W. (1997). Immigration, accultura-

tion, and adaptation. *Applied Psychology: An International Review, 46,* 5–34.

Block, J., Scribner, R., & DeSalvo, K. (2004). Fast food, race/ethnicity, and income: A geographic analysis. *American Journal of Preventive Medicine, 27,* 211–217.

Bogart, L. M., Galvan, F. H., Wagner, G. J., & Klein, D. J. (2011). Longitudinal association of HIV conspiracy beliefs with sexual risk among Black males living with HIV. *AIDS Behavior, 15,* 1180–1186.

Bogart, L. M., Wagner, G., Galvan, F. H., & Banks, D. (2010). Conspiracy beliefs about HIV are related to antiretroviral treatment nonadherence among African American men with HIV. *Journal of Acquired Immune Deficiency Syndrome, 53,* 648–655.

Braveman, P. A., Cubbin, C., Egerter, S., Williams, D. R., & Pamuk, E. (2010). Socioeconomic disparities in health in the United States: What the patterns tell us. *American Journal of Public Health, 100*(S1), S186–S196.

Breslin, T. M., Morris, A. M., Gu, N., Wong, S. L., Finlayson, E. V., Banerjee, M., et al. (2009). Hospital factors and racial disparities in mortality after surgery for breast and colon cancer. *Journal of Clinical Oncology, 27,* 3945–3950.

Broadbent, E., Petrie, K. J., Main, J., & Weinman, J. (2006). The brief Illness Perception Questionnaire. *Journal of Psychosomatic Research, 60,* 631–637.

Brondolo, E. (2011). *Racism and health.* Retrieved December 19, 2011, from *www.health-psych.org/APADivision38Racism.cfm.*

Brondolo, E., Kelly, K. P., Coakley, V., Gordon, T., Thompson, S., Levy, E., et al. (2005). The perceived ethnic discrimination questionnaire: Development and preliminary validation of a community version. *Journal of Applied Social Psychology, 35,* 335–365.

Brotto, L. A., Chou, A. Y., Singh, T., & Woo, J. S. (2008). Reproductive health practices among Indian, Indo-Canadian, Canadian East Asian, and Euro-Canadian women: The role of acculturation. *Journal of Obstetrics and Gynecology Canada, 30,* 229–238.

Buescher, P. A., Gizlice, Z., & Jones-Vessey, K. A. (2005). Discrepancies between published data on racial classification and self-reported race: Evidence from the 2002 North Carolina live birth records. *Public Health Reports, 120*(4), 393.

California Healthcare Interpreters Association. (2002). *California standards for healthcare interpreters: Ethical principles, protocols, and guidance on roles and intervention.* Sacramento, CA: California Endowment.

Castro, F. G., Barrera, M., Jr., & Holleran Steiker, L. K. (2010). Issues and challenges in the design of culturally adapted evidence-based interventions. *Annual Review of Clinical Psychology, 6,* 213–239.

Chen, L., Juon, H. S., & Lee, S. (2011). Acculturation and BMI among Chinese, Korean and Vietnamese adults. *Journal of Community Health, 37*(3), 539–546.

Centers for Disease Control and Prevention. (n.d.) *U.S. Public Health Service Syphilis Study at Tuskegee.* Retrieved December 24, 2011, from *www.cdc.gov/tuskegee/index.html.*

Clark, R., Coleman, A. P., & Novak, J. D. (2004). Brief report: Initial psychometric properties of the everyday discrimination scale in black adolescents. *Journal of Adolescence, 27,* 363–368.

Cole, E. R., & Jacob Arriola, K. R. (2007). Black students on White campuses: Toward a two-dimensional model of Black acculturation. *Journal of Black Psychology, 33,* 379–403.

Comstock, R. D., Castillo, E. M., & Lindsay, S. P. (2004). Four year review on the use of race and ethnicity in epidemiologic and public health research. *American Journal of Epidemiology, 159*(6), 611–619.

Cuellar, I., Arnold, B., & Maldonado, R. (1995). Acculturation rating scale for Mexican-Americans: II. A revision of the original ARMSA scale. *Hispanic Journal of Behavioral Sciences, 17,* 275–304.

Cuellar, I., Harris, L., & Jasso, R. (1980). An acculturation scale for Mexican American and clinical populations. *Hispanic Journal of Behavioral Science, 2,* 199–217.

Davis, L. E., & Engel, R. J. (2011). *Measuring race and ethnicity.* New York: Springer.

Davis, T. C., Long, S. W., Jackson, R. H., Mayeaux, E. J., George, R. B., Murphy, P. W., et al. (1993). Rapid estimate of adult literacy in medicine: A shortened screening instrument. *Family Medicine, 25,* 391–395.

Dawson, E., Crano, W., & Burgoon, M. (1996). Refining the meaning and measurement of acculturation: Revisiting a novel methodological approach. *Intercultural Relations, 20,* 97–114.

Deyo, R. A., Diehl, A. K., Hazuda, H., & Stern, M. (1985). A simple language-based acculturation scale for Mexican Americans: Validation and application to health care research. *American Journal of Public Health, 75,* 51–55.

Do, D. P., Finch, B. K., Basurto-Davila, R., Bird, C., Escarce, J., & Lurie, N. (2008). Does place explain racial health disparities?: Quantifying the contribution of residential context to the black/white health gap in the United States. *Social Science and Medicine, 67,* 1258–1268.

Dodani, S., & Dong, L. (2011). Acculturation, coronary artery disease and carotid intima media thickness in South Asian immigrants: Unique population with increased risk. *Ethnicity and Disease, 21,* 314–321.

Fadiman, A. (1997). *The spirit catches you and you fall down.* New York: Farrar, Straus & Giroux.

Freeman, H. P. (1989). Cancer in the socioeconomically disadvantaged. *CA: A Cancer Journal for Clinicians, 39*(5), 266–288.

Freeman, H. P. (2004). Poverty, culture, and social injustice: Determinants of cancer disparities. *CA: A Cancer Journal for Clinicians, 54,* 72–77.

Gim Chung, R. H., Kim, B. S. K., & Abreu, J. M. (2004). Asian American Multidimensional Acculturation Scale: Development, factor analysis, reliability and validity. *Cultural Diversity and Ethnic Minority Psychology, 10,* 66–80.

Green, A. R., Carney, D. R., Pallin, D. J., Ngo, L. H., Raymond, K. L., Iezzoni, L. I., et al. (2007). Implicit bias among physicians and its prediction of thrombolysis decisions for Black and White patients. *Journal of General Internal Medicine, 22,* 1231–1238.

Guevarra, J. S., Kwate, N. O. A., Tang, T. S., Valdimarsdottir, H. B., Freeman, H. P., & Bovbjerg, D. H. (2005). Acculturation and its relationship to smoking and breast self-examination frequency in African American women. *Journal of Behavioral Medicine, 28,* 191–199.

Hao, Y., Landrine, H., Smith, T., Kaw, C., Corral, I., & Stein, K. (2011). Residential segregation and disparities in health-related quality of life among Black and White cancer survivors. *Health Psychology, 30,* 137–144.

Harris-Kojetin, B. A., & Mathiowetz, N. A. (1998). *The effects of self and proxy response status on the report of race and ethnicity.* Available at *www.amstat.org/sections/srms/proceedings/papers/1998_157.pdf.*

Hooper, M. W., Baker, E. A., de Ybarra, D. R., McNutt, M., & Ahluwalia, J. S. (2011). Acculturation predicts 7-day smoking cessation among treatment-seeking African-Americans in a group intervention. *Annals of Behavioral Medicine, 43*(1), 74–83.

Hunt, L. M., Schneider, S., & Comer, B. (2004). Should "acculturation" be a variable in health research?: A critical review of research on U.S. Hispanics. *Social Science and Medicine, 59,* 973–986.

Kagawa-Singer, M., Dadia, A. V., Yu, M. C., & Surbone, A. (2010). Cancer, culture, and health disparities: Time to chart a new course? *CA: A Cancer Journal for Clinicians, 60,* 12–39.

Kasirye, O. C., Walsh, J. A., Romano, P. S., Beckett, L. A., Garcia, J. A., Elvine-Kreis, B., et al. (2005). Acculturation and its association with health-risk behaviors in a rural Latina population. *Ethnicity and Disease, 15,* 733–739.

Kawachi, I., Daniels, N., & Robinson, D. E. (2005). Health disparities by race and class: Why both matter. *Health Affairs, 24,* 343–352.

Kleinman, A., Eisenberg, L., & Good, B. (1978). Culture, illness, and care: Clinical lessons from anthropologic and cross-cultural research. *Annals of Internal Medicine, 88,* 251–258.

Klonoff, E. A. (2009). Disparities in the provision of medical care: An outcome in search of an explanation. *Journal of Behavioral Medicine, 32,* 48–63.

Klonoff, E. A., & Landrine, H. (1996). Acculturation and cigarette smoking among African-American adults. *Journal of Behavioral Medicine, 19*(5), 501–514.

Klonoff, E. A., & Landrine, H. (1999a). Do Blacks believe that HIV/AIDS is a government conspiracy against them? *Preventive Medicine, 28,* 451–457.

Klonoff, E. A., & Landrine, H. (1999b). Cross-validation of the Schedule of Racist Events. *Journal of Black Psychology, 25,* 231–254.

Klonoff, E. A., & Landrine, H. (2000). Revising and improving the African American Acculturation Scale. *Journal of Black Psychology, 26,* 235–261.

Krieger, N. (1990). Racial and gender discrimination: Risk factors for high blood pressure? *Social Science and Medicine, 30,* 1273–1281.

Krieger, N., Smith, K., Naishadham, D., Hartman, C., & Barbeau, E. M. (2005). Experiences of discrimination: Validity and reliability of a self-report measure for population health research on racism and health. *Social Science and Medicine, 61,* 1576–1596.

Kwok, J., Atencio, J., Ullah, J., Crupi, R., Chen, D., Roth, A. R., et al. (2011). The Perceived Ethnic Discrimination Questionnaire—Community Version: Validation in a multiethnic Asian sample. *Cultural Diversity and Ethnic Minority Psychology, 17,* 271–282.

Landrine, H., & Klonoff, E. A. (1994a). The African American Acculturation Scale: Development, reliability, and validity. *Journal of Black Psychology, 20,* 104–127.

Landrine, H., & Klonoff, E. A. (1994b). Cultural diversity in causal attributions for illness: The role of the supernatural. *Journal of Behavioral Medicine, 17,* 181–193.

Landrine, H., & Klonoff, E. A. (1996). The Schedule of Racist Events: A measure of racist discrimination and a study of its negative physical and mental health consequences. *Journal of Black Psychology, 22,* 144–168.

Landrine, H., Klonoff, E. A., Corral, I., Fernandez, S., & Roesch, S. (2006). Conceptualizing and measuring ethnic discrimination in health research. *Journal of Behavioral Medicine, 29,* 79–94.

Lara, M., Gamboa, C., Kahramanian, M. I., Morales, L. S., & Bautista, D. E. H. (2005). Acculturation and Latino health in the United States: A review of the literature and its sociopolitical context. *Annual Review of Public Health, 26,* 367–397.

Lea, D. H., & Monsen, R. B. (2003). Preparing nurses for a 21st-century role in genomics-based health care. *Nursing Education Perspectives, 24,* 75–80.

Lee, M. A., & Ferraro, K. F. (2007). Neighborhood residential segregation and physical health among Hispanic Americans: Good, bad, or benign? *Journal of Health and Social Behavior, 48,* 131–148.

Link, C., & McKinlay, J. B. (2009). Disparities in the prevalence of diabetes: Is it race/ethnicity or socioeconomic status? Results from the Boston Area Community Health (BACH) survey. *Ethnicity and Disease, 19,* 288–292.

Lucas, F. L., Stukel, T. A., Morris, A. M., Siewers, A. E., & Birkmeyer, J. D. (2006). Race and surgical mortality in the United States. *Annals of Surgery, 243*(2), 281.

Lyles, C. R., Karter, A. J., Young, B. A., Spigner, C., Grembowski, D., Schollinger, D., et al. (2011). Correlates of patient-reported racial/ethnic health care discrimination in the Diabetes Study of Northern California (DISTANCE). *Journal of Health Care for the Poor and Underserved, 22,* 211–225.

Mainous, A. G., III, Smith, D. W., Geesey, M. E., & Tilley, B. C. (2006). Development of a measure to assess patient trust in medical researchers. *Annals of Family Medicine, 4,* 247–252.

Malcarne, V. L., Chavira, D. A., Fernandez, S., & Liu, P. J. (2006). The scale of ethnic experience: Development and psychometric properties. *Journal of Personality Assessment, 86,* 150–161.

Maradiegue, A., & Edwards, Q. T. (2006). An overview of ethnicity and assessment of family history in primary care settings. *Journal of the American Academy of Nurse Practitioners, 18,* 447–456.

Marin, G., & Gamba, R. J. (1996). A new measurement of acculturation for Latinos: The Bidimensional Acculturation Scale for Latinos (BAS). *Hispanic Journal of Behavioral Sciences, 18,* 297–316.

Marin, G., Sabogal, F., Marin, B., Otero-Sabogal, R., & Perez-Stable, E. (1987). Development of a short acculturation scale for Hispanics. *Hispanic Journal of Behavioral Sciences, 18,* 297–316.

Mays, V. M., Cochran, S. D., & Barnes, N. W. (2007). Race, race-based discrimination, and health outcomes among African Americans. *Annual Review of Psychology, 58,* 201–225.

Mays, V. M., Ponce, N. A., Washington, D. L., & Cochran, S. D. (2003). Classification of race and ethnicity: Implications for public health. *Annual Review of Public Health, 24,* 83–110.

Morello-Frosch, R., & Jesdale, B. M. (2006). Separate and unequal: Residential segregation and estimated cancer risks associated with ambient air toxics in U.S. metropolitan areas. *Environmental Health Perspectives, 114,* 386–393.

Morland, K., & Filomena, S. (2007). Disparities in the availability of fruits and vegetables between racially segregated urban neighborhoods. *Public Health Nutrition, 10,* 1481–1489.

Morland, K., Wing, S., Diez Roux, A., & Poole, C. (2002). Neighborhood characteristics associated with the location of food stores and food service places. *American Journal of Preventive Medicine, 22,* 23–29.

Moore, L. V., Diez Roux, A. V., Evenson, K. R., McGinn, A. P., & Brines, S. J. (2008). Availability of recreational resources in minority and low socioeconomic status areas. *American Journal of Preventive Medicine, 34,* 16–22.

Moscou, S., Anderson, M. R., Kaplan, J. B., & Valencia, L. (2003). Validity of racial/ethnic classifications in medical records data: An exploratory study. *American Journal of Public Health, 93*(7), 1084–1086.

Moss-Morris, R., Weinman, J., Petrie, K. J., Horne, R., Cameron, L. D., & Buick, D. (2002). The revised Illness Perception Questionnaire (IPQ-R). *Psychology and Health, 17,* 1–16.

Murguia, A., Zea, M. C., Reisen, C. A., & Peterson, R. A. (2000). The development of the Cultural Health Attributions Questionnaire (CHAQ). *Cultural Diversity and Ethnic Minority Psychology, 6,* 268–283.

Norris, A., Ford, K., & Bova, C. (1996). Psychometrics of a brief acculturation scale for Hispanics in a probability sample of urban Hispanic adolescents and young adults. *Hispanic Journal of Behavioral Sciences, 18,* 29–38.

Omran, A. R. (1971). The epidemiologic transition: A theory of the epidemiology of population change. *Milbank Memorial Fund Quarterly, 49,* 509–538.

Paradies, Y. (2006). A systematic review of empirical research on self-reported racism and health. *International Journal of Epidemiology, 35,* 888–901.

Parker, R. M., Baker, D. W., Williams, M. V., & Nurss, J. R. (1995). The test of functional health literacy in adults: A new instrument for measuring patients' literacy skills. *Journal of General Internal Medicine, 10,* 537–541.

Pascoe, E. A., & Richman, L. S. (2009). Perceived discrimination and health: A meta-analytic review. *Psychological Bulletin, 135,* 531–554.

Phinney, J. S., & Ong, A. D. (2007). Conceptualization and measurement of ethnic identity: Current status and future directions. *Journal of Counseling Psychology, 54*(3), 271–281.

Popescu, I., Cram, P., & Vaughan-Sarrazin, M. S. (2011). Differences in admitting hospital characteristics for Black and White Medicare beneficiaries with acute myocardial infarction. *Circulation, 123,* 2710–2716.

Popkin, B. M. (2006). Global nutrition dynamics: The world is shifting rapidly toward a diet linked with noncommunicable diseases. *American Journal of Clinical Nutrition, 84,* 289–298.

Powell, L. M., Chaloupka, F. J., & Bao, Y. (2007). The availability of fast food and full-service restaurants in the United States: Associations with neighborhood characteristics. *American Journal of Preventive Medicine, 33*(S4), S240–S245.

Powell, L. M., Slater, S., Chaloupka, F. J., & Harper, D. (2006). Availability of physical-activity-related facilities and neighborhood demographic and socioeconomic characteristics: A national study. *American Journal of Public Health, 96,* 1676–1680.

Powers, B. J., Trinh, J. V., & Bosworth, H. B. (2010). Can this patient read and understand written health information? *Journal of the American Medical Association, 304,* 76–84.

Rawson, K. A., Gunstad, J., Hughes, J., Spitznagel, M. B., Potter, V., Waechter, D., et al. (2010). The METER: A brief, self-administered measure of health literacy. *Journal of General Internal Medicine, 25,* 67–71.

Ryder, A. G., Alden, L. E., & Paulhus, D. L. (2000). Is acculturation unidimensional or bidimensional?: A head-to-head comparison in the prediction of personality, self-identity, and adjustment. *Journal of Personality and Social Psychology, 79,* 49–65.

Shariff-Marco, S., Breen, N., Landrine, H., Reeve, B. B., Krieger, N., Gee, G. C., et al. (2011). Measuring everyday racial/ethnic discrimination in health surveys. *Du Bois Review, 8,* 159–177.

Shariff-Marco, S., Gee, G. C., Breen, N., Willis, G., Reeve, B. B., Grant, D., et al. (2009). A mixed-methods approach to developing a self-reported racial/ethnic discrimination measure for use in multiethnic health surveys. *Ethnicity and Disease, 19,* 447–453.

Shea, J. A., Micco, E., Dean, L. T., McMurphy, S., Schwartz, J. S., & Armstrong, K. (2008). Development of a revised Health Care System Distrust Scale. *Journal of General Internal Medicine, 23,* 727–732.

Skloot, R. (2010). *The immortal life of Henrietta Lacks.* New York: Crown.

Smedley, B. D., Stith, A. Y., & Nelson, A. R. (Eds.). (2002). *Unequal treatment: Confronting racial and ethnic disparities in health care.* Washington, DC: National Academies Press.

Smith, F. D., Woo, M., & Austin, B. (2010). "I didn't feel like any of those things were me": Results of a qualitative pilot study of race/ethnicity survey items with minority ethnic adolescents in the USA. *Ethnicity and Health, 15*(6), 621–638.

Snowden, L. R., & Hines, A. M. (1999). A Scale to Assess African American Acculturation. *Journal of Black Psychology, 25,* 36–47.

Stephenson, M. (2000). Development and validation of the Stephenson Multigroup Acculturation Scale (SMAS). *Psychological Assessment, 12,* 77–88.

Street, R. L., Jr., Gordon, H., & Haidet, P. (2007). Physicians' communication and perceptions of patients: Is it how they look, how they talk, or is it just the doctor? *Social Science and Medicine, 65,* 596–598.

Suinn, R. M., Rickard-Figueroa, K., Lew, S., & Vigil, P. (1987). The Suinn–Lew Asian Self-Identity Acculturation Scale: An initial report. *Educational and Psychological Measurement, 47,* 401–407.

Thompson, H. S., Valdimarsdottir, H. B., Winkel, G., Jandorf, L., & Redd, W. (2004). The Group-Based Medical Mistrust Scale: Psychometric properties and association with breast cancer screening. *Preventive Medicine, 38,* 209–218.

Trivedi, A. N., Grebla, R. C., Wright, S. M., & Washington, D. L. (2011). Despite improved quality of care in the Veterans Affairs Health System, racial disparity persists for important clinical outcomes. *Health Affairs, 30,* 707–715.

U.S. Census Bureau. (2012). *The 2012 Statistical Abstract: The National Data Book.* Retrieved December 15, 2011, from *www.census.gov/compendia/statab/cats/income_expenditures_poverty_wealth.html.*

U.S. Department of Health and Human Services. (2011). *The NIH almanac: National Institute on Minority Health and Health Disparities.* Retrieved December 19, 2011, from *www.nih.gov/about/almanac/organization/NIMHD.htm.*

Utsey, S. (1999). Development and validation of a short form of the Index of Race-Related Stress (IRRS)—Brief Version. *Measurement and Evaluation in Counseling and Development, 32,* 149–167.

Utsey, S. O., & Ponterotto, J. G. (1996). Development and validation of the Index of Race-Related Stress (IRRS). *Journal of Counseling Psychology, 43,* 490–501.

Vella, C. A., Ontiveros, D., Zubia, R. Y., & Bader, J. O. (2011). Acculturation and metabolic syndrome risk factors in young Mexican and Mexican-American women. *Journal of Immigrant and Minority Health, 13*(1), 119–126.

Ward, E., Jemal, A., Cokkinides, V., Singh, G. K., Cardinez, C., Ghafoor, A., et al. (2004). Cancer disparities by race/ethnicity and socioeconomic status. *CA: A Cancer Journal for Clinicians, 54,* 78–93.

Weinman, J., Petrie, K., Moss-Morris, R., & Horne, R. (1996). The Illness Perception Questionnaire: A new method for assessing the cognitive representation of illness. *Psychology and Health, 11,* 431–445.

Weiss, B. D., Mays, M. Z., Martz, W., Castro, K. M., DeWalt, D. A., Pignone, M. P., et al. (2005). Quick assessment of literacy in primary care: The newest vital sign. *Annals of Family Medicine, 3,* 514–522.

Williams, D. R., & Mohammed, S. A. (2009). Discrimination and racial disparities in health: Evidence and needed research. *Journal of Behavioral Medicine, 32,* 20–47.

Williams, D. R., Yan, Y., Jackson, J. S., & Anderson, N. B. (1997). Racial differences in physical and mental health: Socio-economic status, stress and discrimination. *Journal of Health Psychology, 2*(3), 335–351.

Yali, A. M., & Revenson, T. A. (2004). How changes in population demographics will impact health psychology: Incorporating a broader notion of cultural competence into the field. *Health Psychology, 23,* 147.

Zea, M., Asner-Self, K., Birman, D., & Buki, L. (2003). The Abbreviated Multidimensional Acculturation Scale: Empirical validation with two Latino/Latina samples. *Cultural Diversity and Ethnic Minority Psychology, 9,* 107–126.

CHAPTER 22

Organ Transplant

Douglas P. Gibson
Kristin Kuntz
Solam Huey
Mary Ellen Olbrisch

The first successful kidney transplant occurred in 1954 between twin brothers living in Boston, Massachusetts. Several years later, in 1962, the first successful kidney transplant was performed using a cadaveric donor (United Network for Organ Sharing [UNOS], 2013a). The first successful kidney-and-pancreas transplant occurred in 1966, followed by a successful liver transplant in 1967 and successful heart and pancreas transplants in 1968 (UNOS, 2013a). Immunosuppression medications evolved over the years; a significant increase in transplantation occurred when cyclosporine, a groundbreaking antirejection drug, was approved for commercial use in 1983. In 1984, Congress passed the National Organ Transplant Act, which, in addition to prohibiting the sale of organs, set up a national transplant network to procure and distribute organs (Organ Procurement and Transplantation Network [OPTN]). This act also served to develop national organ allocation policies to match available organs with transplant candidates. During the first year of the OPTN's existence, more than 10,000 transplants were performed; today, the number of transplants performed per year has almost tripled (OPTN, 2013). Since the OPTN was created, more than 570,000 people have received organ transplants in the United States (OPTN, 2013). The demand for organs has grown continuously as transplantation has become a viable treatment for end-stage organ failure.

Because the biggest barrier to transplantation is the disparity between the number of those who need an organ and the number of cadaveric organs available, living kidney and liver donation is becoming more and more common. Living donation significantly shortens the time spent waiting for a transplant, thus saving more lives (Jakobsen, Holdaas, & Leivestad, 2003). Today, living donor renal transplants make up about 21% of all kidney transplants performed in the United States (OPTN, 2013). Not only does this procedure produce better outcomes compared with cadaveric transplants, but also the risk of death to the donor is estimated to be only about 0.06% (National Kidney Foundation, 2013). In 1989, the first successful living-donor liver transplant was performed (UNOS, 2013a). By the mid-1990s, transplanting the right hepatic lobe from one adult to another with end-stage liver disease was a viable alternative to cadaveric liver transplant (Surman, Fukunishi, Allen, & Hertl, 2005).

Facts about Transplant

In the United States, over 22,000 transplants were performed in 2012 with deceased donor organs; almost 6,000 transplants were performed using organs from living donors (OPTN, 2013). By organ, 16,485 kidney transplants, 6,256 liver transplants, 242 pancreas transplants, 801 kidney/pancreas transplants, 2,378 heart transplants, and 1,754 lung transplants were performed in 2012 (OPTN, 2013). With over 118,000 individuals currently awaiting various organs for transplant in the United States (UNOS, 2013b), it is clear that the demand far outweighs the supply. For patients who are fortunate to receive a transplant, the development of better immunosuppressive agents and enhanced surgical techniques has led to increased patient survival over the years. Survival rates are affected by the recipient's ethnicity, age, and comorbid health conditions, as well as the type of organ transplanted and certain donor characteristics (Ojo et al., 2000).

The Need for Psychosocial Evaluation in Organ Transplant

For multiple reasons, it is important to gather information about a potential transplant recipient's psychosocial status. As stated earlier, there are not enough organs to satisfy the needs of those on the waiting list. Because of this and the responsibility to donors and to society to allot these resources wisely, patients must demonstrate that they are in a position to manage the posttransplant regimen successfully (Collins & Labott, 2007). Various psychosocial issues, including untreated mental illness and poor social support, can lead to complications posttransplant (Levenson & Olbrisch, 1993). It is essential to assess a patient's baseline functioning so that any apparent changes after transplant can be compared with the initial assessment. Various mental health providers such as social workers, psychologists, and psychiatrists might conduct the pretransplant psychosocial evaluation (Collins & Labott, 2007; Olbrisch, Levenson, Fischer, & Kulstad, 2001).

Components of the Psychosocial Evaluation

The psychosocial evaluation consists of multiple sections. A thorough assessment should begin with the patient's medical records. This informs the interviewer about the patient's diagnosis, course of illness, and current treatment. There may be notes in the chart that allude to difficulty with compliance or other psychosocial difficulties (Collins & Labott, 2007) that the patient may not openly offer during the interview. A careful clinical interview is then conducted with the transplant patient and, when possible, his or her support system. Many areas of the patient's life will be assessed during the interview, and these are described in this section. Because certain medications and medical conditions can cause confusion and disorientation at times, a mental status examination should be performed. A collateral interview with the patient's caregiver(s) can be quite informative, as it provides an opportunity to corroborate information obtained in the patient interview or to acquire information not able to be obtained from the patient. It also allows the clinician to assess the adequacy of the caregiver(s).

At the end of the interview, some clinicians may want to add cognitive or personality testing to obtain additional information in a particular domain. Finally, acquiring additional information from other transplant team members, such as the nurse coordinators, social workers, and physicians, is often useful.

Clinical Interview

Medical History

Beginning with the patient's medical history, the patient should be able to explain his or her medical diagnosis, the course of the illness and treatment, and current medications. This part of the history reveals the extent of the patient's involvement in his or her own care and the nature of the patient's relationship with health care providers. It is important that the patient has basic health literacy and is able to form a therapeutic alliance with members of the transplant team.

Knowledge of Transplant

Next, the patient's knowledge of transplant should be assessed, including familiarity with success rates, risks and benefits, and length of time of hospitalization and recovery (Collins & Labott, 2007). The patient's knowledge of the potential for rejection and the subsequent lifetime need for immunosuppressant medication must also be assessed. The risks and benefits of living donation should be discussed when applicable, and the interviewer might assess whether the patient has any potential donors. Within the evaluation of the patient's knowledge of transplant, the patient's expectations for life after transplant and any concerns or hesitations can be discussed. Finally, given the importance of adherence to a rigorous posttransplant regimen, the patient's level of motivation for transplant must be appraised.

Support System

The presence of a good social support network is important for the patient throughout the transplant process. Patients will need tangible, emotional, and informational support. The support system should be identified at this time, as well as the ability of the caregivers to be present before, during, and after the transplant. It is important to learn whether the caregivers work, have limiting health problems of their own, or are responsible for other individuals (e.g., children, other family members or friends). These factors may limit their ability to care for the transplant patient. When possible, this information should be obtained from the individuals in the support system in a separate interview. The perception that adequate support is available contributes to a better quality of life and more satisfaction in posttransplant patients (Goetzmann et al., 2007; Cetingok, Hathaway, & Winsett, 2007).

Psychiatric History

It has been repeatedly documented in the literature that pretransplant psychological functioning may be predictive of posttrans-

plant adjustment and outcome (Favaro et al., 2011; Morana, 2009; Goetzmann et al., 2007; Levenson & Olbrisch, 1993). A study of pretransplant candidates across organ systems found mood and anxiety disorders to be associated with poorer psychosocial adjustment and health status and personality disorders to be associated with medical compliance problems (Chacko, Harper, Kunik, & Young, 1996). More specifically, a major depression episode prior to heart transplantation was found to be a significant independent risk factor for posttransplant malignancies, which significantly contributed to predicting mortality in survival analyses (Favaro et al., 2011). Findings such as these suggest that there are psychiatric contraindications to organ transplantation, supporting the value of assessing a transplant candidate's psychiatric history during the pretransplant evaluation process.

The primary goal of evaluating the psychiatric histories of potential transplant recipients is not to exclude them as candidates for organ transplantation but rather to identify those patients who are likely to exhibit psychiatric, behavioral, and emotional problems throughout the course of the transplantation and recovery process (Huffman, Popkin, & Stern, 2003). For example, adjustment disorders with depression and/or anxiety have been found to be highly prevalent in the transplant population preoperatively (Olbrisch, Benedict, Ashe, & Levenson, 2002). Early identification of these issues allows transplant teams to have the opportunity to develop individualized pre- and posttransplant treatment plans for patients. The ultimate goal is to minimize any negative impact from these psychiatric risk factors, while also optimizing the potential transplant recipient's preparedness for transplantation and maximizing transplant outcome success (DiMartini, Crone, Fireman, & Dew, 2008).

The comprehensive pre–organ transplant psychosocial evaluation should include a detailed assessment of the transplant candidate's baseline level of cognitive and emotional functioning. This often includes documentation of previous psychiatric conditions or excessive emotional difficulties in an attempt to uncover any premorbid psychiatric illnesses in the form of a thought disorder (e.g., acute psychosis, schizophrenia, schizoaffective disorders), major mood disturbance (e.g., major depressive disorder, dysthymic disorder, bipolar disorders), or major anxiety disorder (e.g., generalized anxiety disorder, panic disorder, phobias, posttraumatic stress disorder; Fisher, 2006). Personality traits that mimic a thought disturbance (e.g., schizoid, paranoid types), anxiety distortions (e.g., obsessive–compulsive types), moderate to severe developmental disability, and pervasive patterns of interpersonal/emotional instability raise concerns about potential participation in an organ transplant. The reason is the potential impairment in judgment, decision making, and the ability to work cooperatively with the transplant and support teams. Information about previous suicidal or homicidal ideations and behaviors, psychiatric hospitalizations, and mental health treatment can provide an indication of the general psychiatric stability of the potential transplant recipient. A routine assessment of current psychiatric symptoms, coping and problem-solving ability, and mental status, paired with standardized psychiatric and cognitive measures of functioning (see the later section on psychological testing), is recommended to help determine whether the potential transplant recipient has the emotional stability and cognitive capability to adequately comprehend and adhere to the rigors of an organ transplantation regimen (Huffman et al., 2003). Other factors to consider include family psychiatric history and the patient's current adjustment to medical stressors as a way of early identification of relevant psychiatric risk factors.

Social History

Evaluating a potential transplant recipient's social history provides insights into his or her cognitive, emotional, social, and personality development, as well as current social functioning. This information is important in evaluating whether a potential transplant recipient has the adequate psychosocial resources to successfully adapt to the rigors of the organ transplantation process and adhere to the posttransplant course.

Timely achievement of developmental milestones, academic performance and accomplishments, the presence of any remarkable childhood experiences (e.g.,

unstable family environment, history of abuse or trauma), the ability to develop and maintain stable interpersonal relationships, coping styles, and past reactions to stressful situations are factors that should be considered when evaluating one's early social history. Assessment of marital or relationship status, family composition, and the quality of family and social relationships helps to identify available sources of social support, as well as any relevant social pressures that may unduly affect the transplant recipient's decision making regarding organ transplantation. Information pertaining to work history, disability status, military experience (e.g., type of discharge, disciplinary action), legal or criminal history, engagement in types of social activities, current social stressors, and coping strategies may all be helpful in presenting a more complete picture of one's social functioning and resiliency. As past behavior is the best predictor of future behavior, the presence of any negative health habits or use of maladaptive coping strategies (e.g., substance use or abuse and other risky behaviors) should be routinely assessed. Conversely, the potential transplant recipient's strengths and adaptive behaviors should also be identified and reinforced. This is particularly important because the transplant procedure can be a very demanding and stressful process, which will surely challenge the transplant recipient's coping resources. Any attempt to increase healthy behaviors and adaptive coping are encouraged with the goal of optimizing transplantation outcomes.

Adherence

Of the psychosocial factors, the most common reason for not listing a patient for transplant candidacy is nonadherence (Collins & Labott, 2007). Nonadherence has been described as a complex behavioral variable that is the result of the interaction between multiple enduring and short-term psychiatric and psychosocial factors (Wolcott & Strouse, 1996). The objective of the pretransplant psychological assessment is to identify the potential transplant recipients who could most effectively adhere to the rigorous postoperative transplantation course, because poor outcomes are often a direct result of adherence problems (Stilley et al.,

2010; Mori, Gallagher, & Milne, 2000). Evaluating past and current medical adherence, especially during the pretransplant period, is crucial to the transplant psychological assessment in predicting posttransplant adherence and success.

There are various ways to assess a patient's medical adherence history. Potential transplant recipients may be queried about their record of keeping medical appointments and any problems with following drug, exercise, dietary, or other lifestyle prescriptions. A history of poor follow-up with preventive medical care and ineffective management of other medical or psychiatric conditions are also indicative of adherence problems. Cooperation with the transplant evaluation process and willingness to work collaboratively with members of the transplant team is vital to posttransplant success. Patients who have difficulty dealing with medical professionals or with relationships in general may isolate themselves, withhold important information, or antagonize the medical staff, ultimately affecting their care and posttransplant recovery. Demonstration of the ability to make sound medical decisions (e.g., contacting doctor immediately if experiencing side effects of medications or symptoms of rejection), comprehension of the issues surrounding transplant (medical procedures, risks, potential benefits, and posttransplant regimen), and willingness to commit to making recommended lifestyle changes related to smoking, drinking, drug use, and other high-risk behaviors are extremely important in predicting posttransplant adherence (Stilley et al., 2010). An effort to obtain collateral information from multiple reliable sources to provide further insight into this issue is also desirable.

It is important to highlight that it is often the patient's behaviors, as opposed to psychiatric issues, that ultimately determine his or her appropriateness for organ transplantation from a psychosocial perspective (Mori et al., 2000). Any patient with a recurrent history of nonadherence to previous medical regimens should be considered to be extremely high risk for transplantation (Wilkinson, 1996). Although this does not necessarily preclude one from being placed on the waiting list for transplantation, demonstration of a period of acceptable medical adherence prior to listing should be demanded to maximize posttransplant success and recovery and to avoid unnecessary risks. This is often done in the form of a "compliance contract" that the patient and a transplant team member both sign.

Substance Use

Assessing Alcohol Use, Abuse, and Dependence. Following viral hepatitis, end-stage alcoholic liver disease (ALD) remains the most common indication for liver transplantation. Relapse rates following liver transplantation vary in the literature. Lucey (2001) reviewed the literature and reported that approximately 30–50% of patients returned to some level of alcohol consumption by 5 years posttransplant. Lim and Keeffe (2004) reported a 20% recidivism rate, and Bjornsson et al. (2005) reported a 33% recidivism rate. Whereas the 1- and 5-year survival rates for patients who relapsed and those who abstained have been reported to be similar, the 10-year survival rates differ significantly. Cuadrado, Fabrega, Casafont, and Pons-Romero (2005) reported a 25.9% rate of relapse between 5 and 86.9 months after OLT (orthotopic liver transplant). Although they found no association between relapse and other complications, including graft rejection, infections, associated comorbidities, or compliance, the 5- and 10-year survival rates for patients who relapsed were 92.9% and 45.1%, respectively, compared with 92.4% and 85.5%, respectively, for patients who did not return to using alcohol.

Predicting which patients are most at risk for relapse can be extremely challenging, and to date, no instruments have been shown to reliably do so. Many programs use abstinence of greater than 6 months as a requirement, but this too has not been consistently shown to be a reliable predictor. Pfitzmann et al. (2007) did find abstinence of less than 6 months to be predictive of relapse. Additionally, they reported absence of a companion in life and the presence of young children to be predictive of relapse. Other factors that have been reported to predict relapse include lack of a stable partner, amount per day consumed in the years before assessment for transplant, reliance on family or friends for posttransplant support, tobacco consumption at the time of assessment, and lack of insight into the disease of addiction. Using a multivariate model, these factors reportedly predicted relapse with 89% accuracy.

A thorough assessment of alcohol use in all patients is an integral part of any pretransplant psychosocial evaluation. The clinician must assess alcohol use across the lifetime. Gathering the alcohol use history chronologically may make it easier to organize the information. The types of alcohol consumed, specific amounts, and frequency of consumption need to be solicited. Specific questions aimed at assessing tolerance and withdrawal must be asked. In order to diagnose dependence or abuse, the impact that alcohol use has had on a patient's life must be assessed. The *CAGE* questions (attempts at Cutting down alcohol use, Annoyance by others complaining about one's alcohol use, Guilt associated with alcohol use, and the need for an "*Eye opener*" early in the day) can be quite useful in this regard. It is not unusual for substance abuse to result in illegal behavior, criminal charges, and even incarceration. Inquiries into these areas should always be made, and this should include questions regarding any pending charges, court dates, probation, or issues.

Information on previous attempts at quitting, as well as formal or informal treatment, should be assessed. Specifically, the type, duration, and response to treatment must to be examined. If there have been relapses, then details regarding the frequency, triggers, and responses to relapse has to be gathered.

As many programs stipulate a specified length of abstinence required in order to be listed for transplantation, the date of the last use of alcohol must be determined. Collateral sources can be helpful in narrowing down the time frame and/or validating a patient's report. Finally, the assessment should include an appraisal of the patient's motivation to remain abstinent, as well as his or her confidence level, any self-doubt, and available resources. An assessment of motivation may include a simple query as to what factors (outside of transplantation) are influencing the patient's decision to abstain. These could include relationship improvements, job performance, health, and overall survival. An examination of available resources, patient insight into the potential benefits of abstinence, steps already taken to succeed, and potential barriers (e.g., cost, poor support from family/friends, substance and/or tobacco use) could also prove helpful in the assessment of patient motivation. The psychosocial evaluation itself may prove to be the first phase of abstinence, as it serves to introduce and reinforce the concept. The evaluation may ultimately serve to help direct the course of treatment, and the evaluator should be prepared to play a pivotal role in this regard.

Other Substance Use. The high frequency of substance abuse in the liver transplant population can result in this area of assessment being time-consuming and at times overwhelming. Nonetheless, it is a critical component of the clinician's evaluation, as well as the decision-making process for the transplant team. As with alcohol, drug use must be assessed in every patient being evaluated for transplant, despite age, gender, or medical diagnoses. It is best to assess alcohol and drug use history during the same phase of the evaluation, employing the same queries and considering alcohol to be one of potentially several substances used. Once again, it may be helpful to elicit the history chronologically by substance and include amounts, frequency, evidence of abuse or dependence, impact on one's life, and treatment history. Relapse history, along with perceived triggers and response to relapse, should be assessed. The patient's last reported use of any substance must be determined, and collateral information can be very helpful.

An often-overlooked area of the substance use assessment includes abuse of prescription drugs and over-the-counter (OTC) medications/remedies (including homeopathic and/or herbal remedies). Furthermore, substance *misuse* needs to be assessed, as it, too, can result in negative consequences. Examples of this include taking excessive amounts of acetaminophen, sleep aids, supplements, and other products. Patients are encouraged to inform their transplant team of any medications or remedies used. (See Haller, Acosta, Newville, & Herron, Chapter 6, and Toneatto & Gunaratne, Chapter 7, in this volume for additional information on assessing drug and alcohol use and abuse.)

Tobacco Use. Tobacco use is directly associated with increased morbidity and mortality. Few studies have examined the long-term effect of tobacco use on organ transplant recipients despite the high prevalence of tobacco use in this population. Jain et al. (2000) reported an increased rate of late death (5 years and beyond) in patients who had undergone liver transplantation for alcoholic liver disease compared with those from other disease categories. These deaths were primarily caused by lung and oropharyngeal cancers. Although the investigators did not have data on tobacco use in this study, they suspected that tobacco use contributed to the deaths, pointing to research showing that nearly 90% of alcoholics smoke (Burling & Ziff, 1988). A study by Sanchez-Lazaro et al. (2007) found that among heart transplant recipients, nonsmokers and ex-smokers had a significantly greater survival rate compared with those who smoked up until the time of transplant. Other evidence suggests that smokers and ex-smokers may have a greater risk of complication following transplantation. This includes a higher incidence of difficult-to-manage ascites and encephalopathy, as well as a greater mean length of stay in the hospital and greater overall cost (McConathy et al., 2007). Smokers and ex-smokers also have a greater risk of vascular and arterial complications, and quitting at least 2 years prior to transplantation significantly reduced this risk (Pungpapong et al., 2002). DiMartini et al. (2005) found that smokers resumed smoking quickly after transplantation, with the majority smoking within 3 months. By 18 months, 58% returned to smoking. They noted that these patients not only return to smoking early but also increase their consumption over time and quickly become tobacco dependent.

Sung, Althoen, Howell, Ojo, and Merion (2001), who examined the impact of tobacco use on renal allograft, found that 24% of their sample smoked at time of transplantation and that, of those patients, 90% continued to smoke after transplantation. They found that patients who were smokers at the time of pretransplant evaluation had kidney graft survival of 84%, 65%, and 48% at 1, 5, and 10 years, respectively, compared with graft survival in nonsmokers of 88%, 78%, and 62%. Furthermore, the investigators reported that smoking cessation prior to transplantation had a beneficial effect on graft survival.

Despite what is known about tobacco use and its impact on morbidity and mortality, few transplant programs make tobacco abstinence a requirement for listing. Future research will likely continue to reveal that tobacco use has a detrimental effect on posttransplant survival, complications, and quality of life. Consequently, programs should view tobacco use in the same light as alcohol and other abused substances, and a thorough assessment of past and current tobacco use should be a part of every pretransplant psychosocial evaluation. As with alcohol and drugs, tobacco use assessment should include specifics with regard to amounts, type, frequency, dependence, attempts at cessation, length of abstinence, relapses, triggers to relapse, and last use. Once again, collateral information is useful as it helps to validate patient responses. Finally, the assessment should examine patients' motivation to quit, self-doubt, insight, and plans. Patients should be offered assistance with tobacco cessation. Such assistance could include education, pharmacological interventions, and behavior therapy. Whereas some patients will request assistance, many will opt to "go it on their own." It is best to allow patients this option and to offer assistance as needed. Programs should inform patients that they will be tested for cotinine levels at clinic visits and that continued use of tobacco may affect the team's decision to list. (See Peterson, Brundige, & Houghton, Chapter 5, this volume, for additional information on assessing smoking behavior.)

Substance Abuse Contracts. Transplant programs should strongly consider constructing a substance abuse contract, which outlines in specific but simple terms their policy on alcohol, drug, and tobacco use. Such a contract not only provides each patient with a thorough explanation of the program's policy but also allows documentation of such education, as the patient will also be required to sign and date it. The patient should be provided with a copy of the contract, and the original is placed in his or her medical record. The contract presents the clinician with a good opportunity to enter into a frank and straightforward discussion about substance use and the impact it may have on decisions regarding the patient's care. Finally, the contract conveys the transplant program's strong stance on substance use, misuse, and abuse, as well as its commitment to assisting the patient in overcoming such problems.

Psychological Testing

Psychological and cognitive testing can provide valuable information in the areas of personality and higher cognitive functioning that augment the clinical interview. Cognitive dysfunction is quite common in the pretransplant population and can be the result of numerous factors, including hepatic or metabolic encephalopathy, hypoxia, medication side effects, and depression. Assessing cognitive functioning is an important aspect of the evaluation for several reasons. First, a patient's ability to give informed consent and make informed decisions could be compromised by significant cognitive dysfunction. One's level of intellectual functioning may also affect decision making and should always be assessed during the evaluation. Second, testing may help to identify the presence of other conditions, for example, dementia or delirium, that may sometimes require further evaluation by a neuropsychologist. Third, cognitive testing provides the clinician and team with baseline levels of patient cognitive functioning. This can be useful postoperatively, as it allows the team to gauge progress, as well as further decompensation, by yielding a point of reference.

In addition to intellectual functioning, the cognitive screening should include measures of psychomotor speed, attention/concentration, immediate and delayed recall, language, and visuospatial/constructional praxis. Brief tests of neuropsychological functioning, such as the Repeatable Battery for the Assessment of Neuropsychological Status (RBANS; Randolph, 1998) can provide valid measures in a limited amount of time.

An assessment of personality functioning may be useful in patients suspected of having traits that may become problematic pre- or postoperatively. When questions related to a patient's presentation arise (e.g. suspicion of downplaying emotional factors or exaggeration of symptoms), personality inventories such as the Minnesota Multiphasic Personality Inventory–2 (MMPI-2) may be indicated. Other, briefer measures of psychological functioning can often suffice, particularly when the aim is to capture any reported areas of distress, such as depression or anxiety. Measures such as the Symptom Checklist–90 (SCL-90), the Beck Depression Inventory (BDI), and the Brief Symptom Inventory–18 (BSI-18) can all provide information related to emotional distress and coping. The Millon Behavioral Medicine Diagnostic (MBMD) inventory provides measures of psychiatric distress and coping, as well as other health-related areas of functioning, including coping style, pain sensitivity, and compliance. Thus it lends itself well to the pretransplant evaluation as it provides measures in areas that are more directly related to the transplant process. Finally, measures of quality of life can be valuable in assessing the impact of disease and health deterioration on one's day-to-day functioning. There are a number of health-related quality-of-life measures. The SF-36, for example, is commonly used in the health and medical literature and has been demonstrated to possess solid validity and reliability (see Passchier & Busschbach, Chapter 11, this volume, which discusses quality of life in greater detail).

Psychological testing assists the clinician in determining whether or not a patient possesses the capacity to make an informed decision regarding transplantation and whether the patient truly understands the numerous issues related to transplantation. It also assists the clinician in assessing whether the patient will do what is necessary and expected following transplant. Finally, it provides valuable diagnostic and baseline information related to cognitive and emotional functioning and can assist in both diagnosing and treating conditions.

Transplant Candidate Rating Scales

Two published rating scales are widely used for rating the suitability of candidates for transplantations on psychosocial criteria: the Transplant Evaluation Rating Scale (TERS; Twillman, Manetto, Wellisch, & Wolcott, 1993) and the Psychosocial Assessment of Candidates for Transplantation (PACT; Olbrisch, Levenson, & Hamer, 1989). These scales attempt to quantify the information gathered via the medical record review, patient interview, collateral interviews, and psychological testing that may have been performed, as described earlier, to make a prediction about how well a patient is likely to do following transplant surgery. The scales themselves are of little value without the underlying clinical information, carefully gathered, that is to be weighted in assigning ratings or scores on the scales. These scales have provided a useful shorthand for talking about how a given transplant candidate looks relative to the population of transplant candidates from a psychosocial perspective; the greatest research limitation has been that patients who do not get transplants because of psychological and behavioral problems do not have outcomes to study, leading to a restricted range in the area in which data on the accuracy of predictions would be most vital.

The Report

Reporting the findings of a pretransplant psychosocial evaluation can be challenging given the plethora of information gathered, the numerous issues to address, and the need for accuracy. Before choosing a format, the clinician should consider what the transplant team needs in making a determination. The report should state in straightforward terms whether a patient meets the criteria for transplantation. To this end, the report does not need to be lengthy. In fact, an "executive summary" can be much more valuable to the team, as it outlines the most relevant factors and presents an ultimate finding.

The executive summary should be succinct and to the point. Jargon and "beating around the bush" should be avoided at all costs, as it is of little value to the team and can only serve to complicate decision making. Although it is best to keep the summary short and efficient, this does not have to be done at the expense of being thorough. The summary should adequately address the following areas: presenting problem, medical history, psychiatric history, medications, substance abuse history, tobacco use, social support, compliance, transplant knowledge, mental status, cognitive functioning, behavioral health, impressions, and recommendations. A summary in this format can typically be completed on one page and takes only minutes to produce (see the sample report in Figure 22.1). The semistructured interview form contains the remaining information and is also a part of the medical record, which is, of course, available for review at any time if necessary in the future.

Special Populations

Children and Adolescents

Chronic illness may have a more significant impact on children and adolescents when compared with adults, and this is expected to be even greater in the case of organ transplantation. Given their young age, pediatric patients struggle with their illness for a larger percentage of their lives, and they may not have yet developed the knowledge and coping resources to adapt successfully to their medical conditions. Pediatric transplant recipients who experience psychological difficulties and family dysfunction before and after transplantation had more hospitalizations after transplantation (De Maso, Twente, Spratt, & O'Brien, 1995), and nonadherence to posttransplant treatment regimens is a common cause of graft rejection in children and adolescent transplant recipients (Meade, Creer, & Mahan, 2003).

Much of the literature on pretransplant psychosocial evaluations focuses on adult organ recipients. Although similar assessment guidelines can be applied to the psychosocial evaluation of pediatric transplant patients, special considerations must be given to identify any increased risks for posttransplant nonadherence and poor recovery in this unique population. During the psychosocial evaluation, it is important to first clarify with the family who has the legal or decision-making responsibility for the pediatric patient. The fact that the pediatric patient is a minor requires that the transplant team work closely with those family members who are responsible for the patient. These family members must consent to and be present during the course of the transplant evaluation process. Very often, especially in the case of small children, the psychosocial evaluation focuses more on the adults caring for the pediatric patient than on the patient. The goal is to evaluate whether the caregivers of the pediatric patient can adequately com-

---

Psychological Assessment for Cardiac Transplantation

Patient Name:	A. G.	**Age:**	23 years old
Date of Birth:	censored	**Education:**	high school graduate
Occupation:	Disabled Army Mechanic	**Date of Evaluation:**	censored
Date of Report:	censored	**MR #:**	123456789

- 23-year-old Puerto Rican man referred for pre–heart transplant psychosocial assessment; he was seen with a translator in his hospital room
- **Medical Hx:** diagnosed with non-ischemic cardiomyopathy in 03/20XX, ICD implanted in 06/20XX
- **Psychiatric Hx:** no previous psychiatric diagnosis or treatment; currently experiencing depressed mood with frequent tearfulness; endorsed fear of medical procedures and needles
- **Medications:** patient could not name his medications
- **Substance Use Hx:** history of drinking four drinks/months until 03/XX; no current or past illicit drug use
- **Tobacco Use:** quit smoking in 02/XX after smoking 1 pack/day for three years
- **Family support:** patient has been married for 1 month, his wife visits hospital daily; they have 3 children (ages 4, 3, 9 months) living in Puerto Rico with wife's parents; rest of patient's family is in Puerto Rico
- **Compliance:** with medications and appointments has been good
- **Intellectual/Cognitive Functioning:** range of intelligence appears to be average; attention was good, recall was adequate, psychomotor behavior was normal, speech was of normal rate and volume; English is patient's second language and he needed a translator at times
- **Mental Status:** alert, O x 3; eye contact fair; able to provide sufficient history; no evidence of hallucinations or delusional thought; denied suicidal/homicidal ideation; mood is depressed and affect was flat; judgment appears to be adequate
- **Behavioral Health:** patient reported poor sleep due to discomfort in chest, good appetite, no regular exercise, enjoys playing with his children and listening to music for recreation
- **Impressions:** patient is currently experiencing symptoms consistent with Adjustment Disorder with Depressed Mood; there are no concerns for substance abuse; his support system appears to be adequate; compliance appears to be adequate
- **Recommendations:**
  1) psychiatry consult to assess potential need for antidepressant medication
  2) the psychology team will provide supportive therapy during patient's hospitalization
  3) acceptable candidate for cardiac transplant from a psychosocial perspective

---

Jane Doe, PhD
Clinical Psychologist

FIGURE 22.1. Sample report.

prehend the issues involved in the transplant process and have the ability to assist the pediatric transplant patient in following the rigors of the posttransplant regimen to achieve successful outcomes. A baseline assessment of cognitive and emotional functioning in pediatric transplant patients and/or their legal caregivers should be obtained whenever possible. Additionally, both the pediatric patient and the family's motivation for treatment and expectations of the transplant process should be routinely assessed. Any discrepancies in motivation or expectations should be resolved at the pretransplant stage.

Adherence to medical instructions in pediatric transplant patients remains a challenge, and it is the most complicated problem in all types of pediatric transplants, particularly in the adolescent population (Stuber, 2010). It is important to routinely assess the pediatric patient's previous history of treatment adherence whenever possible when evaluating for transplant candidacy. Poor treatment compliance in adults may suggest ambivalence about survival or depression, and it is likely that the same may be found in pediatric patients (Shaw & Taussig, 1999). The pretransplant psychosocial evaluation can play an important role in the early identification and treatment of any emotional or adjustment difficulties during the pre- and posttransplant course.

A careful assessment of the pediatric patient's medical, psychiatric, coping, and behavioral history should be obtained from as many reliable sources as possible, including family, past and current medical providers, and past treatment records. A detailed family history (medical, psychiatric, social) should also be obtained to assess family stability and adequacy of social support and the presence of any family barriers that could negatively affect the pediatric patient's posttransplant treatment adherence and adjustment.

Sensitivity to developmental issues is also a critical component of the pretransplant psychosocial assessment for pediatric patients. Knowledge of relevant issues in the early developmental stages would be helpful in assessing the level of cognitive and emotional development of the pediatric patient. Issues of body image, modesty and privacy, self-esteem, and social acceptance are common in patients with chronic illness and may take on particular relevance in pediatric patients, especially those in the adolescent age group. It is also important to be sensitive to the inherently traumatic nature of many treatments and of invasive medical procedures for both the pediatric patient and the family, as some studies have found both parents and pediatric organ transplant recipients meeting the criteria for posttraumatic stress disorder following successful transplantation (Stuber, 2010; Shaw & Taussig, 1999). Sensitivity to the preceding psychosocial issues will inform treatment planning and likely reduce treatment nonadherence in this unique population.

Older Adults

Older patients (ages ≥ 65) are currently the fastest growing segment of the population with end-stage organ disease (Wu et al., 2008; Martins et al., 2005). Some studies (e.g., Terasaki, Gertson, Cecka, Takemoto, & Cho, 1997) found that advanced organ transplant recipient age is associated with poor patient survival posttransplant, and the main cause of graft loss is patient death due to a shorter life expectancy as opposed to acute graft rejection. Older patients are believed to have a higher risk of infection, cardiovascular event, and malignancy after organ transplantation than younger patients, and they may also experience more drug toxicity and more drug side effects than their younger counterparts (Huang, Segev, & Rabb, 2009; Wu et al., 2008). However, other studies found similar survival rates and posttransplant outcomes between younger and older patients (Aduen et al., 2009; Mendonça, dos Reis, Sesso, Câmara, & Pacheco-Silva, 2007; Moore et al., 2007; Kuramitsu et al., 2007). This finding suggests that age in and of itself is not a contraindication to organ transplantation, and older patients should not be excluded from transplant candidacy based on age alone. With new advances in surgical techniques, intensive care treatment, and new immunosuppressive drugs, the outcome of transplantation in elderly patients is encouraging, and the age limit of patients eligible for transplantation has increased in many transplant centers (Martins et al., 2005).

To maximize the success of posttransplant outcomes in elderly patients, individual tailoring of immunosuppressive therapy will be crucial due to the consequences of an altered immune response and increased risks of drug toxicity. Careful donor selection and selective use of living donors may also be vital to achieving good posttransplant outcomes. During the psychosocial evaluation, the issue of adequacy of available social support should be considered. Spouses of elderly transplant recipients are often at an advanced age themselves and may present with their own medical illnesses and functional disabilities, making them insufficient caregivers. The availability of alternative sources of social support (e.g., children, siblings, community, or option for home health care aides) should be routinely assessed. Elderly patients are also at an increased risk for cognitive decline, either through advanced age or through disease-specific complications (e.g., hepatic encephalopathy in the case of liver disease). It is important to perform a cognitive assessment during the pretransplant period to obtain a baseline level of cognitive functioning and to evaluate the patient's ability to comprehend the issues surrounding transplant and his or her ability to make sound medical decisions. Elderly patients may elect to decline the option for organ transplantation, as some may feel that they have already lived a full life. Because the posttransplant recovery period is often lengthy and may be plagued with postsurgical complications, some have expressed a preference to live out the rest of their lives with dignity as opposed to being in a debilitated state. As such, knowledge of developmental issues in the older adult stage (e.g., integrity vs. despair, end-of-life issues) is helpful in evaluating elderly patients for organ transplantation. The potential for coercion by family members to have the patient undergo organ transplantation should also be assessed. Evaluators should be alert to any discrepancies in medical decision making between the patient and the family. As motivation for organ transplantation is believed to be associated with posttransplant compliance and success, it is important to determine whether the decision to pursue organ transplantation was carefully made by the patient or whether it was unduly influenced by the family.

Living Donor Evaluation

Psychologists who serve on transplant teams may be called on to serve as evaluators of living donors, as well as of prospective transplant recipients. The issues in donor evaluation are somewhat different, in that these assessments generally involve physically healthy individuals who want to help a family member or friend. However, issues can become quite complex, as in cases in which donors may come forward due to publicity about the recipient or because of a general desire to help other people in need with no specific recipient in mind. In each case, the task of the evaluating clinician is to determine that the prospective donor is psychologically healthy and unlikely to be harmed psychologically by the donation, is adequately informed about the risks, costs, and benefits of living organ donation, and is free from coercion, either from the recipient and the recipient's family and social network or from others in the transplant program who may be motivated to push ahead with surgery in the interest of serving a needy recipient (Olbrisch, Benedict, Haller, & Levenson, 2001).

Psychologists themselves must be aware that their own relationships with recipients might color their views of prospective donors and must guard against any potential bias toward finding a prospective donor suitable because of a wish to help a particular recipient. To this end, objective psychological testing is particularly helpful as a check on the psychologist's personal clinical judgment. Although having two different individuals serve in the role of evaluators of donors and recipients might be desirable, most transplant teams cannot afford to duplicate all of the team roles for all services, and thus for most of the medical, psychosocial, and allied health services provided to transplant patients and donors the same team members will be filling both roles, and only a few individuals will serve as the federally designated "living donor advocates" who are not involved in the day-to-day care of transplant recipients (Medicare Program, 2007).

Ethical Considerations in Organ Transplantation

The scarcity of donor organs and the high cost of transplant create a unique set of circumstances that raise ethical concerns. The absence of national psychosocial selection criteria to assess candidates for organ transplantation further adds to the potential for ethical conflict, with some questioning whether the use of such criteria may have violated the Americans with Disabilities Act (ADA; Orentlicher, 1996). Achieving justice in the allocation of organs is difficult. Psychosocial factors predictive of survival may be confused with judgments of an individual's social worth, and inconsistency in the application of psychosocial criteria across clinicians or transplant centers may create the impression of biased decisions rather than concerns for outcome (Olbrisch, 1996).

A number of ethical concerns involved in the selection of candidates for organ transplantation have been highlighted and discussed by Olbrisch (1996). These include: (1) the patient's right to informed consent and confidentiality; (2) honoring loyalties to multiple parties (individual patients, the pool of all patients needing transplant surgery, and the transplant team); (3) potentially conflicting dual relationships (e.g., psychologist as assessor vs. healer); (4) biases based on social factors unrelated to transplant outcome (e.g., patients with significant alcohol and drug abuse histories, mental retardation, criminal histories, or special privileges such as celebrities, politicians, and foreign nationals) that may affect clinical judgment and raise questions of fair access; (5) judgments based on whether patients have a stable and socially acceptable support network, which might be seen as an unfair imposition of social norms; (6) responsibilities to organ donors; (7) honesty about whether to inform patients that they are poor transplant candidates due to psychosocial issues; and (8) avoidance of imposition of irrelevant moral values. In addition, the ethical issue of organ transplantation in older adults further contributes to the difficulty of achieving equitable organ allocation (Huang et al., 2009).

The ethical issues in the psychosocial evaluation of potential transplant candidates go far beyond the Ethical Principles of Psychologists and the Code of Conduct of the American Psychological Association. Nevertheless, these principles do provide some guidance. Awareness of these ethical issues and challenges leads to an appreciation of the multifaceted concerns involved in the selection of patients for organ transplantation and discourages attempts to reach easy answers or a set of rules and guidelines. The goal is to achieve the best balance in maximizing success for all parties while considering the ethical challenges involved.

Summary

As long as the supply of donor organs fails to meet the demand of patients who need them, careful consideration must be paid to the medical and psychosocial factors that affect outcomes in transplant patients. Though transplant is largely thought of as a surgical procedure, long-term outcomes are often dictated by the degree to which a patient adequately follows the posttransplant regimen. By identifying psychosocial risk factors early in the transplant process, the transplant team and the patient can work together to decrease those risk factors, thus making the psychosocial evaluation a critical part of the transplant experience.

REFERENCES

Aduen, J., Bangarulingam, S., Dickson, R., Heckman, M., Winston, H., Stapelfeldt, W., et al. (2009). Outcomes after liver transplant in patients aged 70 years or older compared with those younger than 60 years. *Mayo Clinic Proceedings, 84*(11), 973–978.

Björnsson, E., Olsson, J., Rydell, A., Fredriksson, K., Eriksson. C., Sjöberg, C., et al. (2005). Long-term follow-up of patients with alcoholic liver disease after liver transplantation in Sweden: Impact of structured management on recidivism. *Scandinavian Journal of Gastroenterology, 40*(2), 206–216.

Burling, T. A., & Ziff, T C. (1988). Tobacco smoking: A comparison between alcohol and drug abuse inpatients. *Addictive Behaviors, 13*(2), 185–190.

Centingok, M., Hathaway, D., & Winsett, R. P. (2007). Contribution of post-transplant social support to the quality of life of transplant recipients. *Social Work in Health Care, 45*(3), 39–56.

Chacko, R. C., Harper, R. G., Kunik, M., & Young, J. (1996). Relationship of psychiatric morbidity and psychosocial factors in organ transplant candidates. *Psychosomatics, 73*, 100–107.

Collins, C. A., & Labott, S. M. (2007). Psychological assessment of candidates for solid organ transplantation. *Professional Psychology: Research and Practice, 38*(2), 150–157.

Cuadrado, A., Fabrega, E., Casafont, F., & Pons-Romero, F. (2005). Alcohol recidivism impairs long-term patient survival after orthotopic liver transplantation for alcoholic liver disease. *Liver Transplantation, 11*(4), 420–426.

De Maso, D. R., Twente, A. W., Spratt, E. G., & O'Brien, P. (1995). Impact of psychologic functioning, medical severity, and family functioning in pediatric heart transplantation. *Journal of Heart and Lung Transplantation, 14*(6), 1102–1108.

DiMartini, A., Crone, C., Fireman, M., & Dew, M. A. (2008). Psychiatric aspects of organ transplantation in critical care. *Critical Care Clinics, 24*(4), 949–981.

DiMartini, A., Javed, L., Russell, S., Dew, M.A., Fitzgerald, M. G., Jain, A., et al. (2005). Tobacco use following liver transplantation for alcoholic liver disease. *Liver Transplantation, 11*(6), 679–683.

Favaro, A., Gerosa, G., Caforio, A., Volpe, B., Rupolo, G., & Zarneri, D., et al. (2011). Posttraumatic stress disorder and depression in heart transplantation recipients: The relationship with outcome and adherence to medical treatment. *General Hospital Psychiatry, 33*, 1–7.

Fisher, M. S. (2006). Psychosocial evaluation interview protocol for pretransplant kidney recipients. *Health and Social Work, 31*(2), 137–144.

Goetzmann, L., Klaghofer, R., Wagner-Huber, R., Halter, J., Boehler, A., Muellhaupt, B., et al. (2007). Psychosocial vulnerability predicts psychosocial outcome after an organ transplant: Results of a prospective study with lung, liver, and bone-marrow patients. *Journal of Psychosomatic Research, 62,* 93–100.

Huang, E., Segev, D., & Rabb, H. (2009). Kidney transplantation in the elderly. *Seminars in Nephrology, 29*(6), 621–635.

Huffman, J. C., Popkin, M. K., & Stern, T., A. (2003). Psychiatric considerations in the patient receiving organ transplantation: A clinical case conference. *General Hospital Psychiatry, 25,* 484–491.

Jakobsen, A., Holdaas, H., & Leivestad, T. (2003). Ethics and safety of living kidney donation. *Transplantation Proceedings, 35,* 1177–1178.

Jain, A., DiMartini, A., Kashyap, R., Youk, A., Rogal, S., & Fung, J. (2000). Long-term follow-up after liver transplantation for alcoholic liver disease under tacrolimus. *Transplantation, 70*(9), 1335–1342.

Kuramitsu, K., Egawa, H., Keeffe, E. B., Kasahara, M., Ito, T., Sakamoto, S., et al. (2007). Impact of age older than 60 years in living donor liver transplantation. *Transplantation, 84*(2), 166–172.

Levenson, J. L., & Olbrisch, M. E. (1993). Psychosocial evaluation of organ transplant candidates. *Psychosomatics, 34,* 314–323.

Lim, J. K., & Keeffe, E. B. (2004). Liver transplantation for alcoholic liver disease: Current concepts and length of sobriety. *Liver Transplantation, 10*(2), S31–S38.

Lucey, M. R. (2001). Liver transplantation in the alcoholic patient. In W. C. Maddrey, E. R. Schiff, & M. F. Sorrel (Eds.), *Transplantation of the liver* (pp. 319–326). Philadelphia: Lippincott Williams and Wilkins.

Martins, P. N. A., Pratschke, J., Pasher, A., Fritsche, L., Frei, U., Neuhaus, P., et al. (2005). Age and immune response in organ transplantation. *Transplantation, 79*(2), 127–132.

McConathy, K., Turner, V., Johnston, T., Jeon, H., Bouneva, I., Koch, A., et al. (2007). Analysis of smoking in patients referred for liver transplantation and its adverse impact of short-term outcomes. *Journal of the Kentucky Medical Center, 105*(6), 261–266.

Meade, M. A., Creer, T. L., & Mahan, J. D. (2003). A self-management program for adolescents and children with renal transplantation. *Journal of Clinical Psychology in Medical Settings, 10*(3), 165–171.

Medicare Program; Hospital Conditions of Participation: Requirements for approval and re-approval of transplant centers to perform organ transplants; Final rule, 42 CFR Parts 405, 482, 488, and 498 (2007).

Mendonça, H. M., dos Reis, M. A., Sesso, R. C. C., Câmara, N. O. S., & Pacheco-Silva, A. (2007). Renal transplantation outcomes: A comparative analysis between elderly and younger patients. *Clinical Transplantation, 21, 755–760.*

Moore, P. S., Farney, A. C., Hartman, E. I., Rogers, J., Doares, W., Gautreaux, M. D., et al. (2007). Experience with deceased donor kidney transplantation in 114 patients over age 60. *Surgery, 142*(2), 514–523.

Morana, J. (2009). Psychological evaluation and follow-up in liver transplantation. *World Journal of Gastroenterology, 15*(6), 694–696.

Mori, D. L., Gallagher, P., & Milne, J. (2000). The structured interview for renal transplantation (SIRT). *Psychosomatics, 41*(5), 393–406.

National Kidney Foundation. (2013). *Q & A on living donation.* Retrieved from *www.kidney. org/transplantation/livingdonors/infoQA. cfm?id=6.*

Ojo, A. O., Hanson, J. A., Wolfe, R. A., Leichtman, A. B., Agodoa, L. Y., & Port, F. K. (2000). Long-term survival in renal transplant recipients with graft function. *Kidney International, 57, 307–313.*

Olbrisch, M. E. (1996). Ethical issues in psychological evaluation of patients for organ transplant surgery. *Rehabilitation Psychology, 41*(1), 53–71.

Olbrisch, M. E., Benedict, S. M., Ashe, K., & Levenson, J. L. (2002). Psychological assessment and care of organ transplant patients. *Journal of Consulting and Clinical Psychology, 70*(3), 771–783.

Olbrisch, M. E., Benedict, S. M., Haller, D. L., & Levenson, J. L. (2001). Psychosocial assessment of living organ donors: Clinical and ethical considerations. *Progress in Transplantation, 11*(1), 40–49.

Olbrisch, M. E., Levenson, J. L., Fischer, B. A., & Kulstad, J. (2001, November). *Psychosocial evaluation of organ transplant candidates: Comparative surveys of process and criteria, 1989–90 and 2000*. Paper presented at the annual meeting of the American Psychosomatic Society, San Antonio, TX.

Olbrisch, M. E., Levenson, J. L., & Hamer, R. (1989). The PACT: A rating scale for the study of clinical decision making in psychosocial screening of organ transplant candidates. *Clinical Transplantation, 3*, 164–169.

Orentlicher, D. (1996). Psychosocial assessment of organ transplant candidates and the Americans with Disabilities Act. *General Hospital Psychiatry, 18*, 5S–12S.

Organ Procurement and Transplantation Network. (2013). *Transplants by donor type* [Data file]. Retrieved from *http://optn.transplant.hrsa.gov/latestData/rptData.asp*.

Pfitzmann, R., Schwenzer, J., Rayes, N., Seehofer, D., Neuhaus, R., & Nussler, N.C. (2007). Long-term survival and predictors of relapse after orthotopic liver transplantation for alcoholic liver disease. *Liver Transplantation, 13*(2), 197–205.

Pungpapong, S., Manzarbeitia, C. Ortiz, J., Reich, D. J., Araya, V., Rothstein, K. D., et al. (2002). Cigarette smoking is associated with an increased risk of vascular complications after liver transplantation. *Liver Transplantation, 8*(7), 582–587.

Randolph, C. (1998). *Repeatable Battery for the Assessment of Neuropsychological Status Manual*. San Antonio, TX: Psychological Corporation/Harcourt Brace.

Sanchez-Lazaro, I. J., Almenar, L., Martinez-Dolz, L., Moro, J., Ortiz-Martinez, V., Izquierdo, M. T., et al. (2007). Impact of smoking on survival after heart transplantation. *Transplantation Proceedings, 39*(7), 2377–2378.

Shaw, R., & Taussig, H. N. (1999). Pediatric psychiatric pretransplant evaluation. *Clinical Child Psychology and Psychiatry, 4*(3), 353–365.

Stilley, C., DiMartini, A., de Vera, M., Flynn, W., King, J., Sereika, S., et al. (2010). Individual and environmental correlates and predictors of early adherence and outcomes after liver transplantation. *Progress in Transplantation, 20*(1), 58–67.

Stuber, M. (2010). Psychiatric issues in pediatric organ transplantation. *Child and Adolescent Psychiatry Clinics of North America, 19*(2), 285–300.

Sung, R. S., Althoen, M., Howell, T. A., Ojo, A. O., & Merion, R. M. (2001). Excess risk of renal allograft loss associated with cigarette smoking. *Transplantation, 71*(12), 1752–1757.

Surman, O. S., Fukunishi, I., Allen, T., & Hertl, M. (2005). Live organ donation: Social context, clinical encounter, and the psychology of communication. *Psychosomatics, 46*(1), 1–6.

Terasaki, P. I., Gertson, D. W., Cecka, J. M., Takemoto, S., & Cho, Y. W. (1997). Significance of the donor age effect on kidney transplants. *Clinical Transplantation, 11*, 366–372.

Twillman, R. K., Manetto, C., Wellisch, D. K., & Wolcott, D. L. (1993). The Transplant Evaluation Rating Scale: A revision of the psychosocial levels system for evaluating organ transplant candidates. *Psychosomatics, 24*(2), 144–153.

United Network for Organ Sharing. (2013a). *History*. Available at *www.unos.org/donation/index.php?topic=history*.

United Network for Organ Sharing. (2013b). *Transplant trends*. Available at *http://unos.org*.

Wilkinson, A. (1996). Evaluation of the transplant recipient. In G. Danovitch (Ed.), *Handbook of kidney transplantation* (2nd ed., pp. 109–122). Boston: Little, Brown.

Wolcott, D., & Strouse, T. (1996). Psychiatric aspects of kidney transplantation. In G. Danovitch (Ed.), *Handbook of kidney transplantation* (2nd ed., pp. 297–309). Boston: Little, Brown.

Wu, C., Shapiro, R., Tan, H., Basu, A., Smetanka, C., Morgan, C., et al. (2008). Kidney transplantation in elderly people: The influence of recipient comorbidity and living kidney donors. *Journal of the American Geriatrics Society, 56*(2), 231–238.

CHAPTER 23

Bariatric Surgery

Mary Ellen Olbrisch
Melanie K. Bean
Karen E. Stewart

Finding successful treatment options for obesity has become increasingly important as the prevalence of the disorder has risen dramatically (Ogden et al., 2006; Ogden, Carroll, Kit, & Flegal, 2012). Obesity is caused by a combination of genetic, metabolic, environmental, cultural, and lifestyle factors; however, the rapid rise in obesity indicates that lifestyle and environmental factors causing energy imbalance are the greatest contributors to the current epidemic (National Heart, Lung, and Blood Institute Obesity Education Initiative Expert Panel, 2000). Currently, the three general approaches to treatment are lifestyle modification (e.g., diet, exercise), pharmacotherapy, and bariatric surgery.

Lifestyle changes are the first step in treating obesity and related comorbidities; lifestyle changes alone, however, are typically not effective for significant, sustained weight loss in the severely obese. Both lifestyle and drug interventions consistently produce about a 7-pound weight loss, sustained for 2 years, which is associated with improvements in diabetes, blood pressure, and/or cardiovascular risk factors (Powell, Calvin, & Calvin, 2007). Although this relatively small weight loss has significant health effects, sustained loss at this level still leaves a patient in the severely obese range with elevated health risks relative to a person of healthy weight. In addition, small weight loss can be difficult for a person with obesity to accept as improving health; benefits in areas such as increased activity, decreased fatigue, and lowered feelings of social stigmatization have not been demonstrated. The greatest potential for sustained significant weight loss in persons with clinically severe obesity is found with surgical intervention (Powell et al., 2007).

Psychologists and other mental health professionals serve an important function in the assessment of bariatric surgery candidates (Bean, Stewart, & Olbrisch, 2008). Presurgical psychological evaluation is recommended in the majority of practices, with several domains deemed important to assess. However, a consensus on how to psychologically assess patients for surgery most effectively in order to predict successful outcomes has not been clearly elucidated. These psychosocial domains and various assessment strategies for bariatric surgery candidates are presented in this chapter.

Obesity

Obesity has reached epidemic proportions in the United States, with one in three adults classified as obese (body mass index [BMI] of ≥ 30.0 kilograms/height in meters squared; Flegal, Carroll, Ogden, & Curtin, 2010). Obesity is the second leading cause of preventable premature death in this country, with some researchers predicting it may eventually outpace smoking and become the leading cause of preventable death (Stein & Colditz, 2004). Overweight, a risk factor for obesity, includes those with a BMI of 25.0–29.0. The obese category is further delineated into Class I (mild) BMI = 30.0–34.9; Class II (moderate) BMI = 35.0–39.0; Class III (severe) BMI ≥ 40.0. Bariatric surgeons sometime classify patients with a BMI > 50 as "superobese." Health consequences of obesity include cardiovascular disease, sleep apnea, hypertension, Type 2 diabetes, and some cancers (Bray, 2004). Psychosocial comorbidities include depression, social stigmatization and discrimination, and poor quality of life (Fabricatore & Wadden, 2006).

Surgical Intervention Guidelines

A consensus conference convened by the National Institutes of Health (NIH) in 1991 recommended bariatric surgery for the treatment of clinically severe obesity and set guidelines for patient selection. Potential candidates must have a BMI ≥ 40.0 or between 35.0 and 40.0 with a weight-related comorbidity, such as cardiopulmonary problems (e.g., sleep apnea or cardiomyopathy), severe diabetes, or other obesity-induced physical health problems. Further, candidates must be "motivated" and must have first attempted and failed at supervised, nonsurgical weight loss approaches (NIH, 1991). The requirement for "failure," in our view, should be rewritten, as the term is misleading and, of course, the goal is easily achieved. What should be required is at least one previous sustained effort at successful weight loss during which the candidate acquired knowledge and skills necessary to be successful with weight loss surgery. Anyone can fail nonsurgical weight loss approaches merely by not putting forth much effort, and this does not prepare or make someone a good candidate for weight loss surgery.

Types of Surgery

The two main contemporary categories of bariatric surgery are restrictive and combined restrictive/malabsorptive. In general, these procedures promote weight loss by altering the digestive process. Currently, over 90% of bariatric procedures are performed laparoscopically (Elder & Wolf, 2007), decreasing the risk of certain complications and shortening recovery time compared with open procedures. With the widespread adoption of laparoscopic techniques, the number of bariatric surgical procedures in the United States increased 800% from 1998 to 2004, with about 121,055 procedures in 2004 (Zhao & Encinosa, 2007). Costs range from $20,000 to $35,000, with varying coverage by state and insurance providers (National Institutes of Health and the National Institute of Diabetes and Digestive and Kidney Diseases, 2004). In a meta-analysis of bariatric surgery outcomes in morbidly obese individuals, Buchwald et al. (2004) reported that surgery reverses, eliminates, or significantly reduces the effects of diabetes, hypertension, hyperlipidemia, and obstructive sleep apnea in the majority of patients, speaking to the great potential for weight loss surgery to significantly improve the health of these patients.

Restrictive

Purely restrictive procedures include adjustable gastric banding and vertical banded gastroplasty (VBG); they promote weight loss by restricting food intake, or limiting the capacity of the stomach to accommodate food. In adjustable gastric banding (such as the Lap-Band System), a synthetic band with a small inflatable inner balloon is placed around part of the stomach. This balloon is inflated by injection of saline into a subcutaneous port to adjust the degree of gastric restriction. This procedure is reversible and is only effective if the band is readjusted as required and on a long-term basis. VBG is a variant of the restrictive approach, which includes placing four rows of staples in the stomach with a band placed on the external gastric surface. Although VBG was a dominant procedure in the 1980s, it is less common today due to low long-term maintenance of weight loss (Elder & Wolfe, 2007). Average weight loss (percentage of excess weight) is about 47.5% for gastric banding and 61.6% for VBG (Buchwald et al., 2004).

Mortality rates are estimated to be 0.1% with restrictive bariatric procedures (Buchwald et al., 2004). Risks include vomiting, band slippage or erosion, leakage, infection, and bleeding. Although these approaches are generally safer than malabsorptive/combined operations (described subsequently), patients lose less weight and are less likely to maintain the weight loss. If health behaviors are not changed to be more consistent with a healthy diet and exercise regimen, this procedure will not be an effective weight loss tool, as success depends on patients' postoperative health behaviors (NIH, 2004).

More recently, the sleeve gastrectomy has become a popular restrictive surgery. In this procedure, the stomach is reduced to the size of a banana or a taco, with the rest of it removed, and there is no bypass of the intestines. Patients frequently report seeking this surgery to avoid the implantation of a foreign object and the inconvenience of returning for band adjustments. Early data indicate that this surgery has higher risk-adjusted morbidity and higher readmission and reoperation/intervention rates compared with gastric banding, but fewer reoperations are needed compared with gastric bypass. Mortality rates were comparable for all surgeries, and effectiveness was somewhat better than for the band but less than for gastric bypass (Hutter et al., 2011).

Combined Restrictive/Malabsorptive

Combined procedures include the gastric bypass and biliopancreatic diversion. The gold standard of weight loss surgery is the Roux en Y gastric bypass procedure (RYGBP), which consists of a stomach reduction to reduce food intake and a bypass of a portion of the small intestine, reducing the amount of calories and nutrients that the body absorbs (Mechanick et al., 2008). For most patients, consumption of sugar results in "dumping syndrome," a highly aversive combination of symptoms that punishes the consumption of sugar in any significant quantity (Tadross & le Roux, 2009). Recent analyses suggest that the gut quickly compensates for malabsorption following RYGBP and that dumping syndrome does not correlate well with weight loss; thus other mechanisms, such as altered entero-endocrine axis responding and changes in taste perception, are being examined as mechanisms of weight loss in this procedure (Tadross & le Roux, 2009). Average weight loss with gastric bypass surgery is about 68% of excess weight (Buchwald et al., 2004).

Biliopancreatic diversion is a less common procedure that promotes the selective malabsorption of fat. Although the average excess weight loss is 70.1% (Buchwald et al., 2004), more complications (e.g., malnutrition and diarrhea) tend to occur with this procedure compared with gastric bypass (Scopinaro et al., 1998). Mortality rates are slightly higher with these combined approaches, with a 0.5% risk of death in gastric bypass and a 1.1% risk with biliopancreatic diversion or duodenal switch (Buchwald et al., 2004). As with the restrictive approaches, successful weight loss is largely a factor of postsurgical patient behaviors, including participation in adequate physical activity and adherence to dietary modifications. Patients must abandon the view that surgery provides a "cure" or an "easy fix" and come to understand surgery as a tool that enables the same healthy and committed behaviors essential to any weight loss program.

Experimental Surgeries

The vagus nerve system is associated with gastric expansion and contraction, release of gastric acid, satiety, and gastric emptying (Schwartz, 2000). Because of these functions, vagus nerve stimulation (VNS) is being investigated for its potential to decrease appetite and promote weight loss. Based on early animal models and VNS for the treatment of epilepsy and treatment-resistant depression, VNS may prove to be effective in promoting weight loss by reducing food cravings (Bodenlos et al., 2007). However, it is premature to suggest that VNS is a safe and effective weight-loss tool. Clinical trials are currently under way to investigate the effects of an implantable vagal nerve blocker on weight loss (Camilleri et al., 2008, 2009). Also under investigation is a similar device called a gastric pacemaker or implantable gastric stimulator (Cigaina & Hirschberg, 2007), which is attached directly to the wall of the stomach. These devices lend themselves to double-blind clinical trials because patients can be randomly assigned to having the device activated or inactive for a period of time.

Patient Characteristics

General characteristics of patients seeking surgery can help to better explain the need for psychological assessment and to shape the assessment process. Overall, about 1% of eligible individuals with morbid obesity receive bariatric surgery (Elder & Wolfe, 2007). These patients have an average BMI of 47.4 (Buchwald, Estok, Fahrbach, Banel, & Sledge, 2007). About 85% of patients are female, with a mean age of 40.0 (Buchwald et al., 2007). Further, European Americans are more likely to seek surgery than African Americans, despite higher prevalence of obesity among African Americans, particularly African American women (Livingston & Ko, 2004). These disparities may reflect differential access to health care and/or cultural differences in acceptance of body size norms.

Common medical comorbidities include Type 2 diabetes, cardiovascular disease, degenerative joint disease, asthma, obstructive sleep apnea, gastroesophageal reflux disease (GERD), hypertension, and hypercholesterolemia (Buchwald et al., 2007; Zhaoping, Bowerman, & Heber, 2005). The high prevalence of medical conditions in this population suggests that many patients will have complicated medical regimens, which may have implications for compliance. Pain and mobility issues may also be factors negatively affecting patients' behavioral and psychosocial status.

Psychological and/or psychiatric difficulties, including depression, eating disorders, anxiety, and personality disorders, are often present (Greenberg, Perna, Kaplan, & Sullivan, 2005; Wadden et al., 2007). An international review suggested that the lifetime presurgical prevalence of DSM-IV Axis I disorders ranged from 27 to 42% (Herpertz et al., 2003). Presence of mood, anxiety, and eating disorders were the most common findings. Patients with Class 3 obesity (BMI ≥ 40) were five times more likely to have experienced an episode of major depression in the preceding year compared with persons of average weight (Onyike, Crum, Lee, Lyketsos, & Eaton, 2003). About 25–30% of patients seeking surgery report clinically significant symptoms of depression at the time of the assessment (Wadden et al., 2007), with about 50% reporting lifetime history of mood or anxiety disorders (Sarwer, Wadden, & Fabricatore, 2005; Wadden et al., 2007). Gender moderates the obesity–depression relationship, with obese women reporting higher rates of depression than obese men (Fabricatore & Wadden, 2006). Lifetime prevalence of DSM-IV Axis II disorders is about 22–24% (Herpertz et al., 2003); psychotic disorders are rare in this population (Glinski, Wetzler, & Goodman, 2001).

Individuals seeking bariatric surgery may present with eating disorders, particularly binge eating disorder (BED) and night-eating syndrome (NES). BED is characterized by binge eating without compensatory behavior (e.g., vomiting, laxative use). Specifically, a binge is defined as the consumption of an amount of food that is "definitely larger" (American Psychiatric Association, 2013, pp. 350–351) than what other people might eat under similar circumstances during a discrete period of time. The binge episode must be characterized by a subjective lack of control and must be associated with three of five additional characteristics: eating rapidly, eating until uncomfortably full, eating in absence of hunger, eating alone out of embarrassment, or feeling disgusted, depressed, or guilty after eating (see American Psychiatric Association, 2013, for full criteria). Proposed diagnostic criteria for NES have included (1) either consuming > 25% of daily calories after the evening meal or nocturnal ingestion (eating during a nighttime waking episode; patient must be aware of and recall the nocturnal ingestion) and (2) the presence of at least three of five of the following symptoms: morning anorexia, strong desire to eat in the evening or during the night, insomnia, belief that eating is required to get back to sleep, and worsening mood during evening hours (see Allison et al., 2010, for full proposed criteria). DSM-5 now includes NES in the category Other Specified Feeding or Eating Disorder, describing NES as "recurrent episodes of night eating as manifested by eating after awakening from sleep, or by excessive food consumption after the evening meal" (American Psychiatric Association, 2013, p. 354; see DSM-5 for full criteria). Reported prevalence rates for these disorders in persons seeking bariatric surgery have been quite variable due to inconsistencies in defining and assessing these conditions. As NES criteria have only recently been formalized, no known studies to date have evaluated the prevalence of NES using these criteria in bariatric surgery candidates. A recent study utilized both self-report and semistructured diagnostic interview and considered varying severity of both BED and NES symptoms. Results indicated that 4.2% of individuals presenting for bariatric surgery met full criteria (according to DSM-IV-TR criteria; American Psychiatric Association, 2000) for BED, while an additional 1.4% reported one binge episode per week (two binges per week are required by DSM-IV-TR; Allison et al., 2006). In assessing NES symptoms in bariatric surgery candidates, Allison et al. (2006) found that the prevalence of evening hyperphagia was 3.7% and that of nocturnal ingestions (three times per week or more) was 3.3% (with an additional 6.5% engaging in nocturnal ingestions less than three times per week). About 18.5% of the sample met criteria for both BED and NES, using the least restrictive definitions of both conditions, and 7% met criteria for both disorders using the strictest definitions (Allison et al., 2006). A diagnosis of BED in this population has been shown to be associated with increased risk of current and lifetime diagnoses of mood and anxiety disorders (Jones-Corneille et al., 2010).

Purpose of the Psychological Assessment

A mental health evaluation was initially required as part of the presurgical comprehensive multidisciplinary assessment to check for psychosocial contraindications to surgery and potential obstacles to postoperative success (NIH, 1991). More recently, the American Society for Bariatric Surgery replaced its statement that evaluation by mental health professionals is not mandatory for all patients with a document outlining "Suggestions for the Pre-Surgical Psychological Assessment of Bariatric Surgery Candidates" (LeMont et al., 2004). Psychological evaluation is the norm as part of a comprehensive multidisciplinary assessment, with over 86% of surgical programs including a psychological assessment as a routine component of the presurgical bariatric surgery evaluation (Bauchowitz et al., 2005; Buchwald & the Consensus Conference Panel, 2005). These assessments are performed primarily by psychologists but also include psychiatrists and master's-level professionals (Bauchowitz et al., 2005).

Psychosocial and psychiatric concerns among candidates and the need to explore motivation and informed consent for surgery are primary reasons for a psychological evaluation as part of the multidisciplinary presurgical assessment. The role of the psychologist is to identify emotional, psychiatric, cognitive, and behavioral factors that may influence surgical success. Multiple behavior changes must be made prior to and for a lifetime after surgery; psychologists can help patients understand their responsibilities and try to anticipate and overcome obstacles to surgical success. The assessment of patients seeking bariatric surgery functions as both assessment and intervention. It also provides an opportunity to educate patients about the surgery and the potential impact of psychological factors on surgery outcomes. Psychologists are thus critical members of the multidisciplinary team for their ability to evaluate behavioral and psychosocial variables influencing treatment outcome and to provide treatment recommendations and behavioral prescriptions that can enhance the likelihood of surgical success.

The role of psychologists is consultative; that is, they identify psychological factors that may require attention prior to surgery and communicate these with the surgeon and others on the multidisciplinary team. Further, it is the psychologist's function to make explicit recommendations to patients based on specific requirements for surgery set by the surgeon and/or the insurer. For example, some surgeons require patients to be abstinent from tobacco for a specified period of time prior to surgery; this message may be communicated to the patient by several members of the multidisciplinary team, with treatment recommendations provided by the psychologist. Some insurers require a medically supervised diet, typically of 6 months' duration, despite the absence of evidence that these are effective over the long term (Ochner, Puma, Raevuori, Teixeira, & Geliebter, 2010). Insurers' requirements often place patients in what patients perceive to be a "Catch-22" situation; they believe that success with presurgical dieting will disqualify them from surgical intervention, thus leading to dishonesty with the health care team and failure to learn from the structure that such programs provide. The psychologist must move the patient from the language and necessity of failure toward an attitude of mastery and success. Emphasis on the risk reduction of presurgical weight loss is also often helpful.

The presurgical evaluation serves to increase the chance of optimal outcomes, such as achieving desired weight loss, improvements in health behavior, adequate coping, and minimal psychosocial concerns. It also serves to reduce the likelihood of postsurgical complications, such as weight gain after an initial period of loss, anorexia or obsessive behaviors surrounding weight loss, malnutrition, failure to achieve adequate weight loss, psychosocial problems, or exacerbation of psychiatric conditions. Alteration in absorption of psychotropic or other medication may occur postoperatively; thus it is essential to communicate with prescribing physicians and to ensure that patients are scheduled for regular psychiatric follow-up in the early months after surgery during the period of most rapid weight loss.

Because there are few absolute psychological contraindications to bariatric surgery, the assessment should focus on risk management, with the goal of improving the patient's postoperative quality of life. Indeed, some psychologists have raised questions about the ethics of denying patients access to surgery when the clinical data do not present a clear picture of the relation between psychiatric status and surgical outcome (Taylor & Misra, 2009; Wadden & Sarwer, 2006). Research efforts to clarify the role of psychosocial factors in long-term outcomes in bariatric surgery and to evaluate assessment procedures are ongoing through the Longitudinal Assessment of Bariatric Surgery (LABS) program sponsored by the National Institute of Diabetes and Digestive and Kidney Diseases at NIH and at a number of surgical programs around the country. Thus it is to be expected that assessment methods in this population will continue to develop in the coming years.

Current methods of assessing patients for bariatric surgery have been developed through a combination of clinical experience working with patients both before and after surgery, review of clinical research focused on bariatric surgery patients, and review of procedures that psychologists are using in other programs. Although specific procedures and measurement tools (both of which are reviewed later in this chapter) vary by site, there appears to be a fair degree of consensus about the domains of psychological functioning that are important to consider in assessing candidates for bariatric surgery.

The Psychological Assessment

Most evaluations consist of a semistructured clinical interview in combination with standardized measures (Fabricatore, Crerand, Wadden, Sarwer, & Krasucki, 2006). The clinical interview assesses the domains described in this section and in Table 23.1. Standardized instruments (also listed in Table 23.1) supplement this interview to formally assess psychopathology, personality, health behaviors, and other domains. Most programs use a semistructured interview, symptom checklist(s) assessing depression, anxiety, and/or eating disorders, and measures of personality/psychopathology. Tests of cognitive function are also used on occasion (Fabricatore et al., 2006).

At this time, there is limited evidence that these assessments have predictive validity for surgical outcomes. Few long-term follow-up studies have been reported. Studies reporting outcomes within the first year after surgery, particularly those focused only on weight loss, are of limited value because most patients will lose weight regardless of success at behavior change or because the opportunity to revert to presurgical behaviors is limited in the early postoperative

TABLE 23.1. Domains Typically Assessed in Psychological Evaluation of Bariatric Surgery Candidates

Domain	Tests administered
Substance abuse	• Clinical Interview • Drug Abuse Screening Test (DAST[a]; Skinner, 1992) • Alcohol Use Disorder Test—Core (AUDIT-C[a]; Babor et al., 1992)
Eating attitudes and behaviors	• Clinical interview • Olbrisch Bariatric Eating Scale (OBESE; Peterson et al., 2012) • Questionnaire on Weight and Eating Patterns—Revised (QEWP-R)[a] (Nangle, Johnson, Carr-Nangle, & Engler, 1994) • Eating Disorder Inventory (Garner, Olmstead, & Polivy, 1983) • Two-Day Food Diaries (Olbrisch et al., 2006) • Eating Disorders Examination—Questionnaire Version (Fairburn & Beglin, 1994)
Health behaviors/ adherence	• Clinical interview—weight and dieting history • Millon Behavioral Medicine Diagnostic (MBMD[a]; Millon, Antoni, Millon, Meagher, & Millon, 2001) • Multidimensional Health Locus of Control (MHLC[a]; Wallston, Wallston, & DeVellis, 1978) • Millon Behavioral Health Inventory (Millon, Green, & Meagher, 1979) • Health and Behavioral Issues Test (HABIT; Heckman et al., 2005) • Medical Outcomes Study, Short Form (SF-36)–Health Status (Ware & Sherbourne, 1992) • Weight and Lifestyle Inventory (WALI; Sandoz Nutrition, 1988)
Personality/ psychopathology	• Minnesota Multiphasic Personality Inventory–2 (MMPI-2; Butcher, Dahlstrom, Graham, Tellegen, & Kaemmer, 1989) • Brief Symptom Index (BSI; Derogatis, 1993) • Structured Clinical Interview of DSM Disorders—I&II (SCID-I & II; First & Gibbon, 2004) • Personality Assessment Inventory (PAI; Morey, 1991) • Symptom Checklist–90 (Derogatis, 1973) • Beck Anxiety Inventory (BAI; Beck, 1993) • State–Trait Anxiety Inventory (STAI; Spielberger, 1983) • Beck Depression Inventory–II (BDI-II; Beck et al., 1996)
Knowledge/ informed consent	• Quiz • Clinical interview
Cognitive function	• Mini Mental Status Examination (Folstein, Folstein, & McHugh, 1975)
Social support	• Clinical interview

[a]Department of Veterans Affairs standard evaluation.

phase, which may last from 1 to 2 years. A systematic review by Livhits et al. (2011) that included 115 articles published on preoperative predictors of weight loss demonstrated that mandatory preoperative weight loss was positively associated with postoperative weight loss and that preoperative BMI, superobesity, and personality disorders were negatively associated with weight loss after surgery. Unfortunately, many of the included studies found conflicting results, which may be related to heterogeneous definitions of predictors and outcome measures and highly variable follow-up periods (Livhits et al., 2011). Thus there is a great need to establish more uniformity in assessment and follow-up of preoperative psychiatric, behavioral, cognitive, and environmental factors that are predicted to be related to postoperative outcomes. In the absence of demonstrated predictive validity, there is little benefit gained from norming instruments on a bariatric population at this time. However, with the additional knowledge expected to be gained through LABS and other large-scale research studies, we may soon be able to identify factors that predict weight loss surgery outcomes, to norm instruments accordingly, and to address factors that predict surgical outcomes. The following section describes each domain assessed in the evaluation and current findings with respect to surgical outcomes.

Knowledge and Informed Consent

Patients should understand the potential risks and complications associated with bariatric surgery, including risk of death, possible conversion to an open procedure (large incision surgery) rather than a laparoscopic surgery, bleeding, infection, pulmonary embolism, and other risks. In addition, patients should also understand the responsibilities of maintaining their health after surgery (taking multivitamins and other supplements, ensuring adequate protein intake, progressing from liquid/pureed to solid foods, reducing fat, avoiding sugar, increasing exercise, avoiding dumping syndrome, etc.). Knowledge of surgery and patient responsibilities can be assessed using a standard quiz (e.g., Madan & Tichansky, 2005) and a clinical interview.

No surgery is risk-free, and many patients acknowledge this in discussion. Patients are often aware of the risk of complications and have already decided that the threat to health caused by their obesity is greater than the risks of surgery. Patients are rarely deemed unable to provide informed consent due to poor understanding of risks (Zimmerman et al., 2007); however, 60% of respondents to a recent survey of mental health professionals ranked knowledge of risks among the most important facets of this type of assessment (Fabricatore et al., 2006). If a patient has inadequate knowledge of the surgery and patient responsibilities, most often the patient can be advised to complete additional reading and attend additional meetings and educational sessions with members of the team to remedy this.

Patients who are cognitively impaired due to mental illness, injury, medical illness, or developmental delay must be considered on a case-by-case basis. In cases of severe mental illness, it may be prudent to advise a patient to enter treatment and achieve and maintain psychological stability for a defined period prior to surgery. A similar approach can be taken with a patient whose medical illness or traumatic injury can be expected to resolve. If cognitive status cannot be expected to improve, surgery should be described to the patient in understandable terms. The patient's support network will be of pivotal importance in determining whether the patient will be able to adhere to behavioral recommendations following surgery. The patient may require extensive support through a day treatment or residential treatment program, although some higher functioning patients can be successful with support from family in the home. If the support network is able to meet the patient's needs, if the patient provides assent, and if a designated medical decision maker provides consent, the patient may in certain cases be an appropriate candidate for surgery. The following case illustrates how the aforementioned factors come into play when deciding the proper course of action.

Case Vignette

A 64-year-old woman from a community 5 hours from our medical center who suffered severe memory, speech, and physical impairment related to a series of strokes 5 years earlier was evaluated for gastric bypass. She had been using a wheelchair for a number of years. Despite her disability, the patient was the primary caregiver for her much older husband, who suffered from dementia but was identified as her main source of support. She had a remote history of successful weight loss with a very low calorie liquid protein diet. The patient was instructed to seek a referral for a physical therapy consultation to determine whether she could begin a supervised aquatic exercise program. She was also provided with instructions for a healthier diet and asked to enlist support from members of her extended family. Finally, the patient was advised that because of her special circumstances, she would be served better by a program closer to her home. The patient followed all of this advice and, after improving her diet and physical conditioning, underwent a successful gastric bypass procedure at a hospital close to her home. The patient was followed by telephone to provide her with support and to assess the value of the recommendations. Her commitment to diet and exercise were maintained for 18 months after surgery when last assessed.

Expectations for Surgery

It is important to determine whether a patient has reasonable expectations for surgery and its short- and long-term outcomes. This factor is primarily assessed by clinical interview, asking questions such as "What are some of your reasons to have this surgery?" "How much weight do you expect to lose?" and "What other ways do you expect surgery/losing weight to affect your life?"

It is critical that a patient understand that surgery is a tool that will help him or her to achieve weight loss through diet and exercise. Patients may also have unrealistic expectations that they will lose 100% of their excess weight, when average weight loss is approximately 70% for gastric bypass and 48% for gastric banding (Buchwald et al., 2004). Discussing realistic weight loss goals may help to prevent patients from feeling like failures if they do not reach their "ideal" body weights following surgery. It can be helpful to frame this weight loss in terms of improvements in health and functioning.

Patients sometimes describe unrealistic expectations in other life domains, such as dramatic improvements in their social lives or greater career success. Although it is likely that people will respond to changes in the patient, patients should be advised that there can be negative as well as positive effects of changing one's appearance. If they have social or career goals that they would like to achieve, they can be counseled in ways in which they may need to change their behavior (e.g., assertiveness training, communication skills). Patients may also be unaware of the potential negative effect of surgery on their existing relationships. Partners may feel threatened by increased sexual attention directed at the patient, and relationships may be challenged as the patient begins to prioritize his or her own health, which others may perceive as "selfish" behavior. Others may resent these changes in the patient as he or she loses weight. Patients should be encouraged to discuss these changes with partners, friends, and family as they consider having surgery. Further, patients should be encouraged to think about how they will feel about

possibly receiving increased attention due to the change in their appearance. This may be particularly relevant for patients who have used their weight as a means of avoiding unwanted social or sexual attention either due to social concerns or history of sexual abuse, harassment, or trauma. Patients with social anxiety disorders or avoidant personality traits may report similar apprehension about changes in appearance.

Eating Attitudes and Behaviors

Ideally, patients will have insight into their dietary and exercise habits and will already have begun these changes as they have contemplated having surgery. Eating attitudes and behaviors can be assessed through a combination of clinical interview, food journals (Olbrisch et al., 2006), and standardized measures.

Current definitions of eating disorders do not adequately encompass the range of eating problems described by obese patients (Olbrisch et al., 2006). It has been believed by many that binge eating prior to surgery would have a deleterious effect on weight loss outcomes, but studies have shown that binge eating does not predict postsurgical weight loss up to 18 months after surgery (Bocchieri-Ricciardi et al., 2006), and one study found weight loss to be greater during the 12 months after surgery among persons with severe symptoms of binge eating (Malone & Alger-Mayer, 2004). Varying rates and effects of binge eating and eating disorders not otherwise specified in bariatric surgery patients are likely due to use of different diagnostic criteria and variable follow-up periods. Binge eating may also fail to consistently relate to weight loss outcomes in short-term follow-up studies because surgery initially causes what some have termed "forced behavior modification" (Elkins et al., 2005, p. 549), and long-term outcomes will depend more heavily on a patient's ability to willingly comply with behavioral recommendations for weight loss and weight management and his or her commitment to lifelong change.

Some have suggested that it is useful to focus on the subjective sense of loss of control over eating rather than the quantity of food consumed, particularly considering that patients will be limited in their ability to eat large quantities of food during a discrete period of time and that binges may shift into grazing-pattern eating after surgery (Saunders, 2004). Focusing on this element of disordered eating also covers a fuller range of eating pathology by including many different types of problem eating (i.e., night eating, grazing, emotional eating, and preference for high-fat and/or high-sugar foods). In support of this approach, a study of patients 2–7 years postsurgery defined binge eaters as people who reported either objective or subjective binge episodes and found that this group had lost comparable amounts of weight postsurgery to non-binge eaters but had experienced greater weight regain than non-binge eaters (Kalarchian et al., 2002).

Some patients mistakenly believe that surgery will solve their eating problems by not allowing them to overeat or binge. Because of the potential for problem eating patterns to resurface in the longer term postsurgery period, patients should be asked to consider entering counseling to learn about and work on their specific eating problems and to develop skills in using alternative coping strategies. Some programs may require that the patient follow through with these recommendations prior to clearing the patient for surgery (Zimmerman et al., 2007).

Psychiatric History and Status/Personality

As described earlier, patients with clinically severe obesity have been shown to suffer greater rates of lifetime psychiatric disorders compared with the general population. A person's psychological stability is important in determining candidacy for surgery. History and current status of suicidal thoughts, intentions, and attempts should be explored, along with a detailed history of prior and current symptoms of clinical disorders. It may be wise to advise patients with a history of, but no current, severe psychopathology to seek support from a mental health professional after surgery to monitor for recurrence of any psychiatric symptoms.

Patients with severe mental illness, such as psychotic disorders, are not necessarily ineligible for surgery, but special attention must be paid to the current status and stability of their symptoms and to possible changes in therapeutic response to their medica-

tions after surgery. Due to uncertainty of the effects of gastric bypass surgery on drug metabolism, patients with severe psychiatric conditions may be better served by having restrictive surgery. Rates of drug absorption and bioavailability (the amount of the administered dose that is delivered into the bloodstream after the drug is metabolized) of orally administered medications may change following gastric bypass due to reductions in hydrochloric acid production and to reduced gastrointestinal surface area necessary for drug absorption. These effects will have differential impacts according to the pharmacokinetic properties of the drug (Miller & Smith, 2006). These changes raise concerns for the postsurgical status of patients whose psychiatric condition(s) are managed by medication. Because pharmacokinetic drug studies do not include patients with altered gastrointestinal systems, the exact effect of the procedure on specific drugs is uncertain; however, certain classes of drugs (nonsteroidal anti-inflammatory drugs [NSAIDs] and salicylates) are not recommended in this population due to potentially increased risk of ulceration. Reductions in bioavailability and drug absorption are more likely to result in poor therapeutic response than increased toxicity; therefore, patients may be able to safely continue using their medications. However, monitoring for therapeutic effectiveness should be increased in the postsurgical period. Immediate release, liquid formulations, and other methods of drug administration may help to improve therapeutic response to medication (Miller & Smith, 2006), and patients should discuss the effects of surgery on all of their medications with the medical professionals who prescribed them. Banding procedures also have the potential to change drug absorption by increasing the amount of time that medications are in the proximal section of the stomach, and close medical supervision is also recommended for these patients (Wilting, 2007).

Studies done with the Minnesota Multiphasic Personality Inventory–2 (MMPI-2; Butcher, Dahlstrom, Graham, Tellegen, & Kaemmer, 1989) have shown that certain personality traits may be associated with poorer weight loss following surgery. Patients with elevations on F, Hysteria (Scale 3), Paranoia (Scale 6), and Health

Concerns scales and who score lower on the Masculinity–Femininity Scale (5) were more likely to belong to a group of patients who lost < 50% of their excess weight with Roux-en-Y gastric bypass than to the group of patients who lost > 50% of their excess weight. Further, a profile with a combination of elevated Health Concerns and low Masculinity–Femininity was the strongest predictor of belonging to this group (Tsushima, Bridenstine, & Balfour, 2004). Even in the < 50% group, these variations were within normal limits, with the exception of mild elevations for Hysteria (T = 65.2) and Hypochondriasis (T = 67.1; Tsushima et al., 2004). These findings suggest the need for further evaluation of the role of personality in postsurgery outcomes and support the use of the MMPI-2 in this population. This study also suggests that personality alone does not warrant exclusion of persons with these traits; however, persons with such a profile may be advised to enter counseling in order to minimize the degree to which behavioral patterns associated with these traits interfere with the patient's postsurgical outcomes.

Social Support

Social support will be important during the immediate postsurgical period and will continue to play a role in the patient's success long term. Patients may underestimate the time of their recovery and the impact of following their recommended postsurgery food plan during the weeks immediately after surgery. Many patients can return to normal physical activity within a week of surgery; however, it is often recommended that they prepare to take 4 weeks off from a full routine of demanding activities at work and at home. This may mean asking family and friends to help with chores in the home for the several weeks following surgery. Meal planning during this time can be time-consuming as patients adjust to a new lifestyle, and this can be a stressful time. This extended period for adjustment also allows patients time to focus their energy on prioritizing their health and setting the stage for a new approach to their health and well-being.

Patients should have a support plan in place for meeting their needs for assistance during the postsurgery period, and patients should be counseled in ways to seek additional support if their existing plans are inadequate. In some cases, patients have presented with negative social support. An example of this would be having a spouse or partner who actively seeks to sabotage the patient's success by making negative comments about the patient's ability to follow the new lifestyle. In cases in which the patient's coping resources are poor and social support is inadequate, clearance for surgery may be delayed to allow time for the patient to improve this support, either through family and friends or by entering individual psychotherapy. Psychotherapy may help patients develop coping resources and a support network to maximize the likelihood of surgical success. Behavioral weight management interventions are often provided in group settings, enhancing social support by providing patients opportunities to discuss challenging behavior change with other individuals who are experiencing similar difficulties. Indeed, patients in our "Back on Track" group for postsurgical patients experiencing weight regain cited social support as a major benefit of participating in the group, and they typically exchange e-mail and phone numbers at the completion of the group to maintain contact with each other (Stewart, Olbrisch, & Bean, 2010).

Substance Use

Rates of current substance abuse and dependence are low among bariatric surgery candidates (Sogg, 2007). However, those who do present with active drug or alcohol abuse will likely be considered high risk for surgery by the surgeon and others on the team. Current tobacco use may similarly be considered an unnecessary high risk by the surgeon, and, as stated earlier, some may require a specified period of abstinence prior to agreeing to surgery. In a recent survey of mental health professionals conducting presurgical assessments for bariatric surgery (Fabricatore et al., 2006), presence of a current substance disorder was the most commonly cited clear contraindication for surgery (listed by 44% of respondents). This is likely due to concerns about reduced tolerance to alcohol and altered metabolism of drugs of abuse following bariatric surgery, which could destabilize the patient's psychosocial functioning. As a result, some programs refer a patient for treatment with the guideline of reevaluating the patient for surgical candidacy once the patient has demonstrated 12 months of abstinence (Grothe, Dubbert, & O'Jile, 2006).

Popular media have paid much attention to the question of substance abuse problems in patients who have had weight loss surgery. The prevailing belief is that patients substitute one addiction (alcohol) for another (food) as part of a phenomenon that has been termed "addiction transfer" (Sogg, 2007). *The Oprah Winfrey Show* (Harpo Productions, 2007) told viewers that "some experts are now estimating that as many as 30 percent of those people who have [gastric bypass] surgery will struggle with new addictions like alcoholism, gambling, compulsive shopping, and sex addiction." This concept relies primarily on the lay usage of the term "addiction," which appears to be synonymous with compulsive behavior, while the scientific community remains uncertain as to whether food constitutes an addictive substance. No empirical evidence validates this claim of increased incidence of alcohol abuse. One recent study that followed up with 60 individuals 6–10 years after surgery found that two individuals without a previous history of alcohol problems developed alcohol dependence after surgery, whereas one individual experienced remission of an existing diagnosis of alcohol dependence following surgery (Ertelt et al., 2008). Similarly, Buffington, Daley, Worthen, and Marema (2006) found that 14% of patients increased their alcohol intake after surgery, while 15% drank less after surgery. Additional studies are needed to establish the rates of substance abuse in post-weight-loss-surgery patients, however; these initial findings do not support this claim. Patients considering surgery should be made aware that although these reports in the media may be premature, they should exercise caution in their use of alcohol because their tolerance will likely decrease after surgery.

Adherence

Patients' past histories of following through with medical appointments and recommendations are important in determining readiness for surgery. Patients must understand that the recommendations of their surgeon are intended to maximize their surgical outcomes in terms of weight loss and minimize long-term health consequences related to changes in their gastrointestinal systems that can lead to nutrient deficiencies. Patient adherence can be assessed through clinical interview or by structured questionnaires that inquire about keeping medical appointments when scheduled, about how patients might respond to a medication side effect, and whether the patients ask questions when they do not understand their doctors' recommendations. Patient adherence may also be assessed by consulting medical records and care providers when appropriate. In working with patients with significant histories of medical nonadherence, it may be advisable to require that the patient demonstrate the ability to adhere to lifestyle recommendations prior to surgery by committing to a period of monitoring with the team.

Conclusions and Recommendations to the Surgeon and the Team

Results from the clinical interview and appropriate assessments are formulated into a recommendation for or against surgery based on psychosocial factors. (See the sample report from the Virginia Commonwealth University [VCU] program in Figure 23.1.) We recommend a brief executive summary format for ease of communication to the team and highlighting main points of concern. In our experience, surgeons do not care for ambiguity; thus we make only two conclusions, "acceptable" or "not acceptable at this time," based on the patient's psychosocial functioning. Others may use a term such as "conditionally acceptable"; we believe, however, that the same information can be conveyed in a "not acceptable at this time" recommendation. This latter recommendation reduces ambiguity, which has sometimes resulted in a poor candidate going to surgery before resolving some serious problems that created difficulties in the recovery process. About 70% of candidates are unconditionally recommended for surgery after the psychological evaluation, with fewer than 4% receiving absolute recommendations against surgery (Fabricatore et al., 2006). Providers recommend postponing surgery until specific issues are

Patient Name:	Patience Prudence
Medical Record #:	987654321
Age:	38
Date of Birth:	November 30. 1974
Sex:	Female
Education:	Associate's degree
Occupation:	Unemployed CNA/part-time student
Date of Evaluation:	September 30, 2013
Date of Report:	September 30, 2013

Confidential Report: Psychological Evaluation for Weight Loss Surgery, Diagnostic Interview, and Psychological Testing

- 38-year-old Caucasian woman with clinically severe obesity, height = 5'8", weight = 320 lbs., BMI = 48.7, comorbidities include diabetes, joint pain, back pain, asthma, dyspnea on exertion, possible sleep apnea, and urinary stress incontinence
- medical history significant for cholecystectomy in 2003, C-section and tubal ligation in 2009, dilatation and curettage procedure in 2011, no complications of any previous surgery; medical history also significant for recent diagnosis of celiac disease
- patient has attempted to cut back on sugar intake following her celiac disease diagnosis and appointment with dietician, reports possible weight loss; past history of significant weight loss on Weight Watchers; exercise limited by significant joint pain; recommended she be seen by a physical therapist to discuss exercise options
- quit 1/2 ppd smoking habit 6 years ago; remote history of a period of several months of alcohol abuse during a stressful time of her life, no alcohol use in last 9 years; past history of experimentation with marijuana (several months) and cocaine (one time), no illicit drug use in the past 8 years; no history of prescription drug abuse
- compliance with medications and medical appointments is adequate; patient reports missing medication doses approximately 1–2x a month; patient reports not being seen by dentist for economic reasons but understands the importance of follow-up
- some social support from church community and adult children and limited support from parents; significant psychosocial stressors related to relationship with ex-husband and traumatic events, financial instability
- psychiatric history significant for posttraumatic stress disorder and depressive episodes; patient denies suicidal ideation and attempts past or present; patient reports increased irritability and anger; describes flashbacks to traumatic events and nightmares; frequent episodes of crying; difficulty concentrating; denies past mania and delusions; some past experience with psychotherapy, terminated with most recent therapist several months ago due to therapist move, some past family therapy; some past work with psychiatrist, no longer sees due to trouble in therapeutic relationship; currently being prescribed Pristiq 100 mg for depression and 0.5 mg Xanax as needed by PCP; reports having been on many other antidepressants with only moderate improvements, reported past hallucinations associated with Abilify; mental status currently dysthymic with significant PTSD symptoms and eating problems
- Diagnostic Impression: 309.81 Posttraumatic Stress Disorder; 307.5, Unspecified Feeding or Eating Disorder, 316; Psychological Factors Affecting Other Medical Conditions; R/O 311, Unspecified Depressive Disorder

(continued)

FIGURE 23.1. Sample bariatric surgery report.

- HABIT indicates problems with general health, nutrition and weight control, exercise, sleep, dental care postponement, compliance, and stress/coping, QoL = 4/10; OBESE indicates eating problems related to preference for high-fat foods, sugar, and fat/sugar/starch combination foods, lack of restraint, time of eating, place of eating, and emotional eating; MMPI-2 profile is valid, indicates significant health concerns with some possible somatization, significant depression, anxiety and PTSD symptoms, feelings of social alienation including suspiciousness of others, high levels of familial discord, concerns about cognitive functioning, high levels of fatigue and lack of motivation, social discomfort, and avoidance
- high expectations for weight loss (80% excess weight with gastric bypass), typical results discussed with patient
- adequate knowledge of weight loss surgery and patient responsibilities following surgery; fair nutritional knowledge
- not an acceptable candidate for weight loss surgery from a psychological perspective at the present time; patient was advised to continue weight loss efforts before surgery, including dietary modification and meeting with a physical therapist to develop a safe and appropriate exercise program; patient advised to begin working with a psychologist and psychiatrist to stabilize PTSD symptoms; patient to return for reevaluation after she has started with new mental heath providers and following 16-pound weight loss required by Dr. Cutter; patient was advised to apply for disability benefits on the basis of her PTSD as she clearly has been disabled for quite some time and it seems quite likely that she will be psychiatrically disabled by this disorder for the next year

I personally interviewed the patient and personally administered, scored, and interpreted all psychological tests reported on herein.

Additional supporting documentation for this note may be found on the Personal History Form and the Patient Interview Form, which have been or will be scanned into the record. Records of psychological test administered are stored in the Department of Psychiatry.

Face to Face Time, 90791: 80 minutes

Testing Time, administration, scoring, interpretation: 2 hours

Report sent to MCV surgeon and faxed to PCP September 30, 2013.

FIGURE 23.1. *(continued)*

addressed for 23% of patients. Those who are deemed "conditionally acceptable" for surgery or "not acceptable at this time" can be advised on specific steps to take to remove these "roadblocks" and are generally able to have surgery later if they are willing and able to follow these recommendations and be reevaluated (e.g., quit smoking and demonstrate cessation with a physiological test; see Peterson, Brundige, & Houghton, Chapter 5, this volume, on tobacco use). In general, it is recommended that patients achieve a period of stability prior to clearance for surgery (medically, psychiatrically, and socially). Recommendations made from the evaluation can help patients work toward this stability. Patients can be reevaluated once this stability is achieved (typically in 3–6 months; Grothe et al., 2006).

Patients who meet program criteria, with each domain assessed as adequate and no concerns found, are deemed acceptable candidates from a psychological perspective. Follow-up to increase motivation or provide additional education about surgery and plans for behavior modification may be recommended, but not required. Patients with inadequate knowledge of risks and responsibilities are often found to be acceptable candidates from a psychological perspective, pending demonstration of knowledge of risks and responsibilities, providing no cognitive barriers to learning exist.

Several situations exist that make candidates acceptable, pending the meeting of certain conditions. To increase surgical safety and to demonstrate the knowledge and skills necessary for long-term behavior change, surgeons often require patients to lose a specific amount of weight prior to surgery. Patients who have not demonstrated behavior changes to promote weight loss but with no other contraindications are often advised to initiate weight loss efforts (e.g., begin an exercise regimen) prior to clearance for surgery. Often, the psychological assessment reveals untreated psychiatric illness, such as depression, anxiety, or other psychopathology. In these cases, recommendations to receive appropriate treatment (psychotherapy or pharmacological treatment) prior to clearance for surgery will be made. Tobacco use is a contraindication for many programs; our surgeons require 90 days of demonstrated tobacco cessation (assessed by cotinine screening). Other conditions that may postpone clearance are an impending stressor (e.g., court appearance) or change in social support system (e.g., divorce) that may necessitate postponing surgery until stressors are reduced or social support has improved.

Clear contraindications endorsed by most programs include active substance abuse, active uncontrolled psychiatric disorder, active suicidal ideation, documented history of medical noncompliance, untreated eating disorder, and severe mental retardation (e.g., inability to give informed consent). Whenever possible, alternative treatments should be discussed with patients and fami-

lies and recommendations provided. Table 23.2 presents a summary of typical recommendations made based on the results of the psychological evaluation.

Special Populations

Children and Adolescents

Pediatric obesity has dramatically increased in the past three decades, representing a public health crisis (Ogden et al, 2012). Currently, about one-third (32%) of children ages 2–19 years are overweight (BMI for age ≥ 85th percentile), and 17% are obese (BMI for age ≥ 95th percentile; Ogden et al., 2012). Alarmingly, 12% of children ages 2–19 years are extremely obese, with a BMI ≥ 97th percentile (Ogden et al., 2012). Multiple comorbidities are associated with pediatric obesity, including glucose intolerance, hypertension, hyperlipidemia, pseudo-tumor cerebri, nonalcoholic fatty liver disease, and Type 2 diabetes (Dietz, 1998). There are also significant psychological comorbidities, such as depression, disordered eating, and impaired quality of life (Bean et al., 2008). Further, overweight children are over 20 times more likely to be obese in adulthood, compared

TABLE 23.2. Summary of Typical Recommendations Made Based on Psychological Evaluation

	Clear contraindication	Relative contraindication
Active substance abuse	X	
Severe mental retardation	X	
Active suicidal ideation	X	
Tobacco use	X	
Inadequate knowledge		x
Inadequate social support		x
Demonstrated nonadherence	X	
Depression		x
Psychiatric hospitalization	X	
Anxiety		x
Current life stressor		x
Untreated thought disorder	X	
No serious past weight-loss attempts	X	
Serious eating disorder (e.g., bulimia)	X	

with their nonoverweight peers, increasing their risk of morbidity and early mortality (Whitaker, Wright, Pepe, Seidel, & Dietz, 1997). Behavioral weight management has been largely unsuccessful in reducing excess weight in the most extremely obese youth, putting these youth at much greater risk of comorbidities in childhood and adulthood. Thus bariatric surgery is becoming more widely accepted as a treatment option for severely obese children, with demonstrated improvements in weight and resolution of comorbidities (Treadwell, Sun, & Schoelles, 2008). Indeed, surgical intervention has had the greatest efficacy among adolescents with severe obesity (Treadwell et al., 2008) and is recommended, in conjunction with lifestyle intervention, for select patients who have not responded to less invasive strategies (Barlow & the Expert Committee, 2007).

Importantly, it is recommended that surgical patients be carefully selected to improve the likelihood of a positive surgical outcome. These criteria are evolving. According to the Best Practice Updates for Pediatric/ Adolescent Weight Loss Surgery from 2009, the American Society for Metabolic and Bariatric Surgery (ASMBS) recommends the following selection criteria for the pediatric population: BMI ≥ 35 kg/m² with major comorbidities (e.g., Type 2 diabetes mellitus, moderate to severe sleep apnea [apnea–hypopnea index > 15], pseudotumor cerebri, or severe nonalcoholic fatty liver disease [NAFLD]) or a BMI ≥ 40 kg/m² with other weight-related comorbidities (e.g., hypertension, insulin resistance, glucose intolerance, substantially impaired quality of life or activities of daily living, dyslipidemia, sleep apnea with apnea–hypopnea index; Pratt et al., 2009; Michalsky et al., 2011). Patients should also have reached their adult height. In addition to the BMI and comorbidity requirements, candidates for surgery must have undergone comprehensive presurgical assessments by a multidisciplinary team including a surgeon, medical pediatric specialist, psychologist, registered dietician, and physical therapist/exercise physiologist and must have participated in at least 6 months of medically observed and attempted nonsurgical weight loss (LeMont et al., 2004; Michalsky et al., 2011).

The psychological evaluation has the same purpose in the adolescent population, with similar contraindications (e.g., unstable psychopathology, substance abuse, poor social support). However, special considerations in the presurgical assessment of adolescents include the clinician's consideration of the adolescent's cognitive, social, and emotional development. Informed consent and assent by both the parent and the adolescent are critical in this assessment to ensure a clear understanding of the risks, benefits, and need for lifetime behavioral modification after surgery (Inge, Xanthakos, & Zeller, 2007).

Older Adults

With the growing population of obese older (≥ 60 years) individuals, assessment issues specific to this population should also be examined. Almost 3% of all bariatric operations at academic health systems are on older patients (Varela, Wilson, & Nguyen, 2006). Mortality and morbidity were found to be higher among older persons undergoing bariatric surgery at these health systems (Varela et al., 2006). Specifically, compared with nonelderly patients, elderly patients had longer lengths of stay (4.9 days vs. 3.8 days), more overall complications (18.9% vs. 10.9%), and higher mortality (0.7 vs. 0.3%). Flum et al. (2005) reviewed the Medicare database and found a mortality rate of 4.8% in patients 65 and older versus 1.7% in Medicare patients under age 65. However, several studies found no increased risk of mortality and morbidity among the elderly (Macgregor & Rand, 1993; Sugerman et al., 2004). To mitigate this potentially increased risk, more careful selection of bariatric surgery candidates has been proposed, in particular with respect to comorbidities (e.g., obstructive sleep apnea and cardiac concerns). Further, greater emphasis on preoperative education and postoperative behavioral management may help lower the risk of complications in the elderly (Hallowell et al., 2007)

Men

Only 20% of patients seeking weight loss surgery are men, and little is known about gender differences in those seeking the surgery. In one study, Mahony (2008) found that men and women differ significantly on suspected psychosurgical risk factors. Male patients seeking weight loss surgery had significantly higher BMIs than women, had tried significantly fewer diets, and were significantly less likely to report a history of depression than women. Females reported significantly higher scores on the PsyBari Depression Index (Mahony, 2008) than males, and females reported significantly higher Beck Depression Inventory–2 (BDI-2; Beck, Steer, & Brown, 1996) scores than males. Women were also significantly more likely to report a history of anxiety than men and scored significantly higher on the PsyBari Social Anxiety Index than men. Whether these differences are related to gender differences in willingness to acknowledge mental health difficulties during the preoperative psychological evaluation or to actual differences in the prevalence of the disorders is unclear at this time. Kolotkin et al. (2008) speculate that because women experience poorer health-related quality of life related to obesity and more depression, they are more likely to seek bariatric surgery. Men tend to have more realistic expectations for weight loss with bariatric surgery than do women (Heinberg, Keating, & Simonelli, 2010).

Cultural Considerations

Ethnic and gender differences exist in overweight and obesity (Cossrow & Falkner, 2004). African American women are at particularly high risk for obesity (Flegal et al., 2010), and African American girls between the ages of 6 and 11 are more likely to be obese than European American girls (Ogden, Carroll, Curtin, Lamb, & Flegal, 2010). Overall, rates of overweight and obesity are higher among African American, Mexican American, and Hispanic youth of all ages than among their European American peers, although prevalence of overweight and obesity among European American youth is indeed significant (Ogden et al., 2010). Moreover, overweight African American youth are more likely than their overweight European American peers to become obese adults (Freedman et al., 2005). Currently, 44% of African American adults are obese, and 74% are overweight (Flegal et al., 2010). African American adult women ages 40–59 (17.7%) are more likely than women

of other ethnic backgrounds to be extremely obese (BMI ≥ 40; Flegal et al., 2010).

Despite the disproportionate numbers of obese African American women, European American women more frequently seek bariatric surgery. Socioeconomic and cultural factors may help explain this discrepancy. It has been proposed that differential access to health care on the basis of socioeconomic disadvantage results in significant health care disparities. Urban residents, persons with private health insurance, younger, healthier, and wealthier patients are all more likely to receive bariatric surgery (Wallace, Young-Xu, Hartley & Weeks, 2010). Cultural norms with respect to body size that contribute to increased rates of body-size dissatisfaction may be a factor in differential desire for surgical intervention. For unclear reasons, African Americans do not lose as much weight as European Americans following bariatric surgery (Harvin, DeLegge, & Garrow, 2008; Kasza et al., 2011). Other ethnic minority groups have not been well studied, although in small studies it appears that Hispanic patients do about as well as European Americans in terms of weight loss and surgical complications. It will be important for scientists to avoid the temptation to aggregate groups that are better separated. For example, there are many subpopulations of Hispanics or Latinos in the United States who have different traditions regarding diet and eating. Aggregating all Hispanic peoples may present a very murky picture of the challenges that individuals from the various subpopulations face in dealing with clinically severe obesity.

Summary

Bariatric surgery is well established as an effective treatment for clinically severe obesity and the comorbid medical conditions that so severely affect the health and life quality of the patients who typically seek these surgeries. Although the mechanisms by which these surgeries enable weight loss are not fully understood, it is increasingly appreciated that long-term success with any weight-loss surgery requires patient adherence to behavior changes that are demanding and difficult. Over time, bariatric surgeons have come to understand the importance of an integrated multidisciplinary team that includes psychologists who can help prepare patients for these changes, identify barriers to change, and learn ways of coping with the stresses and difficulties of new behaviors and the social adjustments related to changes in body and appearance. The presurgical psychological evaluation for bariatric surgery provides an opportunity to evaluate the patients' strengths and weaknesses with regard to the behaviors that result in weight gain, to educate patients about surgery and behavioral and emotional issues in weight loss, and to create an alliance between the surgical program and any existing mental health care practitioners who will be providing ongoing care to the patients after surgery.

REFERENCES

Allison, K. C., Lundgren, J. D., O'Reardon, J. P., Geliebter, A., Gluck, M. E., Vinai, P., et al. (2010). Proposed diagnostic criteria for night eating syndrome. *International Journal of Eating Disorders, 43*(3), 241–247.

Allison, K. C., Wadden, T. A., Sarwer, D. B., Fabricatore, A. N., Crerand, C. E., Gibbons, L. M., et al. (2006). Night eating syndrome and binge eating disorder among persons seeking bariatric surgery: Prevalence and related features. *Surgery for Obesity and Related Diseases, 2,* 153–158.

American Psychiatric Association. (2000). *Diagnostic and statistical manual of mental disorders* (4th ed., text rev.). Washington, DC: Author.

American Psychiatric Association. (2013). *Diagnostic and statistical manual of mental disorders* (5th ed.). Arlington, VA: Author.

Babor, T. F., de la Fuente, J. R., Saunders, J., & Grant, M. (1992). *The Alcohol Use Disorders Identification Test: Guidelines for use in primary care* (WHO Publication No. 92.4). Geneva, Switzerland: World Health Organization.

Barlow, S. E., & the Expert Committee. (2007) Expert committee recommendations regarding the prevention, assessment, and treatment of child and adolescent overweight and obesity: Summary report. *Pediatrics, 120*(Suppl. 4), S164–S192.

Bauchowitz, A. U., Gonder-Frederick, L. A., Olbrisch, M. E., Azarbad, L., Ryee, M. Y., Woodson, M., et al. (2005). Psychosocial evaluation of bariatric surgery candidates: A survey of present practices, *Psychosomatic Medicine, 67*(5), 825–832.

Bean, M. K., Stewart, K., & Olbrisch, M. E., (2008). Obesity in America: Implications for clinical and health psychologists. *Journal of Clinical Psychology in Medical Settings, 15*(3), 214–224.

Beck, A. T. (1993). *Beck Anxiety Inventory (BAI)*. San Antonio, TX: Psychological Corporation.

Beck, A. T., Steer, R. A., & Brown, G. K. (1996). *Beck Depression Inventory—II (BDI-II)*. San Antonio, TX: Harcourt Assessment.

Bocchieri-Ricciardi, L. E., Chen, E. Y., Munoz, D., Fischer, S., Dymek-Valentine, M., Alverdy, J. C., et al. (2006). Pre-surgery binge eating status: Effects on eating behavior and weight outcome after gastric bypass. *Obesity Surgery, 16,* 1198–1204.

Bodenlos, J. S., Kose, S., Borckardt, J. J., Nahas, Z., Shaw, D., O'Neil, P. M., et al. (2007). Vagus nerve stimulation acutely alters food cravings in adults with depression. *Appetite, 48,* 145–153.

Bray, G. A. (2004). Medical consequences of obesity. *Journal of Clinical Endocrinology and Metabolism, 89,* 2583–2589.

Buchwald, H., Avidor, Y., Braunwald, E., Jensen, M. D., Pories, W., Fahrbach,. K., et al. (2004). Bariatric surgery: A systematic review and meta-analysis. *Journal of the American Medical Association, 292,* 1724–1737.

Buchwald, H., & the Consensus Conference Panel. (2005). Consensus conference statement: Bariatric surgery for morbid obesity: Health implications for patients, health professionals, and third-party payers. *Journal of the American College of Surgeons, 200,* 593–604.

Buchwald, H., Estok, R., Fahrbach, K., Banel, D., & Sledge, I. (2007). Trends in mortality in bariatric surgery: A systematic review and meta-analysis. *Surgery, 142,* 632–635.

Buffington, C. K., Daley, D. L., Worthen, M., & Marema, R. T. (2006, June). *Changes in alcohol sensitivity and effects with gastric bypass.* Abstract presented at the annual meeting of the American Society for Bariatric Surgery, San Francisco CA.

Butcher, J. N., Dahlstrom, W. G., Graham, J. R., Tellegen, A., & Kaemmer, B. (1989). *Minnesota Multiphasic Personality Inventory—2 (MMPI-2): Manual for administration and scoring.* Minneapolis: University of Minnesota Press.

Camilleri, M., Toouli, J., Herrera, M. F., Kow, L., Pantoja, J. P., Billington, M. B., et al. (2009). Selection of electrical algorithms to treat obesity with intermittent vagal block using an implantable medical device. *Surgery for Obesity and Related Diseases, 5*(2), 229–230.

Camilleri, M., Toouli, J., Herrera, M. F., Kulseng, B., Kow, L., Pantoja, J. P., et al. (2008). Intraabdominal vagal blocking (VBLOC therapy): Clinical results with a new implantable medical device. *Surgery, 143*(6), 723–731.

Cigaina, V., & Hirschberg, A. L. (2007). Plasma ghrelin and gastric pacing in morbidly obese patients. *Metabolism, 56*(8), 1017–1021.

Cossrow, N., & Falkner, B. (2004). Race/ethnic issues in obesity and obesity related comorbidities. *Journal of Clinical Endocrinology and Metabolism, 89*, 2590–2594.

Derogatis, L. R. (1973). *Symptom Checklist—90 (SCL-90).* Minneapolis, MN: NCS Assessments.

Derogatis, L. R. (1993). *Brief Symptom Inventory (BSI) administration, scoring, and procedures manual* (4th ed.). Minneapolis, MN: National Computer Systems.

Dietz, W. H. (1998). Health consequences of obesity in youth: Childhood predictors of adult disease. *Pediatrics, 101*, 518–525.

Elder, K. A., & Wolf, B. M. (2007). Bariatric surgery: A review of procedures and outcomes. *Gastroenterology, 132*, 2253–2271.

Elkins, G., Whitfield, P., Marcus, J., Symmonds, R., Rodriguez, J., & Cook, T. (2005). Noncompliance with behavioral recommendations following bariatric surgery. *Obesity Surgery, 15*, 546–551.

Ertelt, T. W., Mitchell, J. E., Lancaster, K., Crosby, R. D., Steffen, K. J., & Marino, J. M. (2008). Alcohol abuse and dependence before and after bariatric surgery: A review of the literature and report of a new data set. *Surgery for Obesity and Related Diseases, 4*(5), 647–650.

Fabricatore, A. N., Crerand, C. E., Wadden, T. A., Sarwer, D. B., & Krasucki, J. L. (2006). How do mental health professionals evaluate candidates for bariatric surgery?: Survey results. *Obesity Surgery, 16*(5), 567–573.

Fabricatore, A. N. & Wadden, T. A. (2006). The behavioral evaluation of bariatric surgery candidates. *Obesity Management, 2*(3), 103–109.

Fairburn, C. G., & Beglin, S. J. (1994). The assessment of eating disorders: Interview versus questionnaire. *International Journal of Eating Disorders, 16*, 363–370.

First, M. B., & Gibbon, M. (2004). *The Structured Clinical Interview for DSM-IV—Axis I Disorders (SCID-I) and the Structured Clinical Interview for DSM-IV—Axis II Disorders (SCID-II).* Hoboken, NJ: Wiley.

Flegal, K. M., Carroll, M. D., Ogden, C. L., & Curtin, L. R. (2010). Prevalence and trends in obesity among U.S. adults, 1999–2008. *Journal of the American Medical Association, 303*(3), 235–241.

Flum, D. R., Salem, L., Elrod, J. A. B., Dellinger, E. P., Cheadle, A., & Chan, L. (2005). Early mortality among Medicare beneficiaries undergoing bariatric surgical procedures. *Journal of the American Medical Association, 294*, 1903–1908.

Folstein, M. F., Folstein, S. E., & McHugh, P. R. (1975). Mini-Mental State: A practical method for grading the cognitive state of patients for the clinician. *Journal of Psychiatric Research, 12*(3), 189–198

Freedman, D. S., Khan, L. K., Serdula, M. K., Dietz, W. H., Srinivasan, S. R., & Berenson, G. S. (2005). Racial differences in the tracking of childhood BMI to adulthood. *Obesity Research, 13*, 928–935.

Garner, D. M., Olmstead, M. P., & Polivy, J. (1983). Development and validation of a multidimensional eating disorder inventory for anorexia nervosa and bulimia. *International Journal of Eating Disorders, 2*, 15–34.

Glinski, J., Wetzler, S., & Goodman, E. (2001). The psychology of gastric bypass surgery. *Obesity Surgery, 11*, 581–588.

Greenberg, I., Perna, F., Kaplan, M., & Sullivan, M. A. (2005). Behavioral and psychological factors in the assessment and treatment of obesity surgery patients. *Obesity Research, 13*(2), 244–249.

Grothe, K. B., Dubbert, P. M., & O'Jile, J. R. (2006). Psychological assessment and management of the weight loss surgery patient. *American Journal of the Medical Sciences, 331*(4), 201–206.

Hallowell, P. T., Stellato, T. A., Schuster, M., Graf, K., Robinson, A., & Jasper, J. (2007). Avoidance of complications in older patients and Medicare recipients undergoing gastric bypass. *Archives of Surgery, 142*, 506–512.

Harpo Productions. (2007). *The truth behind bariatric surgery.* Available at *www.oprah.com/tows/pastshows/200610/tows_past_20061024.jhtml.*

Harvin, G., DeLegge, M., & Garrow, D. A. (2008). The impact of race on weight loss after Roux-en-Y gastric bypass surgery. *Obesity Surgery, 18*(1), 39–42.

Heckman, C., Olbrisch, M. E., Rodgers, K., Meador, J. G., DeMaria, E., & Haller, D. L. (2005, August). *The Health and Behavioral Issues Test (HABIT): Psychometric properties in two samples.* Paper presented at the annual meeting of the American Psychological Association, Washington, DC.

Heinberg, L. J., Keating, K., & Simonelli, L. (2010). Discrepancy between ideal and realistic goal weights in three bariatric procedures: Who is likely to be unrealistic? *Obesity Surgery, 20*(2), 148–153.

Herpertz, S., Kielmann, R., Wolf, A. M., Langkafel, M., Senf, W., & Hebebrand, J. (2003). Does obesity surgery improve psychosocial functioning? *International Journal of Obesity, 27*, 1300–1314.

Hutter, M. M., Schirmer, B. D., Jones, D. B., Ko, C. Y., Cohen, M. E., Merkow, R. P., et al. (2011). First report from the American College of Surgeons Bariatric Surgery Center Network: Laparoscopic sleeve gastrectomy has morbidity and effectiveness positioned between the band and the bypass. *Annals of Surgery, 254*, 410–422.

Inge, T. H., Xanthakos, S. A., & Zeller, M. H. (2007). Bariatric surgery for pediatric extreme obesity: Now or later? *International Journal of Obesity, 31*, 1–14.

Jones-Corneille, L. R., Wadden, T. A., Sarwer, D. B., Faulconbridge, L. F., Fabricatore, A. N., Stack, R. M., et al. (2010). Axis I psychopathology in bariatric surgery candidates with and without binge eating disorders: Results of structured clinical interviews. *Obesity Surgery, 22*(3), 389–397.

Kalarchian, M. A., Marcus, M. D., Wilson, G. T., Labouvie, E. W., Brolin, R. E., & LaMarca, L. B. (2002). Binge eating among gastric bypass patients at long-term follow-up. *Obesity Surgery, 12*, 270–275.

Kasza, J., Brody, F., Vaziri, K., Scheffey, C., McMullan, S., Wallace, B., et al. (2011). Analysis of poor outcomes after laparoscopic adjustable gastric banding. *Surgical Endoscopy, 25*(1), 41–47.

Kolotkin, R. L., Crosby, R. D., Gress, R. E., Hunt, S. C., Engel, S. G., & Adams, T. D. (2008). Health and health-related quality of life: Differences between men and women who seek gastric bypass surgery. *Surgery for Obesity and Related Diseases, 4*(5), 651–658.

LeMont, D., Moorehead, M. K., Parish, M. S., Reto, C. S., & Ritz, C. S., & the American Society of Metabolic and Bariatric Surgery. (2004). *Suggestions for the pre-surgical psychological assessment of bariatric surgery candidates.* Available at *http://asmbs.org/2012/06/pre-surgical-psychological-assessment.*

Livhits, M., Mercado, C., Yermilov, I., Parikh, J. A., Dutson, E., Mehran, A., et al. (2011). Preoperative predictors of weight loss following bariatric surgery: Systematic review. *Obesity Surgery, 22*(1), 70–89.

Livingston, E. H., & Ko, C. Y. (2004). Socioeconomic characteristics of the population eligible for obesity surgery. *Surgery, 135*, 288–296.

Macgregor, A. M., & Rand, C. S. (1993). Gastric surgery in morbid obesity: Outcomes in patients aged 55 years and older. *Archives of Surgery, 128*, 1153–1157.

Madan, A. K., & Tichansky, D. S. (2005). Patients postoperatively forget aspects of preoperative patient education. *Obesity Surgery, 15*, 1066–1069.

Mahony, D. (2008). Psychological gender differences in bariatric surgery candidates. *Obesity Surgery, 18*(5), 607–610.

Malone, M., & Alger-Mayer, S. (2004). Binge status and quality of life after gastric bypass surgery: A one-year study. *Obesity Research, 12*(3), 473–481.

Mechanick, J. I., Kushner, R. F., Sugerman, H. J., Gonzalez-Campoy, J. M., Collazo-Clavell, M. L., Guven, S., et al. (2008). American Association of Clinical Endocrinologists, the Obesity Society, and the American Society for Metabolic and Bariatric Surgery medical guidelines for clinical practice for the perioperative nutritional, metabolic, and nonsurgical support of the bariatric surgery patient. *Endocrine Practice, 14*(1), 1–83.

Michalsky, M., Reichard, K., Inge, T., Pratt, J., Lenders, C., & the American Society for Metabolic and Bariatric Surgery. (2011). ASMBS pediatric committee best practice guidelines. *Surgery for Obesity and Related Diseases, 8*, 1–7.

Miller, A. D., & Smith, K. M. (2006). Medication and nutrient administration considerations after bariatric surgery. *American Journal of Health Systems Pharmacists, 62*, 1852–1857.

Millon, T., Antoni, M., Millon, C., Meagher,

S., & Millon, G. S. (2001). *Millon Behavioral Medicine Diagnostic.* Minneapolis, MN: NCS Assessments.

Millon, T., Green, C. J., & Meagher, R. B. (1979). The MBHI: A new inventory for the psycho-diagnostician in medical settings. *Professional Psychology, 10,* 529–539.

Morey, L. C. (1991). *Personality Assessment Inventory (PAI).* Odessa, FL: PAR/Psychological Assessment Resources.

Nangle, D. W., Johnson, W. G., Carr-Nangle, R. E., & Engler, L. B. (1994). Binge-eating disorder and the proposed DSM-IV criteria: Psychometric analysis of the Questionnaire of Eating and Weight Patterns. *International Journal of Eating Disorders, 16,* 147–157.

National Heart, Lung, and Blood Institute Obesity Education Initiative Expert Panel. (2000). *The practical guide: Identification, evaluation, and treatment of overweight and obesity in adults* (NIH Publication No. 00-4084). Bethesda, MD: National Heart, Lung, and Blood Institute.

National Institutes of Health. (1991). Gastrointestinal surgery for severe obesity [National Institutes of Health Consensus Development Conference Draft Statement]. *Obesity Surgery, 1,* 257–265.

National Institutes of Health and the National Institute of Diabetes and Digestive and Kidney Diseases. (2004). Gastrointestinal surgery for severe obesity (NIH Publication No. 04-4006). Bethesda, MD: U.S. Department of Health and Human Services.

Ochner, C. N., Puma, L. M., Raevuori, A., Teixeira, J., & Geliebter, A. (2010). Effectiveness of a prebariatric surgery insurance-required weight loss regimen and relation to postsurgical weight loss. *Obesity, 18,* 287–292.

Ogden, C. L., Carroll, M. D., Curtin, L. R., Lamb, M. M., & Flegal, K. M. (2010). Prevalence of high body mass index in U.S. children and adolescents, 2007–2008. *Journal of the American Medical Association, 303*(3), 242–249.

Ogden, C. L., Carroll, M. D., Curtin, L. R., McDowell, M. A., Tabak, C. J., & Flegal, K. M. (2006). The prevalence of overweight and obesity in the United States, 1999–2004. *Journal of the American Medical Association, 295,* 1549–1555.

Ogden, C. L., Carroll, M. D., Kit, B. K., & Flegal, K. M. (2012). Prevalence of obesity and trends in body mass index among U. S. children and adolescents, 1999–2010. *Journal of*

the American Medical Association, 307*(5), 483–490.

Olbrisch, M. E., Starkcy, J., Ascari, J., Kaplan, E., Meador, J., & Maher, J. W. (2006). Two-day food diaries as tools for assessment of disordered eating behavior in candidates for bariatric surgery. *Bariatric Nursing and Surgical Patient Care, 1*(2), 123–134.

Onyike, C. U., Crum, R. M., Lee, H. B., Lyketsos, C. G., & Eaton, W. W. (2003). Is obesity associated with major depression?: Results from the Third National Health and Nutrition Examination Survey. *American Journal of Epidemiology, 158*(12), 1139–1147.

Peterson, N. D., Olbrisch, M. E., Stewart, K. E., McFarling, K. M., & Gonder-Frederick, L. A. (2012, April). *The Olbrisch Bariatric Eating Style Evaluation (OBESE): A scale to measure subclinical problematic eating behaviors in a surgery-seeking obese patient sample.* Paper presented at the annual meeting and scientific sessions of the Society of Behavioral Medicine, New Orleans, LA.

Powell, L. H., Calvin, J. E., III, & Calvin, J. E., Jr. (2007). Effective obesity treatments. *American Psychologist, 62*(3), 234–246.

Pratt, J. S., Lenders, C. M., Dionne, E. A., Hoppin, A. G., Hsu, G. L., Inge, T. H., et al. (2009). Best practice updates for pediatric/adolescent weight loss surgery. *Obesity (Silver Spring), 17,* 901–910.

Sandoz Nutrition. (1988). *Weight and Lifestyle Inventory (WALI).* Minneapolis, MN: Author.

Sarwer, D. B., Wadden, T. A., & Fabricatore, A. N. (2005). Psychosocial and behavioral aspects of bariatric surgery. *Obesity Research, 13*(4), 639–648.

Saunders, R. (2004). "Grazing": A high-risk behavior. *Obesity Surgery, 14,* 98–102.

Schwartz, G. J. (2000). The role of gastrointestinal vagal afferents in the control of food intake: Current prospects. *Nutrition, 16,* 866–873.

Scopinaro, N., Adami, G. F., Marinari, G. M., Gianetta, E., Traverso, E., Friedman, D., et al. (1998). Biliopancreatic diversion. *World Journal of Surgery, 22,* 936–946.

Skinner, H. A. (1982). The Drug Abuse Screening Test. *Addictive Behavior, 7,* 363–371.

Sogg, S. (2007). Alcohol misuse after bariatric surgery: Epiphenomenon or "Oprah" phenomenon? *Surgery for Obesity and Related Diseases, 3,* 366–368.

Spielberger, C. D. (1983). *State–Trait Anxiety Inventory (STAI)*. Menlo Park, CA: Mind Garden.

Stein, C. J., & Colditz, G. A. (2004). The epidemic of obesity. *Journal of Clinical Endocrinology and Metabolism, 89*(6), 2522–2525.

Stewart, K. E., Olbrisch, M. E., & Bean, M. K. (2010). Back on track: Confronting postsurgical weight gain. *Bariatric Nursing and Surgical Patient Care, 5*(2), 179–185.

Sugerman, H. J., DeMaria, E. J., Kellum, J. M., Sugerman, E. L., Meador, J. G., & Wolfe, L. G. (2004). Effects of bariatric surgery in older patients. *Annals of Surgery, 240*, 243–247.

Tadross, J. A., & le Roux, C. W. (2009). The mechanisms of weight loss after bariatric surgery. *International Journal of Obesity, 33*, S28–S32.

Taylor, V. H., & Misra, M. (2009). Bariatric surgery in patients with bipolar disorder: An emerging issue. *Journal of Psychiatry and Neuroscience, 34*(4), E3.

Treadwell, J. R., Sun, F., & Schoelles, K. (2008). Systematic review and meta-analysis of bariatric surgery for pediatric obesity. *Annals of Surgery, 248*, 763–776.

Tsushima, W. T., Bridenstine, M. P., & Balfour, J. F. (2004). MMPI-2 scores in the outcome prediction of gastric bypass surgery. *Obesity Surgery, 14*, 528–532.

Varela, J. E., Wilson, S. E., & Nguyen, N. T. (2006). Outcomes of bariatric surgery in the elderly. *American Surgery, 72*, 865–869.

Wadden, T. A., & Sarwer, D. B. (2006). Behavioral assessment of candidates for bariatric surgery: A patient-oriented approach. *Surgery for Obesity and Related Diseases, 2*(2), 171–179.

Wadden, T. A., Sarwer, D. B., Fabricatore, A. N., Jones, L., Stack, R., & Williams, N. S. (2007). Psychosocial and behavioral status of patients undergoing bariatric surgery: What to expect before and after surgery. *Medical Clinics of North America, 91*, 451–469.

Wallace, A. E., Young-Xu, Y., Hartley, D., & Weeks, W. B. (2010). Racial, socioeconomic, and rural–urban disparities in obesity-related bariatric surgery. *Obesity Surgery, 20*(10), 1354–1360.

Wallston, K. A., Wallston, B. S., & DeVellis, R. (1978). Development of the Multidimensional Health Locus of Control (MHLC) scales. *Health Education Monographs, 6*, 160–170.

Ware, J. E., Jr., & Sherbourne, C. D. (1992). The MOS 36-Item Short-Form Health Survey (SF-36): I. Conceptual framework and item selection. *Medical Care, 30*(6), 473–483.

Whitaker, R. C., Wright, J. A., Pepe, M. S., Seidel, K. D., & Dietz, W. H. (1997). Predicting obesity in young adulthood from childhood and parental obesity. *New England Journal of Medicine, 337*, 869–873.

Wilting, I. (2007). Effect of gastric banding on pharmacotherapy: Not much known. *Nederlands Tijdschrift Voor Geneeskunde, 151*(20), 1112–1115.

Zhao, Y. & Encinosa, W. (2007). *Bariatric surgery utilization and outcomes in 1998 and 2004: Statistical Brief No. 23*. Rockville, MD: Agency for Healthcare Policy and Research.

Zhaoping, L., Bowerman, S., & Heber, D. (2005). Health ramifications of the obesity epidemic. *Surgery Clinics of North America, 85*, 681–701.

Zimmerman, M., Francione-Witt, C., Chelminski, I., Young, D., Boerescu, D., Attiullah, N., et al. (2007). Presurgical psychiatric evaluations of candidates for bariatric surgery: Part 1. Reliability and reasons for and frequency of exclusion. *Journal of Clinical Psychiatry, 68*, 1557–1562.

CHAPTER 24

Pediatrics

Lisa M. Buckloh
Lisa M. Schilling

Unique Aspects of Assessment of Children and Adolescents

We are often reminded during the course of our training that children are not just small adults and that special consideration must be given to recognizing differences in their cognitive style, behavior, and emotional reactivity. This is particularly important in the area of psychological assessment and in the diagnostic process with children, and there are even more unique aspects to consider within the realm of assessment in child health psychology (generally referred to as pediatric psychology). There are special considerations in assessing each individual health challenge in children, which are discussed later in this chapter, but it is first important to understand the global issues unique to assessment in pediatric psychology. The individual child's progress along the typical trajectory of child development is a critical consideration, as are the impressions of those who know the child well or who have an opportunity to observe directly the problem being assessed. The impact of the child on the environment in which she or he lives, along with the environmental influences of home, school, and community on the child, must be examined. And, most important, thought must be given to the most effective

way to gather this information, based on what the child can understand and communicate, in a nonthreatening manner. The biopsychosocial model is an excellent example of a model that takes into consideration all of these unique aspects of child health.

Taking a Developmental Approach

Age and developmental issues are key concepts that affect all facets of clinical work with children. The presenting problems, type of assessment measures and modalities, diagnoses, and interventions all vary depending on the age, maturity, and general developmental level of the child (Simeonsson & Rosenthal, 2001). Clinicians working with children must have a sufficient background in what constitutes normal development in children and adolescents to understand how behavior, mood, and adaptive functioning are atypical. A number of developmental models exist that explain typical and atypical child development, including behavioral, psychosocial, qualitative-developmental, family life cycle, and psychosexual. Simeonsson and Rosenthal (2001) provide a summary of the basic tenets of each of these developmental models. In addition, the field of developmental psychopathology (Luthar, Burack, Cicchetti, & Weisz, 1997) focuses

427

on the emergence and course of atypical behavior across the life span and draws on these theories, as well as cross-sectional and longitudinal research in the area of child development (Simeonsson & Rosenthal, 2001; Vernberg & Jacobs, 2001).

Adapting the Biopsychosocial Model to Children

In addition to the overlay of developmental factors, children and adolescents function and deal with health problems within a number of systems, including the family (parents, siblings, grandparents), school, peers, neighborhoods, and communities. Because children must depend on their parents and other adults for basic needs, caregiving, and instruction, it is very important to consider the child within the context of the family and to take a family systems approach to assessment and intervention with pediatric populations. Although family systems frameworks are broad and often multidisciplinary, they share the common assumption that human behavior needs to be conceptualized at a level greater than the individual (Kazak, Rourke, & Navsaria, 2009). One such modality, medical family therapy, is a biopsychosocial approach that emphasizes medical illness and its role in the personal life of the patient and the interpersonal relationships of the family, while taking a family systems perspective (McDaniel, Hepworth, & Doherty, 1992). Medical family therapy is especially relevant to pediatric populations, as it argues for a collaborative approach, not only with the family but also with the health care team and related systems (McDaniel et al., 1992).

Ecological theory, a social-ecological theory based on the work of developmental psychologist Urie Bronfenbrenner (1979, 2004), is another framework for understanding assessment issues in pediatric psychology. Ecological theory conceptualizes the child within five systems or concentric spheres of influence, with each becoming more distant from the child (e.g., the family–school–medical team, health care policy, society). When assessing youth, it is important to place the child within these contexts and to identify the factors within the systems that influence the child.

Multimodal Assessment

The use of multiple informants is widely encouraged within clinical practice and research with children and adolescents. Multiple informants (e.g., parents and teachers) are needed to determine some psychological diagnoses in children, such as attention-deficit/hyperactivity disorder (ADHD), in which diagnosis depends on manifestation of symptoms in multiple settings, and the need to seek input from those who interact with the child in each setting is stressed (DSM-5; American Psychiatric Association, 2013). Although it is very important for clinicians to get the perspective of the youth, other informants may be more accurate reporters in certain situations. For example, parents and teachers tend to be more accurate reporters for younger children and for externalizing behaviors such as aggression, defiance, and hyperactivity (Edelbrock, Costello, Dulcan, Kalas, & Calabro-Conover, 1985). As children mature, their accuracy of reporting becomes more reliable (Edelbrock et al., 1985). Youth self-report tends to be more accurate than parent report for internalizing symptoms, such as anxiety and depression, and for attitudes, perceptions, or covert activities, such as alcohol and drug use (e.g. Edelbrock, Costello, Dulcan, Calabro-Conover, & Kalas, 1986; O'Donnell et al., 1998; Valla, Bergeron, Breton, Gaudet, & Berthiaume, 1993). Thus clinicians can maximize reliability and validity of assessment by obtaining information from multiple informants when possible. In addition to using multiple informants, it is important to utilize a variety of modes of assessment to obtain the most accurate evaluation of children. These methods are described in greater detail throughout the chapter but include standardized cognitive-developmental tests, behavioral observations, physiological indicators, and measures specific to the individual's disease management requirements.

Clinical Interview with Youth

A pediatric evaluation should include a clinical interview of parents and other relevant caregivers, as well as the child or adolescent. Interviewing the child gives the clinician a chance to observe behavior directly and assess mental status and capacity to relate to others. It also provides an opportunity to gather information to evaluate the child's level of motivation, coping skills and strategies, and perceptions about his or her problems, family, and social environment (Querido, Eyberg, Kanfer, & Krahn, 2001). Research has shown that children as young as 6 years of age are capable of providing accurate information about their behavior, thoughts, and environment (Hodges & Cools, 1990; La Greca, Kuttler, & Stone, 2001). It is important for the clinician to build rapport with the child and to maintain the child's cooperation throughout the interview through the use of age-appropriate communication (Querido et al., 2001). This may be accomplished through more informal interview techniques or with a structured interview approach. A number of structured interviews have been developed to aid the clinician in the interview and diagnostic process (see review in La Greca et al., 2001). With younger children, the clinician may find it fruitful to gather information and build rapport within the context of play. There are a number of play techniques that the clinician may use, including drawing and other art activities, doll and puppet play, storytelling, and board games (Boyd Webb, 1991).

When working with children and adolescents, there are a number of areas to assess in the parent interview. As with adults, the chief complaint, history of presenting illness, medical history, past psychiatric and psychological history, and strengths and weaknesses of the child and family must be obtained. In addition, clinicians should assess issues related to pregnancy, delivery, birth, and early development. Information should be obtained about cognitive and academic functioning, as well as social functioning within the context of peer and family relationships.

Evidence-Based Assessment in Pediatric Psychology

Although there will probably always remain a subjective component to assessment, investigators have recently focused on the utilization of evidence-based measures in pediatric psychology. The use of reliable and valid instruments with evidence of repeated utility in measuring the condition of interest will allow more consistent comparisons and communication and more effective treatment within the field. To this end, in 2002, the Society of Pediatric Psychology (American Psychological Association Division 54), under the direction of Annette La Greca, assembled a task force to identify, critique, and disseminate information about assessment measures used in pediatric psychology (Cohen, La Greca, et al., 2008). The task force identified eight broad assessment areas of interest: cognitive functioning, psychosocial functioning and psychopathology, quality of life, adherence, stress and coping, pain, family functioning, and social support and peer relations. Measures in each category were reviewed using criteria such as validity and reliability and replication in peer-reviewed studies and were judged based on the following hierarchy: well-established assessment, approaching well-established assessment, and promising assessment (Cohen, La Greca, et al., 2008). Practical information was provided, including name and description of the measure, the central references, psychometric properties, how to obtain the measure, clinical utility, strengths and weaknesses, and the Task Force Criteria Rating (e.g., well-established assessment; Cohen, La Greca, et al., 2008). Reviews of each of the areas of interest can be found in a special issue of the *Journal of Pediatric Psychology* (Cohen, La Greca, et al., 2008). These articles are invaluable resources for pediatric psychologists in choosing assessment tools for their individual purposes. Given space constraints in this chapter, we do not attempt to include information about every available test but plan to focus on both choosing assessment tools and giving consideration to the critical aspects of the biopsychosocial model in using them in clinical practice and research with children. See Table 24.1 for more information about the evidence-based assessment tools discussed in this chapter.

Cognitive Functioning

Comprehensive, standardized assessment of cognitive abilities, academic achievement,

TABLE 24.1. Evidence-Based Assessment in Pediatric Psychology

Domain	Assessment tool or measure	Brief description	References
Family functioning	Self-report measures Family interviews Observational measures	Measures of general family functioning, familial dyadic relationships, illness-related family functioning 29 family assessment measures; 66% "well established"	Alderfer et al. (2008) and supplementary data at *www.jpepsy. oxfordjournals.org*
	Genograms or eco-maps	Qualitative assessment; visual representations of family relationships	Rosenthal, Cohen, & Simeonsson (2001)
Social support and peer relations	Peer measures	Peer nomination, peer reports	Reiter-Purtill & Noll (2003); Reiter-Purtill, Waller, & Noll (2009)
	Parent, teacher, self-report	CBCL and BASC-2 assess social competence and social skills (see description in "Psychosocial Functioning and Psychopathology" below) Use caution in using CBCL with chronically ill children as limitations may affect score	Achenbach (1991); Achenbach & Rescorla (2001); Reynolds & Kamphaus (2004)
Psychosocial Functioning and Psychopathology	Child Behavior Checklist (CBCL)	Broadband rating scales Parent, teacher, and self-rating scales Ages: 1.5–18 years "well established"	Achenbach (1991); Achenbach & Rescorla (2001)
	Behavior Assessment System for Children (BASC) and BASC-2 (2nd edition)	Broadband rating scales Parent, teacher, and self-rating scales BASC ages: 2.5–18 years BASC-2 ages: 2–21 years, 11 months BASC is "well-established"	Reynolds & Kamphaus (1998) Reynolds & Kamphaus (2004)
	Conners' Ratings Scales—Revised (CRS-R)	Broadband rating scale Emphasis on measurement of ADHD symptoms Parent, teacher rating scales Ages: 3–17 parent and teacher 12–17 self-report CRS-R is "well established"	Conners (2001)
	Conners 3	Ages: 6–18 parent and teacher 8–18 self-report	Conners (2008)
	Conners Early Childhood	Ages: 2–6 parent and teacher	Conners (2009)
	Minnesota Multiphasic Personality Inventory—Adolescent (MMPI-A)	Broadband rating scale Self-report measure of adolescent psychopathology Ages: 14–18 "well established"	Butcher et al. (1992)

	Measure	Description	Reference
Pain	Faces Pain Scale—Revised	Self-report measure for acute pain Six cartoon faces from neutral to high pain Ages: 4–16 "well established"	Hicks, von Baeyer, Spafford, van Korlaar, & Goodenough (2001)
	Children's Hospital of Eastern Ontario Pain Scale (CHEOPS)	Observational measure Used for postoperative pain Ages: 1–12 "well established"	McGrath et al. (1985); Beyer, McGrath & Berde (1990)
	Pediatric Pain Questionnaire	Assesses various features of pain in many populations Self-report and parent/physician proxy report Ages: 5–18 "well established"	Varni, Thompson, & Hanson (1987)
Adherence	Self-report	Multiple informants (youth, parent, health care providers) Most accurate with immediate recall and objective questions	Quittner et al. (2008)
	Self-monitoring (diaries)	Written logs, handheld computers (PDAs), phone diaries Poor accuracy with written logs	Quittner et al. (2008)
	Structured interviews	Used with asthma, diabetes, cystic fibrosis, HIV/AIDS	Quittner et al. (2008)
	Medication counts	Removal of pills from blister packs, opening of vials, metered-dose inhalers, blood glucose test results	Quittner et al. (2008)
Stress and Coping	Children's Hassles Scale/Children's Uplifts Scale	Assesses "hassles" and "uplifts" in the past month Self-report Ages: 8–17 years "well established"	Kanner et al. (1987)
	Adolescent Coping Orientation for Problem Experiences	Assesses use of different coping strategies Self-report Ages: 11 and up "well established"	Patterson & McCubbin (1987)
	Kidcope	Respondent is presented with or generates a stressful situation Rate use of coping strategies and how much they helped (Likert scale) Self-report brief screening tool Ages: 7–12 and 13–18 versions "approaching well established"	Spirito, Stark, & Williams (1988)

(continued)

TABLE 24.1. *(continued)*

Domain	Assessment tool or measure	Brief description	References
Health-Related Quality of Life	Child Health and Illness Profile	General measure—not disease-specific Child self-report, adolescent self-report, and parent report versions for children and adolescents Ages: 6–17 "well established"	Starfield, Riley, & Green (1999)
	Pediatric Quality of Life Inventory (PedsQL)	Generic core component and disease-specific modules Self-report and parent report versions, short and long forms Ages: 2–18 (multiple versions) "well established"	Varni, Seid, & Rode (1999)
	Cystic Fibrosis Questionnaire—Revised	English adaptation of scale developed in France Core and disease-specific items Child-report, teen–adult-report, and parent-report versions Ages: 6–adult "well established"	Quittner, Buu, Messer, Modi, & Watrous (2005); Modi & Quittner (2003)
	Pediatric Oncology Quality of Life Scale	Assesses physical function, distress, and reaction to cancer treatment Parent report only Ages: 2–19 "well established"	Goodwin, Boggs, & Graham-Pole (1994)

or processing skills is not always required in pediatric psychology. In fact, time constraints often prevent the use of standardized assessment measures. For inpatient consultations, for example, there is often a brief period of time in which to complete a clinical interview, observe or discuss frequency and severity of symptoms, and consider diagnostic alternatives.

For some patients, however, a basic, or even a comprehensive, assessment of specific abilities may be crucial. It may be necessary to provide a measurement of developmental or cognitive level when the medical staff is questioning whether certain behaviors are age- or developmentally appropriate. Knowledge of the child's reading level may be important if self-report measures are being used (e.g., quality of life ratings or personality evaluations). In some cases, comprehensive testing is required, sometimes repeatedly, to assess treatment impact and determine educational needs (e.g., late effects of cancer treatment). Psychologists often are asked to provide information about the child's ability to understand diagnosis and treatment information and to provide assent related to clinical care or research participation; assessment of cognitive abilities may be necessary to obtain such information (Kupst, 1999). It may be critical to have an accurate measure of the child's current cognitive level when discussing treatment options that are likely to add additional cognitive insult, so that parents may weigh available treatment options or choose not to treat, based on likely medical outcomes.

Pediatric cancer provides the largest body of research examining changes in neurocognitive functioning subsequent to treatment for a medical condition. In this case, treatment involves some combination of surgery, chemotherapy, and radiation therapy. The most extensive research has been in the areas of malignant brain tumors and leukemia, the two most frequent childhood cancers and those in which significant late effects of treatment have been identified (Mulhern & Butler, 2006). Late effects are generally defined as changes in functioning occurring after the completion of active treatment, often 2 or more years following treatment, and are presumed in most cases to be permanent or chronic (Mulhern & Butler,

2006). Although many late effects are medical in nature (e.g., cardiac problems, hearing impairment, secondary malignancies), the focus in pediatric psychology has been on those affecting cognition and learning and on the emotional impact of treatment, acutely and across the life span (Armstrong & Mulhern, 1999). Most typically, declines in IQ have been measured and identified, particularly for those treated with varying degrees of craniospinal radiation and certain combinations of chemotherapy. An additional focus of research has been on defining the specific cognitive processes involved, with deficits most frequently identified in visual–motor integration, processing speed, visual memory, and attention (e.g., Butler, Kerr, & Marchand, 1999; Lockwood, Bell, & Colegrove, 1999).

Cognitive and/or learning deficits have been shown to be associated with a number of common pediatric illnesses, in addition to cancer. The effects of treatment medications on the central nervous system, leading to neurocognitive/learning deficits and/or behavioral issues, and the impact of frequent school absences have been studied in asthma (Lemanek & Hood, 1999). Deficits in language, attention, memory, and motor functioning have been identified in children with HIV infection (Wolters, Brouwers, & Perez, 1999). Neuropsychological evaluation of children with sickle cell disease has identified deficits in IQ, attention and executive function, memory, language, visuomotor abilities, and academic achievement, particularly when there is evidence of stroke or silent infarct (Berkelhammer et al., 2007). These are just a few of the medical conditions in which cognitive deficits have been identified and assessment should be considered.

In many instances, special accommodations must be made in order to accurately assess neurocognitive status in children undergoing treatment for a medical disorder. Testing must be scheduled so that medications that may cause fatigue, confusion, or nausea will have as little impact as possible. Stamina may be limited, so a number of brief testing sessions will likely provide a more accurate measure of functioning. Intravenous (IV) access, mobility limitations, or recent changes in functioning (e.g., vision or hearing loss, loss of the use of the preferred hand, tracheotomy) must all be taken into consideration. Anxiety associated with the medical setting or concern about upcoming medical procedures may also play a role.

General measures of cognitive skills and learning that have been well validated and studied extensively are well known to psychologists working with children and have been reviewed in detail elsewhere (e.g., Sattler, 2008). In the interest of time and space, such measures are not covered in this chapter, and the reader is directed to these resources and others described in this chapter to assist in finding appropriate tools for measuring specific cognitive or learning processes.

The Children's Oncology Group (COG) has recognized that late effects may be studied more consistently by standardizing measures used across member institutions. They have developed a set of core domains to be evaluated, along with suggested measures, forming a comprehensive testing battery appropriate for most baseline evaluations or assessments of treatment impact. Functional domains to be tested include intelligence, language, memory, attention, executive function, academic achievement, and adjustment and quality of life (see Table 14.3 in Mulhern & Butler, 2006). A standardized evaluation is important for conducting multicenter research, but it also allows more consistent communication among professionals who provide clinical treatment to children with a common disorder. This type of suggested standardized evaluation may also be helpful for other childhood medical conditions in which cognitive impact is suspected or has been documented.

Family Functioning

Families have long been recognized as playing a significant role in children's health (Drotar, 1997; Kazak, 1989). Not only does a child's diagnosis of a chronic illness affect other family members, their interactions and relationships, and the overall functioning of the system, but the family also influences the child's chronic condition (Alderfer & Kazak, 2006). In general, families are conceptualized as organized systems that strive to keep balance through assigned roles, affective regulation, and communication (Kazak, Rourke, & Crump, 2003). Important aspects of family functioning include organization (roles, leadership), communication, cohesion (involvement and closeness), affective regulation (expression of feelings and conflict), and problem-solving ability (Alderfer et al., 2008). Most measures of family functioning incorporate one or more of these areas and may include an index of global adaptation.

One consideration in the assessment of the family is that families are made up of subsystems (parent–child, sibling–sibling). When choosing a measure, one needs to consider whether dyadic measurement tools would be of more interest than tools that measure global family functioning. In pediatric populations, a measure that assesses family functioning within the context of the medical condition would be particularly useful (Alderfer et al., 2008).

Family functioning and family relationships can be assessed through self-report measures, family interviews, and observed interactions, or through informal methods such as genograms or eco-maps (Alderfer et al., 2008; Rosenthal, Cohen, & Simeonsson, 2001). Alderfer et al. (2008) reviewed 29 family assessment measures relevant to the field of pediatric psychology and determined that 66% were "well established." They provide detailed information about these measures, which include measures of general family functioning, dyadic family relationships, and family relationships within the context of childhood medical conditions. For detailed tables of information about these family measures, see the supplementary data by Alderfer et al. (2008) referenced at *www.jpepsy.oxfordjournals. org*.

The assessment of family functioning may be particularly critical around the time of diagnosis. Standardized psychosocial risk screening tools are being recognized as important for identifying children and families at highest risk for coping problems in order to provide intervention and support as early as possible and to determine which families are in greatest need of targeted interventions and often limited resources (Kazak et al., 2012). A review of such screening tools and recommendations regarding their integration into clinical practice in pediatric cancer and their utility in enhancing comprehensive care may be found in Kazak et al. (2012).

Social Support and Peer Relations

Social support generally refers to a wide range of social networks and resources available to the individual. For a child, these resources might include peer support, emotional support from family, or physical assistance (Martin & Brantley, 2004). Peer relationships have been considered to be a good measure of social competence and predictive of adjustment (Morison & Masten, 1991; Parker & Asher, 1987).

A number of characteristics of chronic medical conditions and treatment could have an effect on peer relationships in children. Some chronic conditions interfere with daily routines or place restrictions on children's physical activities. Many studies have found that children with chronic medical conditions report fewer social and physical activities than healthy children (e.g., Feldmann, Weglage, Roth, Foell, & Frosch, 2005; Gerhardt, Vannatta, Valerius, Correll, & Noll, 2007; Reiter-Purtill & Noll, 2003). They also have more frequent school absences (Reiter-Purtill, Waller, & Noll, 2009). Certain medical conditions affect physical appearance or cognitive functioning, which may lead to negative self or peer perceptions (La Greca, 1990; Schuman & La Greca, 1999). For example, obese children have reported social difficulties such as victimization, teasing, and stigmatization (Hayden-Wade et al., 2005; Puhl & Latner, 2007; Thompson et al., 2007). There also are data suggesting that obese children are less well liked, have fewer friends, and are perceived by peers to be isolated and sensitive (Strauss & Pollack, 2003; Zeller, Reiter-Purtill, & Ramey, 2008). Reiter-Purtill et al. (2009) reviewed the literature on peer relationships of children with chronic illness and concluded that the majority of the empirical studies suggest that youth with chronic conditions have social difficulties, according to parent report. In contrast, peers did not report peer difficulties in children with chronic conditions unless the condition affected physical appearance or cognitive skills (central nervous system functioning) or was accompanied by somatic complaints (e.g., abdominal pain). Recent meta-analyses also found children and adolescents with chronic physical illness to have on average lower levels of social functioning than their healthy peers (Martinez, Carter, & Legato, 2011; Pinquart & Teubert, 2011), but these findings varied according to individual child factors (e.g., gender, chronic illness type) and measurement factors, such as measure type and informant.

Peer ratings can be considered the best measure of a child's social functioning, as peers generally have the most interactions with the child (Reiter-Purtill et al., 2009). These ratings are often given by multiple raters (e.g., child's classmates), and this provides a more reliable measure than those done by single raters. However, few studies in the pediatric psychology literature have utilized these peer ratings (Reiter-Purtill et al., 2009). Because measures of social skills and peer relationships by peer ratings generally is not realistic in clinical practice, self-report or report by other informants (parents or teachers) on pencil-and-paper measures is a more practical way to assess social competence in children. Self-report measures also are useful in understanding a child's perspective on his or her experiences with peers, social acceptance, and victimization. Reiter-Purtill and colleagues (Reiter-Purtill & Noll, 2003; Reiter-Purtill, Waller, & Noll, 2009) noted that much of the research on peer relationships of children with chronic medical conditions has not utilized measures that primarily assess social functioning. General emotional and behavioral measures such as the Child Behavior Checklist (CBCL; Achenbach, 1991; Achenbach & Rescorla, 2001) and the Behavior Assessment System for Children—2 (BASC-2; Reynolds & Kamphaus, 1998) do assess social competence and social skills. However, it is important to use caution when using the CBCL to assess social competence in chronically ill children because illness-related limitations may influence the score (Drotar, Stein, & Perrin, 1995; Perrin, Stein, & Drotar, 1991). See Reiter-Purtill et al. (2009) and Reiter-Purtill and Noll (2003) for reviews of empirical studies addressing the social functioning of children with chronic medical conditions.

Psychosocial Functioning and Psychopathology

Because children and adolescents are constantly changing and pass through many developmental stages, it is imperative to compare their psychosocial functioning with that of most children of a similar age or developmental level. Psychosocial functioning encompasses adjustment or adaptation across a number of domains, including emotional, behavioral, and social realms. To gain the richest picture of a child's emotional and behavioral adjustment, clinicians should consider the use of structured and informal interview techniques, self-, parent, and teacher report measures, behavioral observations, and review of existing records.

A number of resources are available that review specific measures of psychosocial functioning and psychopathology in both general clinical child psychology (Mash & Hunsley, 2005) and pediatric psychology populations (Rodrigue, Geffken, & Streisand, 2000; Kelley, Reitman, & Noell, 2003). In addition, Holmbeck et al. (2008) provide a comprehensive review of measures of adjustment and psychopathology, as well as perceived self-concept and self-esteem, as part of the Division 54 Task Force on Evidence-Based Assessment in Pediatric Psychology. Their review contains measures of internalizing (e.g. depression, anxiety) or externalizing (e.g. oppositionality, hyperactivity) behavior, broadband rating scales (broad coverage of psychological adjustment concepts), and self-esteem/self-concept scales. More detailed information on the assessment of psychosocial adjustment and psychopathology in pediatric and clinical child populations also is available (Mortweet & Christopherson, 2003; Wallander, Thompson, & Alriksson-Schmidt, 2003; Frick & Kamphaus, 2001).

Holmbeck et al. (2008) concluded that there are a number of excellent measures of psychosocial adjustment and psychopathology that would be relevant to pediatric psychology. Of the 37 measures reviewed, 92% met "well established" evidence-based assessment criteria. "Well established" broadband measures included the Child Behavior Checklist (CBCL; Achenbach, 1991; Achenbach & Rescorla, 2001), the Behavior Assessment System for Children (BASC; Reynolds & Kamphaus, 1998), the Conners Rating Scales—Revised (CRS-R; Conners, 2001), and the Minnesota Multiphasic Personality Inventory—Adolescent (MMPI-A; Butcher et al., 1992; Graham,

Archer, Tellegen, Ben-Porath, & Kaemmer, 2006). Additional detailed broadband measures of specific internalizing–externalizing scales and self-concept measures are also reviewed. Although not reviewed by Holmbeck and colleagues (2008), the Behavior Assessment System for Children–Second Edition (BASC-2: Reynolds & Kamphaus, 2004), the Conners Third Edition (Conners 3; Conners, 2008), and the Conners Early Childhood (Conners EC; Conners, 2009) also are available. When considering measures of psychosocial functioning and psychopathology, clinicians should take into account age of the child, developmental and cognitive levels, and specific factors related to the illness to determine the most appropriate assessment tools. Multiple informants are likely needed to gain the richest, most accurate picture.

Pain

The assessment of acute and chronic pain in pediatric patients is often a particular challenge. Unlike adults, many of whom have experienced childbirth, surgical pain, or an athletic injury, most pediatric patients do not have a reference point for severe or chronic pain. In addition, the perception of pain in children is affected by numerous other factors: other stressors in the child's life (Walker, Garber, Smith, Van Slyke, & Claar, 2001), fear and stress related to the medical setting (McGrath, 1996), parental distress, and, for hospitalized children, possibly even having to adjust to changes in routine and eating issues (e.g., being unable to eat or drink in preparation for tests or surgery, problems with nausea). Although these factors are not necessarily painful, they do contribute to the child's experience of pain and distress.

The measurement of pain has generated considerable research, and a number of good review articles are available, all of which utilized criteria outlined by the Society of Pediatric Psychology Assessment Task Force (Cohen, LaGreca, et al., 2008). The Pediatric Initiative on Methods, Measurement, and Pain Assessment in Clinical Trials (Ped-IMMPACT) has commissioned and published reviews of self-report measures (Stinson, Kavanaugh, Yamada, Gill, & Stevens, 2006) and of observational measures (von Baeyer & Spagrud, 2007), primarily for the purpose of choosing appropriate measures for clinical trials. A focus on identifying appropriate, evidence-based assessment measures for specific populations and individual needs in either clinical practice or research is taken in another recent review commissioned by the American Psychological Association, Division 54, Society of Pediatric Psychology Assessment Task Force (Cohen, Lemanek, et al., 2008).

Standardized measures of pain are most often visual analogue or numerical scales and focus on measuring pain intensity. The Faces Pain Scale—Revised, for example, presents a 6-point scale of pain represented by pictures of faces in varying degrees of pain and distress (Hicks, von Baeyer, Spafford, van Korlaar, & Goodenough, 2001). The child is able to point to the face that best represents his or her current feelings relative to pain. Older children (> 7) are often asked to use numerical scales on which, for example, "1" represents no pain and "10" the worst pain imaginable, as this is an easy, cost-effective monitoring method that does not require assessment tools. Obviously, there remains a significant subjective component to these measurement tools, and they have been noted to lack specificity and to have potential for bias (e.g., McGrath, 1990). Behavioral observation methods in which behaviors such as crying, withdrawal from touch, and facial changes, such as the Children's Hospital of Eastern Ontario Pain Scale (CHEOPS; McGrath et al., 1985), are useful for rating short, sharp pain but are subject to habituation and have not been found to be sensitive to pain even a few hours after surgery (Beyer, McGrath, & Berde, 1990). In choosing tools for assessing pediatric pain, a variety of reliability and validity measures should be considered, including the correlation of the child's ratings with judgments of pain made by the nurse or a parent, the scale's sensitivity to interventions such as analgesics or behavioral pain management, and the consistency of the child's ratings with observed and reported indicators of pain (Dahlquist & Switkin, 2003). Structured interviews such as the Pediatric Pain Questionnaire (Varni, Thompson, & Hanson, 1987) are also available and provide an effective outline for gaining information about the family's pain history, the specific site of the pain (which is often difficult to determine in young children, in particular), and the child's emotional reactivity tendencies.

A variety of physiological/biological measures, primarily of sympathetic and parasympathetic activity, have also been used in the assessment of pediatric pain. Blood pressure, respiration, and electroencephalography (EEG) have been found to be related to pain but lack specificity (McGrath, 1996). Research has examined physiological measures such as heart rate variability, cardiac vagal tone, and salivary cortisol, all of which are generally considered to be valid indicators of pain in certain circumstances (e.g., Walco, Conte, Labay, Engle, & Zeltzer, 2005). Most of these measures, however, tend to habituate when pain becomes more chronic or are also nonspecific to pain. Although physiological measures of pain often are not practical as routine clinical assessment tools, additional research in these areas should help to further define the mechanisms of the pain response.

One of the more challenging aspects of pain assessment occurs when a child exhibits more pain than would be expected based on the extent of injury, typical reactions to the procedure, or amount of tissue damage (McGrath, 1996). In some cases, children with chronic medical problems learn quite quickly that pain is best prevented rather than managed and begin to routinely request medication at the slightest hint of pain in order to prevent what they suspect may become much more uncomfortable. At the other extreme is pain that may be undertreated because of the child's reluctance to report pain that may result in another aversive procedure, such as a needle stick (McGrath, 1996). In all of these cases, the use of multimodal assessment with a variety of raters and sound measurement instruments over a representative period of time is critical in making effective decisions regarding medical and psychological interventions. McGrath (1996) adds that discordance thought to be overreporting of pain is to be expected and should not immediately be considered evidence of malingering or somatization but as a need for both additional assessment and clinical problem solving. McCracken, Zayfert, and Gross (1992) refer to such emotional, behavioral, and cognitive contributions to pain as "pain anxiety," and initial reliability and validity studies of a pediatric measure of pain anxiety have been completed (Pagé, Fuss, Martin, Romero Escobar, & Katz, 2010; Pagé et al., 2011).

Adherence to Medical Treatments

Adherence can be defined as "the extent to which a person's behavior (in terms of taking medications, following diets, or executing lifestyle changes) coincides with medical or health advice" (Haynes, 1979, pp. 1–2). Treatment adherence to medical regimens is a major pediatric health concern (La Greca & Race Mackey, 2009), with estimates of nonadherence as high as 50% in some studies (Carter & Von Weiss, 2005; Rapoff, 1999). Failure to adhere to one's medical regimen is a significant cause of treatment failure, and the consequences of poor adherence are potentially serious. Nonadherence can exacerbate the child's illness or medical complications, which can lead to increased hospitalizations and absences from school (Rapoff, 1999; Sturge, Garralda, Boissin, Doré, & Woo, 1997) and compromised efficacy of medications and treatment regimens (Matsui, 2000). As with adults, failure to adhere to medical regimens has multiple contributing factors, including deficits in education and skills training, problems in understanding the regimen, anxiety and fearfulness, and interference with normal activities and functioning (Carter & Von Weiss, 2005). In addition, family factors, such as parent–child relationship characteristics, and individual characteristics, such as developmental and behavioral problems, can affect adherence (Carter & Von Weiss, 2005).

In general, adolescents have more difficulties with poor adherence than do younger children (Brownbridge & Fielding, 1994; Kovacs, Goldston, Obrosky, & Iyengar, 1992). Adolescents have trouble managing regimens that require major lifestyle adjustments, such as dietary restrictions, exercise, and those that have cosmetic side effects (e.g., taking prednisone) or that interfere with social interactions. With children and adolescents, parents are also at least partly responsible for compliance, so it is important that both youth and parent treatment-related behaviors be assessed in the pediatric population (De Civita & Dobkin, 2005; Watson, Foster, & Friman, 2006). The family's history of adherence is likely an important determinant of how they will manage the disease in the future, as well (Rapoff, 1999).

Treatment adherence or compliance can be measured in a number of ways, depending on the pediatric condition and adherence behavior required. Many investigators have used a categorical cutoff approach using criteria to define groups of adherent or nonadherent patients (La Greca & Race Mackey, 2009). Unfortunately, it is often not known what constitutes an adequate level of adherence for most medical problems, so the cutoff criteria are often arbitrary (La Greca & Race Mackey, 2009). Adherence may be better conceptualized as occurring on a continuum (Quittner, Modi, Lemanek, Ievers-Landis, & Rapoff, 2008), and it may be advisable to consider the multiple aspects involved in a treatment regimen rather than viewing it as a unitary construct (La Greca & Race Mackey, 2009).

Adherence has been assessed using self-report, child and parent monitoring (diary measures), structured interviews, ratings by health care professionals, pill counts, prescription refill histories, electronic monitors, biochemical assays, and measurement of clinical health outcome or status (La Greca & Race Mackey, 2009; Quittner et al., 2008; Siegel & Conte, 2001; Wu et al., 2013). Currently, there is no best practice for measuring adherence in pediatric populations (De Civita & Dobkin, 2005), but technological advances in microprocessors have made available an array of electronic monitors that hold great promise. Quittner and colleagues (2008) provide a comprehensive review of evidence-based adherence assessment measures in pediatric populations.

The most common method for measuring adherence is patient or parent report (De Civita & Dobkin, 2005; Quittner et al., 2008). These measures are relatively easy to obtain, inexpensive, and available for multiple informants (youth, parent, health care providers), and they can assess a complex array of behaviors. Self-reports are most accurate when recall periods are kept to a minimum and when detailed, objective questions are used. Structured interviews to assess adherence also have been used with youth with a number of chronic conditions, including diabetes, asthma, and HIV/AIDS (Quittner et al., 2008).

Self-monitoring using daily diaries has been used to measure adherence to specific regimens. These daily diaries have taken the form of written logs, handheld computers (personal digital assistants [PDAs]), and phone diaries. Unfortunately, research has shown that compliance with completing written logs has been poor, with respondents often completing the diary just prior to the appointment instead of on a daily basis (Quittner et al., 2008). Self-monitoring by mobile device or electronic tablet can increase accuracy, as data are collected in real time or within short periods of recall (e.g., 24 hours).

Recent advances in technology have allowed potentially more accurate measurements of adherence using automated measures. These monitors can record the removal of pills from blister packs, the opening and closing of standard medication vials, the use of metered-dose inhalers, and blood glucose test results. Although the monitors can record continuous and long-term measurement of medication use in real time, there are still disadvantages, such as mechanical malfunctions, overestimates of compliance (medication is recorded only being dispensed, not ingested), and relatively high costs of the devices (Quittner et al., 2008).

It is important to recognize that adherence is a complex and dynamic process that changes over time and must be assessed frequently. It is not an "all or none" process and should be measured in a multidimensional fashion, assessing a number of behaviors, such as taking medication, following dietary guidelines, exercising, and doing self-care tasks (blood glucose sticks, breathing treatments). Understanding the barriers that obstruct adherence is important in designing appropriate interventions (Siegel & Conte, 2001).

Stress and Coping

"Stress" has been defined as "an event or experience that expends the resources of an individual" (Blount et al., 2008, p. 1022), and "coping" has been defined as thoughts and behaviors that are used to manage the internal and external demands of events considered stressful (Lazarus & Folkman, 1984). Both stress and coping can be considered within a risk and resiliency model; coping is considered a dynamic process that changes in responses to changes in demands of the stressor (Blount et al., 2008). Moreover, coping and stress occur within a complex framework, with a dynamic interplay between stress, coping, and biopsychosocial outcomes (Blount et al., 2008). Issues related to stress and coping are relevant for most acute and chronic pediatric medical conditions and for youth dealing with painful and scary medical procedures, including hospitalizations, surgery, and injections (Blount et al., 2008).

Stress includes both objective (chronic medical condition, family death, divorce) and subjective (perceived threat) phenomena (Blount et al., 2008). In general, greater stress is associated with poor outcomes in health (Kiecolt-Glaser, McGuire, Robles, & Glaser, 2002) and psychosocial functioning (Kanner, Feldman, Weinberger, & Ford, 1987; Santa Lucia et al., 2000). Measures of child stress vary in their focus on specific versus general stressors and in assessment format. Blount et al. (2008) identified one inventory of stress, the Children's Hassles Scale/Children's Uplifts Scale (Kanner et al., 1987) as a "well established" assessment measure of stress and two other measures as "approaching well established."

Developmental factors affect children's coping with stressful situations, and independent coping increases with age. As children grow, they become more independent in their ability to cope. Whereas infants and toddlers will need to rely on caregivers to aid in coping by providing distraction and soothing, preschool and young elementary children can utilize some internal coping strategies, such as positive self-talk, imagery, and relaxation skills, with coaching from parents (Harbeck-Weber, Fisher, & Dittner, 2003). Adolescents may be able to use internal coping strategies without the aid of coaching from parents or other adults. Researchers have found that children's use of emotion-focused coping also tends to increase with age (e.g., Band & Weisz, 1988; Compas, Malcarne, & Fondacaro, 1988). In addition, older children are more likely to use a variety of coping strategies and to focus on positive factors (Brown, O'Keeffe, Sanders, & Baker, 1986).

Coping has been conceptualized in a number of ways and across different dimensions, such as information seeking versus information avoidance, emotion-focused versus problem-focused coping, monitoring versus blunting, and approach versus avoidance (Blount, Davis, Powers, & Roberts, 1991; Rudolph, Denning, & Weisz, 1995). As such, coping also has been measured in many ways in pediatric psychology (Siegel & Conte, 2001). One measurement approach has been to identify specific behavioral strategies that children use when dealing with medical procedures or other stressful events (Siegel, 1983; Spirito, Stark, & Tyc, 1994). Another approach has been to assess children's preferences for obtaining or avoiding information about their medical illness or course of treatment (e.g., Field, Alpert, Vega-Lahr, Goldstein & Perry, 1988; Smith, Ackerson, & Blotcky, 1989). Blount et al. (2008) classified four general coping measures as "well established," including the Adolescent Coping Orientation for Problem Experiences (Patterson & McCubbin, 1987) and the Kidcope (Spirito, Stark, & Williams, 1988).

Some childhood illnesses or injuries needing significant medical intervention require frequent, repeated invasive procedures or involve a significant perceived threat to the child's life. Childhood cancer, for example, is generally perceived as potentially life threatening and may involve numerous invasive procedures, potentially devastating side effects, and the need to continue to face stressful medical situations repeatedly over a long period of time. Burn victims have often experienced a terribly traumatic incident (e.g., fire, car accident, physical abuse) and often must endure repeated debridements and potential infections. Research has begun to examine whether circumstances such as these may lead to symptoms of posttraumatic stress disorder, either following treatment or even much later in the child's life.

The diagnosis of posttraumatic stress disorder (PTSD) based on DSM-5 criteria involves assessment of exposure to or threat of a traumatic event; intrusive symptoms (e.g., distressing memories or flashbacks);

avoidance of related stimuli; and alterations in cognition, mood, arousal, and/or reactivity (American Psychiatric Association, 2013). Some criteria specific for children 6 years and younger focus on expression of positive and negative emotion, constriction of play activities, and social withdrawal. Earlier diagnostic criteria required that the patient be exposed to an event "outside of the range of ordinary human experience" (Stuber, 2006). DSM-IV (American Psychiatric Association, 1994); however, first revised diagnostic criteria in recognition of findings that the child's perception of the event is most important in determining the development of PTSD, with DSM-5 providing further guidance in identifying the variety of ways in which traumatic events may be experienced and coping difficulties expressed. For the most part, assessment involves a careful interview (semistructured interviews are used in most research studies) of the child and parent to identify these symptoms, their level of intensity, and the extent to which they interfere with the child's daily functioning. Assessment instruments such as the Post-Traumatic Stress Reaction Index (Kazak et al., 1997) are also used to assess symptom occurrence and severity.

In the pediatric cancer literature, Stuber, Nader, Yasuda, Pynoos, and Cohen (1991) first noted PTSD symptoms such as nightmares, hypervigilance, themes of trauma in play, and avoidance of discussion of their treatment in survivors of bone marrow transplant even 1 year after transplant. A study of 18- to 37-year-old survivors of childhood cancer suggests that late effects occurring long after treatment and chronic health threats may play a role in the development of PTSD, as 20% of these survivors reported symptoms consistent with a diagnosis of PTSD (Hobbie et al., 2000). The majority of studies, however, have found that children and adolescents who have survived cancer adapt quite well and function just as successfully as their peers without a history of cancer (Kazak et al, 1997). Predictors of posttraumatic stress symptoms also have been examined, and it was found that the survivor's retrospective recall of the difficulty of treatment, general level of anxiety, experience of other life stressors, shorter time since treatment completion, female gender, and family and social support were most predictive of the later presence of symptoms (Stuber et al., 1997).

Children and adolescents who have survived burns have also been found to experience PTSD symptoms, during both acute treatment and subsequent rehabilitation (Stoddard & Saxe, 2001). The development of PTSD has also been studied in adolescents with spinal cord injury, with 25% meeting diagnostic criteria in one study (Boyer, Knolls, Kafkalas, & Tollen, 2000) and with a prior history (before the spinal cord injury) of experiencing trauma leading to higher risk (Radnitz, Schlein, & Hsu, 2000).

Further development of standardized assessment methods to study this important illness, injury, and treatment-related reaction will be important in identifying children at risk and studying predictors of successful versus problematic posttreatment courses. This is particularly critical because high self-reports of avoidance in children with health-related PTSD have been associated with nonadherence to their treatment regimens (Shemesh et al., 2000).

Quality of Life

Advancements in medical treatments for serious and chronic diseases in children have necessitated the development of and considerable research on the utility of assessment tools to measure a child's health-related quality of life (HRQoL; Bradlyn et al., 1996). The medical and psychological communities have become increasingly aware of the need to measure the impact of treatment not just on quantity of life and survival but on the quality of those years and the ability to live "normally" after treatment, with assessment including both objective and subjective measures of life satisfaction (Eiser & Morse, 2001).

Once again, assessment of quality of life (QoL) in children is notably different from such assessment in adults, and the relative importance of even childhood QoL factors changes as children move from early to middle childhood and into adolescence and young adulthood (Speith, 2001; Quittner, Davis, & Modi, 2003). QoL in early childhood is primarily related to being able to achieve normal developmental milestones (e.g., walking, speaking, independent toileting), whereas school attendance and social

relationships become more significant in the elementary years. Adolescent QoL is often defined by the ability to complete educational milestones, to be employable in the young adult's field of choice, and to "fit in" physically and interpersonally with peers and potential life partners (Drotar, 2004).

QoL is also a very subjective concept and may be perceived quite differently in various raters considering the same child. A nurse rating a young patient may focus on the child's ability to eat normally and be pain free or on other visible indicators of health (Parsons, Barlow, Levy, Supran, & Kaplan, 1999). Parents have been found to estimate greater impact of disease and to rate their children as functioning more poorly than the children themselves do (e.g., Sawyer, Antoniou, Toogood, & Rice, 1999). The adolescent patient may consider physical attributes and number of friends to be most critical in defining a positive QoL and may be more affected by treatment effects than a younger child (Levi, 2006).

The standardized assessment of HRQoL is critical in both the clinical and research realms in determining the disease burden associated with various diseases, so that appropriate decisions may be made about medical interventions. HRQoL data may also be used to compare two potentially beneficial treatments or medications; if survival outcomes of treatments are similar, benefits and risks also may be defined based on expectations for better HRQoL (Eiser, 2004; Olson, Lara, & Frintner, 2004). Such information may be used in determining standard of care for a specific disease or may be used by individual families in choosing among potentially beneficial treatments based on the family's individual caregiving needs and hopes for the child's future. A comprehensive review of evidence-based assessment measures of QoL and functional impairment in pediatric psychology describes "well established" measures and recommendations for future research needs in this area of assessment (Palermo, Long, Lewandowski, Drotar, Quittner & Walker, 2008).

A number of QoL instruments have been designed and studied to evaluate general HRQoL in pediatric populations (see review in Ravens-Sieberer et al., 2006). The Child Health and Illness Profile (Starfield, Riley,

& Green, 1999) includes self-report and parent versions, can discriminate between children with illnesses and healthy controls, and has been found to correlate with other HRQoL measures. The Pediatric Quality of Life Inventory (PedsQL; Varni, Seid, & Rode, 1999) also includes child and parent versions and an age range extending from 2 to 18 years and has been associated with other HRQoL measures and with daily living measures such as school absences and severity of medical symptoms.

Additional HRQoL measures have been developed and utilized with a variety of chronic illness populations, as well. The PedsQL includes modules for asthma, diabetes, cancer, cardiac problems, arthritis, and other disorders. The Cystic Fibrosis Questionnaire (Quittner, Buu, Messer, Modi, & Watrous, 2005; Modi & Quittner, 2003) and the Pediatric Oncology Quality of Life Scale (Goodwin, Boggs, & Graham-Pole, 1994) are additional examples of disease-specific HRQoL assessments. Instruments are also in development or undergoing further evaluation to address the impact of other chronic medical conditions, such as gastroesophageal reflux disease (Acierno, Chilcote, Edwards, & Goldin, 2010) and epilepsy (Verhey et al., 2009). For detailed tables of information about both general and disease-specific HRQoL measures, see the supplementary data by Palermo et al. (2008) referenced at *www.jpepsy.oxford-journals.org*.

Conclusions

Although standardized assessment of every area described in this chapter is seldom needed in an individual patient, it is important to recognize that each area affects the others and that assessment in one area may be influenced strongly by problems in another area. For example, a child's perception of pain or QoL may influence his or her willingness to adhere to a difficult medical regimen. On the other hand, ratings of QoL may be influenced by cognitive late effects of treatment or by level of stress and poor coping skills.

In assessing pediatric patients for any of these potential challenges, it is most critical to remember that children require special assessment considerations. A developmental approach must be taken that emphasizes the child's level of maturation in comparison with that of typically developing children. The biopsychosocial model should be considered, as it acknowledges the spheres or systems in which a child functions and considers the child's health concerns within these systems. Multiple informants and multimodal assessment will provide the most comprehensive assessment of the child's strengths and weaknesses. Once an assessment need is identified, many well-established measures are available to measure global or disease-specific functioning. Ongoing research in pediatric psychology assessment should focus on further validating existing measures and identifying additional child and family characteristics within these general areas that would provide a clearer picture of the child with health issues. Advancements in medicine will likely pose new challenges in assessment, as well, as we study their impact on children's development, adjustment, and ability to function effectively within their families and communities.

REFERENCES

Achenbach, T. M. (1991). *Manual for the Child Behavior Checklist/4–18 and 1991 profile.* Burlington: University of Vermont, Department of Psychiatry.

Achenbach, T. M., & Rescorla, L. A. (2001). *Manual for the ASEBA school-age forms and profiles.* Burlington: University of Vermont, Research Center for Children, Youth, and Families.

Acierno, S. P., Chilcote, H. C., Edwards, T. C., & Goldin, A. B. (2010). Development of a quality of life instrument for pediatric gastroesophageal reflux disease: Qualitative interviews. *Journal of Pediatric Gastroenterology and Nutrition, 50*(5), 486–492.

Alderfer, M. A., Fiese, B. H., Gold, J. I., Cutuli, J. J., Holmbeck, G. N., Goldbeck, L., et al. (2008). Evidence-based assessment in pediatric psychology: Family measures. *Journal of Pediatric Psychology, 33*(9), 1046–1061.

Alderfer, M. A., & Kazak, A. E. (2006). Family issues when a child is on treatment for cancer. In R. Brown (Ed.), *Pediatric hematology/oncology: A biopsychosocial approach* (pp. 53–74). New York: Oxford University Press.

American Psychiatric Association. (1994). *Diagnostic and statistical manual of mental disorders* (4th ed.). Washington, DC: Author.

American Psychiatric Association. (2013). *Diagnostic and statistical manual of mental disorders* (5th ed.). Arlington, VA: Author.

Armstrong, F. D., & Mulhern, R. K. (1999). Acute lymphoblastic leukemia and brain tumors. In R. T. Brown (Ed.), *Cognitive aspects of chronic illness in children* (pp. 47–77). New York: Guilford Press.

Band, E., & Weisz, J. (1988). How to feel better when it feels bad: Children's perspectives of coping with everyday stress. *Developmental Psychology, 24,* 247–253.

Berkelhammer, L. D., Williamson, A., Sanford, S. D., Dirksen, C. L., Sharp, W. G., Margulies, A. S., et al. (2007). Neurocognitive sequelae of pediatric sickle cell disease: A review of the literature. *Child Neuropsychology, 13*(2), 120–131.

Beyer, J. E., McGrath, P. J., & Berde, C. (1990). Discordance between self-report and behavioral pain measures in 3–7 year old children following surgery. *Journal of Pain and Symptom Management, 5,* 350–356.

Blount, R. L., Davis, N., Powers, S., & Roberts, M. C. (1991). The influence of environmental factors and coping style on children's coping and distress. *Clinical Psychology Review, 11,* 93–116.

Blount, R. L., Simons, L. E., Devine, K. A., Jaaniste, T., Cohen, L. L., Chamber, C. T., et al. (2008). Evidence-based assessment of coping and stress in pediatric psychology. *Journal of Pediatric Psychology, 33*(9), 1021–1045.

Boyd Webb, N. (1991). Play therapy in crisis intervention with children. In N. Boyd Webb (Ed.), *Play therapy with children in crisis: A casebook for practitioners* (pp. 26–42). New York: Guilford Press.

Boyer, B. A., Knolls, M. L., Kafkalas, C. M., & Tollen, L. G. (2000). What is the trauma?: Patients', mothers' and fathers' fear and helplessness related to post-traumatic aspects of pediatric SCI. *Topics in Spinal Cord Injury Rehabilitation, 6*(Suppl.), 134–147.

Bradlyn, A., Ritchey, A., Harris, C., Moore, I., O'Brien, R., Parsons, S., et al. (1996). Quality of life research in pediatric oncology: Research methods and barriers. *Cancer, 78,* 1333–1339.

Bronfenbrenner, U. (1979). *The ecology of human development: Experiments by nature and design.* Cambridge, MA: Harvard University Press.

Bronfenbrenner, U. (2004). *Making human beings human: Bioecological perspectives on human development.* Thousand Oaks, CA: Sage.

Brown, J., O'Keeffe, J., Sanders, S., & Baker, B. (1986). Developmental changes in children's cognition to stressful and painful situations. *Journal of Pediatric Psychology, 11,* 343–357.

Brownbridge, G., & Fielding, D. M. (1994). Psychosocial adjustment and adherence to dialysis treatment regimens. *Pediatric Nephrology, 8,* 744–749.

Butcher, J. N., Williams, C. L., Graham, J. R., Archer, R. P., Tellegen, A., Ben-Porath, Y. S., et al. (1992). *MMPI-A: Minnesota Multiphasic Personality Inventory—Adolescent: Manual for administration, scoring, and interpretation.* Minneapolis: University of Minnesota Press.

Butler, R., Kerr, M., & Marchand, A. (1999). Attention and executive functions following cranial irradiation in children. *Journal of the International Neuropsychological Society, 5,* 108.

Carter, B. D., & Von Weiss, R. T. (2005). Inpatient pediatric consultation-liaison: Applied child health psychology. In R. G. Steele & M. C. Roberts (Eds.), *Handbook of mental health services for children, adolescents, and families* (pp. 63–83). New York: Kluwer Academic/Plenum.

Cohen, L. L., La Greca, A. M., Blount, R. L., Kazak, A. E., Holmbeck, G. N., & Lemanek, K. L. (2008). Introduction to special issue: Evidence-based assessment in pediatric psychology. *Journal of Pediatric Psychology, 33*(9), 911–915.

Cohen, L. L., Lemanek, K., Blount, R. L., Dahlquist, L. M., Lim, C. S., Palermo, T. M., et al. (2008). Evidence-based assessment of pediatric pain. *Journal of Pediatric Psychology, 33*(9), 939–955.

Compas, B., Malcarne, V., & Fondacaro, K. (1988). Coping with stressful events in older children and young adolescents. *Journal of Consulting and Clinical Psychology, 56,* 405–411.

Conners, C. K. (2001). *Conners Rating Scales—Revised: Technical manual.* North Tonawanda, NY: Multi-Health Systems.

Conners, C. K. (2008). *Conners 3rd edition manual.* Toronto, Ontario, Canada: Multi-Health Systems.

Conners, C. K. (2009). *Conners early childhood manual*. Toronto, Ontario, Canada: Multi-Health Systems.

Dahlquist, L. M., & Switkin, M. C. (2003). Chronic and recurrent pain. In M. C. Roberts (Ed.), *Handbook of pediatric psychology* (3rd ed., pp. 198–215). New York: Guilford Press.

De Civita, M., & Dobkin, P. L. (2005). Pediatric adherence: Conceptual and methodological considerations. *Children's Health Care, 34,* 19–34.

Drotar, D. (1997). Relating parent and family functioning to the psychological adjustment of children with chronic health conditions: What have we learned? *Journal of Pediatric Psychology, 22,* 149–165.

Drotar, D. (2004). Validating measures of pediatric health status, functional status, and health-related quality of life: Key methodological challenges and strategies. *Ambulatory Pediatrics, 4*(4, Suppl.), 358–364.

Drotar, D., Stein, R. E. K., & Perrin, E. (1995). Methodological issues in using the Child Behavior Checklist and its related instruments in clinical child psychology research. *Journal of Clinical Child Psychology, 24,* 184–192.

Edelbrock, C., Costello, A. J., Dulcan, M. K., Calabro-Conover, N., & Kalas, R. (1986). Parent–child agreement on child psychiatric symptoms reported via structured interview. *Journal of Child Psychology and Psychiatry, 27,* 181–190.

Edelbrock, C., Costello, A. J., Dulcan, M. K., Kalas, R., & Calabro-Conover, N. (1985). Age differences in the reliability of the psychiatric interview of the child. *Child Development, 56,* 265–275.

Eiser, C. (2004). Use of quality of life measures in clinical trials. *Ambulatory Pediatrics, 4*(4, Suppl.), 395–399.

Eiser, C., & Morse, R. (2001). The measurement of quality of life in children: Past and future perspectives. *Journal of Developmental and Behavioral Pediatrics, 22*(4), 248–256.

Feldmann, R., Weglage, J., Roth, J., Foell, D., & Frosch, M. (2005). Systemic juvenile rheumatoid arthritis: Cognitive function and social adjustment. *Annals of Neurology, 58,* 605–609.

Field, T., Alpert, B., Vega-Lahr, N., Goldstein, S., & Perry, S. (1988). Hospitalization stress in children: Sensitizer and repressor coping styles. *Health Psychology, 1,* 433–445.

Frick, P. J., & Kamphaus, R. W. (2001). Standardized rating scales in the assessment of children's behavioral and emotional problems. In C. E. Walker & M. C. Roberts (Eds.), *Handbook of clinical child psychology* (3rd ed., pp. 190–204). New York: Wiley.

Gerhardt, C. A., Vannatta, K., Valerius, K. S., Correll, J., & Noll, R. B. (2007). Social and romantic outcomes in emerging adulthood among survivors of childhood cancer. *Journal of Adolescent Health, 40,* 462.e9–462.e15.

Goodwin, D. A. J., Boggs, S. R., & Graham-Pole, J. (1994). Development and validation of the Pediatric Oncology Quality of Life Scale. *Psychological Assessment, 6,* 321–328.

Graham, J. R., Archer, R. P., Tellegen, A., Ben-Porath, Y. S., & Kaemmer, B. (2006). *Supplement to the MMPI-A Manual for Administration, Scoring, and Interpretation: The Content/Component Scales; the Personality Psychopathology Five (PSY-5) Scales, and the Critical Items*. Minneapolis: University of Minnesota Press.

Harbeck-Weber, C., Fisher, J. L., & Dittner, C. A. (2003). In M. C. Roberts (Ed.), *Handbook of pediatric psychology* (3rd ed., pp. 99–118). New York: Guilford Press.

Hayden-Wade, H. A., Stein, R. I., Ghaderi, A., Saelens, B. E., Zabinski, M. F., & Wilfley, D. E. (2005). Prevalence, characteristics, and correlates of teasing experiences among overweight children vs. non-overweight peers. *Obesity Research, 13,* 1381–1392.

Haynes, R. B. (1979). Introduction. In R. B. Haynes, D. W. Taylor, & D. L Sackett (Eds.), *Compliance in health care* (pp. 1–7). Baltimore: Johns Hopkins Press.

Hicks, C. L., von Baeyer, C. L., Spafford, P., van Korlaar, I., & Goodenough, B. (2001). The Faces Pain Scale—Revised: Toward a common metric in pediatric pain measurement. *Pain, 93,* 173–183.

Hobbie, W., Stuber, M., Meeske, K., Wissler, K., Rourke, M., Ruccione, K., et al. (2000). Symptoms of posttraumatic stress in young adult survivors of childhood cancer. *Journal of Clinical Oncology, 18,* 4060–4066.

Hodges, K., & Cools, J. N. (1990). Structured diagnostic interviews. In A. M. La Greca (Ed.), *Through the eyes of the child: Obtaining self-reports from children and adolescents* (pp. 109–149). Boston: Allyn & Bacon.

Holmbeck, G. N., Welborn Thill, A., Bachanas, P., Garber, J., Bearman Miller, K., Abad, M., et al. (2008). Evidence-based assessment in pediatric psychology: Measures of psychosocial adjustment and psychopathology. *Journal of Pediatric Psychology, 33*(9), 958–980.

Kanner, A. D., Feldman, S. S., Weinberger, D. A., & Ford, M. E. (1987). Uplifts, hassles, and adaptational outcomes in early adolescents. *Journal of Early Adolescence, 7*, 371–394.

Kazak, A. E. (1989). Families of chronically ill children: A systems and social-ecological model of adaptation and challenge. *Journal of Consulting and Clinical Psychology, 57*, 25–30.

Kazak, A. E., Barakat, L. P., Meeske, K., Christakis, D., Meadows, A. T., Casey, R., et al. (1997). Posttraumatic stress symptoms, family functioning, and social support in survivors of childhood leukemia and their mothers and fathers. *Journal of Consulting and Clinical Psychology, 65*, 120–129.

Kazak, A. E., Brier, M., Alderfer, M. A., Reilly, A., Fooks Parker, S., Rogerwick, S., et al. (2012). Screening for psychosocial risk in pediatric cancer. *Pediatric Blood Cancer, 59*, 822–827.

Kazak, A. E., Rourke, M. T., & Crump, T. A. (2003). Families and other systems in pediatric psychology. In M. C. Roberts (Ed.), *Handbook of pediatric psychology* (3rd ed., pp. 159–175). New York: Guilford Press.

Kazak, A. E., Rourke, M. T., & Navsaria, N. (2009). Families and other systems in pediatric psychology. In M. C. Roberts & R. G. Steele (Eds.), *Handbook of pediatric psychology* (4th ed., pp. 656–671). New York: Guilford Press.

Kelley, M. L., Reitman, D., & Noell, G. H. (Eds.). (2003). *Practitioner's guide to empirically based measures of school behavior.* New York: Kluwer.

Kiecolt-Glaser, J. K., McGuire, L., Robles, T. F., & Glaser, R. (2002). Psychoneuroimmunology: Psychological influences on immune function and health. *Journal of Consulting and Clinical Psychology, 70*, 537–547.

Kovacs, M., Goldston, D., Obrosky, D. S., & Iyengar, S. (1992). Prevalence and predictors of pervasive noncompliance with medical treatments among youth with insulin-dependent diabetes mellitus. *Journal of the American Academy of Child and Adolescent Psychiatry, 31*, 1112–1119.

Kupst, M. J. (1999). Assessment of psychoeducational and emotional functioning. In R. T.

Brown (Ed.), *Cognitive aspects of chronic illness in children* (pp. 25–44). New York: Guilford Press.

La Greca, A. M. (1990). Social consequences of pediatric conditions: Fertile area for future investigation and intervention? *Journal of Pediatric Psychology, 15*, 285–307.

La Greca, A. M., Kuttler, A. F., & Stone, W. L. (2001). Assessing children through interviews and behavioral observations. In C. E. Walker & M. C. Roberts (Eds.), *Handbook of clinical child psychology* (3rd ed., pp. 90–110). New York: Wiley.

La Greca, A. M., & Race Mackey, E. (2009). Adherence to pediatric treatment regimens. In M. C. Roberts & R. G. Steele (Eds.), *Handbook of pediatric psychology* (4th ed., pp. 130–152). New York: Guilford Press.

Lazarus, R. S., & Folkman, S. (1984). *Stress, appraisal, and coping.* New York: Springer.

Lemanek, K. L., & Hood, C. (1999). Asthma. In R. T. Brown (Ed.), *Cognitive aspects of chronic illness in children* (pp. 78–104). New York: Guilford Press.

Levi, R. B. (2006). Quality of life in childhood cancer: Meaning, methods, and missing pieces. In R. T. Brown (Ed.), *Comprehensive handbook of childhood cancer and sickle cell disease* (pp. 170–188). New York: Oxford University Press.

Lockwood, K. A., Bell, T. S., & Colegrove, R. W. (1999). Long-term effects of cranial radiation therapy on attention functioning in survivors of childhood leukemia. *Journal of Pediatric Psychology, 24*, 55–66.

Luthar, S., Burack, J. A., Cicchetti, D., & Weisz, J. R. (Eds.). (1997). *Developmental psychopathology: Perspectives on adjustment, risk, and disorder.* New York: Cambridge University Press.

Martin, P. D., & Brantley, P. J. (2004). Stress, coping, and social support in health and behavior. In J. Raczynski & L. C. Leviton (Vol. Eds.), *Handbook of clinical health psychology: Vol. 2. Disorders of behavior and health* (pp. 233–267). Washington, DC: American Psychological Association.

Martinez, W., Carter, J. S., & Legato, L. J. (2011). Social competence in children with chronic illness: A meta-analytic review. *Journal of Pediatric Psychology, 36*, 878–890.

Mash, E. J., & Hunsley, J. (2005). Special section: Developing guidelines for the evidence-based assessment of child and adolescent disorders. *Journal of Clinical Child and Adolescent Psychology, 34,* 362–379.

Matsui, D. M. (2000). Children's adherence to medication treatment. In D. Drotar (Ed.), *Promoting adherence to medical treatment in chronic childhood illness: Concepts, methods, and interventions* (pp. 135–152). Mahwah, NJ: Erlbaum.

McCracken, L. M., Zayfert, C., & Gross, R. T. (1992). The Pain Anxiety Symptoms Scale: Development and validation of a scale to measure fear of pain. *Pain, 50*(1), 67–73.

McDaniel, S. H., Hepworth, J., & Doherty, W. J. (1992). *Medical family therapy: A biopsychosocial approach to families with health problems.* New York: Basic Books.

McGrath, P. J. (1990). Pain assessment in children: A practical approach. In D. C. Tyler & E. J. Krane (Eds.), *Advances in pain research therapy* (Vol. 15). New York: Raven Press.

McGrath, P. J. (1996). Attitudes and beliefs about medication and pain management in infants and children. *Clinical Journal of Pain, 12,* 46–50.

McGrath, P. J., Johnson, G., Goodman, J., Schillinger, J., Dunn, J., & Chapman, J. (1985). CHEOPS: A behavioral scale for rating postoperative pain in children. *Advanced Pain Research Theory, 9,* 395–402.

Modi, A. C., & Quittner, A. L. (2003). Validation of a disease-specific measure of health-related quality of life for children with cystic fibrosis. *Journal of Pediatric Psychology, 28*(8), 535–545.

Morison, P., & Masten, A. S. (1991). Peer reputation in middle childhood as a predictor of adaptation in adolescence: A seven-year follow-up. *Child Development, 62,* 991–1007.

Mortweet, S. L., & Christophersen, E. R. (2003). Behavior problems in a pediatric context. In M. C. Roberts (Ed.), *Handbook of pediatric psychology* (3rd ed., pp. 599–616). New York: Guilford Press.

Mulhern, R. K., & Butler, R. W. (2006). Neuropsychological late effects. In R. T. Brown (Ed.), *Comprehensive handbook of childhood cancer and sickle cell disease: A biopsychosocial approach* (pp. 262–278). New York: Oxford University Press.

O'Donnell, D., Biederman, J., Jones, J., Wilens, T. E., Milberger, S., Mick, E., et al. (1998). Informativeness of child and parent reports on substance use disorders in a sample of ADHD probands, control probands, and their siblings.

Journal of the American Academy of Child and Adolescent Psychiatry, 37, 752–758.

Olson, L. M., Lara, M., & Frintner, M. P. (2004). Measuring health status and quality of life for U.S. children: Relationship to race, ethnicity, and income status. *Ambulatory Pediatrics, 4*(4, Suppl.), 377–386.

Pagé, M. G., Campbell, F., Isaac, L., Stinson, J., Martin-Pichora, A. L., & Katz, J. (2011). Reliability and validity of the Child Pain Anxiety Symptoms Scale (CPASS) in a clinical sample of children and adolescents with acute postsurgical pain. *Pain, 152,* 1958–1965.

Pagé, M. G., Fuss, S., Martin, A. L., Romero Escobar, E. M., & Katz, J. (2010). Development and preliminary validation of the Child Pain Anxiety Symptoms Scale in a community sample. *Journal of Pediatric Psychology, 35*(10), 1071–1082.

Palermo, T. M., Long, A. C., Lewandowski, A. S., Drotar, D., Quittner, A. L., & Walker, L. S. (2008). Evidence-based assessment of health-related quality of life and functional impairment in pediatric psychology. *Journal of Pediatric Psychology, 33*(9), 983–996.

Parker, J. G., & Asher, S. R. (1987). Peer relations and later personal adjustment: Are low-accepted children at risk? *Psychological Bulletin, 102,* 357–389.

Parsons, S. K., Barlow, S. E., Levy, S. L., Supran, S. E., & Kaplan, S. H. (1999). Health-related quality of life in pediatric bone marrow transplant survivors: According to whom? *International Journal of Cancer, 12*(Suppl.), 46–51.

Patterson, J. M., & McCubbin, H. I. (1987). Adolescent coping style and behaviors: Conceptualization and measurement. *Journal of Adolescence, 10,* 163–186.

Perrin, E. C., Stein, R. E. K., & Drotar, D. (1991). Cautions in using the Child Behavior Checklist: Observations based on research with children with chronic illness. *Journal of Pediatric Psychology, 16,* 411–421.

Pinquart, M., & Teubert, D. (2011, December). Academic, physical, and social functioning of children and adolescents with chronic physical illness: A meta-analysis. *Journal of Pediatric Psychology, 37*(4), 376–389.

Puhl, R. M., & Latner, J. D. (2007). Stigma, obesity, and the health of the nation's children. *Psychological Bulletin, 133,* 557–580.

Querido, J., Eyberg, S., Kanfer, R., & Krahn, G. (2001). The process of the clinical child assessment interview. In C. E. Walker & M.

C. Roberts (Eds.), *Handbook of clinical child psychology* (3rd ed., pp. 75–89). New York: Wiley.

Quittner, A. L., Buu, A., Messer, M. A., Modi, A. C., & Watrous, M. (2005). Development and validation of the Cystic Fibrosis Questionnaire in the United States: A health-related quality-of-life measure for cystic fibrosis. *Chest, 128*(4), 2347–2354.

Quittner, A. L., Davis, M., & Modi, A. (2003). Health-related quality of life in pediatric populations. In M. Roberts (Ed.), *Handbook of pediatric psychology* (3rd ed., pp. 696–709). New York: Guilford Press.

Quittner, A. L., Modi, A. C., Lemanek, K. L., Ievers-Landis, C. E., & Rapoff, M. A. (2008). Evidence-based assessment of adherence to medical treatments in pediatric psychology. *Journal of Pediatric Psychology, 33*(9), 916–936.

Radnitz, C. L., Schlein, I. S., & Hsu, L. (2000). The effects of prior trauma exposure on the development of PTSD following spinal cord injury. *Journal of Anxiety Disorders, 14*, 313–324.

Rapoff, M. A. (1999). *Adherence to pediatric medical regimens.* New York: Kluwer Academic/Plenum.

Ravens-Sieberer, U., Erhart, M., Wille, N., Wetzel, R., Nickel, J., & Bullinger, M. (2006). Generic health-related quality-of-life assessment in children and adolescents: Methodological considerations. *Pharmacoeconomics, 24*(12), 1199–1220.

Reiter-Purtill, J., & Noll, R. B. (2003). Peer relationships of children with chronic illness. In M. C. Roberts (Ed.), *Handbook of pediatric psychology* (3rd ed., pp. 176–197). New York: Guilford Press.

Reiter-Purtill, J., Waller, J. M., & Noll, R. B. (2009). Empirical and theoretical perspectives on the peer relationships of children with chronic conditions. In M. C. Roberts & R. G. Steele (Eds.), *Handbook of pediatric psychology* (4th ed., pp. 672–688). New York: Guilford Press.

Reynolds, C. R., & Kamphaus, R. W. (1998). *Behavior assessment system for children manual.* Circle Pines, MN: American Guidance Service.

Reynolds, C. R., & Kamphaus, R. W. (2004). *Behavior assessment system for children: Second edition manual.* Bloomington, MN: Pearson Assessments.

Rodrigue, J. R., Geffken, G. R., & Streisand, R. M. (2000). *Child health assessment: A handbook of measurement techniques.* Boston: Allyn & Bacon.

Rosenthal, S. L., Cohen, S. S., & Simeonsson, R. J. (2001). Assessment of family context. In R. J. Simeonsson & S. L. Rosenthal (Eds.), *Psychological and developmental assessment: Children with disabilities and chronic conditions* (pp. 141–150). New York: Guilford Press.

Rudolph, K. D., Denning, M. D., & Weisz, J. R. (1995). Determinants and consequences of children's coping in the medical setting: Conceptualization, review, and critique. *Psychological Bulletin, 118*, 328–357.

Santa Lucia, R. C., Gesten, E., Rendina-Gobioff, G., Epstein, M., Kaufmann, D., & Salcedo, O. (2000). Children's school adjustment: A developmental transactional systems perspective. *Journal of Applied Psychology, 21*, 429–446.

Sattler, J. M. (2008). *Assessment of children: Cognitive foundations* (5th ed.). LaMesa, CA: Sattler.

Sawyer, M., Antoniou, G., Toogood, I., & Rice, M. (1999). A comparison of parent and adolescent reports describing the health-related quality of life of adolescents treated for cancer. *International Journal of Cancer, 12*(Suppl.), 39–45.

Schuman, W. B., & La Greca, A. M. (1999). Social correlates of chronic illness. In R. T. Brown (Ed.), *Cognitive aspects of chronic illness in children* (pp. 289–311). New York: Guilford Press.

Shemesh, E., Lurie, S., Stuber, M. L., Emre, S., Patel, Y., Vohra, P., et al. (2000). A pilot study of posttraumatic stress and nonadherence in pediatric liver transplant recipients. *Pediatrics, 105*, E29.

Siegel, L. J. (1983). Hospitalization and medical care of children. In C. E. Walker & M. C. Roberts (Eds.), *Handbook of clinical child psychology* (pp. 1089–1108). New York: Wiley.

Siegel, L. J., & Conte, P. (2001). Hospitalization and medical care of children. In C. E. Walker & M. C. Roberts (Eds.), *Handbook of clinical child psychology* (3rd ed., pp. 895–909). New York: Wiley.

Simeonsson, R. J., & Rosenthal, S. L. (2001). Developmental theories and clinical practice. In C. E. Walker & M. C. Roberts (Eds.),

Handbook of clinical child psychology (3rd ed., pp. 20–33). New York: Wiley.

Smith, K. E., Ackerson, J. D., & Blotcky, A. D. (1989). Reducing distress during invasive medical procedures: Relating behavioral interventions to preferred coping style in pediatric cancer patients. *Journal of Pediatric Psychology, 14*, 405–419.

Speith, L. E. (2001). Generic health-related quality of life measures for children and adolescents. In H. M. Koot & J. L. Wallander (Eds.), *Quality of life in child and adolescent illness: Concepts, methods and findings* (pp. 49–88). New York: Taylor & Francis.

Spirito, A., Stark, L. J., & Tyc, V. L. (1994). Stressors and coping strategies described during hospitalization by chronically ill children. *Journal of Clinical Child Psychology, 23*, 314–322.

Spirito, A., Stark, L. J., & Williams, C. (1988). Development of a brief checklist to assess coping in pediatric patients. *Journal of Pediatric Psychology, 13*, 555–574.

Starfield, B., Riley, A. W., & Green, B. F. (1999). *Manual for the Child Health and Illness Profile: Adolescent edition (CHIP-AE).* Baltimore: Johns Hopkins University.

Stinson, J. N., Kavanagh, T., Yamada, J., Gill, N., & Stevens, B. (2006). Systematic review of the psychometric properties, interpretability and feasibility of self-report pain intensity measures for use in clinical trials in children and adolescents. *Pain, 125*, 143–157.

Stoddard, F. J., & Saxe, G. (2001). Ten-year research review of physical injuries. *Journal of the American Academy of Child and Adolescent Psychiatry, 40*, 1128–1145.

Strauss, R. S., & Pollack, H. A. (2003). Social marginalization of overweight children. *Archives of Pediatrics and Adolescent Medicine, 157*, 746–752.

Stuber, M. L. (2006). Posttraumatic stress and posttraumatic growth in childhood cancer survivors and their parents. In R. T. Brown (Ed.), *Comprehensive handbook of childhood cancer and sickle cell disease: A biopsychosocial approach* (pp. 279–296). New York: Oxford University Press.

Stuber, M. L., Kazak, A. E., Meeske, K., Barakat, L., Guthrie, D., Garnier, H., et al. (1997). Predictors of posttraumatic stress symptoms in childhood cancer survivors, *Pediatrics, 100*, 958–964.

Stuber, M., Nader, K., Yasuda, P., Pynoos, R.

S., & Cohen, S. (1991). Stress responses after pediatric bone marrow transplantation: Preliminary results of a prospective longitudinal study. *Journal of the American Academy of Child and Adolescent Psychiatry, 30*, 952–957.

Sturge, C., Garralda, M. E., Boissin, M., Doré, C. J., & Woo, P. (1997). School attendance and juvenile chronic arthritis. *British Journal of Rheumatology, 36*, 1218–1223.

Thompson, J. K., Shroff, H., Herbozo, S., Cafri, G., Rodriguez, J., & Rodriguez, M. (2007). Relations among multiple peer influences, body dissatisfaction, eating disturbance, and self-esteem: A comparison of average weight, at risk of overweight, and overweight adolescent girls. *Journal of Pediatric Psychology, 32*, 24–29.

Valla, J. P., Bergeron, L., Breton, J. J., Gaudet, N., & Berthiaume, C. (1993). Informants, correlates and child disorders in a clinical population. *Canadian Journal of Psychiatry, 38*, 406–411.

Varni, J. W., Seid, M., & Rode, C. A. (1999). The PedsQL: Measurement model for the pediatric quality of life inventory. *Medical Care, 37*(2), 126–139.

Varni, J. W., Thompson, K. L., & Hanson, V. (1987). The Varni/Thompson pediatric pain questionnaire: I. Chronic musculoskeletal pain in juvenile rheumatoid arthritis. *Pain, 28*, 27–38.

Verhey, L. H., Kulik, D. M., Ronen, G. M., Rosenbaum, P., Lach, L., Streiner, D. L., et al. (2009). Quality of life in childhood epilepsy: What is the level of agreement between youth and their parents? *Epilepsy and Behavior, 14*, 407–410.

Vernberg, E. M., & Jacobs, A. K. (2001). Methods of research in developmental psychopathology and treatment effectiveness. In C. E. Walker & M. C. Roberts (Eds.), *Handbook of clinical child psychology* (3rd ed., pp. 34–47). New York: Wiley.

von Baeyer, C. L., & Spagrud, L. J. (2007). Systematic review of observational (behavioral) measures of pain for children and adolescents aged 3 to 18 years. *Pain, 127*, 140–150.

Walco, G. A., Conte, P. M., Labay, L. E., Engle, R., & Zeltzer, L. K. (2005). Procedural distress in children with cancer: Self-report, behavioral observations, and physiological parameters. *Clinical Journal of Pain, 21*, 484–490.

Walker, L. S., Garber, J., Smith, C. A., Van Slyke,

D. A., & Claar, R. L. (2001). The relation of daily stressors to somatic and emotional symptoms in children with and without recurrent abdominal pain. *Journal of Consulting and Clinical Psychology, 69*, 85–91.

Wallander, J. L., Thompson, R. J., & Alriksson-Schmidt, A. (2003). Psychosocial adjustment of children with chronic physical conditions. In M. C. Roberts (Ed.), *Handbook of pediatric psychology* (3rd ed., pp. 141–158). New York: Guilford Press.

Watson, T. S., Foster, N., & Friman, P. C. (2006). Treatment adherence in children and adolescents. In W. T. O'Donohue (Ed.), *Promoting treatment adherence: A practical handbook for health care providers* (pp. 343–351). Thousand Oaks, CA: Sage.

Wolters, P. L., Brouwers, P., & Perez, L. R. (1999). Pediatric HIV infection. In R. T. Brown (Ed.), *Cognitive aspects of chronic illness in children* (pp. 105–141). New York: Guilford Press.

Wu, Y. P., Rohan, J. M., Martin, S., Hommel, K., Neff Greenley, R., Loiselle, K., et al. (2013). Pediatric psychologist use of adherence assessments and interventions. *Journal of Pediatric Psychology, 38*, 595–604.

Zeller, M., Reiter-Purtill, J., & Ramey, C. (2008). Negative peer perceptions of obese children in the classroom environment. *Obesity, 16*, 755–762.

CHAPTER 25

Older Adults

Christine E. Gould
Merideth D. Smith
Barry A. Edelstein

General Considerations

Demographics of Aging

In 2009, there were 39.6 million adults in the United States ages 65 and older, which represented 12.9% of the U.S. population (Administration on Aging, 2011). By 2030, older adults will represent an estimated 20% of the population (He, Sengupta, Velkoff, & DeBarros, 2005), increasing from 35.9 million to 72 million. Though Americans are living longer with better health, modifiable chronic health problems, such as heart disease, cancer, chronic lower respiratory disease, and stroke, continue to be the leading causes of death (Centers for Disease Control and Prevention [CDC], 2010). Most older adults suffer from at least one chronic health condition, with half of older adults having two or more conditions (He et al., 2005). Moreover, the incidence of risk factors (e.g., obesity) for these conditions is also rising at alarming rates (He et al., 2005). Disability rates are also high among older adults, with 37% reporting some level of disability (Administration on Aging, 2011). Identifying and assessing mental health problems that develop as the result of or exacerbate chronic health problems is imperative.

The Aging Body

The information presented here is a brief overview of normative physical, physiological, and sensory changes that occur as an individual ages. Understanding aging processes is essential to the assessment process and to differential diagnosis in the assessment of older adults.

Physical Changes

Many age-related changes take place in appearance and in mobility. Over time, the skin loses collagen and elasticity and is less able to repair following skin breaks. This leaves wounds open longer and makes older adults more susceptible to infections (Htwe, Mushtaq, Robinson, Rosher, & Khardori, 2007). Changes in mobility occur as muscle mass, bone density, and cartilage degenerate, which increase the risk of falling. These physical changes may influence the symptom presentation, evaluation, and rehabilitation process for older adults.

Physiological Changes

Physiological and structural changes affect the presentation of illness, disease, infection, and other problems in older adults. In the cardiovascular system, cellular changes occur in the ventricles of the heart, and the artery walls become thicker and less flexible. Following these structural changes, the risk of systolic hypertension increases, and the cardiovascular system has more difficulty pumping blood and oxygen throughout the body (Franklin et al., 1997). In response to emotion-evoking laboratory tasks, older adults have lower heart rate reactivity and higher systolic blood pressure reactivity (Uchino, Birmingham, & Berg, 2010). Structural changes in the respiratory system cause decreased lung capacity and less efficient gas exchange across the lung wall (i.e., bronchioles). The resulting lower aerobic capacity and shortness of breath accompanying respiratory problems may mimic panic attack symptoms. In summary, age-related cardiac and respiration changes affect physiological assessments, as well as the presentation of somatic symptoms.

In the digestive system, secretion of gastric acid decreases over time, which slows metabolism of certain nutrients in the small intestine (Whitbourne, 2002). This can lead to malnutrition or deficiencies in various nutrients. Deficiencies in nutrients such as thiamine are associated with reversible cognitive impairment (e.g., delirium). Dehydration or increased toxicity to medications due to decreased kidney functioning and bladder capacity also can cause delirium. Older adults have a lower resistance to infection and are slower to respond to illness because of increased autoimmunity and less effective T-cells. Thus older adults are at an elevated risk of infection, the leading cause of delirium (Inouye & Ferrucci, 2006).

Changes in the autonomic nervous system affect sleep patterns as well. In a meta-analysis, Ohayon, Carskadon, Guilleminault, and Vitiello (2004) examined normative age-related changes in sleep and found that deep or slow-wave sleep decreases linearly with age until about age 60 and then remains constant to age 90. Meanwhile, as older individuals get less "restorative" sleep, it also takes them longer to fall asleep, and they spend more time awake during the night than younger individuals (Ohayon et al., 2004).

Older men and women experience changes in the reproductive system and sexuality as they age, yet 53% of adults ages 65–74 years and 26% of adults ages 75–85 years are sexually active (Lindau et al., 2007). Older men have a decreased number of viable sperm, changes in the prostate, and shorter orgasm duration compared with younger men (Whitbourne, 2002). Among sexually active older men, the three most common sexual problems include difficulty achieving and maintaining an erection (37%), lack of interest in sex (28%), and climaxing too quickly (28%; Lindau et al., 2007). Although most older adult women are postmenopausal and can no longer produce ovum, they are still able to reach orgasm. Sexually active older women report their three most common problems as lack of interest in sex (43%), difficulty with lubrication (39%), and inability to climax (24%; Lindau et al., 2007).

Sensory Changes

Various changes occur in the visual and auditory system as one ages. In the visual system, changes to the lens, retina, and optic nerve affect color perception and the visual field, increase susceptibility to glare changes and light intensity, distort images, and make it more difficult to perceive details. Vision loss ranges from changes that can be corrected so as to not cause impairment in daily functioning to more severe impairments that cannot be corrected by available medications and devices (Whiteside, Wallhagen, & Pettengill, 2006). Age-related macular degeneration, cataracts, glaucoma, and diabetic retinopathy result in significant loss of vision and subsequent impairment in functioning (U.S. Census Bureau, 2010). Impairments in functioning associated with vision loss include increased fall risk, decreased performance in basic activities of daily living (e.g., walking, getting out of bed), decreased performance of independent activities (e.g., getting to outside places, preparing meals, managing medication, driving), and decreased social interactions (Crews & Campbell, 2001). Thus the assessor needs to be mindful of the changes in the visual system that affect assessments.

Clinicians can modify the assessment environment by avoiding the use of high-gloss colored paper for self-report assessments, which decreases contrast between paper and ink and makes it more difficult for older adults to read (Whiteside et al., 2006). Printed, not cursive, larger fonts (14–16 point) may make it easier for older adults to read assessment measures. Glare can be decreased by using higher wattage light-bulbs angled to reduce reflection on objects and direct light shining into the individual's eyes. Darkened glasses and wide-brimmed hats can also decrease glare in bright environments. Devices such as glasses and magnifiers improve vision as well. Low-vision services may help an older adult with vision impairment function independently using technology and other modifications.

Various physiological changes occur in the auditory system with increased age, including hearing loss (e.g., presbycusis). The ability to detect high-frequency noises decreases with age, which makes it more difficult to hear consonants of words during conversational speech or while listening to women and children speak. Of older adults with functional impairments, 15.1% report difficulty with hearing (U.S. Census Bureau, 2010). Hearing problems increase the risk of depression and loneliness among older adults, and in particular among older men and individuals not using hearing aids (Pronk et al., 2011). To help accommodate auditory decrements, clinicians should speak distinctly and pause at the ends of phrases or ideas, but without overexaggeration of words or shouting (Reuben et al., 2011; Storandt, 1994). Clinicians should sit close to the patient, directly face the person when speaking, and decrease any background noise (National Institute on Deafness and Other Communications Disorders, 2001). If need be, clinicians can encourage clients to use hearing aids or a personal amplifier. Providing oral questions in a written form can help older adults with hearing impairments complete assessments with fewer difficulties (Whitbourne, 2002).

Assessment of Functioning

When conducting assessments with older adults, it is necessary to be mindful of the impact of these changes on functioning. Measures of functioning include the assessment of activities of daily living (ADLs), such as physical ambulation, bathing, grooming, and dressing, and assessment of instrumental activities of daily living (IADLs), such as ability to prepare food, manage finances, or use the telephone. Self-report (e.g., Katz,

Downs, Cash & Grotz, 1970; Lawton & Brody, 1969) and performance-based assessment measures (e.g., Independent Living Scales; Loeb, 1996) can be administered. Additionally, the fifth edition of the *Diagnostic and Statistical Manual of Mental Disorders* (DSM-5) includes the World Health Organization Disability Assessment Schedule 2.0 (WHODAS 2.0; World Health Organization, 2010), as a measure of disability, in the cross-cutting assessment measures.

Medication Considerations

Consideration of medications taken by patients is important regardless of the age of the individual. However, consideration of medications and their potential adverse effects is particularly important with older adults. The reason is, in part, the often large number of medications taken by older adults and, in part, age-related changes in pharmacokinetics and pharmacodynamics. In addition, older adults may experience more difficulties in adhering to medical regimens than younger adults. These issues are discussed in this section.

Age-Related Changes in Pharmacokinetics and Pharmacodynamics

In light of the increasing number of medications taken as we age, older adults are at increased risk for adverse drug reactions, which are estimated to be the fourth to sixth greatest cause of death (Lazarou, Pomeranz, & Corey, 1998). A review of the prevalence of adverse drug effects in older adults in ambulatory care revealed a 22.6% prevalence rate, which is a stark contrast to the 8.5% prevalence rate for young adults (Taché, Sönnichsen, & Ashcroft, 2011). Approximately 10% of hospital admissions of older adults are attributed to such reactions, with the number of such problems increasing with age (Bowie & Slattum, 2007). As we age, the body undergoes anatomical and physiological changes that affect drug pharmacokinetics (absorption, distribution, metabolism, excretion) and pharmacodynamics (effect of drug on its target site; Mangoni & Jackson, 2004). Bowie and Slattum (2007) provide a comprehensive review of age-related changes in response to drugs affecting the central nervous system, cardiovascular, and endocrine functions.

Polypharmacy

"Polypharmacy," or the use of multiple medications, is a significant problem for many older adults, as it places them at risk for adverse drug reactions and functional decline (Hajjar & Hanlon, 2006). With the age-related increases in number of chronic diseases, there is an increase in the number of medications taken concurrently and a concomitant increased risk for adverse drug reactions. Older adults constitute 12% of the U.S. population and consume 32% of the medications prescribed in the United States (Hajjar & Hanlon, 2006). Older adults regularly take an average of two to five medications, and 20–40% of older adults take five or more medications (McLean & Le Couteur, 2004). Moreover, between 44 and 57% of older adult patients take one or more unnecessary drugs (Hajjar & Hanlon, 2006). In a study of community-dwelling older adult veterans, Rossi et al. (2007) found that the more medications that were taken by patients, the more likely they were to be taking unnecessary medications.

Medication Adherence

Cooper et al. (2005) studied adherence in more than 3,000 older adults in 11 countries and found that approximately 12.5% of participants reported some level of nonadherence to medication regimens. Other estimates of nonadherence have ranged as high as 45% (Morrow, Leirer, & Sheikh, 1988). Estimates of the percentage of hospitalizations of older adults due to nonadherence have ranged as high as 11% (Campbell et al., 2012).

Medication adherence is a very complex set of behaviors with multiple determinants (physical, cognitive, psychosocial), with no single factor accounting for a substantial amount of variance in predicting adherence (Morrell & Shiffren, 1999). Even the older adult's conceptualization of his or her disease threat can have an impact on adherence (Leventhal, Leventhal, Robitaille, & Brownlee, 1999). Older adults taking multiple medications are at increased risk for nonadherence to their medical regimens (Campbell et al., 2012). However, it is apparently the number of medications and not age per se that is related to nonadherence (Campbell et al., 2012). Among the reasons most often reported by older adults for nonadherence are adverse drug effects and the belief that the medication is not needed (Campbell et al., 2012). Unintentional nonadherence is reportedly due to forgetting to take the medication and unclear information about proper administration. Of the many factors associated with nonadherence, depression is an important and consistent determinant (Vik et al., 2006). In light of the multiple determinants of adherence, a very individualized, behavioral assessment approach that examines the interaction of relevant individual and environmental factors is needed. Finally, age-related decline in cognitive functioning, particularly executive function and working memory, may affect adherence (Insel, Morrow, Brewer, & Figueredo, 2006). The interested reader is referred to Campbell et al. (2012) for a comprehensive review of the literature on measurement and correlates of older adult medication adherence.

Cognitive Processes

Certain normative cognitive abilities such as reaction time decrease as one ages (e.g., memory, reasoning, spatial visualization, speed abilities; Salthouse, 2010), while other abilities remain relatively constant (e.g., vocabulary; Salthouse, 2010), at least until the 80s, or even increase (e.g., creativity; Simonton, 2000). Noticeable changes in memory occur with increased age such that older individuals have more difficulty with working memory and managing irrelevant information in memory, and they experience decreases in perceptual speed during encoding (e.g., speed-deficit hypothesis; Salthouse, 1993). Disease-related cognitive declines are observed in individuals with diabetes, cardiovascular disease, neurological diseases, and related diseases. The assessment of cognitive processes in older adults is essential because cognitive impairments likely influence the presentation of disorders and adherence to recommended treatments or both.

Cognitive Assessment

When assessing older individuals, brief cognitive assessments can be used initially to identify any broad problems in cognitive functioning; however, these brief measures should not be used for diagnosing major and mild neurocognitive disorders. When assessing individuals, the clinician should inquire of the client and any collateral sources who might be able to provide useful information (e.g., spouses, children, family members) about the client's present functioning and changes from previous levels of functioning. In addition to a clinical interview, a clinician can administer a brief cognitive measure to assess an older client's cognitive functioning. Of the available measures, the Mini-Mental State Examination (MMSE; Folstein, Folstein, & McHugh, 1975) is one of the most frequently used and yet often criticized measures. The MMSE does not adequately assess attention and lacks items assessing verbal fluency, reasoning or judgment, and cued verbal recall (Cullen, O'Neill, Evans, Coen, & Lawlor, 2007). It has poor sensitivity for detecting mild cognitive impairment when administered to individuals with higher levels of education (Cullen et al., 2007). (It is important to note that the MMSE is no longer in the public domain, but an improved, longer version of the MMSE is commercially licensed by Psychological Assessment Resources, Inc.)

Two clinician-administered brief cognitive assessments are in the public domain: the Saint Louis University Mental Status Examination (SLUMS; Morley & Tumosa, 2002) and the Montreal Cognitive Assessment (MoCA; Nasreddine et al., 2005). MoCA and SLUMS scores are highly correlated with the MMSE and are suitable replacements for the MMSE depending on the setting and the referral question (Stewart, O'Riley, Edelstein, & Gould, 2012). Both the MoCA and the SLUMS are scored similarly to the MMSE, with 30 total possible points. The SLUMS assesses logical memory, size differentiation, attention, clock drawing to assess executive functioning, and word fluency. It has good sensitivity for identifying individuals with dementia (.983–.998) and mild neurocognitive disorder (MNCD; .927–.941) compared with the MMSE, which had comparable sensitivity for identifying individuals with dementia (.915–.941) but poor sensitivity for detecting MCND (.643–.671; Tariq, Tumosa, Chibnall, Perry, & Morley, 2006). The MoCA is a valid and reliable measure that assesses domains including executive functioning, attention, verbal fluency, abstraction, and

cued recall. Three forms of the MoCA are available, which can counter practice effects in the case of repeat testing. It demonstrates good reliability over a 35-day period ($r = .92$; Nasreddine et al., 2005). Although the MoCA has good sensitivity for detecting mild cognitive impairment and dementia (.90 and 1.00; Nasreddine et al., 2005), some researchers (e.g., Luis, Keegan, & Mullan, 2009) suggested that the original cutoff of 26 is too high, thus resulting in low specificity for detecting cognitive impairment.

The Repeatable Battery for the Assessment of Neuropsychological Status (RBANS; Randolph, 1988) is another cognitive assessment that has norms available for older adults (Duff et al., 2003; Randolph, 1988). The RBANS has two forms, which makes it a good choice when repeat assessments are needed. The RBANS takes longer than the MMSE, SLUMS, or MoCA to administer, but it has added value with the availability of index scores for each subtest. These index scores assist the clinician in detection and characterization of neurocognitive disorders of different etiologies (Randolph, Tierney, Mohr, & Chase, 1998). A measure of executive functioning may be administered alongside the RBANS to obtain a more complete picture of the patient's functioning.

Several considerations should be taken into account when assessing and interpreting cognitive assessments. As education can mask cognitive impairment when using certain brief assessments (e.g., MMSE), normative data adjusted by education should be used (e.g., MMSE, Crum, Anthony, Basset, & Folstein, 1993; MoCA, Nasreddine et al., 2005; SLUMS, Tariq et al., 2005). Assessment of functional abilities should also accompany cognitive assessments. Lastly, neuropsychological assessment should follow significant findings from brief cognitive assessments.

Capacity Assessment

The issue of capacity to make medical decisions becomes more salient as adults age, develop chronic health conditions, and encounter an increasing number of difficult and often complex health care decisions. We are all assumed to be competent to make decisions about our well-being once reaching the age of 21. That competence is often questioned when there are abrupt changes in one's mental state or when one refuses medical treatment. More specifically, one's capacity to consent to treatment is questioned. The term "capacity" is now preferred to the more traditional "competence," as there is now a greater focus on specific capacities or abilities (e.g., medical decision making, financial decision making) as opposed to an overall determination of competence. Medical consent capacity, or health care decision-making capacity, is defined by state statute. The definitions of consent capacity found in these statutes are often similar to that of the Uniform Health Care Decisions Act of 1993 (American Bar Association Commission on Law and Aging & American Psychological Association, 2008), which defines capacity as "an individual's ability to understand the significant benefits, risks, and alternatives to proposed health care and to make and communicate a health-care decision." There remain differences of opinion and confusion regarding how decisional capacity should be operationalized and assessed by clinicians (Moye, Gurrera, Karel, Edelstein, & O'Connell, 2006). A guide for psychologists titled *Assessment of Older Adults with Diminished Capacity: A Handbook for Psychologists,* published by the American Bar Association Commission on Law and Aging and the American Psychological Association, addresses this problem. Copies are available at *www.apa.org/pi/aging/capacity psychologist_handbook.pdf.* There is general agreement among experts in capacity assessment that assessment of medical consent capacity requires formal assessment of cognitive and functional abilities, consideration of the cause(s) of incapacity (e.g., dementia), and the interaction of these elements with the support, or lack thereof, of the environment. The assessment of older adults' diminished capacity is an important and emerging area of practice and research (Moye, Marson, & Edelstein, 2013). The previously mentioned *Handbook* offers an excellent conceptual model to guide the assessment process. The model permits the integration of clinical practice standards, law, and clinical research and comprises five components that define legal competencies: functional, causal, interactive, judgmental, and dispositional components. Moye et al. (2006) offer a review of existing capacity

assessment instruments. The *Handbook* also provides information on various assessment instruments and their use.

Assessment of Anxiety and Depression

Anxiety Assessment

Over a 12-month period, 7% of older adults meet criteria for any anxiety disorder (Gum, King-Kallimanis, & Kohn, 2009). Anxiety measures that incorporate somatic items, such as the Beck Anxiety Inventory (BAI; Beck & Steer, 1993), may have limited utility in identifying anxiety in medically ill older adults due to the high correlation between the somatic items and the physical symptoms of the illness (Wetherell & Gatz, 2005). Other measures designed for use with medical populations or older adults may prove more useful in detecting anxiety. The Hospital Anxiety and Depression Scale (HADS), a 14-item self-report measure of depressive and anxiety symptoms (Zigmond & Snaith, 1983), has been used to assess anxiety in patients with cancer (Mitchell, Meader, & Symonds, 2010), as well as other illnesses. Among patients with cancer, the HADS anxiety scale has lower sensitivity (.49) and specificity (.70) in identifying individuals with anxiety disorders compared with the HADS total scale (.84 and .79). The Geriatric Anxiety Inventory (GAI) is a 20-item measure of late-life anxiety that uses dichotomous responses and contains few somatic symptoms. Pachana and colleagues (2007) found that the GAI is correlated with other measures of anxiety, has good internal consistency (alpha = .91), and has good classification of individuals with generalized anxiety disorder (sensitivity = .75; specificity = .84). However, the GAI was also associated with self-rated health and medical burden (Byrne et al., 2010), which may make the identification of anxiety using the GAI more challenging in a medically ill population. A 5-item GAI has similar psychometric properties to the longer scale (Byrne & Pachana, 2011; Gerolimatos, Gregg, & Edelstein, 2013). Another recently developed measure, the Geriatric Anxiety Scale (GAS), shows promise for the assessment of late-life anxiety (Segal, June, Payne, Coolidge, & Yochim, 2010). The 25-item GAS has good internal consistency for the total scale (alpha = .90–.93) and strong correlations with other measures of anxiety (Segal et al., 2010; Yochim, Mueller, June, & Segal, 2010). Although there is a moderate correlation between the GAS and medical comorbidity (Yochim et al., 2010), the GAS can be broken into its subscales of somatic, cognitive, and affective symptoms, which may help identify somatic symptoms to determine whether they are due to medical conditions, an anxiety disorder, or both.

Depression Assessment

Mood disorders are found in 2.6% of older adults over a 12-month period (Gum et al., 2009); however, depression may be more prevalent in older adults in long-term-care facilities (see Blazer, 2003, for a review). The presentation of depression among older adults differs from that in young adults, with older adults being more likely to report somatic symptoms but less likely to report dysphoria, guilt, and suicide ideation (Fiske & O'Riley, 2008). Several self-report measures are valid and reliable to use to detect depression in older adults. The Geriatric Depression Scale (GDS; Yesavage et al., 1983) is a 30-item measure of depression; a short form consisting of 15 items is also available (Sheikh & Yesavage, 1986). Like the GAI, the GDS has dichotomized responses. The GDS short form has good clinical utility in screening for depression in older adults within a primary care setting due to its quick administration and good sensitivity (.81) and specificity (.78) for the detection of depression (Mitchell, Bird, Rizzo, & Meader, 2010). Some measures (e.g., GDS) exclude somatic symptoms; however, due to the underreporting of depressed mood in older adults, a more inclusive approach that includes somatic symptoms may help clinicians better identify individuals with depressive symptoms. Two other commonly used depression measures, the Patient Health Questionnaire–9 (PHQ-9; Kroenke, Spitzer, & Williams, 2001) and the Beck Depression Inventory–II (BDI-II; Beck, Steer, & Brown, 1996) have been used to identify depression in older adults in primary care (Norris, Arnau, Bramson, & Meagher, 2003). The PHQ-9 is a nine-item self-report measure of depressive symptoms. In groups of adults of mixed ages, the PHQ-9 is correlated with

other measures of depression (r = .73) and has demonstrated reliability (r = .84; Pinto-Meza, Serrano-Blanco, Peñarrubia, Blanco, & Haro, 2005). In a sample of older adults participating in a multisite treatment trial for depression (IMPACT), the change in PHQ-9 scores distinguished between patients identified with depression in remission, in partial remission, and in persistent depression after 6 months (Löwe, Unützer, Callahan, Perkins, & Kroenke, 2004). The BDI-II is a 21-item measure with good internal consistency (alpha = .90) and established validity for use with older adults (Segal, Coolidge, Cahill, & O'Riley, 2008). However, some suggest that the Guttman scale makes the BDI-II difficult for cognitively impaired patients to complete (Edelstein et al., 2008).

Suicide Risk Assessment

In 2011, adults over the age of 65 in the United States had a suicide rate of 15.28 per 100,000, compared with the general population rate of 12.7 per 100,000 (Centers for Disease Control and Prevention, 2011). White males 85 years and older have the highest rate of death by suicide; specifically, this group has a suicide rate of 47.31 per 100,000. Assessment of suicide risk in older adults is important in a medical setting due to the risk for death by suicide, and older adults who have died by suicide are more likely to have had contact with a primary care provider within the month preceding their deaths (Luoma, Martin, & Pearson, 2002). Risk factors to assess for include the presence of a mood disorder, substance abuse, hopelessness, physical illness, limited social support, and access to lethal means (Conwell, 2001; Heisel, 2006).

Of the older adults who have died by suicide, 71–90% had a diagnosable psychiatric disorder (Conwell, 2001), with depression being the most common (Heisel, 2006). Hopelessness and perceived burden to others are cognitions that are associated with increased risk for suicide ideation and suicidal behavior (Conwell, 2001; Cukrowicz, Cheavens, Van Orden, Ragain, & Cook, 2011). Physical illnesses, such as cancer, cardiovascular disease, or neurological disease, contribute to 35–70% of suicides in older adults (Fiske, O'Riley, & Widoe, 2008). In addition, functional disability is significantly related to increased risk for suicide (Conwell et al., 2010). Poor quality of social support is associated with increased depressive symptoms and suicide risk in older adults (Duberstein, Conwell, Conner, Eberly, & Caine, 2004). Finally, access to firearms is a significant suicide risk factor, as older adults are more likely to die by suicide using firearms (Heisel & Duberstein, 2005).

There are few suicide risk assessments specifically validated and standardized for use with older adults. The Geriatric Suicide Ideation Scale (GSIS) is a 31-item measure developed to measure suicide ideation, death ideation, loss of personal and social meaning, and perceived meaning in life in older adults (Heisel & Flett, 2006). This measure is associated with other measures of suicide ideation and has strong internal interitem consistency (alpha = .82 to .93). Additionally, it has good test–retest reliability over a 1- to 2-month period, with scores ranging from $r = .86$ to .75. However, assessing for suicidal ideation alone is not sufficient for identifying suicide risk in older adults because individuals in this age group are less likely to report suicidal ideation prior to attempting suicide (Heisel & Duberstein, 2005).

Measures designed to assess depression and other suicide risk factors such as social disconnection can help clinicians develop a more comprehensive understanding of an older adult's suicide risk. (For a review of social support measures, see Smith and Fiske, Chapter 8, this volume, on social support assessment.) GDS scores differentiate older adults with low levels of suicidal ideation from older adults with high levels of suicidal ideation (Heisel, Flett, & Duberstein, 2005). Heisel et al. (2005) recommend using a cutoff score of 12 or higher on the long form of the GDS and a cutoff score of 6 or greater on the GDS short form to achieve the best sensitivity and specificity in predicting suicide ideation. The Depression and Suicide Screen was derived from five items of the Self-Rating Depression Scale to assess depression and suicide in older adults within a primary care setting (Fujisawa et al., 2005). This measure yielded a sensitivity of .70 and a specificity of .69 when predicting clinician-rated suicide ideation.

To more fully understand suicide risk, it is also important to assess for the protective factors that promote resiliency and decrease the risk for suicidal behavior (Heisel, 2006). The Reasons for Living Scale—Older Adult version (RFL-OA; Edelstein et al., 2009) is a 69-item Likert scale that measures factors that can influence one's decision not to attempt suicide. Reasons for living include, for example, "My religious beliefs forbid it," "I want to see my grandchildren grow up," and "Tomorrow I may feel better." The RFL-OA has high internal consistency (alpha = .98) and good convergent, discriminant, and criterion validity (Edelstein et al., 2009). The DSM-5 includes proposed research criteria for a new diagnosis, suicide behavior disorder, in order to call attention to the importance of assessing suicidal behavior and promote further research. Assessment of suicide behavior and ideation, as well as risk and protective factors within a medical setting, is especially important due to the elevated risk for suicidal behavior within an aging and medically ill population.

End of Life

Psychologists working with older adults will likely encounter patients with terminal illnesses. The assessment of older adults with terminal illnesses should include careful attention to the psychological distress that impairs quality of life and response to care. Individuals receiving end-of-life care are at an increased risk for mental health problems. Of patients with terminal illnesses, 60–75% meet criteria for a depressive disorder (Chochinov, Wilson, Enns, & Lander, 1994; King, Heisel, & Lyness, 2005). Prevalence of anxiety disorders can range from 13 to 20% in terminally ill patients (Mitchell, Meader, & Symonds, 2010; Wilson et al., 2007). Both anxiety and depression include somatic symptoms that overlap with symptoms arising from physical illnesses, such as fatigue, sleep difficulties, changes in appetite, changes in weight, muscle tension, heart palpitations, and gastrointestinal difficulties, which makes the identification of the origins of presenting symptoms difficult (King et al., 2005).

Clinicians can employ several methods to address the overlap in somatic symptoms common at end of life when assessing for depression. One approach is to use self-report assessment instruments for depression that exclude somatic symptoms, such as change in appetite, change in weight, insomnia or hypersomnia, loss of energy or fatigue, and diminished concentration (Noorani & Montagnini, 2007). The GDS, described previously, was developed specifically for older adults and substitutes cognitive symptoms in place of somatic symptoms. The GDS scores had a moderate interrater agreement with clinician-diagnosed depression (kappa = .46) in older adults with terminal illness (Greenberg, Lantz, & Likourezos, 2004). However, excluding items may result in underdiagnosing depression, resulting in a portion of patients with depression not receiving the treatment that could substantially improve their health and quality of life (King et al., 2005). The other approach to assessing depression in patients at end of life is to include all symptoms, regardless of physical or psychological origins. Chochinov and colleagues (1994) found that assessment instruments that used cognitive symptoms in place of somatic symptoms did not produce significantly different results compared with other depression assessments that included somatic items.

A psychologist working with an older adult patient who is terminally ill may find it difficult to differentiate normal grief from depression. The DSM-5 no longer includes the bereavement exclusion criteria with the understanding that, although grief is a normative process, a depressive disorder may also be present in grieving individuals. Several key differences have been identified to distinguish depression from normal grief (Noorani & Montagnini, 2007). Unlike depression, which presents as a persistent depressed mood, grief fluctuates in intensity and will often decrease in intensity over time. Individuals experiencing depression typically withdraw from social interactions and do not find these interactions pleasurable, whereas social interactions with family and friends remain pleasurable for individuals who are grieving. Finally, individuals with grief often express hope, such as hope for comfort at the end of life. Older adults with depression are more likely to express hopelessness and possibly suicidal ideation. The Terminally Ill Grief or Depression Scale (TIGDS) is 42-item measure developed to assess preparatory grief and depression in adults with terminal illness (Periyakoil et al., 2005). The Depression subscale of the

TIGDS has been found to relate to other measures of depression, whereas the Grief subscale has not related to depression measures. The TIGDS has good test–retest reliability (Depression subscale $r = .97$; Grief subscale $r = .86$).

Anxiety is also common in patients with terminal illness and often presents as a free-floating or generalized anxiety (Lyness, 2004). Assessing for anxiety symptoms is important due to the significant impact of anxiety on a patient's response to pain, quality of life, and desire for hastened death (Kelly et al., 2003). As discussed earlier, many anxiety symptoms overlap with symptoms found in medical conditions, and there is limited research on anxiety in patients at end of life (Lyness, 2004; Pessin, Rosenfeld, & Breitbart. 2002) and the use of specific anxiety assessments within this population.

Clinical Problems

There are a variety of psychiatric and medical conditions that present assessment challenges to the clinician working with older adults. Careful assessment and differential diagnosis is critical for determining the best course of treatment.

Differentiating Depression, Dementia, and Delirium

Clinicians working with older adults frequently may face the task of differentiating between dementia and depression and between dementia and delirium. The implications of incorrect diagnoses are considerable. In the DSM-5, dementia should be diagnosed as either major or mild neurocognitive disorder, with the etiology of the impairment specified (e.g., Alzheimer's disease, Lewy body disease). The ICD-10 continues to use the diagnosis of dementia.

Depression and Dementia

Depression and dementia are often comorbid, with about 20–30% of patients with dementia due to Alzheimer's disease experiencing depression (Enache, Winblad, & Aarsland, 2011). The onset of mild cognitive impairment is frequently accompanied by depression, complicating the differential diagnosis (for a review, see Panza et al., 2010). Formal cognitive or neuropsychological assessment is often required to determine whether an individual is experiencing depression, dementia, or both. There are patterns of neuropsychological test performance that can be used in the differential diagnosis process. Individuals with depression are more likely to perform more poorly on tasks that require effort, including memory, attention, confrontational naming, verbal fluency, visuospatial ability, processing speed, and executive functioning (Wright & Persad, 2007). Individuals with dementia due to Alzheimer's disease have more severe impairment, which is likely due to impaired ability rather than decreased effort, as may be present with depression. Specific deficits in dementia include faster rates of forgetting initially recalled material, more false-positive errors on recognition memory tasks, and impairments in temporal orientation, visual recognition, and visuoconstruction (Wright & Persad, 2007).

Dementia and Delirium

Delirium develops in 14–56% of older adults hospitalized for acute medical problems and can be caused by a variety of medical conditions, including infections (Inouye & Ferrucci, 2006). The onset and course of cognitive difficulties represents the major distinction between dementia and delirium. Delirium is an acute, often reversible disorder of attention and cognition that requires immediate attention, as it is life-threatening. In contrast, dementia has a gradual onset, with variations in the course based on the different etiologies of dementia. Another factor to consider when assessing for delirium and dementia is disorientation, which is more often seen early in delirium and in later stages of dementia. Symptoms of delirium tend to be variable from moment to moment, whereas symptoms of dementia tend to be stable over time.

Assessment of Relative Contributions of Each

Clinical interviews with the older adult and other informants (e.g., children, spouses, family members) are an important aspect of the assessment process. The interview can be used to identify the onset and the speed of onset of the cognitive problems. A full medical examination should be completed to identify possible medical causes of cognitive impairment (e.g., thiamine deficiency, infection). To detect cognitive impairment, brief cognitive assessments (e.g., MoCA, SLUMS) can be administered as a preliminary method of determining whether further assessment is necessary. Following positive findings, neuropsychological assessment would be warranted and is considered the gold standard in differentiating cognitive impairment from depression (e.g., Wright & Persad, 2007). Structured and semistructured interviews and several self-report inventories (e.g., GDS) are valid to use to detect depression in older adults (for a review, see Fiske & O'Riley, 2008). A discussion of the psychometric properties of various self-report measures of depression can be found earlier in this chapter.

When delirium is suspected, one of several measures that focus on the detection of delirium could be used. The presence of an infection, particularly respiratory and urinary tract infections, is a risk factor for delirium (Rahkonen et al., 2000). Alertness, cognition, and depression are important domains to assess when infections are present or suspected. In a review of delirium assessments, Jackson and colleagues (2004) identified two measures they recommend using: the Confusion Assessment Method (CAM; Inouye, van Dyck, Alessi, & Balkin, 1990) and the NEECHAM Confusion Scale (Neelon, Champagne, Carlson & Funk, 1996). The sensitivity of the CAM for the detection of delirium ranges from .46 to 1.00, and the sensitivity ranges from .63 to 1.00, across 11 studies (Wei, Fearing, Sternberg, & Inouye, 2008). The sensitivity of the CAM is optimal if used following administration of a brief cognitive screen (Wei et al., 2008). The NEECHAM confusion scale has high internal consistency (alpha = .88), adequate interrater reliability (kappa = .60), high sensitivity (.97), and good specificity (.83) when administered by nurses in an intensive care unit (Immers, Schuurmans, & van de Bijl, 2005).

Arthritis

Osteoarthritis or rheumatoid arthritis often afflict older adults, causing pain and functional limitations. Chibnall and Tait (2001) examined the use of four common pain scales in older hospitalized patients. They concluded that the 21-point Box Scale (BS-21; Jensen, Miller, & Fisher, 1998) was the most reliable and valid assessment self-report scale in their study. The authors found that older patients' average pain experience over a week's period was best captured by the assessment of a patient's worst and usual pain for patients with cognitive impairment and by a patient's least and usual pain ratings for patients without cognitive impairment (Chibnall & Tait, 2001). Disease-specific measures, such as the Arthritis Self-Efficacy Scale (Lorig, Chastay, Ung, Shoor, & Holman, 1989) are alternatives to general pain assessments that have been used with older adults. Another option for evaluating older adults' pain is for nurses and health service workers to use behavior observation scales to evaluate pain. The evaluation of pain is particularly important when working with older adults with dementia, and specific observational measures have been developed, such as the Discomfort Scale for Diseases of Alzheimer's Type (DS-DAT; Hurley, Volicer, Hanrahan, Houde, & Volicer, 1992). A comprehensive and multiple method approach to of the assessment of pain should be used in individuals with dementia (Snow et al., 2004). Assessing depression, anxiety, and sleep difficulties is also important, as these problems are more prevalent among individuals with arthritis (Axford et al., 2010).

Chronic Obstructive Pulmonary Disorder

Chronic obstructive pulmonary disorder (COPD) is a chronic breathing disorder marked by symptoms of shortness of breath, wheezing, and coughing and which is associated with extended hospitalizations (Yellowlees, Alpers, Bowden, Bryant, & Ruffin, 1987) and diminished quality of life (Cully et al., 2006). The average prevalence of depression among patients with COPD is 40%, with a range of 6–80% (Norwood, 2007). The prevalence of clinical anxiety ranges from 13 to 46% among outpatients and from 10 to 55% among hospitalized individuals with COPD (Willgoss & Yohannes, 2013).

COPD symptoms, including dyspnea and hypoxemia, may lead to and also be exacerbated by anxiety and panic symptoms (Maurer et al., 2008). Interoceptive cues such as dyspnea and tachycardia may be misinterpreted by patients with COPD and with high anxiety sensitivity, resulting in anxiety and panic, as well (Simon et al., 2006). Depressive symptoms in COPD are associated with fatigue, shortness of breath, hospitalization, and mortality (for a review, see Maurer et al., 2008). The assessment of anxiety and depression in patients with COPD is prudent. Self-report measures of anxiety and depression, such as the BAI, BDI-II, HADS, and PHQ-9, have been used to assess anxiety and depression in patients with COPD (e.g., Cully et al., 2006).

Parkinson's Disease

Parkinson's disease (PD) is an age-related neurodegenerative disorder with mean age of onset of approximately 70 years (Hindle, 2010). The age-adjusted prevalence of PD is approximately 150 (105–168) cases per 100,000 population, with an age-specific incidence of 10.8 cases of PD per 100,000 population (Hindle, 2010). Major depressive disorder is common among patients with PD, with a prevalence of 19% (Reijnders, Ehrt, Weber, Aarsland, & Leentjens, 2008). Clinically significant symptoms of depression are present in 35% of individuals with PD (Reijnders, et al., 2008). Ehrt, Bronnick, Lentjens, Larsen, and Aarsland (2006) compared the symptoms of depression among older adults with depression with and without PD. Those with PD evidenced less severe sadness, fewer feelings of guilt, slightly less loss of energy, and more difficulty with concentration than those without PD. Depression also can precede the appearance of the motor symptoms of PD. Individuals with PD are 2.4 times more likely to have depression prior to the diagnosis of PD (Leentjens, 2004. The likelihood rises in the 3 years preceding the PD diagnosis (Weintraub, Moberg, Duda, Katz, & Stern, 2003).

Approximately 40% of patients with PD also experience anxiety disorders (Pontone et al., 2009). The most common anxiety diagnoses are panic disorder, generalized anxiety disorder, and simple and social phobia (Aarsland, Marsh, & Schrag, 2009). These symptoms do not appear to be a reaction to the disease or the side effect of treatment but rather a function of the underlying neurochemical changes associated with PD (Cummings & Masterman, 1999). Anxiety and depression tend to be comorbid in patients with PD. In light of the foregoing, one should be alert to the significant risk of both depression and anxiety when working with patients who have PD.

Cancer

Depression diagnosed by a clinician is present in 22–29% of older adults with cancer (Raison & Miller, 2003). Distress associated with cancer varies depending on the type and location of the cancer. Individuals with lung, pancreas, liver, and head and neck cancer have significantly elevated rates of depressive symptoms compared with other types of cancers, such as prostate cancer (Zabora, BrintzenhofeSzoc, Curbow, Hooker, & Piantadosi, 2001). Symptoms of depression may be in evidence before somatic signs of pancreatic cancer are evident, suggesting that depression may be a prodromal symptom of pancreatic cancer (Mayr & Schmid, 2010).

Older adult patients with cancer and depression often have a poor prognosis, poor response to treatment, and increased rate of mortality compared with older adult patients with cancer but without elevated depressive symptoms (Pinquart & Duberstein, 2010; Raison & Miller, 2003). Additionally, a diagnosis of cancer places older adults at increased risk for suicide both at the time of diagnosis and several years after the initial diagnosis (Quan, Arboleda-Flórez, & Fick, 2002; Schairer et al., 2006). Suicidal ideation is more likely in patients with cancer and with depression than in patients with cancer but without depression (Ciaramella & Poli, 2001).

As discussed in the previous section, depression symptoms may overlap with the symptoms experienced due to the cancer or to the side effects of the treatment (Ciaramella & Poli, 2001; Raison & Miller, 2003). Cancer-related fatigue is a common side effect of treatment that may persist after treatment has been completed (Levy, 2008). Treatment of cancer can also have an impact on cognition, specifically in the areas of executive function, information processing speed, verbal memory, and visual memory (Jansen, Miaskowski, Dodd, Dowling, & Kramer, 2005). These cognitive deficits resulting from chemotherapy are sometimes referred to as "chemo brain." Additionally, one treatment option for malignancies, cytokine interferon (IFN)-alpha treatment, can result in depressive symptoms and, less frequently, in mania symptoms (Raison, Demetrashvili, Capuron, & Miller, 2005).

Diabetes

Adults over the age of 65 have consistently had the highest percentage of diagnosed diabetes across all age groups in the United States, and the percentage has increased each year (Centers for Disease Control and Prevention, 2013). Older adults with diabetes are at increased risk for cognitive impairment and depression. Diabetes and poor control of glucose levels over time create an increased risk for cognitive impairment (Stewart & Liolitsa, 1999). Lower cognitive functioning as measured by the MMSE was related to a lower likelihood of engaging in diabetic self-care behaviors, more disability, and more hospitalizations (Sinclair, Girling, & Bayer, 2000). The relation between poor glycemic control and cognitive impairment suggests an ongoing cycle of poor self-care behaviors and increasingly poor health. Individuals with diabetes are at increased risk for depressive and anxiety symptoms. In older adults with diabetes, 26% report elevated depressive symptoms (Anderson, Freedland, Clouse, & Lustman, 2001). Older adults with diabetes who report experiencing distress due to physical symptoms of diabetes also report a higher level of depressive symptoms (Hu, Amoako, Gruber, & Rossen, 2007). Mixed-age adults with diabetes have a higher risk of meeting criteria for an anxiety diagnosis (odds ratio [OR] = 1.2) and expressing elevated anxiety symptoms (OR = 1.48; Smith et al., 2013). The PHQ-9, a nine-item self-report measure of depressive symptoms, has demonstrated good internal consistency (alpha = 0.80) and a sensitivity of .53 and specificity of .94 in predicting depressive symptoms in older adults with diabetes (Lamers et al., 2008).

Sleep

Older adults sleep less deeply, spend more time awake during the night, and have great difficulty maintaining sleep compared with younger adults (Ancoli-Israel & Ayalon, 2006). Age-related changes in the circadian system, as discussed earlier, can be exacerbated by weak environmental cues, such as decreased exposure to light, irregular mealtimes, and less structured daily schedules following retirement (Ancoli-Israel & Ayalon, 2006). The combination of weak environmental cues and circadian rhythm changes may place older adults at risk of developing circadian rhythm sleep–wake disorders, advanced sleep phase type. Age-related changes in sleep may increase the risk of insomnia disorders among older adults.

Insomnia, defined as difficulty falling asleep and staying asleep or waking too early and being unable to fall back to sleep, affects about 12–40% of older adults (Morin et al., 1999). Insomnia is more prevalent among older adults with medical or psychiatric illness. Many older adults have excessive daytime sleepiness (EDS) and nap during the daytime. EDS may be associated with primary sleep disorders (e.g., sleep-disordered breathing, restless-legs syndrome) that are more prevalent among older adults (Ancoli-Israel & Ayalon, 2006). In particular, breathing-related sleep disorders may be more common among older adults due to the changes in the respiratory system that occur with age. Breathing-related sleep disorders are best assessed using laboratory-based polysomnography (PSG) or home-based PSG (Martin, Shocat, & Ancoli-Israel, 2000).

Assessing sleep problems in older adults should include a history of chronic medical and psychiatric problems, medications, and the possible presence of primary sleep disorders. Having patients maintain a sleep diary for a week can provide valuable information regarding bedtimes, waking times, number of nocturnal awakenings, length of nocturnal awakenings, daytime naps, and caffeine and alcohol intake. Sleep diaries can be compared with more objective data collected by wrist actigraphs, which measure sleep and wake by measuring movement (Sivertsen et al., 2006). In addition to collecting sleep diaries and conducting a clinical interview, there are several psychometrically valid instruments used to screen for sleep problems. The Pittsburgh Sleep Quality Index (PSQI; Buysse, Reynolds, Monk, Berman, & Kupfer, 1989; Buysse et al., 1991) and Epworth Sleepiness Scale (Johns, 1991) can be used to screen for general sleep disturbances in older adults. These two measures were found to have adequate internal consistency with older adults (Beaudreau et al., 2012; Buysse et al., 1991). These self-report measures are quick to administer and score and are inexpensive compared with actigraphy and PSG.

Conclusion

The assessment of older adults can present formidable and interesting challenges for mental health professionals, primarily due to the need to sort and integrate the influence of multiple factors (e.g., age-related changes in physiology and cognition, medical disorders, psychiatric disorders) that can contribute to clinical presentations. Assessment requires considerable detective work on the part of the clinician, who must integrate the clues identified through an interdisciplinary approach. We have briefly discussed the most important of those factors to be considered when assessing older adults and attempted to provide the reader with preliminary suggestions for addressing the complexities of the assessment process.

REFERENCES

Aarsland, D., Marsh, L., & Schrag, A. (2009). Neuropsychiatric symptoms in Parkinson's disease. *Movement Disorders, 24,* 2175–2186.

Administration on Aging. (2011). *Profile of older Americans: 2010.* Retrieved November 15, 2011, from *www.aoa.gov/AoARoot/Aging_Statistics/Profile/index.aspx.*

American Bar Association Commission on Law and Aging & American Psychological Association. (2008). *Assessment of older adults with diminished capacity: A handbook for psychologists.* Washington, DC: American Bar Association Commission on Law and Aging and American Psychological Association.

American Psychiatric Association. (2013). *Diagnostic and statistical manual of mental disorders* (5th ed.). Arlington, VA: Author.

Ancoli-Israel, S., & Ayalon, L. (2006). Diagnosis and treatment of sleep disorders in older adults. *American Journal of Geriatric Psychiatry, 14*, 95–103.

Anderson, R. J., Freedland, K. E., Clouse, R. E., & Lustman, P. J. (2001). The prevalence of comorbid depression in adults with diabetes. *Diabetes Care, 24*, 1069–1078.

Axford, J., Butt, A., Heron, C., Hammond, J., Morgan, J., Alavia, A., et al. (2010). Prevalence of anxiety and depression in osteoarthritis: Use of the Hospital Anxiety and Depression Scale as a screening tool. *Clinical Rheumatology, 29*, 1277–1283

Beaudreau, S. A., Spira, A. P., Stewart, A., Kezirian, E. J., Lui, L., Ensrud, K., et al. (2012). Validation of the Pittsburgh Sleep Quality Index and the Epworth Sleepiness Scale in older black and white women. *Sleep Medicine, 13*, 36–42.

Beck, A. T., & Steer, R. A. (1993). *Beck Anxiety Inventory Manual*. San Antonio, TX: Harcourt Brace.

Beck, A. T., Steer, R. A., & Brown, G. K. (1996). *Beck Depression Inventory Manual* (2nd ed.). San Antonio, TX: Psychological Corporation.

Blazer, D. G. (2003). Depression in late life: Review and commentary. *Journal of Gerontology, Medical Sciences, 58A*, 249–265.

Bowie, M. W., & Slattum, P. W. (2007). Pharmacodynamics in older adults: A review. *American Journal of Geriatric Pharmacotherapy, 5*, 263–303.

Buysse, D. J., Reynolds, C. F., III, Monk, T. H., Berman, S. R., & Kupfer, D. J. (1989). The Pittsburgh Sleep Quality Index: A new instrument for psychiatric practice and research. *Psychiatry Research, 28*, 193–213.

Buysse, D. J., Reynolds, C. F., III, Monk, T. H., Hoch, C. C., Yeager, A. L., & Kupfer, D. J. (1991). Quantification of subjective sleep quality in healthy elderly men and women using the Pittsburgh Sleep Quality Index (PSQI). *Sleep, 14*, 331–338.

Byrne, G. J., & Pachana, N. A. (2011). Development and validation of a short form of the Geriatric Anxiety Inventory—The GAI-SF. *International Psychogeriatrics, 23*, 125–131.

Byrne, G. J., Pachana, N. A., Goncalves, D. C., Arnold, E., King, R., & Khoo, S. (2010). Psychometric properties and health correlates of the Geriatric Anxiety Inventory in Australian community-residing older women. *Aging and Mental Health, 14*(3), 247–254.

Campbell, N. L., Boustani, M. A., Skopelja, E. N., Gao, S., Unverzagt, F. W., & Murray, M. D. (2012). Medication adherence in older adults with cognitive impairment: A systematic evidence-based review. *The American Journal of Geriatric Pharmacotherapy, 10*, 165–177.

Centers for Disease Control and Prevention. (2011). *Deaths: Preliminary data for 2011.* Retrieved September 15, 2014, from *www.cdc.gov/nchs/data/nvsr/nvsr61/nvsr61_06.pdf.*

Centers for Disease Control and Prevention. (2013). *Percentage of civilian, noninstitutionalized, population with diagnosed diabetes by age, United States, 1980–2011.* Retrieved from *www.cdc.gov/diabetes/statistics/prev/national/figbyage.htm.*

Chibnall, J. T., & Tait, R. C. (2001). Pain assessment in cognitively impaired and unimpaired older adults: A comparison of four scales. *Pain, 92*, 173–186.

Chochinov, H. M., Wilson, K. G., Enns, M., & Lander, S. (1994). Prevalence of depression in the terminally ill: Effects of diagnostic criteria and symptom threshold judgments. *American Journal of Psychiatry, 151*, 537–540.

Ciaramella, A., & Poli, P. (2001). Assessment of depression among cancer patients: The role of pain cancer type and treatment. *Psycho-Oncology, 10*, 156–165.

Conwell, Y. (2001). Suicide in later life: A review and recommendations for prevention. *Suicide and Life-Threatening Behavior, 31*, 32–47.

Conwell, Y., Duberstein, P. R., Hirsch, J. K., Conner, K. R., Eberly, S., & Caine, E. D. (2010). Health status and suicide in the second half of life. *International Journal of Geriatric Psychiatry, 25*, 371–379.

Cooper, C., Carpenter, I., Katona, C., Schroll, M., Wagner, C., Fialova, D., et al. (2005). The AdHOC study of older adults' adherence to medication in 11 countries. *American Journal of Geriatric Psychiatry, 11*, 1067–1076.

Crews, J. E., & Campbell, V. A. (2001). Health conditions, activity limitations, and participation restrictions among older people with visual impairments. *Journal of Visual Impairment and Blindness, 95*(8), 453–467.

Crum, R. M., Anthony, J. C., Basset, S. S., & Folstein, M. F. (1993). Population-based norms for the Mini-Mental State Examination by age and educational level. *Journal of the American Medical Association, 269*, 2386–2391.

Cukrowicz, K. C., Cheavens, J. S., Van Orden, K. A., Ragain, R., & Cook, R. L. (2011). Perceived burdensomeness and suicide ideation in older adults. *Psychology and Aging, 26,* 331–338.

Cullen, B., O'Neill, B., Evans, J. J., Coen, R. F., & Lawlor, B. A. (2007). A review of screening tests for cognitive impairment. *Journal of Neurology and Neurosurgery Psychiatric, 78,* 790–799.

Cully, J. A., Graham, D. P., Stanley, M. A., Ferguson, C. J., Sharafkhaneh, A., Souchek, J., et al. (2006). Quality of life in patients with chronic obstructive pulmonary disease and comorbid anxiety or depression. *Psychosomatics, 47,* 312–319.

Cummings, J. L., & Masterman, D. L. (1999). Depression in patients with Parkinson's disease. *International Journal of Geriatric Psychiatry, 14*(9), 711–718.

Duberstein, P. R., Conwell, Y., Conner, K. R., Eberly, S., & Caine, E. D. (2004). Suicide at 50 years of age and older: Perceived physical illness, family discord and financial strain. *Psychological Medicine, 34,* 137–146.

Duff, K., Patton, D., Schoenberg, M. R., Mold, J., Scott, J. G., & Adams, R. L. (2003). Age- and education-corrected independent normative data for the RBANS in a community-dwelling elderly sample. *Clinical Neuropsychologist, 17,* 351–366.

Edelstein, B., Woodhead, E., Segal, D., Heisel, M., Bower, E., Lowery, A., et al. (2008). Older adult psychological assessment: Current instrument status and related considerations. *Clinical Gerontologist, 31,* 1–35.

Edelstein, B. A., Heisel, M. J., McKee, D. R., Martin, R. R., Koven, L. P., Duberstein, P. R., et al. (2009). Development and psychometric evaluation of the Reasons for Living—Older Adults Scale: A suicide risk assessment inventory. *Gerontologist, 49,* 736–745.

Ehrt, U., Bronnick, K., Lentjens, A. F. G., Larsen, J. P., & Aarsland, D. (2006). Depressive symptom profile in Parkinson's disease: A comparison with depression in elder patients without Parkinson's disease. *International Journal of Geriatric Psychiatry, 21,* 252–258.

Enache, D., Winblad, B., & Aarsland, D. (2011). Depression in dementia: Epidemiology, mechanisms, and treatment. *Current Opinion in Psychiatry, 24,* 461–472.

Fiske, A., & O'Riley, A. A. (2008). Assessment of depression in late life. In J. D. Hunsley & E. J. Mash (Eds.), *A guide to assessments that work* (pp. 138–157). Oxford, UK: Oxford University Press.

Fiske, A., O'Riley, A. A., & Widoe, R. K. (2008).

Physical health and suicide in late life: An evaluative review. *Clinical Gerontologist, 31,* 31–50.

Folstein, M. F., Folstein, S. E., & McHugh, P. R. (1975). "Mini-mental state": A practical method for grading the cognitive state of patients for the clinician. *Journal of Psychiatric Research, 12,* 189–198.

Franklin, S. S., Gustin, W., Wong, N. D., Larson, M. G., Weber, M. A., Kannel, W. B., & Levy, D. (1997). Hemodynamic patters of age-related changes in blood pressure: The Framingham Heart Study. *Circulation, 96,* 308–315.

Fujisawa, D., Tanaka, E., Sakamoto, S., Neichi, K., Nakagawa, A., & Ono, Y. (2005). The development of a brief screening instrument for depression and suicidal ideation for elderly: The Depression and Suicide Screen. *Psychiatry and Clinical Neurosciences, 59*(6), 634–638.

Gerolimatos, L. A., Gregg, J. J., & Edelstein, B. A. (2013). Assessment of anxiety in long-term care: Examination of the Geriatric Anxiety Inventory (GAI) and its short form. *International Psychogeriatrics, 25,* 1533–1542.

Greenberg, L., Lantz, M. S., & Likourezos, A. (2004). Screening for depression in nursing home palliative care patients. *Journal of Geriatric Psychiatry and Neurology, 17,* 212–218.

Gum, A. M., King-Kallimanis, B., & Kohn, R. (2009). Prevalence of mood, anxiety, and substance-abuse disorders for older Americans in the National Comorbidity Survey—Replication. *American Journal of Geriatric Psychiatry, 17,* 769–781.

Hajjar, E., & Hanlon, J. T. (2006). Polypharmacy in the elderly. In K. Calhoun & D. E. Eibling (Eds.), *Geriatric otolaryngology* (pp. 667–673). New York: Taylor & Francis.

He, W., Sengupta, M., Velkoff, V. A., & DeBarros, K. A. (2005). *Current Population Reports: 65+ in the United States: 2005* (Report No. P23-209). Washington, DC: U.S. Government Printing Office.

Heisel, M. J. (2006). Suicide and its prevention among older adults. *Canadian Journal of Psychiatry, 51*(3), 143–154.

Heisel, M. J., & Duberstein, P. R. (2005). Suicide prevention in older adults. *Clinical Psychology: Science and Practice, 12,* 242–259.

Heisel, M. J., & Flett, G. L. (2006). The development and initial validation of the Geriatric Suicide Ideation Scale. *American Journal of Geriatric Psychiatry, 14,* 742–751.

Heisel, M. J., Flett, G. L., & Duberstein, P. R. (2005). Does the Geriatric Depression Scale (GDS) distinguish between older adults with high versus low levels of suicidal ideation? *American Journal of Geriatric Psychiatry, 13,* 876–883.

Hindle, J. V. (2010). Ageing, neurodegeneration and Parkinson's disease. *Age and Ageing, 39,* 156–161.

Htwe, T. H., Mushtaq, A., Robinson, S. B., Rosher, R. B., & Khardori, N. (2007). Infection in the elderly. *Infectious Disease Clinics of North America, 21,* 711–743.

Hu, J., Amoako, E. P., Gruber, K. J., & Rossen, E. K. (2007). The relationships among health functioning indicators and depression in older adults with diabetes. *Issues in Mental Health Nursing, 28,* 133–150.

Hurley, A. C., Volicer, B. J., Hanrahan, P. A., Houde, S., & Volicer, L. (1992). Assessment of discomfort in advanced Alzheimer patients. *Research in Nursing and Health, 15,* 369–377.

Immers, H. E. M., Schuurmans, M. J., & van de Bijl, J. J. (2005). Recognition of delirium in ICU patients: A diagnostic study of NEE-CHAM confusion scale in ICU patients. *BMC Nursing, 4,* 7–13.

Inouye, S. K., & Ferrucci, L. (2006). Elucidating the pathophysiology of delirium and the interrelationship of delirium and dementia. *Journal of Gerontology: Medical Sciences, 61A*(12), 1277–1280.

Inouye, S. K., van Dyck, C. H., Alessi, C. A., & Balkin, S. (1990). Clarifying confusion: The confusion assessment method: A new method for detection of delirium. *Annals of Internal Medicine, 113,* 141–148.

Insel, K., Morrow, D., Brewer, B., & Figueredo, A. (2006). Executive function, working memory, and medication adherence among older adults. *Journal of Gerontology: Psychological Sciences, 61B*(2), 102–107.

Jackson, J. C., Gordon, S. M., Hart, R. P., Hopkins, R. O., & Ely, E. W. (2004). The association between delirium and cognitive decline: A review of the empirical literature. *Neuropsychology Review, 14,* 87–98.

Jansen, C. E., Miaskowski, C., Dodd, M., Dowling, G., & Kramer, J. (2005). A meta-analysis of studies of the effects of cancer chemotherapy on various domains of cognitive function. *Cancer, 104,* 2222–2233.

Jensen, M. P., Miller, L., & Fisher, L. D. (1998). Assessment of pain during medical procedures: A comparison of three scales. *Clinical Journal of Pain, 14*(4), 343–349.

Johns, M. (1991). A new method for measuring daytime sleepiness: The Epworth Sleepiness Scale. *Sleep, 14*(6), 540–545.

Katz, S., Downs, T. D., Cash, H. R., & Grotz, R. C. (1970). Progress in development of the index of ADL. *Gerontologist, 10*(1), 20–30.

Kelly, B., Burnett, P, Pelusi, D., Badger, S. J., Varghese, F., & Robertson, M. (2003). Factors associated with the wish to hasten death: A study of patients with terminal illness. *Psychological Medicine, 33,* 75–81.

King, D. A., Heisel, M. J., & Lyness, J. M. (2005). Assessment and psychological treatment of depression in older adults with terminal or life-threatening illness. *Clinical Psychology: Science and Practice, 12,* 339–353.

Kroenke, K., Spitzer, R. L., & Williams, J. B. W. (2001). The PHQ-9: Validity of a brief depression severity measure. *Journal of General Internal Medicine, 16,* 606–613.

Lamers, F., Jonkers, C., Bosma, H., Penninx, B., Knottnerus, J., & van Eijk, J. (2008). Summed score of the Patient Health Questionnaire—9 was a reliable and valid method for depression screening in chronically ill elderly patients. *Journal of Clinical Epidemiology, 61,* 679–687.

Lawton, M. P., & Brody, E. M. (1969). Assessment of older people: Self-maintaining and instrumental activities of daily living. *Gerontologist, 9*(3), 179–186.

Lazarou, J., Pomeranz, B. H., & Corey, P. N. (1998). Incidence of adverse drug reactions in hospitalized patients: A meta-analysis of prospective studies. *Journal of the American Medical Association, 279,* 1200–1205.

Leentjens, A. F. G. (2004). Depression in Parkinson's disease: Conceptual issues and clinical challenges. *Journal of Geriatric Psychiatry and Neurology, 17,* 120–126.

Leventhal, E. A., Leventhal, H., Robitaille, C., & Brownlee, S. (1999). Psychosocial factors in medication adherence: A model of the modeler. In D. C. Park, R. W. Morrell, & K. Shifren (Eds.), *Processing of medical information in aging patients* (pp. 145–165). Mahwah, NJ: Erlbaum.

Levy, M. R. (2008). Cancer fatigue: A neurobiological review for psychiatrists. *Psychosomatics: Journal of Consultation Liaison Psychiatry, 49,* 283–291.

Lindau, S. T., Schumm, P., Laumann, E. O.,

Levinson, W., O'Muircheartaigh, C. A., & Waite, L. J. (2007). A study of sexuality and health among older adults in the United States. *New England Journal of Medicine, 357,* 762–774.

Loeb, P. A. (1996). *Independent Living Scales.* San Antonio, TX: Psychological Corporation.

Lorig, K., Chastay, R., Ung, E., Shoor, S., & Holman, H. (1989). Development and evaluation of a scale used to measure perceived self-efficacy in people with arthritis. *Arthritis and Rheumatism, 32,* 37–44.

Löwe, B., Unützer, J., Callahan, C. M., Perkins, A. J., & Kroenke, K. (2004). Monitoring depression treatment outcomes with the Patient Health Questionnaire–9. *Medical Care, 42,* 1194–1201.

Luis, C. A., Keegan, A. P., & Mullan, M. (2009). Cross-validation of the Montreal Cognitive Assessment in community dwelling older adults residing in the southeastern U.S. *International Journal of Geriatric Psychiatry, 24,* 197–201.

Luoma, J. B., Martin, C. E., & Pearson, J. L. (2002). Contact with mental health and primary care providers before suicide: A review of the evidence. *American Journal of Psychiatry, 159,* 909–916.

Lyness, J. M. (2004). End-of-life care: Issues relevant to the geriatric psychiatrist. *American Journal of Geriatric Psychiatry, 12,* 457–472.

Mangoni, A. A., & Jackson, S. H. D. (2004). Age-related changes in pharmacokinetics and pharmacodynamics: Basic principles and practical applications. *British Journal of Clinical Pharmacology, 57,* 6–14.

Martin, J., Shocat, T., & Ancoli-Israel, S. (2000). Assessment and treatment of sleep disturbances in older adults. *Clinical Psychology Review, 20,* 783–805.

Mayr, M., & Schmid, R. (2010). Pancreatic cancer and depression: Myth and truth. *BMC Cancer, 10,* 569–575.

McLean, A. J., & Le Couteur, D. G. (2004). Aging biology and geriatric clinical pharmacology. *Pharmacological Reviews, 56,* 163–184.

Maurer, J., Rebbapragada, V., Borson, S., Goldstein, R., Kunik, M. E., Yohannes, A. M., et al. (2008). Anxiety and depression in COPD: Current understanding, unanswered questions, and research needs. *Chest Journal, 134,* 43S–56S.

Mitchell, A. J., Bird, V., Rizzo, M., & Meader, N. (2010). Diagnostic validity and added value of the Geriatric Depression Scale for depression in primary care: A meta-analysis of GDS_{30} and GDS_{15}. *Journal of Affective Disorders, 125,* 10–17.

Mitchell, A. J., Meader, N., & Symonds, P. (2010). Diagnostic validity of the Hospital Anxiety and Depression Scale (HADS) in cancer and palliative settings: A meta-analysis. *Journal of Affective Disorders, 126,* 335–348.

Morin, C. M., Hauri, P. J., Espie, C. A., Spielman, D. J., Buysse, D. J., & Bootzin, R. R. (1999). Nonpharmacologic treatment of chronic insomnia. *Sleep, 22,* 1134–1156.

Morley, J. E., & Tumosa, N. (2002). Saint Louis University Mental Status Examination (SLUMS). *Aging Successfully, 12,* 4.

Morrell, R. W., & Shifren, K. (1999). Issues in the measurement of medication adherence. In D. C. Park, R. W. Morrell, & K. Shifren (Eds.), *Processing of medical information in aging patients* (pp. 185–198). Mahwah, NJ: Erlbaum.

Morrow, D. G., Leirer, V. O., & Sheikh, J. (1988). Adherence and medication instructions: Review and recommendations. *Journal of the American Geriatrics Society, 36*(12), 1147–1160.

Moye, J., Gurrera, R. J., Karel, M. J., Edelstein, B. A., & O'Connell, C. (2006). Empirical advances in the assessment of the capacity to consent to medical treatment: Clinical implications and research needs. *Clinical Psychology Review, 26,* 1054–1077.

Moye, J., Marson, D. C., & Edelstein, B. (2013). Assessment of capacity in an aging society. *American Psychologist, 68,* 158–171.

Nasreddine, Z. S., Phillips, N. A., Bédirian, V., Charbonneau, S., Whitehead, V., Collin, I., et al. (2005). The Montreal Cognitive Assessment: A brief screening tool for mild cognitive impairment. *Journal of the American Geriatrics Society, 53,* 695–699.

National Institute on Deafness and Other Communications Disorders. (2001). Hearing loss and older adults. Retrieved November 23, 2011, from *www.nidcd.nih.gov/health/hearing/Pages/older.aspx.*

Neelon, V. J., Champagne, M. T., Carlson, J. R., & Funk, S. G. (1996). The NEECHAM Confusion Scale: Construction, validation, and clinical testing. *Nursing Research, 45,* 324–330.

Noorani, N. H., & Montagnini, M. (2007). Recognizing depression in palliative care patients. *Journal of Palliative Medicine, 10,* 458–464.

Norris, M. P., Arnau, R. C., Bramson, R., & Meagher, M. W. (2003). The efficacy of somatic symptoms in assessing depression in older primary care. *Clinical Gerontologist, 27*, 43–57.

Norwood, R. J. (2007). A review of etiologies of depression in COPD. *International Journal of Chronic Obstructive Pulmonary Disease, 2*(4), 485–491.

Ohayon, M. M., Carskadon, M. A., Guilleminault, C., & Vitiello, M. V. (2004). Meta-analysis of quantitative sleep parameters from childhood to old age in healthy individuals: Developing normative sleep values across the human lifespan. *Sleep, 27*(7), 1255–1273.

Pachana, N. A., Byrne, G. J., Siddle, H., Koloski, N., Harley, E., & Arnold, E. (2007). Development and validation of the Geriatric Anxiety Inventory. *International Psychogeriatrics, 19*, 103–114.

Panza, F., Frisardi, V., Capirso, C., D'Introno, A., Colacicco, A. M., Imbimbo, B. P., et al. (2010). Late-life depression, mild cognitive impairment, and dementia: Possible continuum? *American Journal of Geriatric Psychiatry, 18*, 98–116.

Periyakoil, V. S., Kraemer, H. C., Noda, A., Moos, R., Hallenbeck, J., Webster, M., et al. (2005). The development and initial validation of the Terminally Ill Grief or Depression Scale (TIGDS). *International Journal of Methods in Psychiatric Research, 14*, 202–212.

Pessin, H., Rosenfeld, B., & Breitbart, W. (2002). Assessing psychological distress near the end of life. *American Behavioral Scientist, 46*, 357–372.

Pinquart, M. M., & Duberstein, P. R. (2010). Depression and cancer mortality: A meta-analysis. *Psychological Medicine, 40*, 1797–1810.

Pinto-Meza, A., Serrano-Blanco, A., Peñarrubia, M. T., Blanco, E., & Haro, J. M. (2005). Assessing depression in primary care with the PHQ-9: Can it be carried out over the telephone? *Journal of General Internal Medicine, 20*, 738–742.

Pontone, G. M., Williams, J. R., Anderson, K., Chase, G., Goldstein, S., Grill, S., et al. (2009). Prevalence of anxiety disorders and anxiety subtypes in patients with Parkinson's disease. *Movement Disorders, 24*, 1333–1338.

Pronk, M., Deeg, D. J. H., Smits, C., van Tilburg, T. F., Kuik, D. J., Festen, J. M., et al. (2011). Prospective effects of hearing status on loneliness and depression in older persons: Identifi-

cation of subgroups. *International Journal of Audiology, 50*, 887–896.

Quan, H., Arboleda-Flórez, J., & Fick, G. H. (2002). Association between physical illness and suicide among the elderly. *Social Psychiatry and Psychiatric Epidemiology, 37*, 190–197.

Rahkonen, T., Mäkelä, H., Paanila, S., Halonen, P., Sivenius, J., & Sulkava, R. (2000). Delirium in elderly people without severe predisposing disorders: Etiology and 1-year prognosis after discharge. *International Psychogeriatrics, 12*, 473–481.

Raison, C., Demetrashvili, M., Capuron, L., & Miller, A. (2005). Neuropsychiatric adverse effects of interferon-alpha: Recognition and management. *CNS Drugs, 19*, 105–123.

Raison, C., & Miller, A. H. (2003). Depression in cancer: New developments regarding diagnosis and treatment. *Biological Psychiatry, 54*, 283–294.

Randolph, C. (1998). *Repeatable Battery for the Assessment of Neuropsychological Status Manual.* San Antonio, TX: Psychological Corporation.

Randolph, C., Tierney, M. C., Mohr, E., & Chase, T. N. (1998). The Repeatable Battery for the Assessment of Neuropsychological Status (RBANS): Preliminary clinical validity. *Journal of Clinical and Experimental Neuropsychology, 20*, 310–319.

Reijnders, J. S. A. M., Ehrt, U., Weber, W. E. J., Aarsland, D., & Leentjens, A. F. G. (2008). A systematic review of prevalence studies of depression in Parkinson's disease. *Movement Disorders, 23*, 183–189.

Reuben, D. R., Herr, K. A., Pacala, J. T., Pollock, B. G., Potter, J. F., & Semla, T. P. (2011). *Geriatrics at your fingertips: 2011* (13th ed.). New York: American Geriatrics Society.

Rossi, M. I., Young, A., Maher, R., Rodriquez, K. L., Appelt, C. J., Perera, S., et al. (2007). Polypharmacy and health beliefs in older outpatients. *American Journal of Geriatric Pharmacotherapy, 5*, 317–323.

Salthouse, T. A. (1993). Speed and knowledge as determinates of adult age differences in verbal tasks. *Journal of Gerontology: Psychological Sciences, 48*, 29–36.

Salthouse, T. A. (2010). *Major issues in cognitive aging.* New York: Oxford University Press.

Schairer, C., Brown, L. M., Chen, B. E., Howard, R., Lynch, C. F., Hall, P., et al. (2006). Suicide after breast cancer: An international population-based study of 723,810 women.

Journal of the National Cancer Institute, *98*(19), 1416–1419.

Segal, D. L., Coolidge, F. L., Cahill, B. S., & O'Riley, A. A. (2008). Psychometric properties of the Beck Depression Inventory-II (BDI-II) among community-dwelling older adults. *Behavior Modification, 3,* 3–20.

Segal, D. L., June, A., Payne, M., Coolidge, F. L., & Yochim, B. (2010). Development and initial validation of a self-report assessment tool for anxiety among older adults: The Geriatric Anxiety Scale. *Journal of Anxiety Disorders, 24,* 709–714.

Sheikh, J. I., & Yesavage, J. A. (1986). Geriatric Depression Scale (GDS): Recent evidence and development of a shorter version. *Clinical Gerontologist: The Journal of Aging and Mental Health, 5* (1–2), 165–173.

Simon, N. M., Weiss, A. M., Kradin, R., Evans, K. C., Reese, H. E., Otto, M. W., et al. (2006). The relationship of anxiety disorders, anxiety sensitivity and pulmonary dysfunction with dyspnea-related distress and avoidance. *Journal of Nervous and Mental Disease, 194,* 951–957.

Simonton, D. K. (2000). Creativity, cognitive, social, and personal aspects. *American Psychologist, 55,* 151–158.

Sinclair, A. J., Girling, A. J., & Bayer, A. J. (2000). Cognitive dysfunction in older subjects with diabetes mellitus: Impact on diabetes self-management and use of care services: All Wales research into elderly (AWARE) study. *Diabetes Research and Clinical Practice, 50*(3), 203–212.

Sivertsen, B., Omvik, S., Havik, O. E., Pallesen, S., Bjorvatn, B., Neilsen, G. H., et al. (2006). A comparison of actigraphy and polysomnography in older adults treated for chronic primary insomnia. *Sleep, 29*(10), 1353–1358.

Smith, K. J., Béland, M., Clyde, M., Gariépy, G., Pagé, V., Badawi, G., et al. (2013). Association of diabetes with anxiety: A systematic review and meta-analysis. *Journal of Psychosomatic Research, 74*(2), 89–99.

Snow, A. L., O'Malley, K. J., Cody, M., Kunik, M. E., Ashton, C. M., Beck, C., et al. (2004). A conceptual model of pain assessment for noncommunicative persons with dementia. *Gerontologist, 44,* 807–817.

Stewart, R., & Liolitsa, D. (1999). Type 2 diabetes mellitus, cognitive impairment, and dementia. *Diabetic Medicine, 6,* 93–112.

Stewart, S., O'Riley, A., Edelstein, B., & Gould,

C. (2012). A preliminary comparison of three cognitive screening instruments in long term care: The MMSE, SLUMS, and MoCA. *Clinical Gerontologist, 35,* 57–75.

Storandt, M. (1994). General principles of assessment of older adults. In M. Storandt & G. R. VandenBos (Eds.), *Neuropsychological assessment of dementia and depression in older adults: A clinician's guide.* Washington, DC: American Psychological Association.

Taché, S. V., Sönnichsen, A., & Ashcroft, D. M. (2011). Prevalence of adverse drug events in ambulatory care: A systematic review. *Annals of Pharmacotherapy, 45,* 977–989.

Tariq, S. H., Tumosa, N., Chibnall, J. T., Perry, M. P., & Morley, J. E. (2006). Comparison of the Saint Louis University Mental Status Examination and the Mini-Mental State Examination for detecting dementia and mild neurocognitive disorder: A pilot study. *American Journal of Geriatric Psychiatry, 14*(11), 900–910.

U.S. Census Bureau. (2010). *Disability characteristics: 2010 American community survey 1-year estimates.* Retrieved from *http://factfinder2. census.gov/faces/tableservices/jsf/pages/ productview.xhtml?pid=ACS_10_1YR_ S1810&prodType=table.*

Uchino, B. N., Birmingham, W., & Berg, C. A. (2010). Are older adults less or more physiologically reactive?: A meta-analysis of age-related differences in cardiovascular reactivity to laboratory tasks. *Journals of Gerontology: B. Psychological Sciences and Social Sciences, 65B,* 154–162.

Vik, S. A., Hogan, D. B., Patten, S. B., Johnson, J. A., Romonko-Slack, L., & Maxwell, C. J. (2006). Medication nonadherence and subsequent risk of hospitalization and mortality among older adults. *Drugs and Aging, 23,* 345–356.

Wei, L. A., Fearing, M. A., Sternberg, E. J., & Inouye, S. K. (2008). The Confusion Assessment Method: A systematic review of current usage. *Journal of the American Geriatrics Society, 56,* 823–830.

Weintraub, D., Moberg, P. J., Duda, J. E., Katz, I. R., & Stern, M. B. (2003). Recognition and treatment of depression in Parkinson's disease. *Journal of Geriatric Psychiatry and Neurology, 16,* 178–183.

Wetherell, J. L., & Gatz, M. (2005). The Beck Anxiety Inventory in older adults with generalized anxiety disorder. *Journal of Psycho-*

pathology and Behavioral Assessment, *27*, 17–23.

Whitbourne, S. K. (2002). *The aging individual: Physical and psychological perspectives* (2nd ed.). New York: Springer.

Whiteside, M., Wallhagen, M., & Pettengill, E. (2006). Sensory impairment in older adults: Part 2. Vision loss. *American Journal of Nursing*, *106*(11), 52–61.

Willgoss, T. G., & Yohannes, A. M. (2013). Anxiety disorders in patients with COPD: A systematic review. *Respiratory Care*, *58*, 858–866.

Wilson, K. G., Chochinov, H., Skirko, M., Allard, P., Chary, S., Gagnon, P. R., et al. (2007). Depression and anxiety disorders in palliative cancer care. *Journal of Pain and Symptom Management*, *33*, 118–129.

World Health Organization. (2010). Measuring health and disability: Manual for WHO Disability Assessment Schedule (WHODAS 2.0). Geneva, Switzerland: Author.

Wright, S. L., & Persad, C. (2007). Distinguishing between depression and dementia in older persons: Neuropsychological and neuropatho-

logical correlates. *Journal of Geriatric Psychiatry and Neurology*, *20*, 189–198.

Yellowlees, P. M., Alpers, J. H., Bowden, J. J., Bryant, G. D., & Ruffin, R. E. (1987). Psychiatric morbidity in patients with chronic airflow obstruction. *Medical Journal of Australia*, *146*, 305–307.

Yesavage, J. A., Brink, T. L., Rose, T. L., Lum, O., Huang, V., Adey, M. B., et al. (1983). Development and validation of a geriatric depression screening scale: A preliminary report. *Journal of Psychiatric Research*, *17*, 37–49.

Yochim, B. P., Mueller, A. E., June, A., & Segal, D. L. (2010). Psychometric properties of the Geriatric Anxiety Scale: Comparison to the Beck Anxiety Inventory and Geriatric Anxiety Inventory. *Clinical Gerontologist*, *34*, 21–33.

Zabora, J., BrintzenhofeSzoc, K., Curbow, B., Hooker, C., & Piantadosi, S. (2001). The prevalence of psychological distress by cancer site. *Psycho-Oncology*, *10*, 19–28.

Zigmond, A. S., & Snaith, R. P. (1983). The Hospital Anxiety and Depression Scale. *Acta Psychiatrica Scandinavica*, *67*, 361–370.

CHAPTER 26

Primary Care

Christopher L. Hunter

Over 30% of individuals in the United States in a given year meet diagnostic criteria for a behavioral health or substance-related disorder (Kessler et al., 2005). These disorders account for one-half as many disability days as "all" physical conditions measured in a recent U.S. population comorbidity survey (Merikangas et al., 2007). In fact, the top five conditions driving overall health costs (work-related productivity + medical + pharmacy costs) are depression, obesity, arthritis, back and neck pain, and anxiety (Loeppke et al., 2009). Data suggest that approximately one-half of all behavioral health disorders are being treated exclusively in primary care by a primary care provider (PCP) without additional behavioral health assistance (Kessler et al., 2005). Unfortunately, standard primary care services for the treatment of behavioral health problems are consistently less effective than enhanced primary care services that incorporate behavioral health support (Butler et al, 2008; Craven & Bland, 2006; Gilbody, Bower, & Whitty, 2006; Hunter, Goodie, Oordt, & Dobmeyer, 2009; Williams et al., 2007).

The specialty care health psychology model has structured itself in a manner consistent with the idea that "if we build it (behavioral health care) they will come." But does that actually happen? Do the vast majority of individuals who would benefit from a health psychologist's services receive those services? The answer is clearly "no." The process of the PCP knowing how a health psychologist can assist, convincing his or her patient to see a "psychologist," and getting the patient to follow through on that consultation is full of barriers. Over 50% of the 6,586 physicians in a survey examining primary care physicians and mental health services reported that they can only "sometimes," "rarely," or "never" get high-quality referrals for outpatient behavioral health care (Trude & Stoddard, 2003, p. 444). Data also suggest that 30–50% of the patients referred from primary care to a specialty mental health provider never make the first appointment (Fisher & Ransom, 1997; Hoge, Auchterlonie, & Miliken, 2006).

To better meet the overall needs of those in primary care, various models of behavioral health care have been developed and implemented over the last 20 years with varying degrees of success (Blount, 2003; Blount et al., 2007; Collins, Hewson, Munger, & Wade, 2010). These models fall on a continuum to include coordinated, colocated, and integrated models. *Coordinated care* involves providing behavioral health and primary care in different locations, using different records with separate treatment plans. However, information is exchanged between primary care and behavioral health care when the patient is being treated in both settings. Typically large-scale efforts to promote coordinated care have been unsuccessful (Blount, 2003). A *colocated care* model involves behavioral health care that is provided at the same site as primary medical care. Behavioral health and primary care providers are typically located in the same office area, with a shared waiting room and staff (Blount, 2003). Patients usually are referred from the medical side to the behavioral health side, and separate treatment records and treatment plans are maintained. The proximity of the service can enhance the exchange of information, make referrals easier, and increase percentage of initial behavioral health appointments that are kept (Blount et al., 2007; Gatchel & Oordt, 2003). *Integrated care* has medical and behavioral health components together, with a behavioral health provider working as a member of the primary care team (Blount et al., 2007). There is one treatment plan targeting the patient's needs and a shared medical record, and the patient is likely to perceive this as medical care (Blount et al., 2007). A growing base of research suggests that an integrated model of care provides the opportunity for far more individuals to have access to behavioral health assessment and intervention services than do other models (Blount, 2003; Collins et al., 2010).

The primary care behavioral health (PCBH) model of integrated care has been on the cutting edge of the integrated care movement and has been employed as the model of integrated care by such large health care systems as Kaiser Permanente, Veterans Administration, federally qualified health centers, and the United States Air Force, Army, and Navy (Strosahl & Robinson, 2008). In sum, the components of the PCBH model are:

1. Population health focus includes access to all enrollees, secondary prevention, acute care, and disease management.
2. Health psychologists are part of the primary care team who see patients where other primary care providers see patients.
3. Health psychologists function as consultants to the primary care provider/team (primary customer).
4. Health psychologists see patients in 15- to 30-minute consultations with the goal of comanaging the patient to improve functioning, decrease symptoms, and improve quality of life.
5. Treatment emphasis on psychoeducation and home-based practice of skills.

For a more comprehensive review of the PCBH model, see Robinson and Reiter (2007), Strosahl and Robinson (2008), and Collins et al. (2010).

Working within this integrated model requires the health psychologist to make significant changes to traditional assessment. The health psychologist, on average, is likely to see 10–12 patients a day in 15- to 30-minute consultation appointments and will be expected to document and provide feedback to the PCP that day. Time limitations do not allow for standard health psychology assessment practices. A focused biopsychosocial assessment geared toward what the PCP sees as the main problem by default has to be different from what most health psychologists have been trained to do. However, by adapting skills to this fast-paced setting, health psychologists can bring about functional improvement and symptom change over a short period of time for many primary care patients. Because other authors (e.g., Linton, 2004) have detailed practice changes for "coordinated" and "colocated" care, this chapter focuses exclusively on assessment within a PCBH model, detailing how to conduct a focused and effective 15-minute biopsychosocial assessment. It provides a retooling of what and how to gather information, including guidance on a semistructured biopsychosocial functional assessment and the use of screening and assessment measures designed for primary care.

The assessment methods described in this chapter can be extended and used in the five A's (Assess, Advise, Agree, Assist, Arrange) model format for assessment and intervention in primary care (Whitlock, Orleans, Pender, & Allan, 2002). The five A's format has been "strongly" (Goldstein, Whitlock, & DePue, 2004, p. 74) recommended as an effective strategy for assessment and intervention across a range of problems in primary care. Specific information for behavioral health providers working in primary care on the Advise, Agree, Assist, and Arrange portions of this model for a host of problem health psychology areas can be found in Hunter et al. (2009).

How Can I Complete a Biopsychosocial Functional Assessment in 15 Minutes?

The assessment in primary care must be more focused than a traditional health psychology assessment. This holds true for the clinical interview and any screening or instrument used. This more focused assessment can unfold in the following way:

1. Introduction (1–2 minutes)
2. Identifying/clarifying consultation problem (10–60 seconds)
3. Conducting a functional analysis of the problem (12–15 minutes)

Introduction

For both the health psychologist and the patient, the first minute of interaction often sets the tone for a successful or unsuccessful primary care visit. It is essential to provide the patient with information about who the health psychologist is and his or her role in the clinic and to set an agenda within the first 1–2 minutes. If the health psychologist skips this step, clinical experience suggests that the patient may have more difficulty answering questions and may be more likely to believe the health psychologist is going to provide a service that he or she cannot provide (i.e., traditional tertiary health psychology services).

The health psychologist should start by making the following clear: (1) his or her profession and training; (2) his or her role in the clinic; (3) the amount of time he or she will be spending with the patient during the appointment; (4) who will have access to the information discussed; and (5) what the health psychologist is going to do to try to help the patient. To assist with this process, the health psychologist may want to provide the patient with an educational pamphlet detailing what he or she has just described. An information sheet example is provided in Appendix 26.1.

Verbal Explanation Example

"Before we start I'd like to give you this [hand the patient the pamphlet]. It explains who I am and my role in the clinic, and I'd like to briefly describe what is in the pamphlet before we start.

"I'm the behavioral health consultant for the clinic, and I'm a health psychologist. I work with the providers when good health care involves paying attention to physical health, emotional health, habits, behaviors, and how those things might interact with each other.

"When your provider wants, she or he can call me in as a consultant. In this consultative role, my job is to help the two of you better manage your current concerns and problems.

"To help with this, I'm going to spend about 30 minutes with you in a consultation appointment. I want to get a good idea of what's working well and what's not working so well, then take the information you give me and together we'll come up with a plan or set of recommendations to help better manage the problems you're having.

"I'm going to write a note that will go into your medical record, and I'm going to give your provider some feedback on the plan we come up with. So don't be surprised if your provider or any other health care team member asks you how parts of the plan are going.

"Do you have any questions before we begin?"

Identifying/Clarifying Consultation Problem

After the health psychologist has provided an introduction, described his or her role in the clinic, and answered any questions the patient has, he or she should go immediately to identifying the presenting problem. This information can be elicited rather quickly in most patients by saying something like the following:

"[Medical provider's name] is concerned about [reason PCP has brought you in to assist]. Is that what you see as the main reason for coming to see me, or is it something different?"

If the patient says "no," then the health psychologist should ask what the patient sees as the main problem. Sometimes PCPs misunderstand what the patient sees as the main problem, or the PCP and the patient disagree about the main problem. Attempting to assess a problem the patient is not concerned about may increase the chances of creating an unproductive assessment. If the patient agrees that the PCP's main concern is also his or her main concern, then begin the functional assessment.

Conducting a Functional Assessment of the Problem

A common mistake at the beginning of the functional assessment is to start with an ambiguous, open-ended question. Although open-ended questions are certainly useful in a specialty health psychology setting, time limitations make use of this strategy impractical as a primary way to gather information in primary care. Patients often respond to open-ended questions with open-ended ambiguous responses. As such, a health psychologist may find him- or herself at the 15-minute mark without the necessary information for evidence-based interventions or recommendations.

Using questions that are menu-driven (i.e., providing patients with several choices to pick when answering) or closed-ended (yes–no) improves the chances that the health psychologist will collect specific, relevant information in an effective and efficient manner. This does not mean that open-ended questions could not be asked. Open-ended questions can yield valuable information that is more difficult to obtain with closed-ended questions. Use of open-ended questions is recommended once the health psychologist believes he or she has gathered all the information he or she thinks is needed in order to understand the patient's problem from a biopsychosocial perspective.

For instance, open-ended questions like the following might be used:

"What haven't I asked you about that you think is important for me to know?"
"Take me through what a typical day [workday if the patient works] looks like for you."
"What does your nonwork day look like?"

Functional Assessment Areas

There are several areas the health psychologist may want to consider assessing with each patient regardless of the referral problem. Assessing these areas is likely to yield

clinically rich information in a short period of time.

1. Nature of the referral problem
2. Duration of problem
3. Triggering events
4. Frequency and intensity of the problem
5. Factors that make the problem better or worse
6. Functional impairment
7. Changes in sleep, interest, energy, concentration, appetite
8. Substance use
9. Mood and suicidal/homicidal ideation

Examples of closed-ended or menu-type questions one might ask for each category—using irritable bowel syndrome as the example—are presented in Appendix 26.2. Individual responses on some questions (in **bold italics** inside quotation marks) are included to demonstrate follow-up questions that might be asked.

Using this format increases the chances of effective and efficient information collection that can provide a good understanding of the frequency, duration, and severity of symptoms and functional impairments for that individual.

Measures

The use of psychological screening and assessment measures in primary care can pose a unique challenge for the health psychologist. There must be a shift from the traditional health psychology assessment practice, which typically consists of longer assessment time, scoring, and write-up to the use of screening and assessment measures that fit the pace and focus of primary care. In order to be useful, screening and assessment measures in primary care have to be quickly and easily completed and scored and yield information that is clinically useful in evaluating symptom severity and functional impairment or that improves diagnostic accuracy and case identification. Although some instruments can be used as both screening and assessment measures (e.g., the Patient Health Questionnaire [PHQ-9]), knowing the differences between the goals of each and how and when to use them is important.

TABLE 26.1. Self-Report Screening and Assessment Measures in Primary Care

Measure	Content assessed/Time frame	No. of items/Time to administer	Psychometric data
Beck Depression Inventory—Primary Care (BDI-PC; Steer, Cavalieri, Leonard, & Beck, 1999)	Depression/In last 2 weeks	7 self-administered items/ Less than 5 minutes	Sensitivity = 97% Specificity = 99% Score of ≥ 4
Patient Health Questionnaire–9 (PHQ-9; Kroenke, Spitzer, & Williams, 2001).	Depression/In last 2 weeks	9 self-administered items/ Less than 5 minutes	Sensitivity = 88% Specificity = 88% Score of ≥ 10
Patient Health Questionnaire–2 (PHQ-2; Kroenke, Spitzer, & Williams, 2003)	Depression/In last 2 weeks	2 self-administered items/ Less than 3 minutes	Sensitivity = 83% Specificity = 92% Score of ≥ 3
Edinburgh Postnatal Depression Scale (EPDS; Cox, Holden, & Sagovsky, 1987; Murray & Carothers, 1990)	Postpartum depression/In the last week	10 self-administered items/ Less than 5 minutes	Sensitivity = 68–86% Specificity = 78–96% Score of ≥ 13
Generalized Anxiety Disorder–7 (GAD-7; Spitzer, Kroenke, Williams, & Lowe, 2006; Kroenke, Spitzer, Williams, Monahan, & Lowe, 2007)	Generalized anxiety/In last 2 weeks	7 self-administered items/ Less than 5 minutes	Sensitivity = 89% Specificity = 82% Score of ≥ 10
Primary Care PTSD Screen (PC-PTSD; Prins et al., 2004)	PTSD/In the last month	4 self-administered items/ Less than 5 minutes	Sensitivity = 78% Specificity = 87% Score of ≥ 3
My Mood Monitor (M3; Gaynes et al., 2010)	Depression, any anxiety disorder, history symptoms of bipolar spectrum disorder, functional impairment/In last 2 weeks	27 self-administered items/ Less than 5 minutes	Any mood/anxiety disorder Sensitivity = 83% Specificity = 76%
Alcohol Use Disorders Identification Test—Consumption (AUDIT-C; Bradley, DeBenedetti, Volk, Williams, & Kivlahan, 2007)	Alcohol misuse/In the last week, month, year	3 self-administered items/ Less than 5 minutes	Sensitivity = 86% Specificity = 89% Score of ≥ 4 in men Sensitivity = 73% Specificity = 91% Score of ≥ 3 in women
Quick Psychodiagnostics Panel (QPD; Shedler, Beck, & Bensen, 2000)	Major depression, dysthymic, bipolar, generalized anxiety, panic, and obsessive–compulsive disorders. Also bulimia, substance abuse, and somatization disorder/	59 self-administered questions on a handheld computer unit/Just over 6 minutes	Sensitivity range 69–98% Specificity range 90–97%

Measure	Construct measured/Time frame	Format/Administration time	Psychometric properties
Behavioral Health Measure–20 (BHM-20 [previously the Behavioral Health Questionnaire–20]; Kopta & Lowry, 2002)	(1) Well-being (distress, life satisfaction, motivation), (2) psychological symptoms (depression, anxiety, panic disorder, mood swings associated with bipolar disorder, eating disorder, alcohol/drug abuse, suicidal tendencies, risk of violence), (3) life functioning (work/school, intimate relationships, social relationships, life enjoyment/In the last 2 weeks	20 self-administered items via World Wide Web or personal digital assistant (PDA)/2.5 minutes; Scored automatically	Internal consistency global mental health = .89–90 Well-being = .65–.74; Symptoms = .85–.86; Life functioning = .72–.77; Test–retest reliability = .71–.83
Patient Health Questionnaire (PHQ)–15 (Kroenke, Spitzer, & Williams, 2002)	15 somatic symptoms that account for more than 90% of physical complaints/In the last 4 weeks	15 self-administered items/Less than 5 minutes	Internal consistency = .80; Significant association with increased score and functional disability
Outcome Questionnaire Short Form (OQ-10; Seelert, Hill, Rigdon, & Schewenzfeier, 1999)	General psychological functioning, including positive and negative affect/In the last week	10 self-administered items/Less than 5 minutes	Internal consistency = .88; Significantly correlated with the Duke self-esteem, well-being and perceived health and anxiety and depression scores
Duke Health Profile (Parkerson, 2002)	Quality of life/health/In the last week	17 self-administered items/Less than 5 minutes	Internal consistency = generally between .60s and .70s for multi-item scales; Test–retest reliability generally between .40s and .50s for single-item scales.
Short Form–12 (SF-12; Ware, Kosinski, & Keller, 1996)	Quality of life/health functioning: physical and mental health summary scores/In the last 2 weeks	12 self-administered items/Less than 5 minutes	Correlated with SF-36 scores averaged .91; Test–retest reliability averaged .82
Health Anxiety Inventory Short Version (HAIS; Salkovskis, Rimes, Warwick, & Clark, 2002)	Health anxiety/In the last 6 months	18 self-administered items/Less than 10 minutes	No sensitivity/specificity given; Score above 31 more likely to denote health anxiety
Athens Insomnia Scale (AIS; Soldatos, Dikeos, & Paparrigopoulos, 2000)	Sleep difficulty/In the last month	8 self-administered items/Less than 5 minutes	Internal consistency =.90; Test–retest reliability = .90; External validity = .90 with Sleep Problems Scale
Insomnia Severity Index (ISI; Bastien, Vallieres, & Morin, 2001)	Insomnia severity/In the last 2 weeks	7 self-administered items/Less than 5 minutes	Internal consistency = .74; Sensitivity = 94%; Specificity = 94% (Smith & Trinder, 2001); Score of ≥ 14 distinguished those with and without insomnia

Time frame based on time parameters for DSM-IV diagnoses.

Scored automatically

Screening

Screening measures are typically used to help the PCPs identify groups of individuals in the population who might benefit from additional evaluation or intervention or who might not otherwise be recognized based on initial clinical presentation alone. In other words, screening is a case-finding method used to improve the detection of behavioral health symptoms or factors (e.g., poor life quality) that might be affecting the patient's functioning and quality of life or perpetuating or exacerbating a medical problem. For instance, a depression screening measure might be given to all patients enrolled in the clinic once a year. It could also be geared toward a subgroup of individuals who are at greater risk for depression (e.g., those with diabetes or chronic pain conditions). Other screening tools that target quality of life and functioning can be used in a similar manner. Screening tools should be highly sensitive (limited false negatives) but especially specific (limited false positives) to avoid creating unnecessary work for the primary care team, the health psychologist, and the patient. A primary role that the health psychologist might play regarding screening measures is to introduce new screeners that PCPs can efficiently and effectively incorporate into standard practice. A particular score on a screening measure might be used as a cue to prompt the PCP to consult with a health psychologist for assistance with additional assessment and intervention.

Assessment

Assessment measures can be used to assist with diagnosis, but more typically they will be used in the planning of interventions and evaluating response to intervention. There are a number of assessment instruments that focus on one area (e.g., the Insomnia Severity Index) and other instruments that focus on global distress (e.g., the Behavioral Health Measure–20) or health-related quality of life (e.g., SF-12). A balance must be made between the time it takes for completion and scoring of the measure and the other tasks that must take place during focused appointments. Assessment measures can also be used to demonstrate the effectiveness of the health psychologist's interventions and to help jus-tify his or her value to the clinic. It may take some trial and error to deduce what assessment measures work best for a particular clinic enrollment and operating structure. There can be vast differences from clinic to clinic, and a measure that worked well in one clinic might work poorly in another. Health psychologists should experiment with multiple measures to determine what works best. As chapter limits do not allow for a detailed and comprehensive review of all measures available, a list of common screening and assessment measures are provided in Table 26.1 on pp. 474–475.

Summary

Working as a health psychologist in primary care can be challenging and rewarding. In order to work efficiently and effectively in the fast pace of primary care, and specifically the PCBH model of integrated care, a different set of assessment skills is necessary. Using the format and following the guidance in this chapter can help the health psychologist adapt well to this ever-evolving environment, one that he or she is sure to be a part of with more frequency in the coming years.

AUTHOR'S NOTE

The opinions and statements in this chapter are the responsibility of the author, and such opinions and statements do not necessarily represent the policies of the Department of Defense, the United States Department of Health and Human Services, or their agencies.

REFERENCES

Bastien, C., Vallieres, A., & Morin, C. M. (2001). Validation of the Insomnia Severity Index as a clinical outcome measure for insomnia research. *Sleep Medicine, 2,* 297–307.

Blount, A. (2003). Integrated primary care: Organizing the evidence. *Families, Systems, and Health, 21,* 121–133.

Blount, A., Shoenbaum, M., Kathol, R., Rollman, B. L., Thomas, M., O'Donohue W., et al. (2007). The economics of behavioral health services in medical settings: A summary of the evidence. *Professional Psychology: Research and Practice, 38,* 290–297.

Bradley. K. A., DeBenedetti, A. F., Volk, R. J., Williams, E. C., Frank, D., & Kivlahan, D. R. (2007). AUDIT-C as a brief screen for alcohol misuse in primary care. *Alcoholism: Clinical and Experimental Research, 31,* 1208–1217.

Butler, M., Kane, R. L., McAlpine, D., Kathol, R. G., Fu, S. S., Hagedorn, H., et al. (2008). *Integration of mental health/substance abuse and primary care* (AHRQ Publication No. 09-E003). Rockville, MD: Agency for Healthcare Research and Quality.

Collins, C., Hewson, D. L., Munger, R., & Wade, T. (2010). *Evolving models of behavioral health integration in primary care.* New York: Milbank Memorial Fund.

Cox, J. L., Holden, J. M., & Sagovsky, R. (1987). Detection of postnatal depression: Development of the 10-item Edinburgh Postnatal Depression Scale. *British Journal of Psychiatry, 150,* 782–786.

Craven, M., & Bland, R. (2006). *Better practices in collaborative mental health care: An analysis of the evidence base.* Mississauga, Ontario, Canada: Canadian Collaborative Mental Health Initiative.

Fisher, L., & Ransom, D. C. (1997). Developing a strategy for managing behavioral health care within the context of primary care. *Archives of Internal Medicine, 6,* 324–333.

Gatchel, R. J., & Oordt, M. S. (2003). *Clinical health psychology and primary care: Practical advice and clinical guidance for successful collaboration.* Washington, DC: American Psychological Association.

Gaynes, B. N., Deveaugh-Geiss, J., Weir, S., Gu, H., MacPherson, C., Schulberg, H. D., et al. (2010). Feasibility and diagnostic validity of the M-3 checklist: A brief, self-rated screen for depressive, bipolar, anxiety and posttraumatic stress disorders in primary care. *Annals of Family Medicine, 8,* 160–169.

Gilbody, S., Bower, P., & Whitty, P. (2006). Costs and consequences of enhanced primary care for depression: Systematic review of randomised economic evaluations. *British Journal of Psychiatry, 189,* 484–493.

Goldstein, M. G., Whitlock, E. P., & DePue, J. (2004). Multiple behavioral risk factor interventions in primary care. *American Journal of Preventive Medicine, 27*(S2), 61–79.

Hoge, C. W., Auchterlonie, J. L., & Miliken, C. S. (2006). Mental health problems, use of mental health services, and attrition from military service after returning from deployment to Iraq or Afghanistan. *Journal of the American Medical Association, 295,* 1023–1032.

Hunter, C. L., Goodie, J. L., Oordt, M. S., & Dobmeyer, A. C. (2009). *Integrated behavioral health in primary care: Step-by-step guidance for assessment and intervention.* Washington, DC: American Psychological Association.

Kessler, R. C., Demler, O., Frank, R. G., Olfson, M., Pincus, H. A., Walters, E. E., et al.(2005) Prevalence and treatment of mental disorders, 1990 to 2003. *New England Journal of Medicine, 352,* 2515–2523.

Kopta, S. M., & Lowry, J. L. (2002). Psychometric evaluation of the Behavioral Health Questionnaire–20: A brief instrument for assessing global mental health and the three phases of psychotherapy outcome. *Psychotherapy Research, 12,* 413–426.

Kroenke, K., Spitzer, R. L., & Williams, J. B. (2001). The PHQ-9: Validity of a brief depression severity measure. *Journal of General Internal Medicine, 16,* 606–613.

Kroenke, K., Spitzer, R. L., & Williams, J. B. (2002). The PHQ-15: Validity of a new measure of evaluating the severity of somatic symptoms. *Psychosomatic Medicine, 64,* 258–266.

Kroenke, K., Spitzer, R. L., & Williams, J. B. (2003). The Patient Health Questionnaire–2: Validity of a two-item depression screener. *Medical Care, 41,* 1284–1292.

Kroenke, K., Spitzer, R. L., Williams, J. B. W., Monahan, P. O., & Lowe, B. (2007). Anxiety disorders in primary care: Prevalence, impairment, comorbidity, and detection. *Annals of Internal Medicine, 146,* 317–325.

Linton, J. (2004). Psychological assessment in primary care. In L. J. Haas (Ed.), *Handbook of primary care psychology* (pp. 35–45). New York: Oxford University Press.

Loeppke, R., Taitel, M., Haufle, V., Parry, T., Kessler, R. C., Jinnett, K. (2009). Health and productivity as a business strategy: A multiemployer study. *Journal of Occupational and Environmental Medicine, 51,* 411–428.

Merikangas, K. R., Ames, M., Cui, L., Stang, P. E., Ustun, T. B., Von Korff, M., et al. (2007). The impact of comorbidity of mental and physical conditions on role disability in the U.S. adult household population. *Archives of General Psychiatry, 64,* 1180–1188.

Murray, L., & Carothers, A. D. (1990). The validation of the Edinburgh Postnatal Depression Scale on a community sample. *British Journal of Psychiatry, 157,* 288–290.

Parkerson, G. R. (2002). *User's guide for Duke Health Measures*. Durham, NC: Duke University Medical Center.

Prins, A., Ouimette, P., Kimerling, R., Cameron, R. P., Hugelshofer, D. S., Shaw-Hegwer, J., et al. (2004). The Primary Care PTSD Screen (PC–PTSD): Development and operating characteristics. *Primary Care Psychiatry, 9*, 9–14.

Robinson, P. J., & Reiter, J. T. (2007). *Behavioral consultation and primary care: A guide to integrating services*. New York: Springer.

Seelert, K. R., Hill, R. D., Rigdon, M. A., & Schwenzfeier, E. (1999). Measuring patient distress in primary care. *Family Medicine, 31*, 483–487.

Salkovskis, P. M., Rimes, K. A., Warwick, H. M. C., & Clark, D. M. (2002). The Health Anxiety Inventory: Development and validation of scales for the measurement of health anxiety and hypochondriasis. *Psychological Medicine, 32*, 843–853.

Shedler, J., Beck, A., & Bensen, S. (2000). Practical mental health assessment in primary care: Validity and utility of the quick psychodiagnostics panel. *Journal of Family Practice, 49*, 614–621.

Smith, S., & Trinder, J. (2001). Detecting insomnia: Comparison of four self-report measures of sleep in a young adult population. *Journal of Sleep Research, 10*, 229–235.

Soldatos, C. R., Dikeos, D. G., & Paparrigopoulos, T. G. (2000). Athens Insomnia Scale: Validation of an instrument based on ICD-10 criteria. *Journal of Psychosomatic Research, 48*, 555–560.

Spitzer, R. L., Kroenke, K., Williams, J. B. W., & Lowe, B. (2006). A brief measure for assessing generalized anxiety disorder: The GAD-7. *Archives of Internal Medicine, 166*, 1092–1097.

Steer, R. A., Cavalieri, T. A., Leonard, D. M., & Beck, A. T. (1999). Use of the Beck Depression Inventory for primary care to screen for major depression. *General Hospital Psychiatry, 21*, 106–111.

Strosahl, K., & Robinson, P. (2008). The primary care behavioral health model: Application to prevention, acute care and chronic condition management. In R. Kessler & D. Stafford (Eds.), *Collaborative medicine case studies: Evidence in practice* (pp. 85–95). New York: Springer.

Trude, S., & Stoddard, J. J. (2003). Referral gridlock: Primary care physicians and mental health services. *Journal of General Internal Medicine, 18*, 442–449.

Ware, J. E., Kosinski, M. M., & Keller, S. D. (1996). A 12-item short-form health survey: Construction of scales and preliminary tests of reliability and validity. *Medical Care, 34*, 220–233.

Whitlock, E. P., Orleans, C. T., Pender, N., & Allan, J. (2002). Evaluating primary care behavioral counseling interventions: An evidence-based approach. *American Journal of Preventive Medicine, 22*, 267–284.

Williams, J. W., Gerrity, M., Holsinger, T., Dobscha, S., Gaynes, B., & Dietrich, A. (2007). Systematic review of multifaceted interventions to improve depression care. *General Hospital Psychiatry, 29*, 91–116.

APPENDIX 26.1. Behavioral Health Consultation Information Handout

What Is the Behavioral Health Consultation Service?

The Behavioral Health Consultation Service offers assistance when habits, behaviors, stress, worry, or emotional concerns about physical or other life problems are interfering with someone's daily life and/or overall health. The Behavioral Health Consultant (BHC) works with your Primary Care Provider (PCP) to evaluate the mind–body–behavior connection and provide brief, solution-focused interventions.

The BHC has specialty training in the behavioral management of health problems. Together, the BHC and your PCP can consider all of the physical, behavioral, and emotional aspects of your health concern and help you determine a course of action that will work best for you.

What Kinds of Health Concerns Do We See?

The BHC can help you reduce symptoms associated with various chronic medical conditions or help you cope better with these conditions. A few of these are:

Headaches	Asthma	Chronic pain
Sleep	Diabetes	Irritable Bowel Syndrome
High Blood Pressure	Obesity	

The BHC can help you and your PCP develop behavioral change plans for smoking cessation, weight loss, alcohol use, exercise, or other lifestyle modifications. The BHC can also help you and your PCP develop skills to effectively manage emotional or behavioral difficulties such as:

Depression	Family/ relationship problems	Bereavement
Anxiety	Stress	Anger

Who Is Eligible to Receive These Services?

The service is available to all patients within the Family Health Center as a part of good overall health care.

What Should I Expect When I See the BHC?

You can expect the BHC to ask you specific questions about your physical symptoms, any emotional concerns you are experiencing, your behaviors, and how all of these might be related. You can expect your appointments to be no longer than 30 minutes, in general, and for the BHC to provide brief solution-focused assessment and treatment. You can also expect to be seen in this clinic and for the BHC to have a close working relationship with your PCP. Remember: You and your PCP remain in charge of your health care—the BHC's primary job is to help you and your PCP develop and implement the best integrated health care plan for YOU!

How Is this Service Different from Mental Health Services?

The services provided by the BHC are simply another part of your overall health care and are *not* specialty mental health care. Documentation of your assessment and recommendations from the BHC will be written in your medical record. A separate mental health record will not be kept when you see the BHC.

Communications with your BHC may not be entirely confidential as required by state law. Your BHC will make every effort to protect your privacy. But, like *all* providers, they *may* have to report information regarding child or spouse abuse or share information regarding those at risk to harm or kill themselves or others.

You will be seen in the Family Health Center, and the BHC will not provide traditional psychotherapy. If you request, or if the BHC thinks you would benefit from specialty mental health services, the BHC will recommend that you and your PCP consider specialty mental health services.

How Do I Schedule a BHC Appointment?

Discuss with your PCP the desire to access this service. If you and your provider agree that this service would be helpful, call the Family Health Center at 301-555-1234 to schedule a BHC appointment.

APPENDIX 26.2. Functional Analysis Questions for a Focused IBS Assessment in Primary Care

Physical/Medical Factors

Frequency and Intensity of the Problem

- Symptoms of IBS can be different for different people and may include bloating, cramping, diarrhea, constipation, or other physical symptoms. What are your IBS symptoms?
- Which of those symptoms bothers you the most?
- How many times a day/week/month would you say that _____ [*the most bothersome symptom*] is occurring?
- On a scale of 0–10, with 0 meaning the symptom is gone and 10 being the most bothersome/painful it has ever been, what would be the average number you would give to _____ [*the most bothersome symptom*] over the last 2 weeks?
- What is the highest number you would give _____ [*the most bothersome symptom*] in the last 2 weeks?
- What is the lowest number you would give _____ [*the most bothersome symptom*] in the last 2 weeks?

Duration

- Have your IBS symptoms been going on for just the last few months, or has it been longer or shorter than that?
- About how long ago was it that you first noticed your IBS symptoms?

Changes in Sleep, Energy, Concentration, Appetite

- Do you feel rested when you get out of bed in the morning?
- What is the average number of hours you are asleep while in bed?
- Are you sleeping about the same, more, or less than is typical for you over the past month? *If less, then ask . . .*
  - Are you having trouble falling asleep, staying asleep, or both? *"Both."*
  - Over the past month on average, how long does it take you to fall asleep?
  - Over the past month on average, how many times do you wake up at night?
  - About how long does it take you to fall back asleep?
- Have you noticed a decrease, an increase, or has your energy been about the same as usual over the last month? *"About the same."*
- Do you feel like you have reasonable energy, or does it feel like you're dragging through your day? *"Dragging."*
- Has your ability to concentrate decreased?
- Have you seen any increase or decrease in your appetite, or is it about the same as usual?
- Have you lost or gained any weight over the last year?

Medication/Substance Use

a. **Medications or Supplements**
  - Are you taking any medications or supplements? *"Yes."*
  - What are you taking, how much are you taking, and what are you taking it for?

b. **Caffeine Use**
  - Do you drink caffeinated drinks? *"Yes."*
  - What kind: tea, coffee, soda?
  - How many in a typical day?
  - How many ounces in each drink?

c. **Alcohol Use**
  - Do you drink alcoholic drinks? *"Yes."*
  - What kind: beer, wine, mixed drinks?
  - How many in a drinks in a typical day, week, or month?
  - How many ounces in each drink?

d. **Tobacco Use**
  - Do you use tobacco products? *"Yes."*
  - What do you use?
  - How many/much on a typical day?

Psychosocial Factors

Triggering events

- Was there anything different going on in your life or anything that happened, good or not so good, that seems to be associated with your IBS, or did the symptoms just seem to be there one day not related to anything in particular?

Factors That Make the Symptom/s Better or Worse

- Is there anything that you do or that seems to happen that decreases the intensity or frequency of your symptom(s)?
- Is there anything that you do or that seems to happen that seems to increase the intensity or frequency of your symptom(s)?

Functional Impairment

a. **Changes in Work Performance**

   - Have you noticed any changes or decreases in your ability to do your job in response to your symptoms or as your symptoms get worse? *If yes, then ask what those changes are.*

b. **Changes in Work Relationships:**

   - Have you noticed any changes in your work relationships in response to your symptoms or as your symptoms get worse? *If yes, then ask what those changes are.*

c. **Changes in Significant Familial Relationships (i.e., spouse, children, etc.)**

   - Have your symptoms been affecting your relationships with your [spouse/partner/fiancé/girlfriend/boyfriend, children, friends]? *If yes, then ask what those changes are.*

d. **Changes in Social Activities (e.g., going out with friends, church):**

   - Often people with IBS will decrease or stop their social activities. Has that happened for you? *If yes, then ask . . .*
     o What have you cut back on or stopped?
     o How often did you used to _____ [*the activity cut back on or stopped*]?

e. **Changes in Fun/Recreational/Relaxing/Meaningful Activities:**

   - Sometimes people with IBS cut back on or stop meaningful or enjoyable activities. Have you cut back on or stopped enjoyable or meaningful activities? *If yes, then ask . . .*
     o What have you cut back on or stopped?
     o How often did you used to _____ [*the activity cut back on or stopped*]?

f. **Change in Exercise**

   - Are you exercising right now? *If yes, assess frequency and duration.*
   - Is this the same level of exercise that you usually do, or does it go up and down depending on the severity of your symptoms?
   - If not exercising now:
     o Have you exercised in the past? *If yes, assess frequency and duration and why it was stopped.*
     o When you were exercising before, what benefits did you get from it?

Relationship with Significant Other

   - Would you describe your relationship with your spouse/partner/fiancé/girlfriend/boyfriend as "poor," "OK, but could be better," "good," or "excellent"?
   - On a scale of 0–10, with 0 being not satisfied at all and 10 being the most satisfied you can imagine, what number would represent your satisfaction in this relationship?

How Others Respond to Symptoms

   - How do members of your family, coworkers, or close friends respond to your symptoms?

Relations with Others

   - Do you find it difficult to make decisions?
   - Can you be openly critical of others' ideas, opinions, or behaviors?
   - Do you generally express what you feel?
   - Do have difficulty refusing requests made by a friend if you don't want to do what is being asked?

Life Stress, Negative Life Event

   - If you were to rate your average stress level over the last month on a scale of 0–10, with 0 being no stress, completely relaxed, and 10 being the most stressed you could imagine, what number would you give as your average stress level?
   - What is the highest your stress level has gone in the last month?
   - Does anything seem to be associated with your highest stress level?
   - What is your lowest stress level?
   - Does anything seem to be associated with your lowest stress level?
   - Have you noticed any changes in your IBS symptoms as your stress level changes?
   - Is there anything unpleasant, bothersome, or distressing happening in your life right now besides your IBS symptoms that you would like to see be changed or different?
   - Is there anything unpleasant, bothersome, or distressing that happened in your past (e.g. physical/sexual assault, physical/sexual/emotional abuse, near-death experience, or being that you were going to die) besides your symptoms that is distressing/bothersome to you now?

Mood Over Past 2 Weeks

- Over the past 2 weeks would you describe your mood as good, normal, happy, down, sad, depressed, anxious, worried, angry, frustrated, stressed, something different, or is it a combination of things? *If good, normal, happy are reported, skip the rest of the questions in this section.*

- How many days a week would you say you have been feeling _____ [*e.g., depressed*]?

- When you are feeling this way, what are the kinds of thoughts you have that are leading you to feel this way?

- On a scale of 0–10, with 0 being not being _____ [*e.g., depressed*] at all and 10 being the most _____ [*e.g., depressed*] you've ever felt in your life, what would you say your average level of _____ [*e.g., depression*] has been over the last 2 weeks?

- How often do you feel _____ [*e.g., depressed*]?

Maladaptive Thoughts about Symptoms

- When your symptoms are flaring up, what are the thoughts that run through your mind?

Suicidal Thoughts

- In the last month have you had any thoughts, plans, or intent to kill yourself?

Open-Ended Questions as Time Allows

- Is there anything I haven't asked you about that you think is important for me to know?

- What is a typical weekday like for you from the time you get up to the time you go to bed?

- What do you typically do on your nonwork days (or weekend)?

Author Index

Subject Index

An *f* following a page number indicates a figure; a *t* following a page number indicates a table.